FROM THE EXPERTS IN ENDOCRINOLOGY

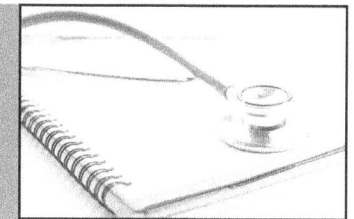

ENDO 2024
MEET THE PROFESSOR

REFERENCE EDITION

ENDOCRINE
CASE MANAGEMENT

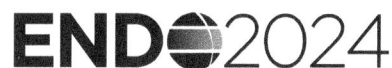

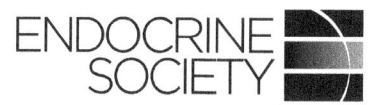
ENDOCRINE SOCIETY

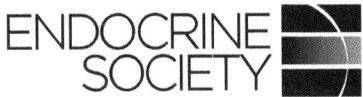

2055 L Street, NW, Suite 600
Washington, DC 20036
www.endocrine.org

Other Publications:
endocrine.org/publications

The Endocrine Society is the world's largest, oldest, and most active organization working to advance the clinical practice of endocrinology and hormone research. Founded in 1916, the Society now has more than 18,000 global members across a range of disciplines.

The Society has earned an international reputation for excellence in the quality of its peer-reviewed journals, educational resources, meetings, and programs that improve public health through the practice and science of endocrinology.

Clinical Practice Chair, ENDO 2024
Selma Feldman Witchel, MD

ISBN: 978-1-936704-35-4
Library of Congress Control Number: 2024935369

On the Cover: © Shutterstock. Close up stethoscope on blank notepad as medical concept. (By Singha Songsak P).

FROM THE EXPERTS IN ENDOCRINOLOGY

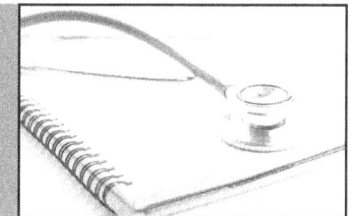

ENDO 2024
MEET THE PROFESSOR

REFERENCE EDITION

ENDOCRINE
CASE MANAGEMENT

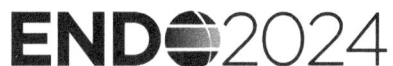

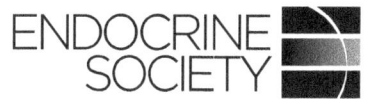

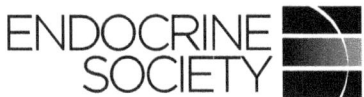

2055 L Street, NW, Suite 600
Washington, DC 20036
www.endocrine.org

Other Publications:
endocrine.org/publications

The Endocrine Society is the world's largest, oldest, and most active organization working to advance the clinical practice of endocrinology and hormone research. Founded in 1916, the Society now has more than 18,000 global members across a range of disciplines.

The Society has earned an international reputation for excellence in the quality of its peer-reviewed journals, educational resources, meetings, and programs that improve public health through the practice and science of endocrinology.

Clinical Practice Chair, ENDO 2024
Selma Feldman Witchel, MD

ISBN: 978-1-936704-35-4
Library of Congress Control Number: 2024935369

On the Cover: © Shutterstock. Close up stethoscope on blank notepad as medical concept. (By Singha Songsak P).

ENDO 2024 CONTENTS

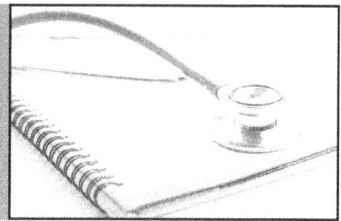

CARDIOVASCULAR ENDOCRINOLOGY

DIABETES MELLITUS AND GLUCOSE METABOLISM

GENERAL ENDOCRINOLOGY

NEUROENDOCRINOLOGY AND PITUITARY

PEDIATRIC ENDOCRINOLOGY

REPRODUCTIVE ENDOCRINOLOGY

THYROID

TUMOR BIOLOGY

APPENDIX

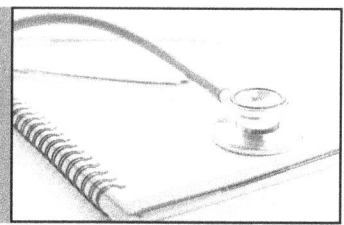

2024 Endocrine Case Management: Meet the Professor Faculty

Layla Abushamat, MD, MPH
Baylor College of Medicine

Saumya Agrawal, MD
*Creighton University
School of Medicine*

Mona Al Mukaddam, MD, MS
*University of Pennsylvania
Health System*

Grazia Aleppo, MD
Northwestern University

Nasreen Alfaris, MD, MPH
King Fahad Medical City

Dalal S. Ali, MD, MSc
McMaster University

Trevor E. Angell, MD
*Keck School of Medicine of
University of Southern California*

Ambika P. Ashraf, MD
*University of Alabama
at Birmingham*

Natalie Hecht Baldauff, DO, MBA
*University of Pittsburgh
Medical Center Children's
Hospital of Pittsburgh*

Linda A. Barbour, MD, MSPH
*University of Colorado School
of Medicine and Anschutz
Medical Campus*

Cesar Luiz Boguszewski, MD, PhD
Federal University of Parana

A. Enrique Caballero, MD
*Brigham and Women's Hospital
and Harvard Medical School*

Frederic Castinetti, MD, PhD
Aix Marseille University

Layal Chaker, MD, PhD
Erasmus University Medical Center

Uriel Clemente-Gutierrez, MD
*University of Texas MD
Anderson Cancer Center*

**Roderick Clifton-Bligh,
BSc (med), MBBS, PhD**
*Royal North Shore Hospital
and University of Sydney*

Kevin Colclough, DClinSci
*Royal Devon University
Healthcare National Health
Service Foundation Trust*

Martine Cools, MD, PhD
*Ghent University Hospital
and Ghent University*

Kenneth Cusi, MD
The University of Florida

Francesco d'Aniello, MD
*Bambino Gesù Children's
Hospital and Queen Mary
University of London*

**Nancy Samir Elbarbary,
MBBCh, MSc, MD, PhD**
Ain Shams University

Tobias Else, MD
University of Michigan

James W. Findling, MD
Medical College of Wisconsin

Maria Fleseriu, MD
Oregon Health & Science University

Joseph Henske, MD
*University of Arkansas
for Medical Sciences*

Sasha R. Howard, MBBS, PhD
Queen Mary University of London

Bernice L. Huang, MD
*University of Texas MD
Anderson Cancer Center*

Christopher Hvisdas, PharmD
*University of Pennsylvania
Medical Center*

Sean J. Iwamoto, MD
*University of Colorado School of
Medicine, Anschutz Medical Campus
and Rocky Mountain Regional
Veterans Affairs Medical Center*

Malavika Kesavan, MD
University of Virginia Health

Aliya A. Khan, MD
McMaster University

Alexandra N. Krez, BA
Hospital for Special Surgery

Amanda La Greca, MD
*University of Colorado
School of Medicine*

Carol J. Levy, MD, CDCES
*The Icahn School of
Medicine at Mount Sinai*

E. Michael Lewiecki, MD
*University of New Mexico
Health Sciences Center*

Sarah E. Mayson, MD
*University of Colorado
School of Medicine*

Alon Y. Mazori, MD
*The Icahn School of
Medicine at Mount Sinai*

Michael T. McDermott, MD
*University of Colorado Denver
School of Medicine*

Moisés Mercado, MD
National Autonomous
University of México

Alia Munir, MBBCh, PhD
Sheffield Teaching Hospitals National
Health Service Foundation Trust

Lynnette K. Nieman, MD
National Institute of Diabetes and
Digestive and Kidney Diseases,
National Institutes of Health

Kashyap A. Patel, PhD
Royal Devon University Healthcare
National Health Service
Foundation Trust and University
of Exeter Medical School

Robin Peeters, MD, PhD
Erasmus University Medical Center

Nancy D. Perrier, MD
University of Texas MD
Anderson Cancer Center

JoAnn V. Pinkerton, MD
University of Virginia Health

Tamar Reisman, MD
Weill Cornell Medicine

Jane E. B. Reusch, MD
University of Colorado,
Anschutz Medical Campus

Eyal Robenshtok, MD
Rabin Medical Center

Micol S. Rothman, MD
University of Colorado
School of Medicine

Omair A. Shariq, MD, MS
Mayo Clinic

Jennifer A. Sipos, MD
The Ohio State University

Emily M. Stein, MD, MS
Hospital for Special Surgery

Anand Vaidya, MD, MMSc
Brigham and Women's Hospital
and Harvard Medical School

Elena V. Varlamov, MD
Oregon Health & Science University

Joseph G. Verbalis, MD
Georgetown University
Medical Center

Danica M. Vodopivec, MD
University of Texas MD
Anderson Cancer Center

Margaret E. Wierman, MD
University of Colorado
Anschutz Medical Center

Annual Meeting Steering Committee (AMSC)

Lauren Fishbein, MD,
PhD – AMSC Chair
University of Colorado
School of Medicine

Selma Feldman Witchel, MD –
Clinical Practice Chair
University of Pittsburgh
Medical Center Children's
Hospital of Pittsburgh

Niki Karavitaki, MSc PhD –
Clinical Science Chair
University of Birmingham

Daniel E. Frigo, PhD –
Basic Science Chair
University of Texas MD
Anderson Cancer Center

Annual Meeting Steering Committee Clinical Peer Reviewers

Ana Paula Abreu Metzger, MD, PhD

Olga Astapova, MD, PhD

Irina Bancos, MD

Ernesto Bernal-Mizrachi, MD

Laura Boucai, MD

Barbara Gisella Carranza Leon, MD

Stephanie Anne Fish, MD

Christa E. Flueck, MD

Ole-Petter Hamnvik, MBBCh
BAO, MMSc, MRCPI

Edward Chiaming Hsiao, MD, PhD

Hebatullah M. Ismail, MD

Katja Kiseljak-Vassiliades, DO

Raghavendra Mirmira, PhD, MD

Gabrielle Page-Wilson, MD

Yumie Rhee, MD, PhD

W. Edward Visser, MD, PhD

Bu Beng Yeap, MBBS, PhD

Jun Yang, MBBS, PhD

Elaine Wei-Yin Yu, MD

PEDIATRIC ENDOCRINOLOGY

REPRODUCTIVE ENDOCRINOLOGY

THYROID

TUMOR BIOLOGY

APPENDIX

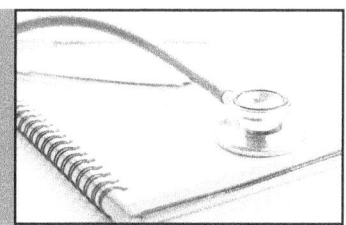

OVERVIEW

The *Endocrine Case Management: Meet the Professor* reference book is intended primarily for consultation relating to endocrinology. As a reference book, educational credits are not available. For information on educational products that include educational credit, please visit endocrine.org/store.

LEARNING OBJECTIVES

Endocrine Case Management: Meet the Professor will allow learners to assess their knowledge of all aspects of endocrinology, diabetes, and metabolism.

Completion of this educational activity enables learners to accomplish key objectives:

- Recognize clinical manifestations of endocrine and metabolic disorders and select among current options for diagnosis, management, and therapy.

- Identify risk factors for endocrine and metabolic disorders and develop strategies for prevention.

- Evaluate endocrine and metabolic manifestations of systemic disorders.

- Use existing resources pertaining to clinical guidelines and treatment recommendations for endocrine and related metabolic disorders to guide diagnosis and treatment.

TARGET AUDIENCE

Endocrine Case Management: Meet the Professor provides case-based education to clinicians interested in improving patient care.

STATEMENT OF INDEPENDENCE

The Endocrine Society has a policy of ensuring that the content and quality of this educational activity are balanced, independent, objective, and scientifically rigorous. The scientific content of this activity was developed under the supervision of the Endocrine Society's Annual Meeting Steering Committee.

DISCLOSURE POLICY

The faculty, committee members, and staff who are in position to control the content of this activity are required to disclose to the Endocrine Society and to learners any relevant financial relationship(s) of the individual or spouse/partner that have occurred within the last 12 months with any commercial interest(s) whose products or services are related to the content. Financial relationships are defined by remuneration in any amount from the commercial interest(s) in the form of grants; research support; consulting fees; salary; ownership interest (e.g., stocks, stock options, or ownership interest excluding diversified mutual funds); honoraria or other payments for participation in speakers' bureaus, advisory boards, or boards of directors; or other financial benefits. The intent of this disclosure is not to prevent planners with relevant financial relationships from planning or delivery of content, but rather to provide learners with information that allows them to make their own judgments of whether these financial relationships may have influenced the educational activity with regard to exposition or conclusion. The Endocrine Society has reviewed all disclosures and resolved or managed all identified conflicts of interest, as applicable.

The Endocrine Society has reviewed these relationships to determine which are relevant to the content of this activity and resolved any identified conflicts of interest for these individuals.

The faculty reported the following relevant financial relationship(s) during the content development process for this activity:

Mona Al Mukaddam, MD, MS Grant Recipient: Ipsen, Incyte Pharmaceutical.

Grazia Aleppo, MD Consulting Fee: Insulet Corporation, Dexcom; Research Investigator: Insulet Corporation, Fractyl Laboratories, Tandem Diabetes Care, Welldoc.

Nasreen Alfaris, MD, MPH Advisory Board Member: Eli Lilly & Company; Consulting Fee: Eli Lilly & Company, Novo Nordisk; Speaker: Eli Lilly & Company.

Trevor E. Angell, MD Research Investigator: Immunovant, Inc.

Ambika P. Ashraf, MD Moderator, AMRYT PES Webinar in October 2023; Consultant, BioMarin, one time commitment.

Cesar Luiz Boguszewski, MD, PhD Consulting Fee: Novo Nordisk, Ipsen; Research Investigator: Crinetics; Speaker: Ipsen, Novo Nordisk, Recordati.

Frederic Castinetti, MD, PhD Advisory Board Member: HRA Pharmaceuticals; Grant Recipient: HRA Pharmaceuticals.

Layal Chaker, MD, PhD Grant Recipient: Abbott Diabetes Care.

Roderick Clifton-Bligh, BSc (med), MBBS, PhD Advisory Board Member: Kirin Brewery, Ipsen.

Kenneth Cusi, MD Consulting Fee: Arrowhead, Novo Nordisk, Boehringer Ingelheim, Bristol-Myers Squibb, Aligos Therapeutics, Prosciento, Terns Pharma, Sagimet Biosciences, Eli Lilly, AstraZeneca, 89Bio, Covance, Siemens USA; Research Investigator: Boehringer Ingelheim, Echosens, Inventiva, LabCorp, Perspectum, Target-NASH.

Tobias Else, MD Advisory Board Member: Merck.

Maria Fleseriu, MD Consulting Fee: Amryt, Camurus, Crinetics, Ipsen, Recordati; Research Investigator: Amryt, Crinetics, Ionis, Recordati.

Sasha R. Howard, MBBS, PhD Speaker: Pfizer, Inc, Novo Nordisk.

Aliya A. Khan, MD Grant Recipient: Alexion Pharmaceuticals, Inc, Takeda, Ascendis, Amolyt, Calcilytix; Speaker: Amgen Inc, Alexion Pharmaceuticals, Inc, Ascendis.

Carol J. Levy, MD, CDCES Advisory Board Member: Dexcom; Grant Recipient: Dexcom, Abbott Diabetes, Novo Nordisk; Research Investigator: Tandem, Insulet, Dexcom, Mannkind, Eli Lilly.

E. Michael Lewiecki, MD Advisory Board Member: Amgen, Inc, Radius Health, Inc; Research Investigator: Amgen Inc, Radius Health, Inc; Speaker: Amgen, Inc.

Alia Munir, MBBCh, PhD Grant Recipient: Neuroendocrine Cancer UK Charity for practice changing grant; Speaker: Ipsen; Other: Rhado none pharma family LTD company.

Lynnette K. Nieman, MD Grant Recipient: Crinetics Pharmaceuticals; Other: UpToDate.

Jane E. B. Reusch, MD Advisory Board Member: Medtronic Diabetes.

Eyal Robenshtok, MD Advisory Board Member: CTS Pharmaceutical Industries; Consulting Fee: Merck.

Emily M. Stein, MD, MS Grant Recipient: Radius Health, Inc, Novartis Pharmaceuticals.

Elena V. Varlamov, MD Grant Recipient: Recordati, Lumiio/Pfizer.

Margaret E. Wierman, MD Research Investigator: Crinetics.

The following faculty reported no relevant financial relationships:

Layla Abushamat, MD, MPH; Saumya Agrawal, MD; Dalal S. Ali, MD, MSc; Natalie Hecht Baldauff, DO, MBA; Linda A. Barbour, MD, MSPH; A. Enrique Caballero, MD; Uriel Clemente-Gutierrez, MD; Kevin Colclough, DClinSci; Martine Cools, MD, PhD; Francesco d'Aniello, MD; Nancy Samir Elbarbary, MBBCh, MSc, MD, PhD; James W. Findling, MD; Joseph Henske, MD; Bernice L. Huang, MD; Christopher Hvisdas, PharmD; Sean J. Iwamoto, MD; Malavika Kesavan, MD; Alexandra N. Krez, BA; Amanda La Greca, MD; Sarah E. Mayson, MD; Alon Y. Mazori, MD; Michael T. McDermott, MD; Moisés Mercado, MD; Kashyap A. Patel, PhD; Robin Peeters, MD, PhD; Nancy D. Perrier, MD; JoAnn V. Pinkerton, MD; Tamar Reisman, MD; Micol S. Rothman, MD; Omair A. Shariq, MD, MS; Jennifer A. Sipos, MD; Anand Vaidya, MD, MMSc; Joseph G. Verbalis, MD; and **Danica M. Vodopivec, MD**

The following AMSC peer reviewers reported relevant financial relationships:

Irina Bancos, MD Advisory Board: Adrenas, HRA Pharma, Corcept, Recordati; Consulting: HRA Pharma, Corcept, Sparrow Pharmaceutics, Recordati; Writer: Elsevier, Funding for Investigator Initiated Award: Recordati, NIH; Reviewer: Dynamed

Barbara Gisella Carranza Leon, MD Co-investigator: Novartis, IONIS Pharmaceutical Inc, NIH, FH Foundation, Regenxbio, Inc; Member of the Maintenance of Certification Committee: American Board of Obesity Medicine

Stephanie Anne Fish, MD Advisory Board: American Thyroid Association, Other: American Board of Internal Medicine, write questions for endocrine maintenance of certification.

Lauren Fishbein, MD, PhD Advisory Board: A5, PheoPara Alliance; Consulting: Lantheus/Azedra.

Christa E. Flueck, MD Advisory Board: European Society Paediatric Endocrinology; Grant Recipient: Novo Nordisk, Merck, Pfizer, Sandoz, Swiss National Science Foundation, European Society Paediatric Endocrinology; Consulting: Novo Nordisk, Pfizer, EffRx; Speaker: Sandoz; Editor: Hormone Research Paediatrics.

Ole-Petter Hamnvik, MB BCh BAO, MMSc, MRCPI Education Editor: *New England Journal of Medicine.*

Edward Chiaming Hsiao, MD, PhD Advisory Board: International FOP Association, FD/MAS Alliance, International Clinical Council on FOP; Editor: *Endocrine Journal, Journal of Bone and Mineral Research*; Research Investigator: Clementia Pharmaceuticals/Ipsen Pharmaceuticals, Ultragenyx.

Niki Karavitaki, MSc, PhD Advisory Board: European Neuroendocrine Association; Editor: HRA Pharma; Speaker: Recordati Rare Diseases, HRA Pharma, Pfizer, Ipsen, Conselient Health.

Katja Kiseljak-Vassiliades, DO Advisory Board: HRA Pharma.

Raghavendra Mirmira, PhD, MD; Editor: *Journal of Clinical Endocrinology and Metabolism,* Advisory Board: Veralox Therapeutics; Investigator-Initiated Award: Veralox Therapeutics, HiberCell, Inc.

Gabrielle Page-Wilson, MD Advisory Board: Strongbridge Biopharma, Recordati Rare Diseases, Inc, Xeris BioPharma; Consultant: Xeris BioPharma.

Yumie Rhee, MD, PhD Ambassador: American Society of Bone and Mineral Research; Committee: Korean Endocrine Society, Korean Society of Bone and Mineral Research; Editor: *JCEM Case Reports.*

W. Edward Visser, MD, PhD Royalties (Institution): Egetis Therapeutics

Selma Feldman Witchel, MD Editor: *Journal of the Endocrine Society, Sex Development, Steroids*; Research Investigator: Neurocrine Sciences; Contributor: UpToDate; Speaker: Canadian Society of Endocrinology and Metabolism, EndoBridge Conference.

Bu Beng Yeap, MBBS, PhD Advisory Board: Novo Nordisk, Bayer, Lilly; Research Support: Lawley Pharmaceuticals; Advisor: Lawley Pharmaceuticals; Speaker: AstraZeneca, Besins, Philippine Society for Endocrinology, Diabetes and Metabolism, View Street Medical; Past-President: Endocrine Society of Australia; Editor: *Asian Journal of Andrology, Journal of Gerontology Medical Sciences*; Editorial Board: *Journal of Gerontology Medical Sciences, Journal of Clinical Endocrinology and Metabolism, Maturitas.*

Elaine Wei-Yin Yu, MD Grant Recipient: Amgen.

The following AMSC members reported no relevant financial relationships:

Ana Paula Abreu Metzger, MD, PhD; Olga Astapova, MD, PhD; Ernesto Bernal-Mizrachi, MD; Laura Boucai, MD; Hebatullah M. Ismail, MD; and Jun Yang, MBBS, PhD

DISCLAIMERS
The information presented in this activity represents the opinion of the faculty and is not necessarily the official position of the Endocrine Society.

USE OF PROFESSIONAL JUDGMENT:
The educational content in this activity relates to basic principles of diagnosis and therapy and does not substitute for individual patient assessment based on the health care provider's examination of the patient and consideration of laboratory data and other factors unique to the patient. Standards in medicine change as new data become available.

DRUGS AND DOSAGES:
When prescribing medications, the physician is advised to check the product information sheet accompanying each drug to verify conditions of use and to identify any changes in drug dosage schedule or contraindications.

POLICY ON UNLABELED/OFF-LABEL USE
The Endocrine Society has determined that disclosure of unlabeled/off-label or investigational use of commercial product(s) is informative for audiences and therefore requires this information to be disclosed to the learners at the beginning of the presentation. Uses of specific therapeutic agents, devices, and other products discussed in this educational activity may not be the same as those indicated in product labeling approved by the Food and Drug Administration (FDA). The Endocrine Society requires that any discussions of such "off-label" use be based on scientific research that conforms to generally accepted standards of experimental design, data collection, and data analysis. Before recommending or prescribing any therapeutic agent or device, learners should review the complete prescribing information, including indications, contraindications, warnings, precautions, and adverse events.

ACKNOWLEDGMENT OF COMMERCIAL SUPPORT

The activity is not supported by educational grant(s) or other funds from any commercial supporters.

PUBLICATION DATE: June 2024

COMMON ABBREVIATIONS

ACTH = corticotropin

ACE inhibitor = angiotensin-converting enzyme inhibitor

ALT = alanine aminotransferase

AST = aspartate aminotransferase

BMI = body mass index

CNS = central nervous system

CT = computed tomography

DHEA = dehydroepiandrosterone

DHEA-S = dehydroepiandrosterone sulfate

DNA = deoxyribonucleic acid

DPP-4 inhibitor = dipeptidyl-peptidase 4 inhibitor

DXA = dual-energy x-ray absorptiometry

FDA = Food and Drug Administration

FGF-23 = fibroblast growth factor 23

FNA = fine-needle aspiration

FSH = follicle-stimulating hormone

GH = growth hormone

GHRH = growth hormone–releasing hormone

GLP-1 receptor agonist = glucagonlike peptide 1 receptor agonist

GnRH = gonadotropin-releasing hormone

hCG = human chorionic gonadotropin

HDL = high-density lipoprotein

HIV = human immunodeficiency virus

HMG-CoA reductase inhibitor = 3-hydroxy-3-methylglutaryl coenzyme A reductase

inhibitor

IGF-1 = insulinlike growth factor 1

LDL = low-density lipoprotein

LH = luteinizing hormone

MCV = mean corpuscular volume

MIBG = *meta*-iodobenzylguanidine

MRI = magnetic resonance imaging

NPH insulin = neutral protamine Hagedorn insulin

PCSK9 inhibitor = proprotein convertase subtilisin/kexin 9 inhibitor

PET = positron emission tomography

PSA = prostate-specific antigen

PTH = parathyroid hormone

PTHrP = parathyroid hormone–related protein

SGLT-2 inhibitor = sodium-glucose cotransporter 2 inhibitor

SHBG = sex hormone–binding globulin

T$_3$ = triiodothyronine

T$_4$ = thyroxine

TPO antibodies = thyroperoxidase antibodies

TRH = thyrotropin-releasing hormone

TRAb = TSH-receptor antibodies

TSH = thyrotropin

VLDL = very low-density lipoprotein

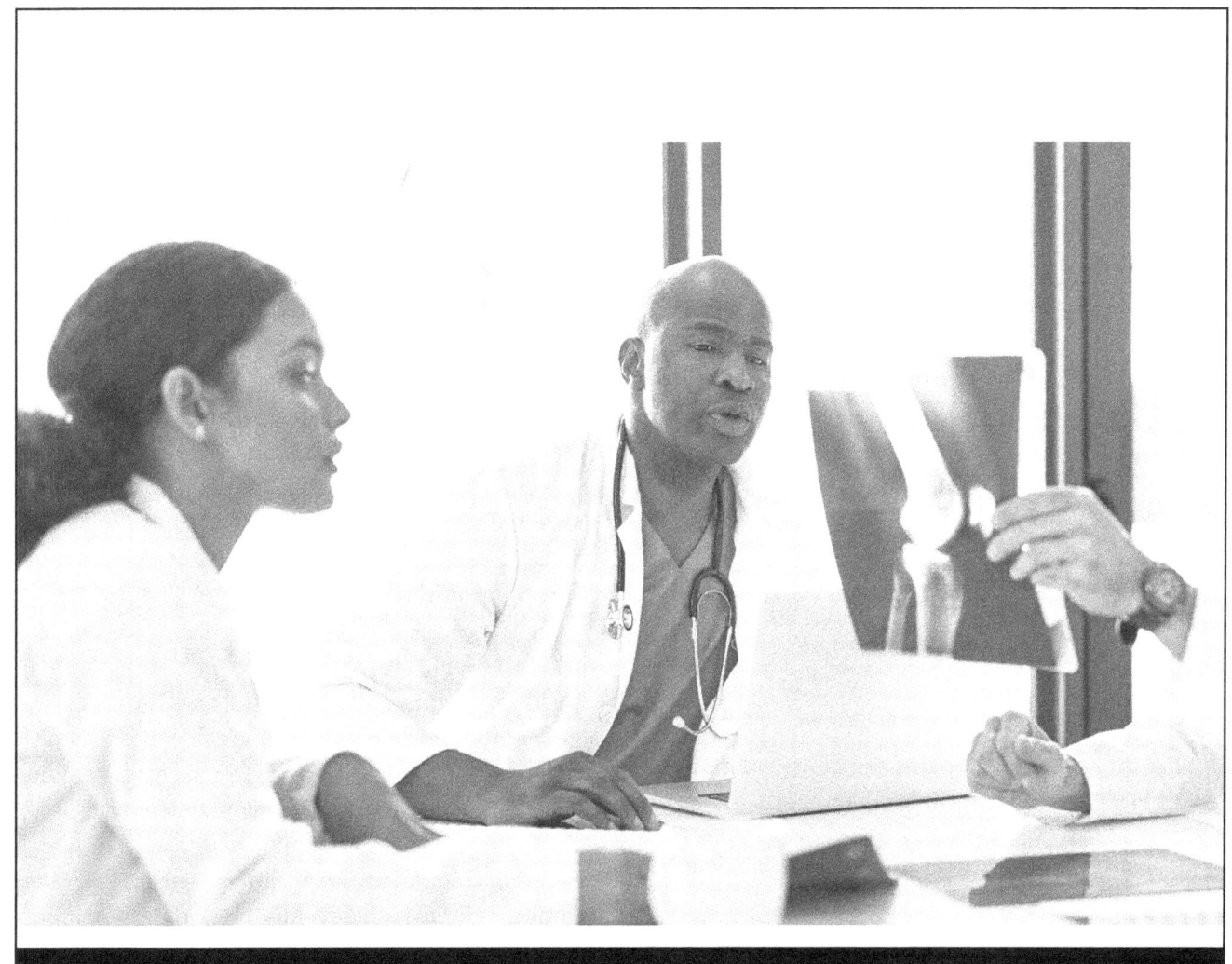

ADIPOSE TISSUE, APPETITE, OBESITY, AND LIPIDS

Primer on Weight-Loss Medications

Nasreen Alfaris, MD, MPH. Obesity Medicine Department, Obesity, Endocrine, and Metabolism Center, King Fahad Medical City, Riyadh, Saudi Arabia; Email: Nasreen.alfaris@gmail.com

Educational Objectives

After reviewing the chapter, learners should be able to:

- Identify the patient population that should be treated with antiobesity medications (AOMs).

- Describe the current evidence-based pharmacotherapeutic agents used to treat individuals living with obesity.

- Identify potential benefits of obesity treatment in individuals living with the disease.

- Describe the use of AOMs in children and adolescents.

Significance of the Clinical Problem

Obesity is the most common chronic disease globally. Multiple epidemiologic studies have identified preobesity (BMI = 25-29.9 kg/m^2) and obesity (BMI $\geq$30 kg/m^2) as predisposing factors to a number of noncommunicable diseases, including type 2 diabetes mellitus (T2DM), cardiovascular disease, and cancer. Obesity contributes significantly to the burden of disease, accounting for 120 million disability-adjusted life-years.[1]

Despite efforts focused on behavioral modifications such as alterations in diet and increased physical activity, these interventions have not demonstrated consistent, clinically meaningful, and sustainable weight-loss outcomes.[2] Historically, pharmacotherapy for obesity faced skepticism due to concerns about effectiveness and safety, leading to the withdrawal of several medications from the market due to potential serious adverse effects. Coupled with the pervasive stigma surrounding obesity as a chronic condition, AOMs garnered a controversial reputation.[3]

However, a shift has occurred recently, with AOMs emerging as pivotal, safe, and effective tools in the treatment of obesity. The US FDA has approved multiple AOMs for weight management based on several randomized controlled trials (RCTs) demonstrating their efficacy and safety. Ongoing research is further investigating numerous AOMs in development, underscoring a changing landscape where AOMs are increasingly recognized as valuable components in the multifaceted approach to treating obesity.

Practice Gaps

- There is a lack of awareness among many health care providers regarding the potential advantages of using AOMs in the treatment of obesity.

- It is crucial for clinicians to tailor treatments for obesity to distinct patient populations, as there is a variety (AOMs) with diverse mechanisms of action.

- There is a lack of awareness of the complexity and chronicity of obesity treatment in both children and adults.

Discussion

Obesity is a chronic, progressive, relapsing, multifactorial, heterogenous disease requiring a multifaceted, transdisciplinary approach to treatment. Lifestyle intervention has been shown to cause modest weight loss with more than 80% of the weight lost regained at 5 years.[4] Therefore, the use of effective, safe treatments is an essential tool in the management of this disease. Several AOMs have been approved as an adjunct to lifestyle intervention in the long-term treatment of obesity in both children 12 years and older and adults (*Figure*). These medications are approved for use in individuals with a BMI of 27 kg/m² or higher with an obesity-related complication, such as T2DM, hypertension, or obstructive sleep apnea, and in individuals with a BMI of 30 kg/m² or higher with or without obesity-related complications. These medications have different mechanisms of action.

AOMs Currently Approved for Long-Term Treatment of Obesity

Phentermine

Phentermine is a centrally acting noradrenergic agent that reduces appetite by increasing activation of adrenergic and dopaminergic receptors. Phentermine was approved for the short-term treatment of obesity (≤12 weeks duration) in 1959. It is important to note that this drug was approved before the necessity of long-term treatment for obesity was established. Therefore, there are limited studies exploring the long-term use of phentermine. Weight loss in those limited trials was about 5% of total body weight, with adverse effects being reported as symptoms of central nervous system stimulation such as insomnia, irritability, and anxiety.[5]

Orlistat

Orlistat is a gastrointestinal lipase inhibitor that was approved for weight management in 1999. In an RCT, orlistat (120 mg 3 times daily) as an adjunct to a reduced-calorie diet over a period of 2 years resulted in 7.6% total body weight loss. The most common adverse effects reported with the medication were gastrointestinal symptoms.[6]

Figure. Percentage Total Body Weight Loss in RCTs of Approved AOMs

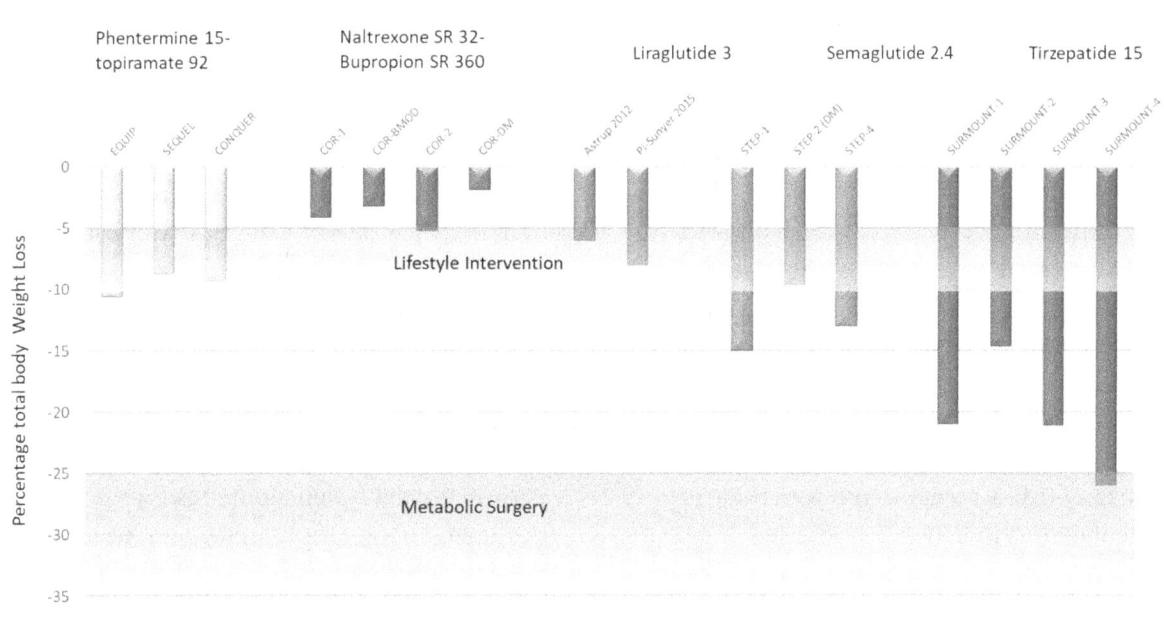

[Color—Print (Color Gallery page CG3) or web & ePub editions]

Phentermine/Topiramate

Phentermine plus topiramate extended release was approved for long-term use for weight management in adults living with obesity in 2012 and in children 12 years and older in 2022. This combination therapy comprises of phentermine, a centrally acting noradrenergic agent, and topiramate, a carbonic anhydrase inhibitor with neurotransmitter-mediated appetite suppression and the ability to enhance satiety. This combination was studied in 3 RCTs: the EQUIP, CONQUER, and SEQUEL trials. At its highest dosage of 15/92 mg, the combination drug resulted in 10.6% total body weight loss over 1 year. The most common adverse effects reported with the combination drug were dysgeusia, paresthesia, dry mouth, disturbance in attention, hypoesthesia, constipation, and dizziness.[6]

Naltrexone/Bupropion

Naltrexone plus bupropion extended release is a combination AOM approved for weight management in adults in 2014. This formulation acts through stimulating the pro-opiomelanocortin (POMC) and blocking the autoinhibitory feedback that is associated with a decline in weight reduction. Additionally, the combination drug also regulates the mesolimbic reward pathways, potentially promoting further weight reduction by modulating reward values and goal-oriented behaviors. This formulation has been studied in in the COR program. These RCTs demonstrated weight loss up to 6.1% total body weight at 1 year, with 60% of participants reaching clinically meaningful weight loss of at least 5%. The most common adverse effects reported with the combination drug were gastrointestinal in nature including nausea and constipation. Other reported adverse events were headaches, dizziness, and dry mouth.[5]

Liraglutide 3.0 mg

Liraglutide is a GLP-1 receptor agonist taken as a daily subcutaneous injection. Liraglutide 3 mg was approved for weight management in adults in 2014 and in children 12 years and older in 2020.

GLP-1 receptors are expressed in hypothalamic nuclei involved in the regulation of appetite such as the paraventricular and arcuate nuclei resulting in reduced energy intake. In addition, liraglutide slows gastric emptying resulting in a feeling of fullness.[7]

In the SCALE program, liraglutide demonstrated 8% total body weight loss in individuals taking the drug for 1 year. The most common adverse effects associated with liraglutide were nausea and vomiting. These effects occurred in the first 4 to 8 weeks of treatment initiation. Gall bladder–related events were also reported in some participants who lost more weight. Additionally, pancreatitis was a rare adverse effect that was reported with the use of GLP-1 receptor agonists.[7] These drugs should be used with caution in patients with a history of pancreatitis.

Semaglutide 2.4 mg

Semaglutide is a long acting GLP-1 receptor agonist that is administered as a once-weekly subcutaneous injection. It was approved for weight management in adults in 2021 and for children 12 years and older in 2022. Semaglutide surpasses liraglutide in reducing energy intake, with a notable difference of 35% vs 16%. Additionally, semaglutide is associated with a decrease in food cravings. This enhanced efficacy may be attributed to structural distinctions between semaglutide and liraglutide enabling semaglutide to target a broader spectrum of GLP-1 receptors than liraglutide.

In the STEP program, semaglutide demonstrated weight loss reaching 15% of total body weight at 68 weeks. Adverse effects associated with the drug are gastrointestinal and similar to those associated with other GLP-1 receptor agonists.[8]

Tirzepatide

Tirzepatide is a dual GLP-1/glucose-dependent insulinotropic polypeptide (GIP) receptor agonist. It is a once-weekly subcutaneous injection that was approved for weight management in adults in 2023. In addition to its GLP-1 effect, this molecule acts on GIP. GIP regulates energy balance through cell surface receptor signaling in the brain and adipose tissue. GIP activation appears to act synergistically with GLP-1 receptor activation to allow greater weight reduction. The SURMOUNT program reported weight loss reaching 21.5% at 72 weeks with adverse effects including gastrointestinal disturbances similar to those of other incretin-based therapies.[9]

Finally, there are conflicting reports regarding the potential link between GLP-1 receptor agonists and thyroid cancer, particularly medullary thyroid cancer. Following a thorough review of various publications and systematic reviews addressing this association, the European Medicine Agency's Pharmacovigilance Risk Assessment Committee reached the conclusion that the available evidence does not substantiate a causal connection between GLP-1 receptor agonists and thyroid cancer.[10]

Despite this conclusion, caution is advised when prescribing liraglutide, semaglutide, and tirzepatide, as they still include a warning regarding the risk of thyroid C-cell tumors based on rat studies. Consequently, GLP-1 receptor agonists are contraindicated in individuals with a personal or family history of medullary thyroid cancer or multiple endocrine neoplasia type 2.

Setmelanotide

Setmelanotide is a melanocortin 4 receptor agonist approved for the treatment of monogenic obesity resulting from proopiomelanocortin (POMC) deficiency, proprotein convertase subtilisin and kexin type 1 (PCSK1) deficiency, leptin receptor (LEPR) deficiency, and Bardet-Biedl syndrome. Setmelanotide reinstates the functionality of the melanocortin 4 receptor pathway, leading to decreased appetite and facilitating weight loss. This is achieved by reducing caloric intake and boosting energy expenditure. In open-label studies, setmelanotide resulted in weight loss of about 10% within 1 year for individuals affected by these conditions.[11]

Future Direction

In addition to the aforementioned AOMs, several agents are currently undergoing phase 2 and phase 3 trials for obesity management. These newer agents include oral formulations of GLP-1 receptor agonists (oral semaglutide and orforglipron) demonstrating weight loss up to 15% in phase 3 trials[6]; triple agonists retatrutide (GLP-1 receptor agonist/GIP/glucagon) with weight loss reported up to 30% in phase 2 trials; and dual agonists (GLP-1 receptor agonist/glucagon) pemvidutide, cagrilintide (an amylin analogue) in combination with semaglutide, and GLP-1 receptor agonist combined with GIP antagonist.[6] Other molecules being investigated are the newer activin receptor agonists such as bimagrumab, which is a monoclonal antibody that binds to muscle activin-2 receptors with greater affinity than its natural ligands activin and myostatin, which function as negative regulators of muscle growth. These activin receptor agonists may help in preserving lean muscle mass with agents resulting in greater weight loss.[12]

Clinical Case Vignettes
Case 1

A 32-year-old woman with class I obesity (weight = 135 lb [61 kg]; BMI = 33 kg/m²) is seeking treatment of her obesity. She does not currently have any obesity-related complications, and she has no contraindications to the use of AOMs. While discussing her symptoms, she reports increased hunger throughout the day, often leading her to consume a second serving at meals, as one serving is typically insufficient to satisfy her.

Following a thorough review of available AOMs and their potential adverse effects, she conveys a desire for "the most effective treatment available."

On average, considering RCTs, which FDA-approved medication exhibits the highest efficacy for obesity treatment?

A. Semaglutide, 2.4 mg weekly

B. Phentermine 15 mg/topiramate 92 mg daily

C. Tirzepatide, 15 mg weekly

D. Bupropion 360 mg/naltrexone 32 mg twice daily

E. Liraglutide, 3 mg daily

Answer: C) Tirzepatide, 15 mg weekly

Several FDA-approved medications for obesity are currently available and they differ in administration route (oral vs subcutaneous injections) and efficacy. The SURMOUNT RCT investigated tirzepatide (Answer C), a once-weekly GLP-1/GIP receptor agonist, with documented weight loss up to 21.5% of total body weight at 72 weeks in the tirzepatide group compared with 3.1% in the placebo group.[9] This establishes tirzepatide as the most effective weight-loss medication to date. In the STEP trials, semaglutide 2.4 mg (Answer A) a GLP-1 receptor administered once weekly through subcutaneous injection, demonstrated 15% total body weight loss at 68 weeks in the semaglutide group compared with 2.4% in the placebo group.[8] Conversely, liraglutide 3 mg (Answer E), a GLP-1 receptor agonist administered once daily through subcutaneous injection, is the least effective among GLP-1 receptor agonists, with a mean total body weight loss of 8% compared with 2% in the placebo group at 56 weeks.[7]

Among oral AOMs, phentermine/topiramate 15 mg/92 mg (Answer B) emerged as the most effective, as indicated by the EQUIP trial, showcasing a 10.6% total body weight loss in the drug arm compared with 1.6% in the placebo arm at 56 weeks.[5] The least-effective oral agent is bupropion/naltrexone 360 mg/32 mg (Answer D), exhibiting 6.1% total body weight loss in the drug arm vs 1.3% in the placebo arm at 56 weeks.[5]

It is crucial to emphasize that when selecting an AOM, effectiveness should not be the sole deciding factor. Obesity is a chronic, complex, and heterogenous disease, with individuals showing varying responses to different interventions. The disease's heterogeneity implies differences in how individuals respond to treatments. When choosing an AOM, considerations should extend beyond efficacy to encompass other parameters, including complications associated with the disease such T2DM, hypertension, and polycystic ovary disease.

Moreover, factors such as patient preferences (oral vs injectable options), medication costs—especially given that obesity treatment may not be universally covered by insurance—potential drug interactions, and adverse effects should all be considered. Therefore, in the treatment of individuals living with obesity, it is essential to comprehensively consider the aforementioned aspects to ensure that patients receive the most suitable and sustainable option for their unique circumstances.

Case 2

A 46-year-old man with class II obesity currently weighs 239 lb (108.5 kg) (BMI 37.5 kg/m^2) with a waist circumference of 59 in (150 cm). He has a history of hypertension and experienced a myocardial infarction 3 years ago. He has no other chronic diseases. He is worried about having another heart attack if he does not treat his obesity.

Which of the following AOMs is the most appropriate choice for this patient?

A. Liraglutide, 3 mg daily

B. Semaglutide, 2.4 mg weekly

C. Tirzepatide, 15 mg weekly

D. Orlistat, 120 mg daily

E. Phentermine 15 mg/topiramate 92 mg daily

Answer: B) Semaglutide, 2.4 mg weekly

Overweight and obesity are linked to a heightened risk of cardiovascular events, even when considering metabolic cardiovascular risk factors associated with excess weight. There is established evidence supporting the reduction of cardiovascular disease risk through treating dyslipidemia, hypertension, and diabetes. GLP-1 receptor agonists such as liraglutide and semaglutide have been studied for secondary prevention of cardiovascular disease in patients with T2DM.[13] But until recently, no AOM had been evaluated in the treatment of individuals living with obesity with preexisting cardiovascular disease but without T2DM. The SELECT trial assessed whether semaglutide 2.4 mg (Answer B) could reduce excess cardiovascular risk associated with overweight or obesity in patients without diabetes. Among 17,604 patients with a BMI of 27 kg/m² or higher and preexisting cardiovascular disease but without diabetes, treatment with once-weekly subcutaneous semaglutide at 2.4 mg reduced the risk of cardiovascular events by 20% over a mean duration of 33 months. The trial included patients with preexisting cardiovascular disease, and the effects of semaglutide on primary prevention in individuals without prior atherosclerotic disease were not studied.[14]

Currently, there is no evidence supporting the efficacy of tirzepatide (Answer C) or orlistat (Answer D) in the secondary prevention of cardiovascular events for individuals living with obesity. Available data do not indicate any increased cardiovascular risk associated with phentermine/topiramate (Answer E), but also no additional benefit in secondary prevention of cardiovascular events for individuals living with obesity.[15]

Case 3

A 13-year-old girl is accompanied by her mother seeking advice for treatment of obesity. The patient's weight today is 175 lb (79 kg), placing her above the 95th percentile with a BMI of 34 kg/m². The mother reports that her daughter started gaining weight at age 9 years and that her current weight represents the highest recorded. The girl underwent thorough evaluation for secondary causes of obesity, including genetic testing conducted by her pediatrician, which did not reveal any genetic factors contributing to

her condition. Despite a year-long collaborative effort with the pediatrician focusing on lifestyle modifications, such as adopting healthier school lunches and engaging in 30 minutes of aerobic exercise 3 times weekly, the mother perceives limited success in addressing her daughter's obesity. The girl reports experiencing hunger, particularly at night, and discloses persistent bullying from peers at school because of her weight.

Which of the following is the best advice to give this mother and her daughter?

A. Intensify lifestyle intervention to achieve weight loss

B. Start tirzepatide, 15 mg weekly

C. Recommend watchful waiting given her age

D. Start semaglutide, 2.4 mg weekly

E. Start setmelanotide, 3 mg daily

Answer: D) Start semaglutide, 2.4 mg weekly

The World Obesity Federation predicts that more than 250 million children and adolescents will have obesity by 2030.[1] Historically, the approach to childhood obesity leaned towards watchful waiting (Answer C) and lifestyle interventions (Answer A) that only resulted in modest weight loss that was difficult to maintain in the long run. However, recent recommendations from the American Academy of Pediatrics signify a shift away from this stance to offer treatment options early and at the highest available intensity. This has been fueled by the availability of effective pharmacotherapy for this age group, and the understanding of obesity as a complex, chronic, progressive, relapsing disease that requires lifelong multimodal intervention.[11]

In recent years, several medications have been studied in RCTs and approved for the long-term treatment of obesity (BMI ≥95th percentile) in children and adolescents 12 years and older. These include phentermine/topiramate combination therapy, which was studied in a 56-week RCT. On a dosage of 15/92 mg, weight loss was reported at 10.44%. On this dosage, 53% of participants lost

5% or more of their body weight, 48% lost 10% or more, and 32% lost 15% or more.[11]

Liraglutide 3 mg, a GLP-1 receptor agonist, was also studied in this age group. Results from a 56-week RCT demonstrated a 6% total body weight loss in participants taking the drug where 45% of participants lost at least 5% of their total body weight.[11]

Semaglutide 2.4 mg (Answer D) gained approval for weight management in the same age group based on the STEP-TEENS trial, showcasing 16% total body weight loss. Over 68 weeks within the trial, total body weight loss was 5% or more in 73% of participants, 10% or more in 62% of participants, 15% or more in 53% of participants, and 20% or more in 37% of participants.[11]

Trials of tirzepatide (Answer B) in children and adolescents are still ongoing, and the drug has not yet received approval for use in this age group.

Setmelanotide (Answer E), a melanocortin 4 receptor agonist, is approved for managing conditions such as proopiomelanocortin (POMC) deficiency, proprotein convertase subtilisin and kexin type 1 (PCSK1) deficiency, leptin receptor (LEPR) deficiency, and Bardet-Biedl syndrome. Although rare, these conditions pose significant challenges for health care professionals. In cases where setmelanotide has been used, it demonstrated a notable weight reduction of up to 10% within 1 year for individuals affected by these conditions, characterized by early-onset obesity and hyperphagia.[11]

Key Learning Points

- Obesity is a chronic, progressive, multifactorial, heterogeneous, relapsing disease that requires long-term treatment. AOMs are safe and effective tools for the treatment of obesity. Unfortunately, data from the ACTION-IO study show that this tool is underused.

- Different AOMs have different mechanisms of action and different efficacies. Incretin-based therapies are the most effective available AOMs so far.

- Semaglutide 2.4 mg has shown potential for secondary prevention of cardiovascular disease in patients without T2DM, demonstrating a reduced risk for cardiovascular events by 20% over 33 months.

- Several AOMs have been approved for the long-term treatment of obesity in children 12 years and older. Healthcare providers should shift from the watchful waiting stance when managing childhood obesity and follow a more evidence-based approach.

References

1. Alfaris N, Alqahtani AM, Alamuddin N, Rigas G. Global impact of obesity. *Gastroenterol Clin North Am.* 2023;52(2):277-293. PMID: 37197873

2. Look AHEAD Research Group; Wing RR, Bolin P, et al. Cardiovascular effects of intensive lifestyle intervention in type 2 diabetes. *N Engl J Med.* 2013;369(2):145-154. PMID: 23796131

3. Kaplan LM, Golden A, Jinnett K, et al. Perceptions of barriers to effective obesity care: results from the National ACTION Study. *Obesity (Silver Spring).* 2018;26(1):61-69. PMID: 29086529

4. Anderson JW, Konz EC, Frederich RC, Wood CL. Long-term weight-loss maintenance: a meta-analysis of US studies. *Am J Clin Nutr.* 2001;74(5):579-584. PMID: 11684524

5. Yanovski SZ, Yanovski JA. Long-term drug treatment for obesity: a systematic and clinical review. *JAMA.* 2014;311(1):74-86. PMID: 24231879

6. Chakhtoura M, Haber R, Ghezzawi M, Rhayem C, Tcheroyan R, Mantzoros CS. Pharmacotherapy of obesity: An update on the available medications and drugs under investigation. *EClinicalMedicine.* 2023;58:101882. PMID: 36992862

7. Pi-Sunyer X, Astrup A, Fujioka K, et al. A randomized, controlled trial of 3.0 mg of liraglutide in weight management. *N Engl J Med.* 2015;373(1):11-22. PMID: 26132939

8. Wilding JPH, Batterham RL, Calanna S, et al. Once-weekly semaglutide in adults with overweight or obesity. *N Engl J Med.* 2021;384(11):989-1002. PMID: 33567185

9. Jastreboff AM, Aronne LJ, Ahmad NN, et al; SURMOUNT-1 Investigators. Tirzepatide once weekly for the treatment of obesity. *N Engl J Med.* 2022;387(3):205-216. PMID: 35658024

10. European Medicines Agency. Meeting highlights from the Pharmacovigilance Risk Assessment Committee (PRAC) 23-26 October 2023. GLP-1 receptor agonists: available evidence not supporting link with thyroid cancer. October 27, 2023. https://www.ema.europa.eu/en/news/meeting-highlights-pharmacovigilance-risk-assessment-committee-prac-23-26-october-2023.

11. Wong G, Srivastava G. Obesity management in children and adolescents. *Gastroenterol Clin North Am.* 2023;52(2):443-455. PMID: 37197885

12. Heymsfield SB, Coleman LA, Miller R, et al. Effect of bimagrumab vs placebo on body fat mass among adults with type 2 diabetes and obesity: a phase 2 randomized clinical trial. *JAMA Netw Open.* 2021;4(1):e2033457. PMID: 33439265

13. Kristensen SL, Rørth R, Jhund PS, et al. Cardiovascular, mortality, and kidney outcomes with GLP-1 receptor agonists in patients with type 2 diabetes: a systematic review and meta-analysis of cardiovascular outcome trials. *Lancet Diabetes Endocrinol.* 2019;7(10):776-785. PMID: 31422062

14. Lincoff AM, Brown-Frandsen K, Colhoun HM, et al. Semaglutide and cardiovascular outcomes in obesity without diabetes. *N Engl J Med.* 2023;389(24):2221-2232. PMID: 37952131

15. Jordan J, Astrup A, Engeli S, Narkiewicz K, Day WW, Finer N. Cardiovascular effects of phentermine and topiramate: a new drug combination for the treatment of obesity. *J Hypertens.* 2014;32(6):1178-1188. PMID: 24621808

Practical Approach to Patients With Metabolic Dysfunction-Associated Steatotic Liver Disease

Kenneth Cusi, MD. Division of Endocrinology, Diabetes, and Metabolism, The University of Florida, Gainesville, Florida; Email: kcusi@ufl.edu

Educational Objectives

After reviewing this chapter, learners should be able to:

- Explain the link between metabolic dysfunction-associated steatotic liver disease (MASLD) and cirrhosis, and why individuals with obesity or type 2 diabetes mellitus (T2DM) are at the highest risk of cirrhosis if unidentified and untreated.

- Describe recent clinical practice guideline recommendations for screening/risk-stratifying individuals at risk for metabolic dysfunction-associated steatohepatitis (MASH) and clinically significant hepatic fibrosis (those with moderate-to-advanced liver fibrosis [≥F2] and at high risk of developing cirrhosis) and determine when to refer to a specialist.

- Apply strategies to manage intermediate-to-advanced liver fibrosis (≥F2), especially for patients with obesity or T2DM, using recommended lifestyle approaches and pharmacological treatments that reverse steatohepatitis and slow fibrosis progression.

- Recognize the higher risk of T2DM and of cardiovascular disease in people with MASLD and how to intervene to prevent or treat.

*The term *nonalcoholic fatty liver disease (NAFLD)* has been replaced with the term *metabolic dysfunction-associated steatotic liver disease (MASLD),* and the term *nonalcoholic steatohepatitis (NASH)* has been replaced with the term *metabolic dysfunction-associated steatohepatitis (MASH).*

Significance of the Clinical Problem

The epidemics of obesity and T2DM have made MASLD the most common chronic liver condition across the globe.[1] Its impact is reaching epidemic proportions but has just recently been more appreciated by primary care clinicians and endocrinology specialists. In the United States, an estimated 70% to 80% of people with obesity and T2DM have steatosis.[2-5] About 30% to 50% of patients with T2DM and steatosis have MASH,[6] the progressive kind of the disease associated with ballooning (ie, hepatocyte injury) and lobular inflammation. People with obesity or T2DM and MASH are at a high risk of developing not only cirrhosis but hepatocellular carcinoma. About 12% to 20% of all patients with T2DM have clinically significant fibrosis (histological stage ≥F2), meaning that they are on a path to cirrhosis if unidentified and untreated.[1] Patients with T1DM, believed to not be at risk of cirrhosis from steatohepatitis, are also at risk if they have obesity. Cirrhosis from steatohepatitis is becoming the most common cause of liver transplantation in the United States. If identified early, such patients could receive nutritional and lifestyle counseling, be considered for metabolic surgery, or be offered pharmacological treatments such as a GLP-1 receptor agonist or pioglitazone with the dual goal of treating steatohepatitis and associated comorbidities (ie, obesity and/or T2DM).

The nomenclature of NAFLD and NASH has recently changed to MASLD and MASH.[7] In addition to steatosis, to meet the definition of MAFLD, individuals must at least have 1 cardiometabolic risk factor associated with insulin resistance (ie, prediabetes or T2DM, obesity, hypertension, atherogenic dyslipidemia). A new category labeled MetALD encompasses people with significant alcohol intake greater than in MASLD, but not to levels observed in alcoholic liver disease. The nomenclature modification aimed to take away any potential patient stigma from the term "fatty" (for steatosis) and to make a "positive" diagnosis by including at least 1 cardiometabolic risk factor that could be associated with insulin resistance or "metabolic dysfunction." The new definition correlates well with NAFLD for patients in hepatology or endocrinology clinics who have T2DM and several features of the metabolic syndrome. The new definition also appears to do so in the general population, because approximately 75% of people in the United States already have overweight or obesity, and 85% have 1 cardiometabolic risk factor even without steatosis, although it may miss younger adults with insulin resistance and steatosis but without cardiometabolic risk factors.[8] Still, different cardiometabolic risk factors need more validation as surrogates for insulin resistance (eg, low for essential hypertension but high for T2DM). For instance, hypertension is caused by multiple pathways beyond insulin resistance. Another caveat is that diabetes as a MASLD criterion is not always associated with insulin resistance (ie, malabsorption in cystic fibrosis, T1DM, post pancreatectomy, or other secondary causes), leading steatosis to potentially be caused by other conditions. In summary, more work is needed to validate and add greater precision to the definition of MASLD in the future.

Practice Gaps

- Few patients in primary care or endocrine/diabetes clinics are risk-stratified for liver fibrosis from MASLD.

- Most individuals with MASLD who would benefit from treatment are unidentified and on a pathway of developing cirrhosis because of clinician unawareness, missed diagnoses, and/or inaction.

- Contrary to current clinical practice guidelines, statins are often not prescribed to individuals with MASLD (who have a very high risk of cardiovascular disease) or are discontinued when patients have mildly elevated plasma aminotransferases.

Discussion

Several recent clinical practice guidelines have recommended screening for fibrosis with the FIB-4 index in individuals at high-risk for steatohepatitis.[2-5] The highest-risk groups include people with T2DM (also prediabetes), people with overweight or obesity with cardiometabolic risk factors, and people with elevated plasma aminotransferases or steatosis on imaging. Normal ALT cutoffs are lower than those reported in most clinical laboratories (29-33 U/L [0.48-0.55 μkat/L] for males and 19-25 U/L [0.32-0.42 μkat/L] for females), as higher concentrations are associated with increased liver-related mortality.[2] In these high-risk groups, the initial screening/fibrosis risk-stratification strategy is based on using FIB-4, calculated from age, ALT, AST, and platelet count (risk calculator: https://www.mdcalc.com/calc/2200/fibrosis-4-fib-4-index-liver-fibrosis). The rationale for the use of FIB-4 as first-line screening is based on its low cost, simplicity, and specificity, although its sensitivity is far from ideal. When the index is less than 1.3, most individuals have a low risk of advanced liver fibrosis (stages F3 [precirrhosis] or F4 [cirrhosis]). A value greater than 2.67 suggests a high probability of advanced fibrosis and end-stage liver disease.[2-5]

Values between 1.3 and 2.67 are considered of intermediate risk or "indeterminate" to make a diagnosis of advanced fibrosis (F3-F4). The FIB-4 also assists clinicians with monitoring changes in hepatic fibrosis over time and has been reported to even predict future hepatic decompensation and liver-related mortality, as well as future cardiovascular disease. If a patient's FIB-4 index is greater than 1.3, clinical practice guidelines recommend a second risk-stratification test: either transient elastography or, alternatively, a second blood test—the enhanced liver fibrosis (ELF) test. Given the effect of age in the FIB-4 calculation, it should not be used in people younger than 35 years and used with caution in people 65 years or older where higher cutoffs should be considered. Having MASLD also increases the risk of developing T2DM and cardiovascular disease. People with obesity and T2DM usually have severe insulin resistance that worsens the natural history of steatohepatitis and likely accelerates the likelihood of developing end-stage liver disease.[2-5]

People with overweight or with obesity and MASLD should be encouraged to introduce lifestyle changes that lead to weight loss, as well as consider bariatric surgery when indicated, as it can reverse steatohepatitis and reverse fibrosis (or slow its progression). The Mediterranean diet is the most commonly recommended diet for long-term liver and cardiometabolic health, but any diet that promotes weight loss has beneficial effects on MASLD.

Pharmacological approaches are available to reverse MASH, although none are approved specifically to treat MASH (*Table, following page*). Among them, GLP-1 receptor agonists take advantage of human physiology to promote weight loss, with liraglutide and semaglutide being the best studied drugs in this class in MASH.[9] Combined with lifestyle changes, GLP-1 receptor agonists often lead to a weight reduction that is associated with significant histological improvement of steatohepatitis.[9,10] GLP-1 receptor agonists improve glycemic control and atherogenic dyslipidemia and reduce cardiovascular risk. Pioglitazone has also been incorporated into all clinical practice recommendations to treat steatohepatitis.[2-5] Several paired-biopsy randomized controlled trials have consistently reported a reversal of MASH in people with obesity, prediabetes, or T2DM.[11-16] A recent meta-analysis confirms that pioglitazone reverses steatohepatitis, and in a minority of patients, also fibrosis. Pioglitazone improves insulin sensitivity, glucose and lipid metabolism, and many cardiometabolic parameters present in persons with obesity and T2DM (endothelial function, systemic inflammation, dyslipidemia, low adiponectin).[10] The 2024 American Diabetes Association guidelines also suggest its use to lower the risk of cerebrovascular events and myocardial infarction in people with a medical history of stroke who also have prediabetes and insulin resistance.[4] Pioglitazone significantly decreases the risk of cardiovascular risk in patients with or without T2DM, as well as progression of atherosclerosis.[10]

Clinical Case Vignettes
Case 1

A 66-year-old man with obesity (BMI = 39 kg/m²), atherogenic dyslipidemia, hypertension, and cardiovascular disease has a routine follow-up appointment for hypothyroidism. However, his greatest concern is his risk of steatohepatitis. Steatosis was diagnosed on ultrasonography performed to evaluate right upper-quadrant discomfort.

On physical examination, he has central obesity and acanthosis nigricans, but findings are overall unremarkable.

A recent routine laboratory panel was within normal limits, except for the following:

> Plasma AST = 26 U/L (20-48 U/L) (SI: 0.43 μkat/L [0.33-0.80 μkat/L])
> Plasma ALT = 49 U/L (10-40 U/L) (SI: 0.82 μkat/L [0.17-0.67 μkat/L])
> Platelet count = 250 × 10³/μL (150-450 × 10³/μL) (SI: 250 × 10⁹/L [150-450 × 10⁹/L])

Secondary causes of liver disease have been ruled out by his primary care provider on the basis of history, physical examination, and pertinent laboratory values.

Table 1. Summary of Antihyperglycemic Drugs Used in Randomized Controlled Trials for Treatment of Adults With Nonalcoholic Fatty Liver Disease

	NAFLD	Other benefits	Contraindications	Side effects
Pioglitazone (91–9591–95)	Improves steatohepatitis; improves liver fibrosis in some studies (92, 94)	Cardiometabolic benefit	Caution if history of osteoporosis	Lower-extremity edema (5%-8%)
		Prevents development of T2D	Avoid if history of heart failure or bladder cancer	Dose-dependent weight gain: 15 mg/d: 1%-2% 30-45 mg/d: 3%-5%
GLP-1 receptor agonists (78, 102, 103) (liraglutide, semaglutide)	Liraglutide and semaglutide ameliorate inflammation and progression of fibrosis	Cardiometabolic benefit	Cholelithiasis	Gastrointestinal side effects
		Weight loss	Pancreatitis (?) At risk of medullary thyroid cancer	
Dual GIP-GIP-1 receptor agonist (tirzepatide) (107)	Reduces steatosis	Weight loss	At risk of medullary thyroid cancer	Gastrointestinal side effects
SGLT2 inhibitors (111–113111–113)	Reduces steatosis (unknown effect on steatohepatitis)	Cardiometabolic benefit	CKD (eGFR 20-30 depending on SGLT2i)	Genital infections
		Prevention of ESRD		Volume depletion, hypotension Diabetic ketoacidosis (rare)
Metformin (1, 19, 109)	No effect on steatohepatitis	Cardiometabolic benefit	CKD (eGFR < 30)	Gastrointestinal side effects
			Heart failure	B_{12} deficiency
			Cirrhosis	Risk of lactic acidosis (rare)
DPP-4 inhibitors (108, 109)	No effect on steatosis (unknown if steatohepatitis benefit)	Weight neutral	Pancreatitis	
Insulin (114, 115)	Reduces steatosis (unknown effect on steatohepatitis)	Cardiometabolic benefit (controversial)	Caution in patients at high risk of hypoglycemia	Hypoglycemia (more in patients with cirrhosis)

Abbreviations: CKD, chronic kidney disease; DPP-4, dipeptidyl dipetidaase-4; eGFR, estimated glomerular filtration rate; ESRD, end-stage renal disease; GIP, glucose-dependent insulinotropic polypeptide; GLP-1, glucagon-like peptide 1; NAFLD, nonalcoholic fatty liver disease; SGLT2i, sodium glucose cotransporter 2 inhibitor; T2D, type 2 diabetes.

Reprinted from Belfort-DeAguiar R et al. J Clin Endocrinol Metab, 2023; 108(2): 483-495. © The Authors. Published by Oxford University Press on behalf of the Endocrine Society.[17]

[Color—Print (Color Gallery page CG4) or web & ePub editions]

Which of the following is the best initial test to determine his risk of having steatohepatitis with clinically significant liver fibrosis (≥F2 or moderate-to-advanced fibrosis)?

A. CT of the liver

B. Liver biopsy

C. Calculation of FIB-4 index

D. Lifestyle changes and measurement of plasma aminotransferases in 3 months

E. GLP-1 receptor agonist therapy and liver ultrasonography in 3 months

Answer: C) Calculation of FIB-4 index

As shown in the *Figure* (*following page*), the first risk-stratification test recommended by current clinical practice guidelines is not CT (Answer A) or liver biopsy (Answer B) but calculation of the FIB-4 index (Answer C) (https://www.mdcalc.com/calc/2200/fibrosis-4-fib-4-index-liver-fibrosis). More than 70% of people with obesity or T2DM have steatosis.[6] Therefore, liver CT or liver biopsy would not be cost-effective and would expose patients to unnecessary radiation (CT) or to the risks of an invasive procedure (liver biopsy).

Secondary causes of elevated liver enzymes should be considered and ruled out (eg, alcohol abuse, viral hepatitis, hemochromatosis, medications). Prescribing lifestyle changes (Answer D) or a GLP-1 receptor agonist (Answer E) and repeating measurement of plasma aminotransferases or ultrasonography in 3 months is wrong because whether this patient has advanced liver fibrosis and cirrhosis has not been established. If he has advanced fibrosis and cirrhosis, a liver specialist should be engaged within a multidisciplinary team.

This patient's FIB-4 index was 0.98 (low risk <1.3) placing him in the low-risk category for liver fibrosis (*Figure*). He most likely has steatohepatitis given his elevated plasma aminotransferase concentrations but without significant fibrosis.

Case 1 (continued)

Should this patient be referred to a hepatologist?

A. Yes, because he has steatosis on imaging

B. Yes, because he likely has steatohepatitis

C. Yes, because he should have a liver biopsy as soon as possible

D. No, because the calculated FIB-4 index is <1.3

E. No, because we weight loss should be tried as a strategy first

Answer: D) No, because the calculated FIB-4 index is <1.3

Although this patient is likely to have steatohepatitis (secondary causes of liver disease were ruled out and the calculated FIB-4 index is <1.3), it is unlikely he has advanced fibrosis or needs a liver biopsy. Referral to a hepatologist

Figure. Approach to Patients at Risk of Clinically Significant Liver Fibrosis

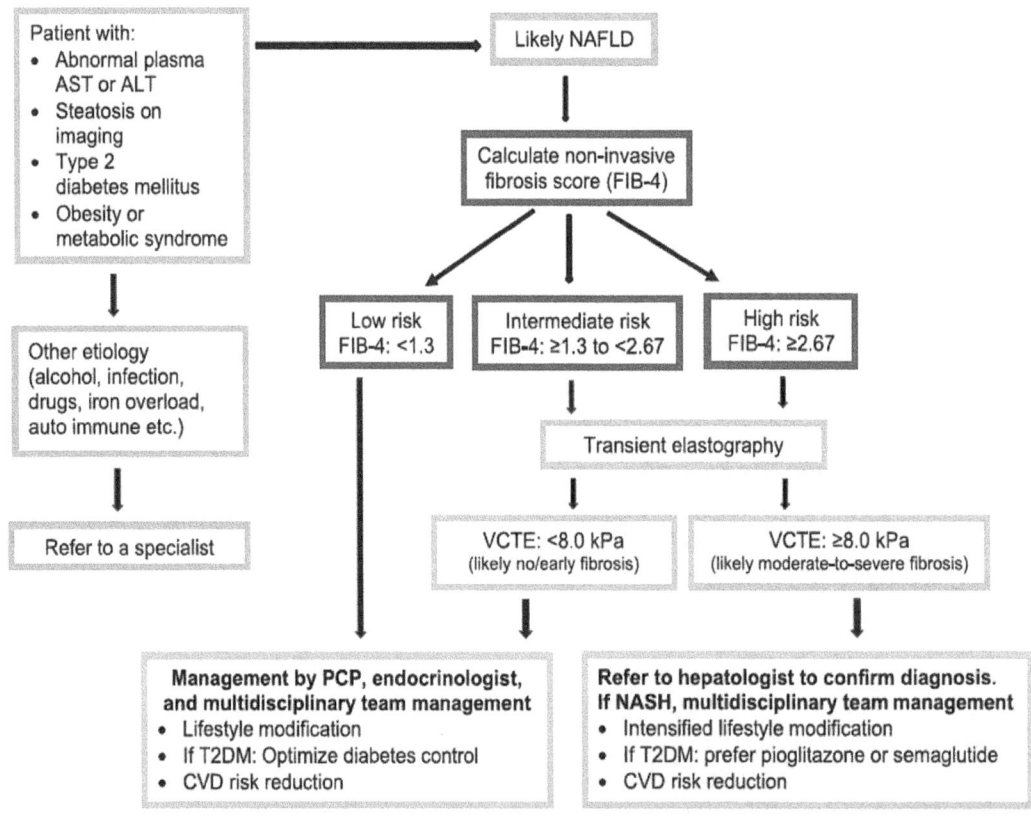

Reprinted from Chavez CP et al. *J Clin Endocrinol Metab*, 2022; 107(1):29-38. © The Authors. Published by Oxford University Press on behalf of the Endocrine Society.[11]

[Color—Print (Color Gallery page CG5) or web & ePub editions]

is unnecessary. The primary care physician or endocrinologist should recommend management. However, referral to hepatology is recommended if findings from the workup (ie, FIB-4 >1.3 and better if confirmed by transient elastography and/or plasma enhanced liver fibrosis testing) suggest "at risk" (of cirrhosis) steatohepatitis with moderate-to-advanced fibrosis (stages F2-F3) or if he already has cirrhosis (stage F4). Individuals with persistently elevated or worsening ALT or AST concentrations for longer than 6 months with hepatic steatosis on imaging should be referred to a gastroenterologist or hepatologist for further assessment, especially if they are at indeterminate risk (FIB-4, 1.3-2.67; liver stiffness measurement, 8-12 kPa; or enhanced liver fibrosis test, 7.7-9.8) or high risk (FIB-4, >2.67; liver stiffness measurement, >12 kPa; or enhanced liver fibrosis test, >9.8).

Treatment should be directed to lifestyle changes that promote weight loss, and the patient should be referred to a nutritionist and enrolled in a structured weight-loss program. Consideration should be given to bariatric surgery and eventual use of a GLP-1 receptor agonist. Taken together, these measures are likely to lead to weight loss, normalization of plasma aminotransferase values, and reversal of steatohepatitis.

Case 2

A 55-year-old woman seeks your care. She is frustrated by recurrent weight-loss attempts, having had in the past only partial success that has been followed by weight regain. She is worried about the medical implications of having obesity (current BMI = 39.2 kg/m^2) and is bothered by chronic fatigue (has obstructive sleep apnea on continuous positive airway pressure), uncontrolled T2DM (hemoglobin A$_{1c}$ = 7.9% [63 mmol/mol]), atherogenic dyslipidemia, and hypertension. Her mother had T2DM and died of cardiovascular disease at age 53 years. Her diabetes is treated pharmacologically with metformin, a sulfonylurea, and an SGLT-2 inhibitor.

Laboratory test results:

AST = 36 U/L (20-48 U/L) (SI: 0.60 μkat/L [0.33-0.80 μkat/L])
ALT = 32 U/L (10-40 U/L) (SI: 0.53 μkat/L [0.17-0.67 μkat/L])
Platelet count = 203 × 10^3/μL (150-450 × 10^3/μL) (SI: 203 × 10^9/L [150-450 × 10^9/L])

Because she is in a group at high risk for MASH with advanced fibrosis (ie, obesity, T2DM) her FIB-4 index is calculated, and it is 1.72 (considered indeterminate for advanced fibrosis; normal ≤1.3). Liver elastography is ordered (vibration-controlled transient elastography), and it reveals hepatic steatosis (controlled attenuation parameter of 311 dB/m [normal ≤274 dB/m]) and clinically significant fibrosis (liver stiffness measurement of 11.0 kPa or stage F3 fibrosis). She is referred to a hepatologist for further workup and management within a multidisciplinary team.

Which of the following approaches has the best evidence for reversing steatohepatitis, slowing fibrosis progression, and promoting cardiometabolic health?

A. Intermittent fasting diet

B. Low-fat or low-carbohydrate diet

C. Mediterranean diet

D. Ketogenic diet

E. Aerobic exercise

Answer: C) Mediterranean diet

The consensus is that all patients with overweight or obesity and MASLD must lose weight to reverse steatohepatitis and prevent cirrhosis, as well as T2DM and cardiovascular disease.[2,17,18] All of the listed diets can induce weight loss and significantly reverse steatosis. However, the recommended approach in current guidelines[2-5] based on the strongest evidence is to reverse steatohepatitis and promote cardiometabolic health by adopting the Mediterranean diet (Answer C). This diet is low in simple carbohydrates, saturated fat, and processed meats, while favoring vegetables, fruits, seeds, nuts, minimally processed foods, healthier fats (ie, omega-3 fatty acids, olive oil), whole grains, and seafood. Although any approach that promotes patient adherence to a weight-loss program is acceptable, the evidence for intermittent fasting, low-fat, low-carbohydrate diets, or ketogenic diets as a means to reverse steatohepatitis comes from small, short-term studies, and few studies having done paired liver biopsies.

Of note, about 60% of individuals who achieve 5% or more body weight loss with lifestyle modification have resolution of steatohepatitis at 1 year, which rises to 90% if weight loss is 10% or more.[19] More weight loss is often thought to be associated with regression of hepatic fibrosis, but this may not always be the case.[2] Of interest, both aerobic and resistance training can reduce steatosis if of similar intensity. An increase in physical activity decreases/reverses hepatic steatosis, even without weight loss. Structured weight-loss program are more effective in achieving weight loss, especially if combined with 150 to 300 minutes per week of moderate intensity exercise or 75 to 150 minutes per week of vigorous-intensity exercise.[2,4] A meta-analysis including 2809 participants from 26 behavioral weight-loss programs, 9 pharmacotherapy-based programs, and 8 surgery-based programs reported a clear dose-response between magnitude of weight loss and resolution of steatohepatitis, although the same was not true for fibrosis.[2]

Clinicians must always consider obesity pharmacotherapy as adjunctive therapy to lifestyle modification for individuals with obesity and MASLD. Medications approved for the treating obesity are orlistat (an oral lipase inhibitor), oral combinations phentermine/topiramate ER or naltrexone/bupropion ER (acting in the CNS), and subcutaneous formulations of GLP-1 receptor agonists such as liraglutide (titrated up to 3 mg daily) or semaglutide (titrated up to 2.4 mg weekly).[2] Most antiobesity medications are associated with a reduction in plasma aminotransferase concentrations, but their effect on liver histology in MASH (ie, paired liver biopsies) has not been well studied. Current clinical practice guidelines recommend GLP-1 receptor agonists for weight loss in patients with obesity and steatohepatitis,[2,4] with semaglutide having the strongest evidence from clinical trials.[20]

Case 2 (continued)

Which of the following is true about bariatric surgery for this individual with obesity, cardiometabolic risk factors, and steatohepatitis?

A. It is not recommended for patients with steatohepatitis

B. It is not recommended for patients with steatohepatitis and advanced fibrosis

C. It is never recommended for patients with cirrhosis

D. It would be recommended for this patient

E. It would be recommended even in the presence of decompensated cirrhosis

Answer: D) It would be recommended for this patient

Many studies report improvement of steatohepatitis, even of fibrosis, after bariatric surgery.[2,17] Bariatric surgery is recommended for people with a BMI 35 kg/m² or greater (≥32.5 kg/m² if of Asian ancestry), especially if T2DM is also present. Bariatric surgery is also indicated in the presence of MASH and cardiometabolic risk factors in patients with a BMI of 30 to 34.9 kg/m² (≥27.5-32.4 kg/m² if of Asian ancestry). A large retrospective study compared 650 patients who underwent bariatric surgery (537 Roux-en-Y gastric bypass and 113 sleeve gastrectomy) vs 508 patients assigned to be nonsurgical controls.[21] Bariatric surgery significantly reduced the absolute risk of liver outcomes (progression to cirrhosis, liver transplantation, liver cancer, or liver-related death). There was also an approximate 14% decrease in major adverse cardiovascular events.

However, in steatohepatitis with compensated cirrhosis, clinicians should individualize the use of bariatric surgery and recommend it only if an experienced surgical center is available.[2-5] In decompensated cirrhosis, the evidence of benefit for bariatric surgery is minimal and is associated with increased morbidity and mortality, and is therefore not currently recommended.[2-5]

Case 3

A 68-year-old woman with T2DM (hemoglobin A$_{1c}$ = 8.0% [64 mmol/mol]), obesity (BMI = 29.1 kg/m^2), cardiovascular disease, and atherogenic dyslipidemia is referred for management. Her current medications are metformin; a DPP-4 inhibitor; and atorvastatin, 10 mg daily.

Laboratory test results:

AST = 35 U/L (20-48 U/L) (SI: 0.58 µkat/L [0.33-0.80 µkat/L])
ALT = 45 IU/L (10-40 U/L) (SI: 0.75 µkat/L [0.17-0.67 µkat/L])
Platelet count = 127 × 10^3/µL (150-450 × 10^3/µL) (SI: 127 × 10^9/L [150-450 × 10^9/L])
FIB-4 = 2.79 (normal ≤1.3)

Vibration-controlled transient elastography documents hepatic steatosis (controlled attenuation parameter of 345 dB/m [normal ≤274 dB/m]) and clinically significant fibrosis (liver stiffness measurement of 12.0 kPa or stage F3). The patient is referred to a hepatologist, and MRI confirms elevated liver fat of 10.4% (normal ≤5.5%). Magnetic resonance elastography documents advanced liver fibrosis (3.8 kPa [stage F3: 3.62-4.69 kPa]). Liver biopsy confirms steatohepatitis: NAFLD activity score 6 (steatosis 3 [severe], inflammation 2 [moderate, with 2 to 4 foci per 200 field], and ballooning 1 [few balloon cells], and fibrosis stage 3 [advanced fibrosis]).

Which of the following agents for the treatment of type 2 diabetes have been proven in randomized controlled trials to reverse steatohepatitis?

A. Metformin

B. GLP-1 receptor agonists

C. SGLT-2 inhibitors

D. Pioglitazone

E. B and D

Answer: E) GLP-1 receptor agonists and pioglitazone

Current recommendations are that primary care providers and endocrinologists treat patients with T2DM with lifestyle modification and pharmacotherapy with proven efficacy to reverse steatohepatitis (*Table*). Pharmacotherapy for MASH in T2DM is based on the following rationale: (a) T2DM and steatohepatitis often coexist (ie, about 1 in 6 individuals with T2DM has moderate-to-advanced fibrosis [stage F ≥2]), so both pioglitazone and GLP-1 receptor agonists can be used with a "dual goal" to treat T2DM and steatohepatitis; (b) the presence of MASH with moderate-to-advanced fibrosis (stages F2-F3) is associated with higher risk of cirrhosis and liver-related mortality and can be prevented with early treatment; (c) patients with T2DM progress more rapidly to cirrhosis ("rapid progressors") and need a more aggressive approach; (d) weight loss alone is rarely successful, unless it occurs within a structured weight-loss program and with close follow-up. In addition, weight loss alone does not always reverse hepatic fibrosis.

No medication for obesity or T2DM is currently FDA-approved for the treatment of steatohepatitis. Steatohepatitis has not been reported to improve with metformin (Answer A) in randomized controlled trials with paired liver biopsy as the primary outcome. Insulin and SGLT-2 inhibitors (Answer C), while they may reduce hepatic steatosis on imaging, lack data regarding liver histological outcomes and are not recommended to reverse steatohepatitis. In contrast, pioglitazone (Answer D) and GLP-1 receptor agonists (Answer B) are safe and effective to treat both T2DM and MASH (and may also reduce cardiovascular disease, the main cause of death in MASH).

Six randomized controlled trials have reported that pioglitazone improves steatohepatitis in a significant number of patients, either with or without T2DM.[11-16] Recent meta-analysis confirms that pioglitazone reverses steatohepatitis and, in a minority of patients, also fibrosis. Pioglitazone reduces cardiovascular disease and the development of T2DM in people with insulin resistance or prediabetes, as reviewed elsewhere.[10] Adverse effects include weight gain (~1% with pioglitazone 15 mg/day and ~2%-5% with 45 mg daily in long-term studies), bone loss (potentially ameliorated with calcium and vitamin D supplementation; avoid in individuals with osteoporosis), and a perhaps small but controversial risk of bladder cancer (avoid if such a history).[10] Heart failure may occur if fluid retention happens in an individual with preexisting heart failure (pioglitazone does not cause per se heart failure). Increased rates of congestive heart failure have not been observed in randomized controlled trials studying MASH. Pioglitazone should be avoided if lower-extremity edema is already present, or in patients using very high insulin doses or amlodipine, as both medications are associated with lower-extremity edema. Pioglitazone, 15 mg daily, improves glucose and lipid metabolism in T2DM and reduces elevated plasma aminotransferases and steatosis,[22] so starting at 15 mg daily and up-titrating to 30 mg daily during follow-up is advisable, although the efficacy of 15 mg daily for reversing steatohepatitis on liver histology (biopsies) remains to be established.

A number of relatively small studies have reported benefit in MASLD with GLP-1 receptor agonists.[9,10] The best evidence supporting the role of GLP-1 receptor agonists in MASH comes from a 72-week phase 2 randomized controlled trial in 320 patients with MASH (~70% having stages F2-F3 liver fibrosis).[20] The highest dosage of semaglutide equivalent to 2.4 mg weekly led to significantly more patients having resolution of steatohepatitis (primary outcome) compared with placebo (59% vs 17% on placebo). Thus, GLP-1 receptor agonists can simultaneously treat MASH, diabetes, obesity, and cardiovascular disease and eventually be combined with other effective agents for MASH, such as pioglitazone. In 296 individuals from a substudy of the SURPASS-3 trial, participants assigned to tirzepatide (a dual GLP-1 and glucose-dependent insulinotropic polypeptide receptor agonist) at a dosage of 10 mg or 15 mg had a significant reduction in ALT and AST and in liver steatosis by MRI.[23] Recently, a randomized controlled trial with histology as the primary outcome established the role of tirzepatide in patients with MASH and stage 2 or 3 fibrosis (SYNERGY-NASH phase 2 study). In a preliminary report, all dosages of tirzepatide led to improvement in steatohepatitis and fibrosis, with the highest dosage causing resolution of MASH without progression of fibrosis in 73.9% of participants compared with 12% in participants taking placebo (https://investor.lilly.com/static-files/ecfe166b-dd40-45df-afd7-ddb81fe2cb33https://investor.lilly.com/static-files/ecfe166b-dd40-45df-afd7-ddb81fe2cb33, slide number 17; accessed March 7, 2024). Finally, survodutide, a glucagon/GLP-1 receptor dual agonist, in another preliminary report of their phase 2 study paired-liver biopsy study that up to 83% of adults achieved a significant improvement in steatohepatitis compared to 18.2% with placebo. Hepatic fibrosis was also improved (https://www.boehringer-ingelheim.com/human-health/metabolic-diseases/survodutide-top-line-results-mash-fibrosis; accessed March 7, 2024). Of note, resmetirom, a thyroid hormone β-receptor agonist, is undergoing FDA review and, if approved, would be the first FDA-approved treatment for patients with steatohepatitis (Harrison SA, et al. A phase 3, randomized, controlled trial of resmetirom in NASH with liver fibrosis. *N Engl J Med.* 2024;390[6]:497-509).

Case 3 (continued)

The patient is also concerned about having cardiovascular disease and major risk factors for a recurrent cardiovascular event. However, she is hesitant about taking statins because she has elevated plasma aminotransferases.

Laboratory test results:

> Total cholesterol = 190 mg/dL (SI: 4.92 mmol/L)
> LDL cholesterol = 90 mg/dL (SI: 2.33 mmol/L)
> Triglycerides = 250 mg/dL (SI: 2.83 mmol/L)
> HDL cholesterol 50 mg/dL (SI: 1.30 mmol/L)
> Non-HDL cholesterol = 140 mg/dL
>   (SI: 3.63 mmol/L)

Should this patient be prescribed a statin?

A. No; LDL cholesterol is already below 100 mg/dL (<2.59 mmol/L)

B. No; statins are not recommended in patients with steatohepatitis

C. No; the patient has advanced liver fibrosis and statins would be unsafe

D. Yes; statins have proven to be generally safe in patients with steatohepatitis

E. Yes; statins can reverse steatohepatitis and hepatic fibrosis

Answer: D) Yes; statins have proven to be generally safe in patients with steatohepatitis

Statins have proven to be generally safe in patients with steatohepatitis and are recommended by all clinical practice guidelines (thus, Answer D is correct and Answers A, B, and C are incorrect).[2-5] Unfortunately, too often statins are not prescribed or are discontinued with modest increases in ALT or AST, although individuals with MASLD are at a higher risk of cardiovascular disease than individuals with comparable risk factors without steatosis. Statins reduce overall mortality in people with steatohepatitis and compensated cirrhosis but should be avoided in decompensated cirrhosis.[2-5]

An LDL-cholesterol concentration of 90 mg/dL (2.33 mmol/L) is above the target for a patient with T2DM and cardiovascular disease based on current guidelines that recommend high-dosage statin therapy (should be <55 mg/dL [<1.42 mmol/L] for a patient with T2DM and established cardiovascular disease) (thus, Answer A is incorrect).

Although statins have many beneficial effects on liver metabolism and hepatocyte function, studies have not shown that they can reverse steatohepatitis and hepatic fibrosis (thus, Answer E is incorrect). Finally, caution should be given to an increased risk of myalgias, myopathy, and rhabdomyolysis when statins are given to individuals after liver transplant who are on immunosuppressants, especially with cyclosporine, although most liver transplant recipients today receive tacrolimus that is safer than cyclosporine when combined with statins.[17]

Key Learning Points

- Patients in primary care or endocrine/diabetes clinics should be risk-stratified for liver fibrosis from MASLD.

- Most individuals with MASLD benefit from treatment, including lifestyle changes, proper management of pharmacotherapy for obesity (eg, GLP-1 receptor agonists) and T2DM (eg, pioglitazone and/or GLP-1 receptor agonists), or bariatric surgery when indicated.

- Current clinical practice guidelines recommend the prescription of statins to individuals with MASLD, as they are safe and can prevent cardiovascular events in this population at very high risk of cardiovascular disease.

References

1. Stefan N, Cusi K. A global view of the interplay between non-alcoholic fatty liver disease and diabetes. *Lancet Diabetes Endocrinol*. 2022;10(4):284-296. PMID: 35183303

2. Cusi K, Isaacs S, Barb D, et al. American Association of Clinical Endocrinology clinical practice guideline for the diagnosis and management of nonalcoholic fatty liver disease in primary care and endocrinology clinical Settings: co-sponsored by the American Association for the Study of Liver Diseases (AASLD). *Endocr Pract*. 2022;28(5):528-562. PMID: 35569886

3. Kanwal F, Shubrook JH, Adams LA, et al. Clinical care pathway for the risk stratification and management of patients with nonalcoholic fatty liver disease. *Gastroenterology*. 2021;161(5):1657-1669. PMID: 34602251

4. American Diabetes Association Professional Practice Committee. 4. Comprehensive medical evaluation and assessment of comorbidities: standards of care in diabetes-2024. *Diabetes Care*. 2024;47(Suppl 1):S52-S76. PMID: 38078591

5. Rinella ME, Neuschwander-Tetri BA, Siddiqui MS, et al. AASLD practice guidance on the clinical assessment and management of nonalcoholic fatty liver disease. *Hepatology*. 2023;77(5):1797-1835. PMID: 36727674

6. Lomonaco R, Godinez Leiva E, Bril F, et al. Advanced liver fibrosis is common in patients with type 2 diabetes followed in the outpatient setting: the need for systematic screening. *Diabetes Care*. 2021;44(2):399-406. PMID: 33355256

7. Rinella ME, Lazarus JV, Ratziu V, et al; NAFLD Nomenclature Consensus Group. A multisociety Delphi consensus statement on new fatty liver disease nomenclature. *J Hepatol*. 2023;79(6):1542-1556. PMID: 37364790

8. Cusi K, Younossi Z, Roden M. From NAFLD to MASLD: promise and pitfalls of a new definition. *Hepatology.* 2024;79(2):E13-E15. PMID: 38112428

9. Patel Chavez C, Cusi K, Kadiyala S. The emerging role of glucagon-like peptide-1 receptor agonists for the management of NAFLD. *J Clin Endocrinol Metab.* 2022;107(1):29-38. PMID: 34406410

10. Gastaldelli A, Cusi K. From NASH to diabetes and from diabetes to NASH: mechanisms and treatment options. *JHEP Rep.* 2019;1(4):312-328. PMID: 32039382

11. Belfort R, Harrison SA, Brown K, et al. A placebo-controlled trial of pioglitazone in subjects with nonalcoholic steatohepatitis. *N Engl J Med.* 2006;355(22):2297-2307. PMID: 17135584

12. Aithal GP, Thomas JA, Kaye PV, et al. Randomized, placebo-controlled trial of pioglitazone in nondiabetic subjects with nonalcoholic steatohepatitis. *Gastroenterology.* 2008;135(4):1176-1184. PMID: 18718471

13. Sanyal AJ, Chalasani N, Kowdley KV, et al. Pioglitazone, vitamin E, or placebo for nonalcoholic steatohepatitis. *N Engl J Med.* 2010;362(18):1675-1685. PMID: 20427778

14. Cusi K, Orsak B, Bril F, et al. Long-term pioglitazone treatment for patients with nonalcoholic steatohepatitis and prediabetes or type 2 diabetes mellitus: a randomized trial. *Ann Intern Med.* 2016;165(5):305-315. PMID: 27322798

15. Bril F, Biernacki DM, Kalavalapalli S, et al. Role of vitamin E for nonalcoholic steatohepatitis in patients with type 2 diabetes: a randomized controlled trial. *Diabetes Care.* 2019;42(8):1481-1488. PMID: 31332029

16. Huang JF, Dai CY, Huang CF, et al. First-in-Asian double-blind randomized trial to assess the efficacy and safety of insulin sensitizer in nonalcoholic steatohepatitis patients. *Hepatol Int.* 2021;15(5):1136-1147. PMID: 34386935

17. Belfort-DeAguiar R, Lomonaco R, Cusi K. Approach to the patient with nonalcoholic fatty liver disease. *J Clin Endocrinol Metab.* 2023;108(2):483-495. PMID: 36305273

18. Bril F, Sanyal A, Cusi K. Metabolic syndrome and its association with nonalcoholic steatohepatitis. *Clin Liver Dis.* 2023;27(2):187-210. PMID: 37024202

19. Vilar-Gomez E, Martinez-Perez Y, Calzadilla-Bertot L, et al. Weight loss through lifestyle modification significantly reduces features of nonalcoholic steatohepatitis. *Gastroenterology.* 2015;149(2):367-378. PMID: 25865049

20. Newsome PN, Buchholtz K, Cusi K, et al; NN9931-4296 Investigators. A placebo-controlled trial of subcutaneous semaglutide in nonalcoholic steatohepatitis. *N Engl J Med.* 2021;384:1113-1124. PMID: 33185364

21. Aminian A, Al-Kurd A, Wilson R, et al. Association of bariatric surgery with major adverse liver and cardiovascular outcomes in patients with biopsy-proven nonalcoholic steatohepatitis. *JAMA.* 2021;326(20):2031-2042. PMID: 34762106

22. Della Pepa G, Russo M, Vitale M, et al. Pioglitazone even at low dosage improves NAFLD in type 2 diabetes: clinical and pathophysiological insights from a subgroup of the TOSCA.IT randomised trial. *Diabetes Res Clin Pract.* 2021;178:108984. PMID: 34311022

23. Gastaldelli A, Cusi K, Fernández Landó L, Bray R, Brouwers B, Rodríguez Á. Effect of tirzepatide versus insulin degludec on liver fat content and abdominal adipose tissue in people with type 2 diabetes (SURPASS-3 MRI): a substudy of the randomised, open-label, parallel-group, phase 3 SURPASS-3 trial. *Lancet Diabetes Endocrinol.* 2022;10(6):393-406. PMID: 35468325

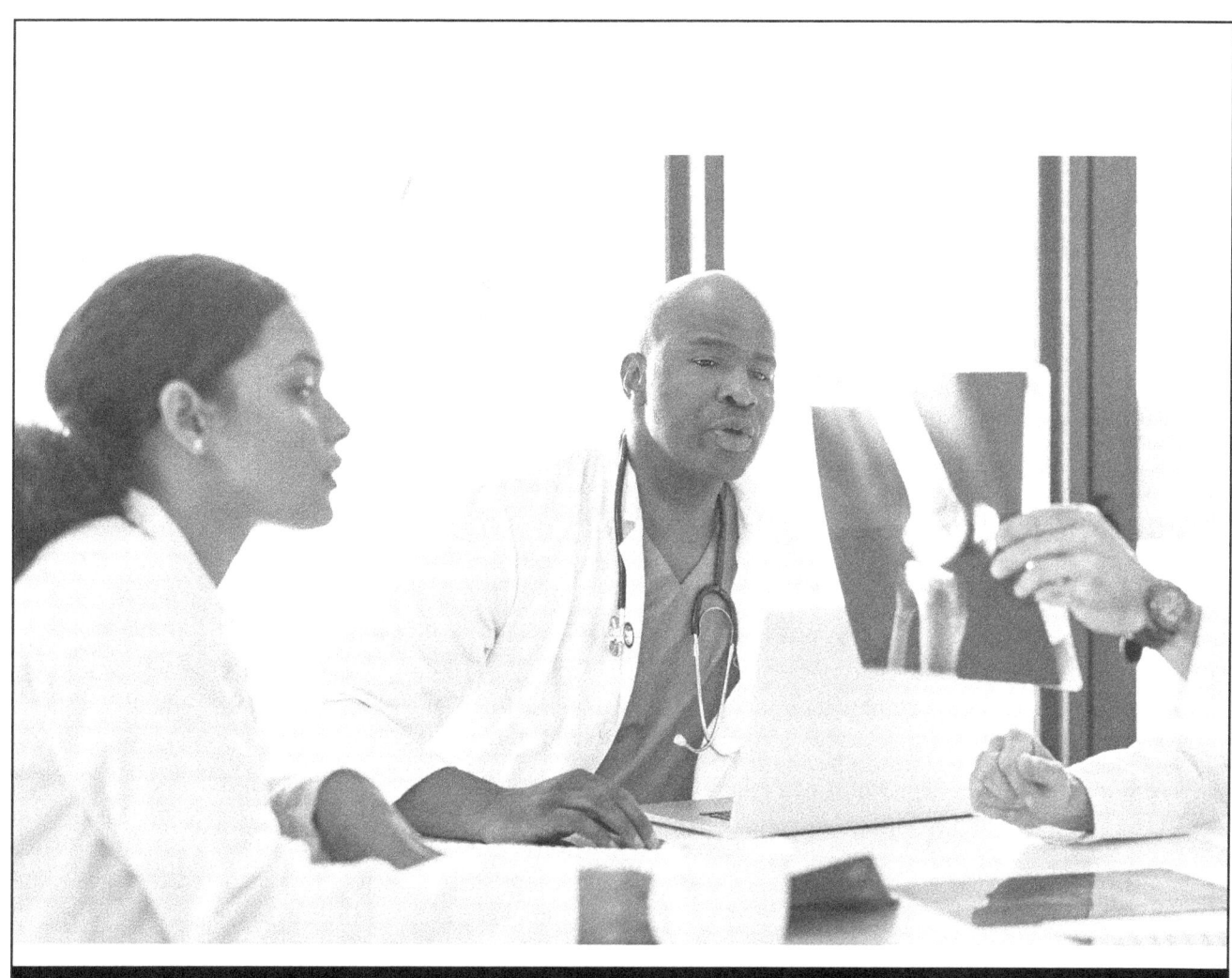

ADRENAL

Management of Hereditary Pheochromocytoma/ Paraganglioma Syndromes

Roderick Clifton-Bligh, BSc (med), MBBS, PhD. Department of Endocrinology, Royal North Shore Hospital, Sydney, NSW, Australia, and University of Sydney, NSW, Australia. Email: Roderick.cliftonbligh@sydney.edu.au

Educational Objectives

After reviewing this chapter, learners should be able to:

- Diagnose hereditary pheochromocytoma/ paraganglioma (PPGL) syndromes and arrange appropriate genetic testing.

- Recommend appropriate strategies to test at-risk family members for hereditary PPGL syndromes.

- Recommend appropriate surveillance for patients with pathogenic variants in hereditary PPGL genes.

- Identify syndromic but nonhereditary forms of PPGL due to mosaicism.

Significance of the Clinical Problem

Hereditary PPGL syndromes are autosomal dominant disorders characterized by familial predisposition to PPGLs and a variety of other neoplasms. Pheochromocytomas are tumors of the adrenal medulla that usually secrete epinephrine and/or norepinephrine; paragangliomas (PGLs) arising in extra-adrenal sympathetic chromaffin tissue often secrete norepinephrine; and head and neck parasympathetic PGLs may secrete dopamine or be biochemically silent.[1] Surgery is the only curative option for PPGLs, and it is most successful for smaller tumors (<5 cm). Failure to recognize a hereditary PPGL syndrome therefore exposes the patient to risks of delayed diagnoses of relevant syndromic features, including second primary tumors or metastases, and exposes their family members to late diagnosis of potentially incurable PPGLs.

PPGLs are rare tumors with an annual incidence of 5 to 8 cases per million.[1] Nevertheless, they are the most highly heritable of all tumors in humans, with 30% to 40% associated with germline pathogenic variants in 1 of 16 genes.[2] The most common genetic causes of PPGLs are pathogenic variants in the genes encoding the 4 subunits (A-D) of the Krebs cycle enzyme succinate dehydrogenase (SDH). Indeed, pathogenic variants in *SDHB* are found in approximately 10% of all PPGLs.[2] By comparison, the next most commonly associated genes are *VHL* (4%-10%), *RET* (1%-5%), *NF1* (1%-5%), *FH* (3%), *TMEM127* (1%), and *MAX* (1%). Newer genetic associations with *EGLN1, DNMT3A, MDH2, GOT2, DLST, SLC25A11,* and *SUCGL2* emphasize the complexity of the genetic architecture of PPGLs, albeit with rarer and likely low-penetrance alleles.[2] Recognizing these hereditary PPGL syndromes is important for the patient, their reproductive decisions, and their family members. A pathway for managing hereditary PPGL syndromes is shown in *Figure 1* (*following page*).

Figure 1. Management of Hereditary PPGL Syndromes

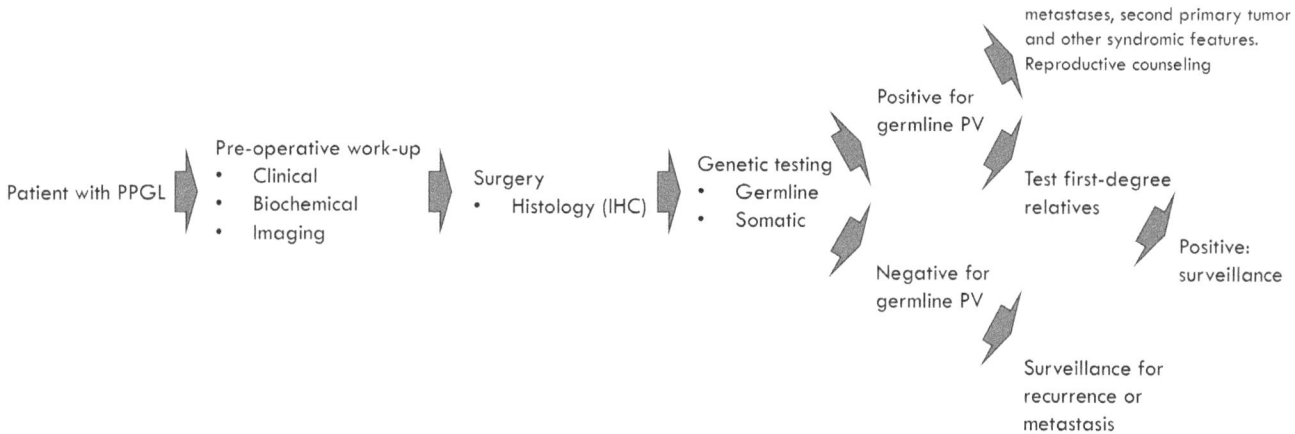

[Color—Print (Color Gallery page CG5) or web & ePub editions]

Practice Gaps

- The recognition of hereditary PPGL syndromes, which is crucial to provide appropriate surveillance for recurrent and/or metastatic disease in the patient, and as the starting point for cascade testing of first-degree relatives.

- Efficient identification of at-risk relatives, which is typically the provenance of genetic specialists working in a multidisciplinary team, who identify first-degree relatives and encourage them to come forward for counseling and genetic testing.

- Implementation of surveillance programs for carriers of pathogenic variants in PPGL genes, with mechanisms to encourage adherence to monitoring so tumors are detected early enough for optimal outcomes.

- The recognition of syndromic but nonhereditary PPGL syndromes, which can appear identical to hereditary PPGL syndromes, but which require specific patient-centered care.

Discussion

Diagnosis of Hereditary PPGL Syndromes

Diagnosis of hereditary PPGL syndromes requires careful clinical assessment, histology review, and genetic testing after appropriate counseling. Risk factors increasing the likelihood of a hereditary cause being discovered in a patient presenting with PPGL include younger age, sympathetic (thoraco-abdominal) PGL, multiple PGLs, absent SDHB immunohistochemical staining in a resected tumor, presence of syndromic features, and family history of PPGL. Importantly, absence of these features does not eliminate the possibility of an underlying genetic diagnosis; index cases of older individuals with apparently solitary pheochromocytomas may still lead to diagnoses with major importance to their family members. The *Table (following page)* lists each hereditary PPGL syndrome according to gene, associated tumor spectrum, and suggested surveillance for carriers of pathogenic variants. It is important to recognize that the specific nature of follow-up depends on a precise genetic diagnosis.

Clinical assessment of a patient presenting with PPGL should always include age of onset; nature and frequency of symptoms relevant to PPGL; history of hypertension and antihypertensive medication use; personal or

Table. Genes Associated With Hereditary PPGL and Associated Syndromes

Syndrome	Gene	Tumors	Suggested screening for PPGL in carriers*
MEN2	*RET*	MTC PC HPT	From age 11-16 y (depending on risk category of *RET* PV): annual medical review and blood pressure; annual fasting free plasma metanephrines or 24 hour urine metanephrines*
VHL	*VHL*	Retinal angioma Cerebellar, spinal HB PPGL RCC PanNET	From age 2 y: annual physical examination with BP From age 5 y: annual fasting free plasma metanephrines (if plasma unavailable 24-hour urine free metanephrines). From aged 10-15 y: abdominal MRI 2nd yearly with abdominal ultrasound in intervening years*
NF1	*NF1*	Cutaneous NFs Plexiform NFs Optic glioma PC	From age 10 y: Annual blood pressure measurement; consider measuring biogenic amines if there is unexplained hypertension*
Hereditary PGL type 1	*SDHD*	PPGL RCC GIST	For paternal inheritance only From age 10-15 y: annual clinical assessment and biennial plasma or urinary metanephrines (yearly after age 18 y) From age 10-15 y: MRI base of skull to coccyx every 2-3 years From age 18 y: DOTATATE-PET (baseline; not available in all countries)
Hereditary PGL type 2	*SDHAF2*	PGL (HN)	For paternal inheritance only From age 18 y: annual clinical assessment and plasma or urinary metanephrines From age 18 y: MRI base of skull to coccyx every 2-3 years From age 18 y: DOTATATE-PET (baseline; not available in all countries)
Hereditary PGL type 3	*SDHC*	PPGL	From age 10-15 y: annual clinical assessment and biennial plasma or urinary metanephrines (yearly after age 18 y) From age 10-15 y: MRI base of skull to coccyx every 2-3 years From age 18 y: DOTATATE-PET (baseline; not available in all countries)
Hereditary PGL type 4	*SDHB*	PPGL RCC GIST pitNET	From age 6-10 y: annual clinical assessment and biennial plasma or urinary metanephrines (yearly after age 18 y) From age 6-10 y: MRI base of skull to coccyx every 2-3 years From age 18 y: DOTATATE-PET (baseline; not available in all countries)
Hereditary PGL type 5	*SDHA*	PPGL GIST	From age 10-15 y: annual clinical assessment and biennial plasma or urinary metanephrines (yearly after age 18 y) From age 10-15 y: MRI base of skull to coccyx every 2-3 years From age 18 y: DOTATATE-PET (baseline; not available in all countries)
MEN5	*MAX*	PPGL PitNET Ganglioneuroma HPT	UNK
-	*TMEM127*	PPGL RCC	UNK
*	*FH*	PPGL	UNK
-	*DNMT3A*	PPGL (HN)	UNK
-	*MDH2*	PPGL	UNK
-	*GOT2*	PPGL	UNK
-	*SLC25A11*	PPGL	UNK
-	*DLST*	PPGL	UNK
-	*SUCGL2*	PPGL	UNK
-	*EGLN1*	PPGL	UNK

Abbreviations: GIST, gastrointestinal stromal tumor; HPT, hyperparathyroidism; MTC, medullary thyroid cancer; NF, neurofibromatosis; panNET, pancreatic neuroendocrine tumor; pitNET, pituitary neuroendocrine tumor; PC, pheochromocytoma; PPGL, pheochromocytoma and paraganglioma; RCC, renal cell cancer; UNK, unknown (no consensus yet).

*Recommendations for surveillance of carriers to detect PPGLs, noting these may differ from country to country and that for VHL, MEN 2, and NF1 additional surveillance is required for other tumors associated with these syndromes. Data drawn from Amar L, Pacak K, Steichen O, et al. International consensus on initial screening and follow-up of asymptomatic SDHx mutation carriers. Nat Rev Endocrinol. 2021;17(7):435-444, VHL Alliance (https://www.vhl.org), Cancer.NET (https://www.cancer.net), and https://www.eviq.org.au/cancer-genetics.

[Color—Print (Color Gallery page CG6) or web & ePub editions]

family history of other tumors, including PPGLs, renal cell cancer, gastrointestinal stromal tumors (GISTs), pituitary neuroendocrine tumors (NETs), pancreatic NETs, thyroid cancer (medullary), plexiform neurofibromas, optic gliomas, and retinal angiomas or hemangioblastomas; and family history of sudden death attributed to cardiovascular causes. Careful physical examination is crucial and clinical features alone might be sufficient for diagnosis. For instance, a patient with pheochromocytoma who also has cerebellar or spinal hemangioblastoma and/or retinal angioma is highly likely to have von Hippel-Lindau (VHL) syndrome. Conversely, a patient with pheochromocytoma, a neck mass, and elevated calcitonin is likely to have multiple endocrine neoplasia type 2 (MEN 2). Remember some patients with VHL present with only pheochromocytoma (type 2C pattern), and as many as 10% of patients with MEN 2 present with pheochromocytoma as their index tumor.

Biochemical assessment should include measurement of supine fasting plasma metanephrine, normetanephrine, and (if available) 3-methoxytyramine by liquid chromatography with tandem mass spectrometry. Urinary metanephrine and normetanephrine measurements are reasonable if plasma measurements are not available for an individual patient.

Imaging assessment should include structural imaging directed at the index tumor (eg, adrenal). Preoperative functional imaging (eg, somatostatin receptor targeted PET) may be appropriate when the chance of finding a second tumor or metastases is high, for instance, if the patient is already known to carry an *SDHx* pathogenic variant. If the index tumor is a head/neck PGL, then the possibility of also having a biochemically functioning tumor (eg, thoraco-abdominal PGL or pheochromocytoma) should be investigated.

Histological assessment is a vital part of diagnosing hereditary PPGL syndromes. Although traditional appearance with hematoxylin and eosin stain is similar for all genetic subtypes of PPGL, immunohistochemical deficiency of SDHB identifies tumors with a high likelihood of an underlying pathogenic variant in any of the SDH genes or occasionally in the *VHL* gene.[3] When such variants are not identified, SDHB deficiency becomes the cornerstone of diagnosing Carney triad (see below).[4] Loss of SDHA staining is helpful in identifying patients with an *SDHA* pathogenic variant; loss of FH and gain of 2SC staining identifies patients likely carrying an *FH* pathogenic variant.[5]

Referral for genetic testing is usually performed after resection of the index PPGL, although selected patients may benefit from preoperative genetic diagnosis where the surgical approach would change, (eg, adrenocortical-sparing surgery in patients with MEN 2 or VHL and bilateral pheochromocytoma). There is still some controversy regarding whether all patients presenting with PPGL should have germline genetic testing. In the absence of the moderating risk factors noted above, the risk of finding a pathogenic variant in a patient with adrenal pheochromocytoma is low after age 70 years. However, for patients with PGL, the risk of finding a pathogenic variant remains greater than 10% even at older ages.

Genetic testing is usually performed on germline DNA isolated from peripheral blood leukocytes, after appropriate counseling. Genetic testing on tumor tissue, however, offers the following advantages:

- Somatic pathogenic variants in *HRAS, CSDE1, FGFR1, BRAF,* or *MAML3* fusions identify patients with sporadic disease in whom no additional germline testing is required (pathogenic variants in these genes are purely somatic and mutually exclusive to germline pathogenic variants).[6]

- Diagnosis of pathogenic variants in *RET, VHL, NF1,* or *SDHx* genes identifies patients for whom targeted testing of germline DNA is appropriate (tumor pathogenic variants in these genes may be either somatic or germline).

- Identification of pathogenic variants in *EPAS1* or *H3F3A* diagnoses specific syndromic but nonhereditary forms of PPGL syndromes.

Genetic testing should ideally be performed using next-generation sequencing methods, supplemented as needed by techniques sensitive to copy-number pathogenic variants (eg, multiplex ligation-dependent probe amplification) that occur in the *VHL, NF1,* and *SDHx* genes.[7]

After a positive genetic diagnosis, the patient should receive posttest counseling that includes their risk for a second PPGL and associated syndromic features (*Table*); risk to first-degree relatives of inheriting the pathogenic variant; and reproductive counseling where appropriate, which may include discussion of preimplantation genetic diagnosis. For instance, for patients newly diagnosed with a germline *SDHB* pathogenic variant, up to 25% have a synchronous primary tumor and a lifetime risk of developing metastases of 35% to 40%.[8] Comprehensive initial diagnostic evaluation is therefore essential to plan appropriate follow-up. If not performed preoperatively, the patient should have imaging to identify other tumors (*Table*). For *SDHx* syndromes, imaging should encompass the skull base to the pelvis and include MRI or CT in adults and MRI in children; functional imaging with somatostatin receptor targeted PET (performed either as PET-CT or PET-MRI) is highly sensitive to detect additional PPGLs.[8,9]

A trap to be aware of is to adjust the plasma (or urinary) metanephrine reference range downwards by approximately 50% during follow-up of a patient after unilateral adrenalectomy, as recurrent pheochromocytoma in the contralateral gland may present with seemingly normal metanephrine values.

Finally, PPGL may be part of a syndrome due to mosaic pathogenic variants without being hereditary. Two noteworthy examples are Carney triad (the syndromic but nonhereditary association of PPGL, GIST, and/or pulmonary chondroma associated with mosaic hypermethylation of the *SDHC* promoter)[4] and Pacak-Zhuang syndrome (encompassing PPGLs, congenital polycythemia, and duodenal somatostatinomas associated with mosaic pathogenic variants in *EPAS1*)[10] Recognizing these syndromes is important to identify patients for whom specific follow-up

management plans are required, even though their first-degree relatives are not at risk (ie, germline DNA testing is negative).

Familial Testing and Surveillance

All at-risk family members of patients with hereditary PPGL syndromes should be counseled about the risks of inheriting these variants.[11] Despite several potential barriers, including cost, parental concern about testing children, burden of a lifetime surveillance program, and concerns about accessing life insurance, early diagnosis and surveillance in carriers of pathogenic variants has now been shown to improve survival in MEN 2, VHL, and hereditary PGL type 4 (*SDHB*).[12,13] Absence of a family history of PPGLs due to relatively low penetrance of many PPGL syndromes may lull family members into false optimism. Surveillance programs should carefully balance benefits of early tumor detection against risks, including the use of ionizing radiation and psychological consequences inherent to tumor predisposition syndromes.

The methods and frequency of follow-up vary between different syndromes (*Table*). For MEN 2 and VHL, annual clinical examination and plasma metanephrine measurement is recommended, with adrenal imaging reserved for when metanephrines become elevated (noting patients with VHL will have abdominal imaging surveillance to detect renal cell carcinoma). For *SDHx* syndromes, in which recurrent PPGLs may be biochemically silent, annual biochemical assessment should be supplemented with whole-body imaging every 2 to 4 years. Whole-body imaging with MRI or CT is also sensitive to detecting renal cell cancers and larger GISTs; current consensus is that endoscopy is not routinely required to screen for smaller GISTs. There is some controversy as to whether imaging in *SDHx* carriers should include the pituitary; a handful of case reports illustrate a definite association between *SDHx* pathogenic variants and pituitary NETs, although the risk seems low. Notably, *SDHD* and *SDHAF2* are imprinted such that disease expression occurs commonly when a pathogenic variant is paternally inherited and very rarely when maternally inherited.

Counseling of family members is ideally provided by genetic counselors and cancer genetics specialists, who will then systematically contact at-risk family members, engage carriers of pathogenic variants in surveillance programs, and provide reproductive counseling. Of note, although these syndromes are autosomal dominant, recent evidence suggests preferential inheritance of pathogenic variants in *SDHB* and *SDHD*—a phenomenon known as transmission ratio distortion. Accordingly, carriers of these pathogenic variants should be counseled that the risk their offspring will inherit the allele with the variant is approximately 60% (rather than 50%).[14]

The following clinical case vignettes each highlight a particular issue in the management of hereditary PPGL syndromes. The first case occurred after missed opportunities for predictive testing and surveillance; the second case highlights the particular challenges of managing patients with *SDHD* pathogenic variants; and the third case is a cautionary tale after surveillance fatigue on the part of the patient.

Clinical Case Vignettes

Case 1

A 26-year-old woman presents with a 3-month history of right-sided chest pain. She has chronic, paroxysmal sweating and palpitations and intermittent headaches. She was treated for hypertension during her only pregnancy 6 years ago; her blood pressure has been normal since without treatment. Her medical history is otherwise unremarkable. Her family history includes a maternal cousin with a bladder PGL diagnosed at age 18 years and a maternal uncle with head/neck PGL.

Imaging identifies an 8-cm right upper posterior mediastinal mass with destruction of the adjacent T4 vertebral body and posterior right fourth rib and associated mild narrowing of the right side of the spinal canal at T4 without cord compression. Representative CT and MRI images are shown (*Figure 2*).

Figure 2. Axial CT (left) and Coronal MRI (right) Showing a Mediastinal Mass

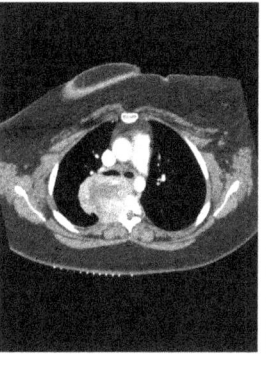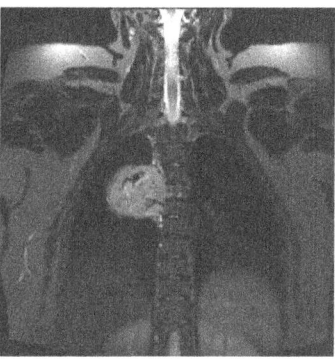

DOTATATE-PET scan shows uptake in this thoracic lesion, and no other sites of DOTATATE-avid disease. Her plasma metanephrine concentration is normal (19.9 pg/mL [<88 pg/mL] [SI: 101 pmol/L [<447 pmol/L]) and normetanephrine is normal (39 pg/mL [<106 pg/mL] [SI: 214 pmol/L [<580 pmol/L]).

The patient proceeds to resection of the thoracic lesion via bilateral extended thoracotomies with en bloc resection of T3, T4, and T5 and spinal reconstruction. Histopathology confirms a 72-mm mediastinal paraganglioma, completely excised (R0), pT3N1 (stage III), extension into bone, metastatic in 1 of 5 lymph nodes, and SDHB immunochemistry negative (abnormal).

The patient consents for genetic testing of DNA from peripheral blood leukocytes, and a pathogenic variant is found in *SDHB*.

Which of the following individuals should initially be offered predictive testing for this *SDHB* pathogenic variant?

A. Her daughter (aged 6 years) and her parents

B. Only her daughter

C. Only her parents

D. Only her mother

E. Her mother and the maternal cousin with the history of bladder PGL

Answer: A) Her daughter (aged 6 years) and her parents

First-degree relatives should be offered predictive testing for the *SDHB* pathogenic variant after appropriate counseling. It is appropriate to test her daughter, since a positive result would lead to recommendation for surveillance starting at age 6 years. It is appropriate to test both parents even though the family history strongly suggests the pathogenic variant has been inherited from the mother. Surprises do occasionally occur in cascade testing. If the mother is confirmed to carry the *SDHB* pathogenic variant, then genetic testing would in turn be recommended for her first-degree relatives.

Case 1 (continued)

The patient's mother is confirmed to carry the *SDHB* pathogenic variant.

Which of the following is appropriate now for the patient's mother?

A. Reassurance in the absence of symptoms and signs, as her risk of having a PPGL is low

B. Biochemical assessment only, including plasma normetanephrine, metanephrine, and (if available) 3-methoxytyramine

C. Structural imaging, but only if plasma metanephrines are elevated

D. Clinical and biochemical assessment and DOTATATE-PET imaging

E. MRI of the head and neck

Answer: D) Clinical and biochemical assessment and DOTATATE-PET imaging

The mother should have gene-appropriate surveillance for PPGLs, which for *SDHB* includes clinical assessment, plasma metanephrine measurement, and DOTATATE-PET imaging.[11] If PET imaging is unavailable, then whole-body structural imaging should be performed with CT or MRI.

DOTATATE-PET discovered an intensely DOTATATE-avid, 15-mm, soft-tissue lesion in the upper abdomen anterior to the inferior vena cava, likely representing a PGL. No other sites of disease were identified. Plasma normetanephrine was mildly elevated at 152 pg/mL (830 pmol/L). The mother

underwent successful surgical resection of the PGL. Both patients (proband and her mother) remain in a surveillance program that includes annual clinical and biochemical assessment and biennial whole-body MR imaging. The proband was recently discovered to have a small GIST on the lesser curvature of the stomach, which is being monitored.

Case 2

A 42-year-old woman presents with paroxysmal palpitations, sweating, and headaches associated with new-onset hypertension. She had resection of a left thoracic PGL at age 20 years and a right jugular PGL at age 21 years. Her plasma normetanephrine concentration is elevated at 260 pg/mL (1420 pmol/L). Abdominal CT identifies a 10-mm lesion at the bifurcation of the aorta. This is surgically resected, and histopathology confirms a PGL with absent (abnormal) staining for SDHB.

Which genetic test is appropriate for this patient?

A. *SDHB*

B. *VHL*

C. *RET*

D. A panel (or exome) including at least *SDHB, SDHC, SDHD, SDHAF2, VHL, RET, TMEM127, MAX,* and *FH*

E. Multiplex ligation-dependent probe amplification (MLPA)

Answer: D) A panel (or exome) including at least SDHB, SDHC, SDHD, SDHAF2, VHL, RET, TMEM127, MAX, and FH

Absent SDHB staining in PPGL is consistent with a pathogenic variant in any of the *SDHx* genes and is occasionally observed with *VHL* pathogenic variants. Full panel testing is therefore the most expeditious manner to arrive at the correct genetic diagnosis. Multiplex ligation-dependent probe amplification may be required to detect larger copy-number variants in the *SDHx* genes if no pathogenic variants are identified on panel/exome testing.

Case 2 (continued)

The patient undergoes genetic testing and is found to have an *SDHD* pathogenic variant.

Which of the following is the most correct statement?

A. The patient's son (aged 15 years) does not need genetic testing because he is unlikely to express the phenotype, even if positive

B. The patient should continue to have annual clinical and biochemical assessment and whole-body imaging every 2 to 3 years

C. The patient should have ongoing imaging, but only of the head/neck, which is the area most at risk for recurrent PPGLs associated with *SDHD* pathogenic variants

D. The patient has had 3 PGLs already and is unlikely to develop additional PGLs

E. If the patient's parents are clinically unaffected, then they do not need to undergo genetic testing

Answer: B) The patient should continue to have annual clinical and biochemical assessment and whole-body imaging every 2 to 3 years

This patient remains at risk for developing additional PGLs, renal cell cancer, and GIST, so ongoing surveillance with whole-body imaging is appropriate. If her son has inherited the *SDHD* pathogenic variant, then his lifetime risk of developing PPGL is less than 5% (due to imprinting of the *SDHD* locus). Nevertheless, if he has children, then they would be at risk of disease expression if they inherit the pathogenic variant, and reproductive counselling would be appropriate. It is likely the patient has inherited the *SDHD* pathogenic variant from her father. If he is clinically unaffected, then we can assume he had inherited the pathogenic variant from his mother. Other family members may be at risk, and cascade genetic testing of first-degree family members is still appropriate.

She underwent DOTATATE-PET, which identified bilateral carotid body tumors that were subsequently resected. Two additional head/neck PGLs remain under surveillance: a 4-mm PGL just anteromedial to the left inferior vena cava at the C3 level and a 2-mm PGL just anteromedial to the right internal jugular vein, just below the skull base.

Case 3

A 50-year-old woman presents with a right occipital headache and palpitations. She has a history of an abdominal PGL (organ of Zuckerkandl) resected 10 years ago and a second abdominal PGL resected in 7 years ago. DOTATATE-PET 5 years ago did not identify any abnormalities. She had consented to genetic testing and a pathogenic variant was identified in *SDHA*. She was then lost to follow-up/surveillance until now.

On physical examination, her blood pressure is 192/102 mm Hg. She has a right-sided hypoglossal nerve palsy. Her plasma normetanephrine concentration is markedly elevated at 2084 pg/mL (11,380 pmol/L) and her 3-methoxytyramine concentration is 18.3 pg/mL (110 pmol/L).

MRI (*Figure 3*) shows a right jugular PGL measuring 37 × 44 mm invading the occipital condyle and petrous temporal bone, with marked succinate accumulation on MR spectroscopy (not yet readily available).

Figure 3. MRI Axial Image Showing Right Jugular PGL (*top left*); and MR Spectroscopy Showing Succinate Peak (*bottom*)

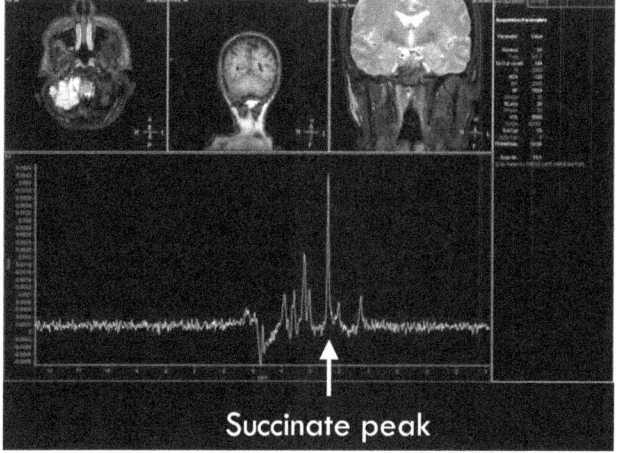

Succinate peak

[Color—Print (Color Gallery page CG7) or web & ePub editions]

Which of the following is the most accurate statement?

A. DOTATATE-PET is indicated

B. The jugular PGL is the likely source of her elevated plasma normetanephrine

C. Her first-degree relatives are at high risk for developing PPGLs if they have inherited the *SDHA* pathogenic variant

D. Her phenotype of recurrent PPGLs is inconsistent an *SDHA* pathogenic variant and an alternative genetic diagnosis should be sought

E. The patient should be offered urgent surgical debulking of her jugular PGL

Answer: A) DOTATATE-PET is indicated

Head/neck PGLs rarely secrete high levels of norepinephrine, and another PPGL should be sought to explain her markedly elevated normetanephrine. DOTATATE-PET has very high sensitivity for PPGLs associated with *SDHx* pathogenic variants and would be the imaging modality of first choice; structural imaging with CT or MRI can then be used for more precise anatomic definition of any PPGL discovered on PET. Her phenotype is consistent with *SDHA* pathogenic variants—such patients are at risk for recurrent, often aggressive PPGLs[15]; moreover, the elevated succinate level in her jugular PGL confirms this is related to *SDH* deficiency. Despite this aggressive phenotype in probands, penetrance in carriers of SDHA pathogenic variants appears to be low (≤5%); indeed, there is controversy about the frequency of surveillance required for carriers of *SDHA* pathogenic variants that are discovered during predictive testing in first-degree family members.

DOTATATE-PET showed intense uptake in the right jugular PGL and another focus of uptake in an abdominal lesion at the level of the aortic bifurcation measuring 17 mm. On the basis that the abdominal PGL was the likely source of elevated norepinephrine, this was resected first (after α-adrenergic blockade). Surprisingly, her plasma normetanephrine remained markedly elevated and she continued α-blockade until surgical debulking of the right jugular PGL was performed. She is now undergoing adjuvant treatment with external beam radiotherapy and considering additional treatment with Lutate peptide receptor radionuclide therapy.

Key Learning Points

- Diagnosis of hereditary PPGL syndromes is based on clinicopathological risk factors and appropriately targeted genetic testing.

- A patient with a newly diagnosed hereditary PPGL syndrome requires appropriate education about syndrome-specific follow-up and management of associated syndromic features.

- Family members at risk for inheriting pathogenic variants in hereditary PPGL genes require counseling to discuss appropriate genetic testing; this is best accomplished by a multidisciplinary team, including genetic specialists.

- Carriers of pathogenic variants in hereditary PPGL genes require surveillance to detect PPGLs (and other syndrome-associated tumors) early enough for optimal outcomes.

- Patients with syndromic but nonhereditary PPGL syndromes (such as Carney triad or the Pacak-Zhuang syndrome) require syndrome-specific follow-up, although their first-degree relatives are not at risk.

References

1. Lenders JWM, Kerstens MN, Amar L, et al. Genetics, diagnosis, management and future directions or research of phaeochromocytoma and paraganglioma: a position statement and consensus of the Working Group on Endocrine Hypertension of the European Society of Hypertension. *J Hypertens.* 2020;38(8):1443-1456. PMID: 32412940

2. Cascón A, Calsina B, Monteagudo M, et al. Genetic bases of pheochromocytoma and paraganglioma. *J Mol Endocrinol.* 2023;70:e220167. PMID: 36520714

3. Papathomas TG, Oudijk L, Persu A, et al. SDHB/SDHA immunohistochemistry in pheochromocytomas and paragangliomas: a multicenter interobserver variation analysis using virtual microscopy: a multinational study of the European Network for the Study of Adrenal Tumors (ENS@T). *Mod Pathol.* 2015;28(6):807-821. PMID: 25720320

4. Pitsava G, Settas N, Faucz FR, Stratakis CA. Carney triad, Carney-Stratakis syndrome, 3PAS and other tumors due to SDH deficiency. *Front Endocrinol (Lausanne).* 2021;12:680609. PMID: 34012423

5. Fuchs TL, Luxford C, Clarkson A, et al. A clinicopathologic and molecular analysis of fumarate hydratase-deficient pheochromocytoma and paraganglioma. *Am J Surg Pathol.* 2023;47(1):25-36. PMID: 35993574

6. Fishbein L, Leshchiner I, Walter V, et al. Comprehensive molecular characterization of pheochromocytoma and paraganglioma. *Cancer Cell.* 2017;31(2):181-193. PMID: 28162975

7. NGS in PPGL (NGSnPPGL) Study Group, Toledo RA, Burnichon N, et al. Consensus statement on next-generation-sequencing-based diagnostic testing of hereditary phaeochromocytomas and paragangliomas. *Nat Rev Endocrinol.* 2017;13(4):233-247. PMID: 27857127

8. Taïeb D, Nolting S, Perrier ND, et al. Management of phaeochromocytoma and paraganglioma in patients with germline SDHB pathogenic variants: an international expert consensus statement. *Nat Rev Endocrinol.* 2023;20(3):168-184. PMID: 38097671

9. Taïeb D, Wanna GB, Ahmad M, et al. Clinical consensus guideline on the management of phaeochromocytoma and paraganglioma in patients harbouring germline SDHD pathogenic variants. *Lancet Diabetes Endocrinol.* 2023;11(5):345-361. PMID: 37011647

10. Zhuang Z, Yang C, Lorenzo F, et al. Somatic HIF2A gain-of-function mutations in paraganglioma with polycythemia. *N Engl J Med.* 2012;367:922-930. PMID: 22931260

11. Amar L, Pacak K, Steichen O, et al. International consensus on initial screening and follow-up of asymptomatic SDHx mutation carriers. *Nat Rev Endocrinol.* 2021;17(7):435-444. PMID: 34021277

12. Buffet A, Ben Aim L, Leboulleux S, et al. Positive impact of genetic test on the management and outcome of patients with paraganglioma and/or pheochromocytoma. *J Clin Endocrinol Metab.* 2019;104(4):1109-1118. PMID: 30698717

13. Davidoff DF, Benn DE, Field M, et al. Surveillance improves outcomes for carriers of SDHB pathogenic variants: a multi-center study. *J Clin Endocrinol Metab.* 2022;107(5):e1907-e1916. PMID: 35037935

14. Davidoff DF, Lim ES, Benn DE, et al. Distortion in transmission of pathogenic SDHB- and SDHD-mutated alleles from parent to offspring. *Endocr Relat Cancer.* 2023;30:e220233. PMID: 36786389

15. Jha A, de Luna K, Balili CA, Millo C, Paraiso CA, et al. Clinical, diagnostic and treatment characteristics of *SDHA*-related metastatic pheochromocytoma and paraganglioma. *Front Oncol.* 2019;9:53. PMID: 30854332

What Every Endocrinologist Should Know About Interpreting PET Scans in the Diagnosis of Ectopic ACTH Syndrome

Lynnette K. Nieman, MD. Diabetes, Endocrinology, and Obesity Branch, National Institute of Diabetes and Digestive and Kidney Diseases, National Institutes of Health, Bethesda, MD; Email: NiemanL@nih.gov

Educational Objectives

After reviewing this chapter, learners should be able to:

- Individualize the approach to imaging to detect an ectopic ACTH-secreting tumor.

- Identify potential false-positive results on PET/CT and determine how to further evaluate those lesions.

- Communicate effectively with nuclear medicine physicians and radiologists about PET/CT results.

Significance of the Clinical Problem

Cushing syndrome is a potentially lethal disease, with a mortality rate of approximately 3% over time. Persons with ectopic ACTH secretion (EAS) are disproportionately at risk, having a mortality rate of approximately 20%.[1] Surprisingly, in a study of 89 patients with EAS, death occurred within 90 days of treatment initiation in 12 patients, mostly of infection. Later deaths usually related to tumor progression.[1]

Ideally, prompt diagnosis of EAS and identification of the causal tumor allows for surgical resection, which decreases the risk of mortality by normalizing cortisol levels and reducing the risk of metastatic progression. Unfortunately, up to 50% of affected patients do not achieve successful surgical resection after initial imaging because the tumor remains occult. Of the latter group, up to 25% remain occult, while the tumor is eventually discovered in the others, often after bilateral adrenalectomy has been required for normalization of cortisol.[2] It is critical to begin treatment with steroidogenesis inhibitors as soon as the diagnosis of EAS is confirmed. Adequate treatment to normalize cortisol will not interfere with the diagnostic accuracy of imaging and should not be withheld pending imaging results.

Many EAS tumors can be detected by structural imaging with CT or MRI (individual sensitivities, 66% and 54%, respectively, in one large review).[3] However, the addition of functional imaging with PET provides useful adjunctive information. Functional imaging refers to approaches that take advantage of molecular and cellular characteristics of tumor cells. Nearly all EAS tumors are neuroendocrine neoplasms (NENs), primarily neuroendocrine tumors (NETs) (although some are neuroendocrine cancers).

NENs often express somatostatin receptor types 2 and 5, and/or the large neutral amino acid transporters of the L-type; these characteristics underlie the potential utility of somatostatin radioligands (eg, ^{68}Ga-DOTATATE/DOTATOC/DOTANOC)[4] and ^{18}F-DOPA,[5] respectively. By contrast, they are less likely to overexpress glucose transporters or to have high proliferation and metabolic rates, characteristics that promote update of ^{18}F-fluorodeoxyglucose (FDG).

There is little guidance in the literature about how best to localize EAS tumors, probably because of their rarity and a paucity of prospective clinical trials. Much of the available information is collated from case reports or small series that do not directly compare the modalities. Additionally, while the US FDA approved DOTATATE for detection of NETs in 2016, F-DOPA is not approved for this indication in the United States. Both agents, as well as other somatostatin receptor radioligands, are approved in Europe.

Practice Gaps

- Failure to obtain scans in a discrete time frame.
- Failure to obtain the most useful scans.
- Failure to look at the scans—alone or with a radiologist/nuclear medicine physician.
- Failure to correlate the results of all scans.
- Lack of recognition of false-positive findings.

Discussion

Multimodal imaging is essential for optimal localization of an EAS tumor. A cost-minimizing approach synthesizes clinical and laboratory information with the probable location of these tumors. In contrast to initial reports in the 1970s, currently, most EAS tumors are noncancerous pulmonary NETs usually 1 cm or larger in diameter (*Table 1*). Because of this, if the history and physical exam do not suggest hypertension (pheochromocytoma), thyroid mass (medullary thyroid cancer), cachexia (cancer), or anemia of

Table 1. Types of Noncorticotrope Tumors Reported to Secrete ACTH

Type of EAS tumor	Reference					
	Salgado et al (ref. #7) (n = 25)	Aniszewski et al (ref. #8) (n = 106)	Ilias et al (ref. #9) (n = 73)	Isidori et al (ref. #2) (n = 40)	Ejaz et al (ref. #10) (n = 43)	Total No. (%)
Pulmonary NET	10	28	35	12	9	94 (32)
Occult	2	17	17	5	...	41 (14)
Small cell lung cancer	...	12	3	7	9	31 (10)
Nonspecific NET	...	7	13	2	3	25 (8)
Other tumors[a]	1	9	3	5	6	24 (8)
Pancreatic NET	3	17	1	3	...	24 (8)
Medullary thyroid cancer	...	9	2	3	5	19 (6)
Thymic NET	4	5	5	2	3	19 (6)
Pheochromocytoma	5	3	5	1	...	14 (5)
Gastrinoma	...	...	6	...	...	6 (2)

[a] Other tumors include olfactory esthesioneuroblastoma, mesothelioma, glomus tumor, other NET tumors (hepatic, appendix, tumorlets, disseminated GEP-NET), tumors of the esophagus, stomach, pancreas, larynx, trachea, salivary gland, Leydig cell, breast, ovary, cervix, kidney, gallbladder, prostate, hepatocellular carcinoma, melanoma, leukemia, lymphoma, osteomyeloma. Adapted from Nieman LK. Imaging of ACTH-Dependent Cushing's Syndrome. In: Taïeb D, Pacak K, eds. *Current Diagnostic and Therapeutic Approaches in Nuclear Endocrinology.* Cambridge Scholars Publishing, 2020.[6]

chronic disease (cancer), one might begin with a thin-slice CT and MRI of the thorax.

Conversely, if cancer, pheochromocytoma, or medullary thyroid cancer is possible, specific laboratory results, such as increased co-secreted hormones/peptides or elevated liver function tests, may indicate the need for neck-, adrenal-, or liver-directed imaging. If initial studies are inconclusive, F-DOPA and/or DOTATATE scans may point to a thoracic lesion that was not appreciated initially, or to other sites, which should then be assessed with CT and MRI. PET with [18]FDG can identify highly proliferative tumors with a high metabolic glucose requirement. However, these tumors are generally evident on structural imaging, so the adjunctive use of [18]FDG-PET is not needed.[9]

Few clinical studies have examined use of these PET agents in EAS. In the sole prospective comparative study, of 21 patients, F-DOPA and DOTA were significantly more sensitive (91% and 86%, respectively) than octreotide (31%).[11] In another study, DOTATATE identified the primary tumor in 11 of 17 patients.[12] In systematic literature reviews, histologically confirmed tumors were identified in 51 of 67 patients (76%) by various ^{68}Ga-somatostatin receptor ligands[13] and in 18 of 22 (81%) patients by DOTATATE.[3]

Ways to Improve PET Results

Most centers now obtain CT with PET, so they can be co-registered. This vastly improves the ability to pinpoint the anatomic location of any lesion on PET. CT is generally not sufficiently detailed to identify small tumors.

Carbidopa is given to improve ^{18}F-DOPA uptake into tumors. It inhibits the action of aromatic amino acid decarboxylase and the conversion of L-DOPA to dopamine. By inhibiting conversion of ^{18}F-DOPA to ^{18}F-dopamine, ^{18}F-DOPA blood concentrations are higher and NET uptake is greater. However, pancreatic uptake is reduced.

False-Positive and False-Negative Results

The physiologic uptake of F-DOPA and somatostatin-binding radionuclides are shown in *Table 2* (*following page*). Any reported "lesion" should be viewed with skepticism, as nontumor cells can potentially take up the radionuclide. The shape of the lesion (round vs amorphous) and its standardized uptake view (SUV) relative to background (eg, the liver) provide helpful clues as to the importance of the finding, with round, bright lesions being more suspicious. The adrenal glands may take up each ligand, but generally do so symmetrically with an SUV less than that of the liver. The presence of intense, round uptake suggests a suspicious lesion.

Failure to identify a lesion may occur for a variety of reasons. In the lungs, the vasculature appears round, as does a small NET. When viewing such scans, it is helpful to move through cross-sectional (axial) sections (up and down) to determine if the round lesion has a tubular structure (ie, a vessel) or diminishes in diameter and ends (a tumor). If a lesion has an SUV close to background (eg, a metastasis in the liver), it may not be obvious on PET. Similarly, if the lesion is adjacent to a structure with a higher SUV (eg, a liver lesion next to the gallbladder), it may not appear significant. Finally, because many lesions are small, they may not be recognized as potential tumors.

Ways to Improve PET Interpretation

1. Obtain all imaging in a discrete time frame, perhaps within 2 weeks. If a sequential approach is used, such as initial structural imaging of the thorax, ideally any needed PET should be scheduled soon thereafter. This is important because CT and MRI should be read with the PET scans, and the utility of this comparison can degrade if a new confounding lesion occurs in the interim, such as infection.

2. Review all the scans together to correlate the results. In our center, scans are read individually by staff radiologists who may be

part of the research team and who have access to any previous scans. However, the final review for management decisions is done by a multidisciplinary team (endocrinology, surgery, nuclear medicine/radiology) that evaluates all pertinent images. We strongly prefer to operate only on lesions that are positive on both structural and functional imaging.

3. For patients with occult disease with a new lesion, review the previous scans to determine if the lesion was present, but not appreciated, or if there is some reason that the lesion was not seen. This assists in assessing the pace of tumor growth, and it is also a learning opportunity to see how lesions progress. Sometimes, we retrospectively see a small abnormality that was either overlooked or discounted earlier.

4. Consider whether any lesion is a false-positive reading. This is facilitated greatly by review of the other scans, by knowledge of the medical history and, potentially, review of lesions on temporally distant imaging. Additional imaging (x-rays, ultrasonography, nuclear medicine studies [hemangiomas]) may facilitate understanding of the new PET finding.

5. When PET scans show uptake near the heart, but standard CT and MRI are negative, consider a gated cardiac CT. A gated cardiac CT is done by obtaining CT with simultaneous electrocardiography; images can then be reconstructed by retaining only those acquired during systole to reduce the effects of cardiac motion to obscure a pericardiac lesion.

6. Consider looking at your patient's scans, especially if your radiologist is pressed for time and only does a fast zip-zip up and down, looking for large lesions. Small lesions can be missed with a quick review. If no one has sufficient time (we may spend 30 minutes or more) to look at all the studies carefully, it may be time to send your patient to a center with more experience!

Table 2. Physiologic and Nonphysiologic Uptake of Radionuclides

Somatostatin-binding radionuclides[4]	F-DOPA[5]
Physiologic uptake of radionuclides	
Pituitary gland	Basal ganglia
Greatest: spleen	Spleen (mild)
Liver	Liver
Pancreas (variable)	Pancreas (especially uncinate process)
Adrenal glands	Adrenal glands: variable; should be symmetric and less intense than liver
Stomach wall, bowel	Gallbladder and biliary tract
Urinary system	Urinary system
Growth plate (children)	Growth plate (children)
White blood cells (inflammation): nodes, post radiation, infection, prostatitis, tuberculosis, sarcoidosis, infection	Acute or subacute brain ischemia, abscess
Normal thyroid	
Salivary glands	Salivary glands
Breast, prostate: mild and diffuse	Myocardium[a]
Osteoblast activity: fracture, fibrous dysplasia, degenerative bone disease, vertebral hemangioma	Lungs[a]
Nonphysiologic uptake of radionuclides	
Incidental non-NETs: meningioma, neuroblastoma, mesenchymal tumors causing tumor-induced osteomalacia	Pancreatic serous adenoma
NETs: gastroenteropancreatic, pheochromocytoma, paraganglioma, pulmonary, thymic	Pheochromocytoma, paraganglioma
Medullary thyroid cancer, esthesioneuroblastoma, nonavid thyroid Cancer	Medullary thyroid cancer

[a] With carbidopa pretreatment.

Data from Hofman MS et al. *Radiographics*, 2015; 35(2): 500-16. © Radiological Society of North America; Calabria FF et al. *Clin Nucl Med*, 2016;41(10): 753-60. © Wolters Kluwer Health, Inc.[4]

Clinical Case Vignettes

Case 1

A 57-year-old woman presents with florid Cushing syndrome. Evaluation findings suggest EAS. F-DOPA scan shows a small retrocardiac lesion that is not noted on chest CT or MRI. No lesions are seen on CT/MRI of the neck, abdomen, or pelvis.

Which of the following is the best step?

A. Perform bronchoalveolar lavage; this is likely a false-positive lesion, possibly due to infection

B. Perform bilateral adrenalectomy because she has florid Cushing syndrome

C. Obtain a gated cardiac CT

D. Treat medically and rescan in 6 months; since there is no lesion on structural imaging, the F-DOPA finding should be discounted as important

E. Obtain a DOTATATE scan

Answer: C) Obtain a gated cardiac CT

The issue posed by this vignette is the need to obtain structural evidence of a surgically resectable lesion. A gated cardiac CT (Answer C) gives better delineation of the retrocardiac space by diminishing cardiac motion artifact. It was done in this case and demonstrated a clear 5-mm lesion that was subsequently resected.

An inflammatory/infectious lesion (Answer A) is less likely because nothing is seen on CT/MRI.

A DOTATATE scan (Answer E) could confirm that the lesion is likely an NET, but it may not help to identify an anatomic target.

Bilateral adrenalectomy (Answer B) and treating medically and rescanning in 6 months (Answer D) are second-line approaches. However, treatment before additional scanning has drawbacks: adrenalectomy requires lifelong hormone replacement and may be associated with diminished quality of life; medical therapy may not normalize cortisol, so Cushing syndrome comorbidities might not be addressed. Furthermore, tumors may progress or metastasize in the interim.

Case 2

A 27-year-old woman is referred with a 4-year history Cushing syndrome. She is currently treated for amenorrhea, diabetes, and hypertension. Initial evaluation (done 4 weeks after urinary free cortisol excretion was 10 times the upper normal limit) included a midnight serum cortisol value of 6.7 μg/dL (184.8 nmol/L), a basal morning ACTH value of 34.9 pg/mL (7.7 pmol/L), a 25% increase in cortisol after corticotropin-releasing hormone, an 82.7% decrease in cortisol after 8 mg of dexamethasone, and a urinary free cortisol excretion of 8.1 μg/24 h (22.4 nmol/d). One month later, midnight serum cortisol is 22.9 μg/dL (631.8 nmol/L), with an ACTH value of 64.4 pg/mL (14.2 pmol/L). Cortisol increases 8.3% after corticotropin-releasing hormone and is suppressed by 12.4% after high-dose dexamethasone administration. The highest central-to-peripheral gradient in inferior petrosal sinus sampling is 2.3, with a normal venogram and prolactin-normalized ACTH values, indicating normal catheterization. Pituitary MRI shows partially empty sella. Torso and neck CT and MRI and octreotide scintigraphy are negative. DOTATATE and F-DOPA scans show a lesion in the lower abdomen, just to the right of midline.

Which of the following is the best next step?

A. Proceed to surgery for an exploratory laparotomy to "run the gut" and look for a lesion

B. Treat medically and rescan in 6 months

C. Review CT and MRI in hopes of finding something in the abdomen

D. Obtain an MIBG scan

E. Measure catecholamine and calcitonin

Answer: C) Review CT and MRI in hopes of finding something in the abdomen

This vignette illustrates difficulties in interpretation of biochemical data pertaining to the presence of hypercortisolism and the differential diagnosis of Cushing syndrome. This patient had cyclic Cushing syndrome, as shown by normal urinary free cortisol excretion and midnight cortisol concentration during initial evaluation. Those test results reflect normal corticotrope responses due to lack of suppression but might be interpreted as indicative of Cushing disease. The second set of tests clearly reflect EAS during a hypercortisolemic phase. Certainty about the correct differential diagnosis is important: if the initial test results had been interpreted as the patient having Cushing disease, the EAS tumor would not have been found.

This vignette also tests how to proceed when initial imaging fails to identify a putative lesion. As in the first case, the choices are to proceed to therapy or perform further biochemical tests or scans. Another option, unique to this vignette, is to re-review the scans (Answer C), which is the best option. It is phrased in a slightly "desperate" way, but in reality, it should be a given that all scans are read by an interdisciplinary team with experience in EAS tumors before any additional testing or treatment is done. (Except of course in the case of a severely ill patient who may need immediate intervention, perhaps with etomidate.) In this case, the initial scans were interpreted as they were obtained and were not correlated. The research radiologist overlaid the CT and PET scans, pinpointed the lesion on CT and then used 3-dimensional rotation of the scan to determine that there was a mass, connected to a tube, which could be followed to the junction of the small and large intestine. As expected, an appendiceal NET was resected at laparoscopic surgery. Histology revealed a well-differentiated, intermediate grade NET with 13 mitotic figures per 50 high-power field and subserosal and lymphovascular tissue invasion without involvement of visceral peritoneum.

Treating medically and rescanning in 6 months (Answer B), has the downsides as discussed in Case 1.

Exploratory laparotomy (Answer A) might not find a very small lesion, so the risk-benefit ratio of this approach is unsatisfactory.

The position of the lesion does not suggest a pheochromocytoma or medullary thyroid cancer,

and the F-DOPA scan does not show other lesions, so there is no justification to perform an MIBG scan (Answer D) or to measure catecholamine and calcitonin levels (Answer E).

Case 3

A 76-year-old man is referred for evaluation of hypokalemia discovered at the time of a cervical laminectomy 5 months earlier. His medical history is notable for a prostate carcinoma with a high burden of bone metastases (diagnosed 4 years ago). He underwent androgen-deprivation therapy, followed by radiation to the spine and prostate and treatment with sipuleucel-T and ^{177}lutetium, which ended about 9 months before the laminectomy. Urinary free cortisol excretion was about 4 times the upper normal limit, with a normal volume and creatinine excretion of 900 mg/24 h. He has no symptoms of Cushing syndrome, and he has lost about 5 lb (2.3 kg).

On physical examination, he has profound generalized weakness and a liver edge 2 cm below the right costal margin. When comparing his appearance with a driver's license photo, his face seems fuller.

Biochemical testing documents high cortisol and ACTH concentrations and hypokalemia, consistent with severe EAS. CT and MRI (neck, chest, abdomen, pelvis) shows multiple hepatic and bony lesions, a bulky lesion at the prostate, and some intra-abdominal lymphadenopathy. DOTATATE scan is positive in some, but not all, of the hepatic lesions.

Which of the following is the most likely cause of this patient's EAS?

A. Gut NET

B. Pulmonary NET

C. Pancreatic NET

D. Prostate carcinoma

Answer: D) Prostate carcinoma

Transformation of prostate carcinoma (Answer D) to a neuroendocrine carcinoma is an uncommon occurrence that is usually associated with androgen-deprivation therapy.[14] The presence of DOTATATE in some but not all nodules may indicate that some of the nodules represent the original prostate cancer. It is possible that he could have developed a gut or pancreatic NET (Answers A and C), as these metastasize to the liver, but this seems quite unlikely, both in terms of a second cancer and also since there was no other signal in the intestine or pancreas. Pulmonary NETs (Answer B) metastasize to the hilum before further spread; the absence of PET uptake or structural masses in the chest argue against this possibility.

Case 3 (continued)

Which of the following is the best way to establish the etiology of the hepatic masses?

A. CT-guided biopsy

B. Laparoscopy with multiple biopsies

C. Prostate-specific membrane antigen PET

D. F-DOPA PET

Answer: A) CT-guided biopsy

A CT-guided biopsy (Answer A) is the least invasive way to establish the etiology of the hepatic masses, which can be used to determine further management. In this case, the biopsy showed neuroendocrine carcinoma with 80% mitotic index, consistent with neuroendocrine clonal transformation of his known prostate carcinoma.

Laparoscopy with multiple biopsies (Answer B) is less attractive because it is more invasive.

Prostate-specific membrane antigen PET (Answer C) could differentiate whether some of the masses were prostate carcinoma. This was done—the prostate-specific membrane antigen–positive lesions were not positive on DOTATATE scan, suggesting prostate carcinoma metastases. However, this would not help direct further management.

F-DOPA PET (Answer D) would not provide additional information beyond what was known from the DOTATATE scan.

Key Learning Points

- DOTATATE and F-DOPA are useful adjunctive imaging modalities; they complement information on structural imaging with CT and MRI, and positive uptake may prompt closer scrutiny of structural images.

- All scans should be reviewed and correlated to maximize their collective value.

- Ideally, imaging for EAS tumors should be reviewed by a multidisciplinary team (radiology, nuclear medicine, endocrinology, surgery) with expertise in the field.

- Additional radiologic studies may be needed to evaluate suspect lesions or those that may represent a false-positive result.

- Knowledge of the physiologic and nonphysiologic uptake of radioligands should guide interpretation of results.

- Imaging is critical to successful management of EAS. If your group does not have extensive experience with this condition, consider referral to others who see it frequently and have a track record of successful localization.

References

1. Valassi E. Clinical presentation and etiology of Cushing's syndrome: data from ERCUSYN. *J Neuroendocrinol.* 2022;34(8):e13114. PMID: 35979717

2. Isidori AM, Sbardella E, Zatelli MC, et al; ABC Study Group. Conventional and nuclear medicine imaging in ectopic Cushing's syndrome: a systematic review. *J Clin Endocrinol Metab.* 2015;100(9):3231-3244. PMID: 26158607

3. Isidori AM, Kaltsas GA, Pozza C, et al. The ectopic adrenocorticotropin syndrome: clinical features, diagnosis, management, and long-term follow-up. *J Clin Endocrinol Metab.* 2006;91(2):371-377. PMID: 16303835

4. Hofman MS, Lau WF, Hicks RJ. Somatostatin receptor imaging with 68Ga DOTATATE PET/CT: clinical utility, normal patterns, pearls, and pitfalls in interpretation. *Radiographics.* 2015;35(2):500-516. PMID: 25763733

5. Calabria FF, Chiaravalloti A, Jaffrain-Rea ML, et al. 18F-DOPA PET/CT Physiological Distribution and Pitfalls: Experience in 215 Patients. *Clin Nucl Med.* 2016;41(10):753-760. PMID: 27454592

6. Nieman LK. Imaging of ACTH-Dependent Cushing's Syndrome. In: Taïeb D, Pacak K, eds. *Current Diagnostic and Therapeutic Approaches in Nuclear Endocrinology*. Cambridge Scholars Publishing, 2020.

7. Salgado LR, Fragoso MC, Knoepfelmacher M, et al. Ectopic ACTH syndrome: our experience with 25 cases. *Eur J Endocrinol*. 2006;155(5):725-733. PMID: 17062889

8. Aniszewski JP, Young WF, Thompson GB, Grant CS, van Heerden JA. Gushing syndrome doe to ectopic adrenocorticotropic hormone secretion. *World J Surg*. 2001;25(7):934-940. PMID: 11572035

9. Ilias I, Torpy DJ, Pacak K, Mullen N, Wesley RA, Nieman LK. Cushing's syndrome due to ectopic corticotropin secretion: twenty years' experience at the National Institutes of Health. *J Clin Endocrinol Metab*. 2005;90(8):4955-4962. PMID: 15914534

10. Ejaz S, Vassilopoulou-Sellin R, Busaidy NL, et al. Cushing syndrome secondary to ectopic adrenocorticotropic hormone secretion: the University of Texas MD Anderson Cancer Center Experience. *Cancer*. 2011;117(19):4381-4389. PMID: 21412758

11. Elenius H, McGlotten R, Nieman LK. THU538 use of multiple functional and structural imaging modalities improves detection of ectopic ACTH tumors. *J Endocr Soc*. 2023;7(1).

12. Wannachalee T, Turcu AF, Bancos I, et al. The clinical impact of [⁶⁸Ga]-DOTATATE PET/CT for the diagnosis and management of ectopic adrenocorticotropic hormone - secreting tumours. *Clin Endocrinol (Oxf)*. 2019;91(2):288-294. PMID: 31066920

13. Varlamov E, Hinojosa-Amaya JM, Stack M, Fleseriu M. Diagnostic utility of gallium-68-somatostatin receptor PET/CT in ectopic ACTH-secreting tumors: a systematic literature review and single-center clinical experience. *Pituitary*. 2019;22(5):445-455. PMID: 31236798

14. Iravani A, Mitchell C, Akhurst T, Sandhu S, Hofman MS, Hicks RJ. Molecular imaging of neuroendocrine differentiation of prostate cancer: a case series. *Clin Genitourin Cancer*. 2021;19(4):e200-e205. PMID: 33678552

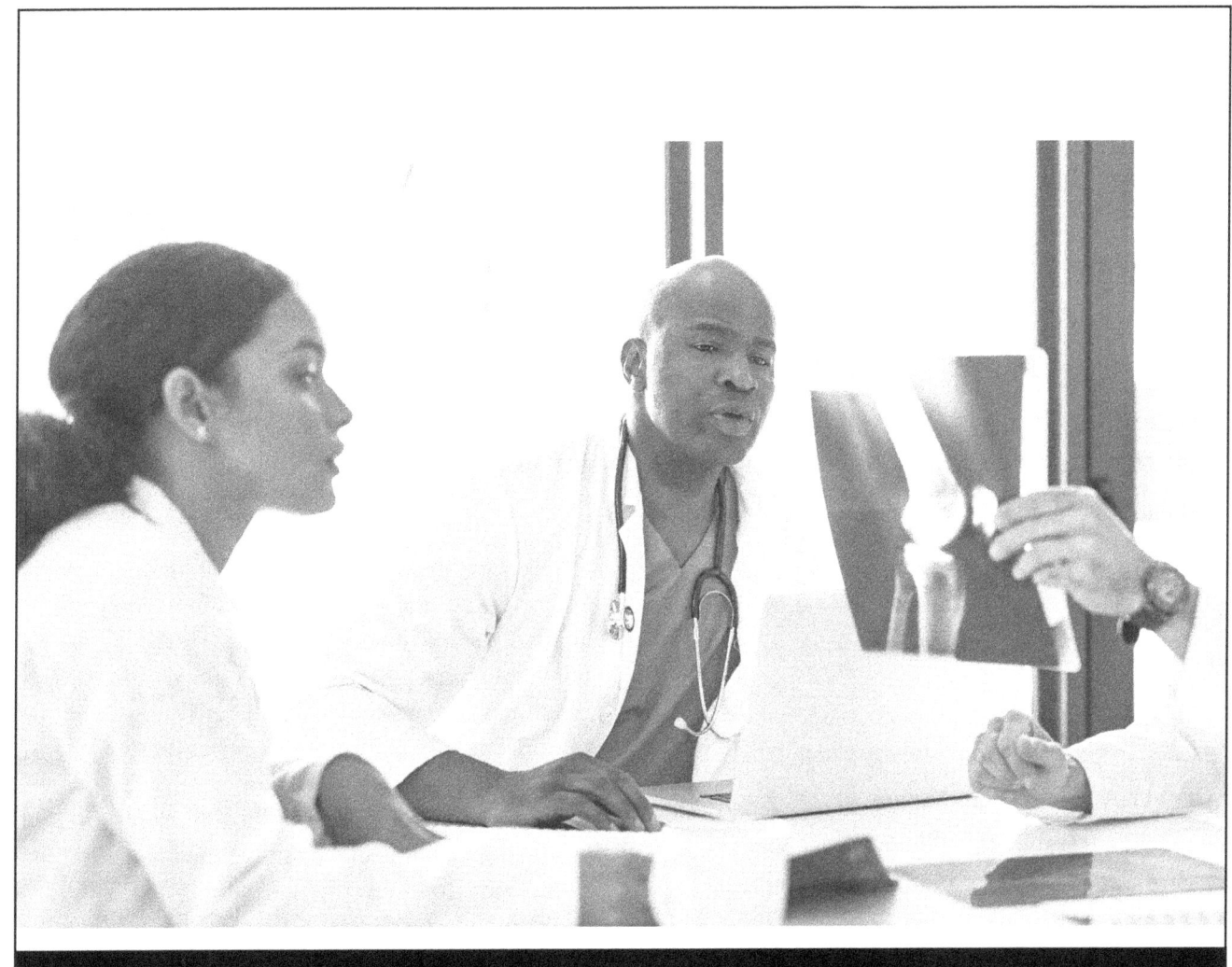

BONE AND MINERAL METABOLISM

Strategies for Osteoporosis Treatment: Risk Stratification and Treatment Sequence Matter

Mona Al Mukaddam, MD, MS. University of Pennsylvania Health System, Philadelphia, PA; Email: Mona.almukaddam@pennmedicine.upenn.edu

Christopher Hvisdas, PharmD. Penn Presbyterian Medical Center, University of Pennsylvania Medical Center, Philadelphia, PA; Email: Christopher.Hvisdas@pennmedicine.upenn.edu

Educational Objectives

After reviewing this chapter, learners should be able to:

- Identify appropriate initial osteoporotic therapy based on risk stratification.

- Review evidence for sequential therapy in patients with osteoporosis.

- For patients at very-high risk, recommend osteoanabolic treatments and consider long-term treatment goals in all treatment decisions, including fracture risk reduction, bone mineral density targets, minimization of short- and long-term adverse drug events.

- Apply treatment recommendations to clinical case vignettes.

Significance of the Clinical Problem

Pharmacologic recommendations for osteoporosis treatment vary considerably based on many clinical and nonclinical factors, including individual prescriber preferences, familiarity with advanced treatment options, varying treatment guideline recommendations, global availability, and ability to overcome access issues such as cost and insurance restrictions. Many different treatment guidelines from national and international societies recommend varying approaches for medication management of postmenopausal osteoporosis. Emerging literature continues to suggest that risk stratification and pharmacologic treatment sequences matter to achieve optimal patient outcomes. However, the generalizability of guideline recommendations and lack of robust clinical data make the incorporation of individualized treatment sequence recommendations in guidelines difficult. This creates confusion among health care professionals and patients, and justifiably allows the creation of insurance compendium requirements that preferentially dictate certain therapy that may be inappropriate based on individual patient factors.

Practice Gaps

- Many initial prescribers of osteoporosis medications are not comfortable screening for, stratifying, and subsequently treating osteoporosis with advanced injectable treatments. Current guidelines do not provide specific treatment recommendations based on individual risk.

- Some clinical guidelines do not tier treatment approaches and broadly list bisphosphonates as preferred first-line treatment options even for patients with very severe osteoporosis.

Treatment considerations include severity, sequences, and impact on the next therapy.

- Overcoming insurance restrictions and tier criteria requires specialized knowledge and dedication of time to ensure appropriate treatment is received.

Discussion

Numerous postmenopausal osteoporosis guidelines exist with notable differences throughout the world. The references are not all-inclusive but demonstrate an explanation for common prescribing variance observed in clinical practice. For the purposes of this educational content, the focus will remain on 5 treatment guidelines for postmenopausal osteoporosis, including Endocrine Society, American Academy of Endocrinology (AACE), International Osteoporosis Foundation (IOF) and European Society for Clinical and Economic Aspects of Osteoporosis (ESCEO), American College of Physicians (ACP), and Bone Health and Osteoporosis Foundation (BHOF). Other guidelines are also commonly referenced depending on the country of origin for clinical practice and specialty prescribing location but are outside the scope of the content presented herein. The Table (*following page*) summarizes the 5 guidelines for risk stratification from each society along with corresponding treatment recommendations.[1-5]

The importance of risk stratification is summarized in the 2019 IOF and ESCEO guidelines and for the fracture to be expressed as an absolute risk probability with occurrence over time, commonly 10 years.[5] It is important to understand that fracture risk varies by country and that multiple risk assessment tools differ in predictive value.[5]

Patient-specific properties that contribute to bone strength include bone mineral density (BMD), bone geometry and mineralization, the microarchitecture of the bone commonly assessed with trabecular bone scores, and markers of bone turnover, such as C-telopeptide (CTX). BMD correlates to fracture risk with increasing risk inversely related to decreasing BMD.[6] Assessment of bone microarchitecture requires methodologies not routinely used in clinical practice. Non-BMD factors that increase fracture risk include advancing age, sex, low BMI, history of fragility fracture or other previous atraumatic fractures, parental history of hip fracture, glucocorticoid therapy, cigarette smoking status, and alcohol use. Incorporating these risk factors independent of BMD increases the sensitivity of fracture risk assessment, which should improve and optimize treatment intervention strategies.[6] These are reflected in treatment guidelines but remain nonspecific without reference of risk factors to guide specific treatment recommendations in some guidelines.

Consider the current structure of the 5 guidelines summarized in the *Table*. Similarities and differences are observable. There is a degree of risk stratification for most guidelines; however, the definition of low vs high risk varies, as do the corresponding treatment recommendations. Currently, all but one guideline recommends denosumab as a potential first-line treatment option. ACP is the only societal organization to the author's knowledge that recommends denosumab as the preferred second-line option given risks of interruption, impacts on future treatments, and reversibility. Likewise, 3 of the 5 treatment guidelines (BHOF, IOF, ESCEO, and ACP) recommend osteoanabolic treatment as the preferred initial treatment in patients at very high risk for fracture or those with a history of osteoporotic fracture based on observed treatment differences.[2,4,5]

Multiple guidelines highlight the differences in cost-effectiveness among the agents with a note of lack of proven difference in efficacy among the major treatment options for postmenopausal osteoporosis. There are limited head-to-head comparisons of interventions which is why a resulting hierarchy of treatments has not been developed; however, data suggest treatment sequences matter.

Table. Summarized Guideline Risk Stratification and Treatment Recommendations

	Endocrine Society	AACE	IOF and ESCEO	ACP	BHOF
Date published	2020	2020	2019	2023	2022
Low Risk	• No prior hip or spine fracture • BMD T-score at hip and spine both above –1.0 • 10-year hip fracture <3% and 10-year risk factor of major osteoporotic fracture <20%	Not defined	Not defined	Baseline fracture risk assessment is based on diagnosis of osteoporosis, history of osteoporotic fractures (clinical or incidental) multiple risk factors for fractures or failure or intolerability of osteoporosis medications rather than scores from available tools	No previous spine or hip fracture; T-score at hip and spine above –1.0; FRAX below treatment threshold
Moderate risk	• No prior hip or spine fracture • BMD T-score at hip and spine both above –2.5 • 10-year hip fracture <3% and 10-year risk factor of major osteoporotic fracture <20%	Not defined			No previous spine or hip fracture; T-score between –1 and –2.5; FRAX above treatment threshold
High risk	• Prior hip or spine fracture • BMD T-score at hip and spine below –2.5 • 10-year hip fracture ≥3% and 10-year risk factor of major osteoporotic fracture ≥20%	• Lumbar spine or femoral neck or total hip T-score of –2.5 or below, or a history of fragility fracture, or high FRAX fracture probability defined as 10-year major osteoporotic fracture risk ≥20% or hip fracture risk ≥3% (nonuse regions may have different thresholds) • No prior fractures but risk factors present such as advanced age, frailty, glucocorticoids, very low T-scores, or increased fall risk			Prior spine or a hip fracture or lumbar spine or hip T-score of –2.5 or below; FRAX 10-year absolute fracture risk above the treatment threshold
Very high risk	Multiple spinal fractures and a BMD T-score at the hip or spine of –2.5 or below	Very high-risk factors include advanced age, frailty, glucocorticoids, very low T-scores, or increased fall risk		Very high risk based on older age, a recent fracture (eg, within the past 12 months), history of multiple clinical osteoporotic fractures, multiple risk factors for fracture, or failure of other available osteoporosis therapy	Multiple spine fractures/hip fracture and T-score of –2.5 or lower at lumbar spine or hip

	Endocrine Society	AACE	IOF and ESCEO	ACP	BHOF
Treatment recommendations	• Low risk: reassess fracture risk in 2-4 years • Moderate risk: reassess fracture risk in 2-4 years or bisphosphonate (oral or intravenous) • High very high risk: bisphosphonates, denosumab, teriparatide or abaloparatide, romosozumab	• Low and moderate risk: no recommendation for treatment • High risk or no prior fractures: bisphosphonates, denosumab • Very high risk or prior fractures: denosumab, abaloparatide, teriparatide, romosozumab, zoledronic acid	High risk: anabolic agent	• First-line: bisphosphonates • Second line: denosumab • Primary osteoporosis with very high risk of fracture: use romosozumab teriparatide or abaloparatide followed by a bisphosphonate	• Low and moderate risk: reassess fracture risk in 2-4 years • High risk: initial treatment with bisphosphonates or denosumab • Very high risk: teriparatide, abaloparatide, or romosozumab
Recommends bisphosphonates first line	Yes	Yes	Yes	Yes	Yes
Recommends denosumab first-line	Yes	Yes	Yes	No	Yes
Prioritizes osteoanabolic therapy as initial therapy for patients with a history of fracture or very high-risk	No	No	Yes	Yes	Yes

Treatment Sequence

Bisphosphonates are the most consistently recommended first-line therapy for postmenopausal osteoporosis treatment secondary to their broad-spectrum antifracture efficacy data. Additionally, these are the only oral medications with robust antifracture data and are often preferred by patients due to route of administration. Oral bisphosphonates are associated with limited patient and prescriber obstacles for accessing therapy such as insurance prior authorization requirements and complicated office administration billing or instructions for use. They are associated with little to no patient out-of-pocket expense. Most societal guidelines recommend bisphosphonates as first-line therapy; however, there are treatment concerns when considering long-term effects on patient care and the efficacy and safety of treatment sequence.

Bisphosphonates are embedded in the bone matrix and are associated with recirculation for many years. This recirculation impacts bone resorption, a part of the therapeutic process that PTH analogues depend on, particularly during the initial phase of anabolic therapy where biomarkers are increased. Most studies and guidelines support the finding that bisphosphonates blunt the effect of osteoanabolic therapy.[1-5] Based on the impairment of biomarkers in patients receiving PTH analogues after receiving bisphosphonates compared with PTH analogue alone, it is hypothesized that the ability of osteoanabolic medications to increase BMD optimally is reduced. Confirmation of this finding is further supported by more recent romosozumab studies, where BMD gains in the hip and spine were significantly less in patients pretreated with bisphosphonates 1 year before romosozumab initiation.[7] This finding supports the need to identify and treat appropriately selected patients with osteoanabolic medications prior to bisphosphonates but is only reflected in certain guideline recommendations.

Denosumab is a fully human monoclonal antibody to the receptor activator of nuclear factor–kappa β (RANKL) that blocks osteoclast differentiation and decreases bone resorption. In the 36-month, prospective placebo-controlled FREEDOM Trial, denosumab did the following: (1) decreased CTX by 86% at 1 month and by 72% at 36 months; (2) increased BMD by 9.2% in the spine and 6.0% in the total hip; and (3) decreased fracture risk by 68% in the spine, 40% in the hip, and 20% for nonvertebral locations compared with placebo.[8] In the FREEDOM extension trial, denosumab resulted in sustained incremental increases in BMD by 22% at the spine and 9% at the total hip over 10 years.[9] After stopping denosumab, preosteoclasts rapidly mature into osteoclasts, which results in increases in bone resorption markers and is associated with BMD decline to pretreatment levels within 2 years. This increases the risk of developing vertebral fractures as evidenced by a larger proportion of patients experiencing multiple vertebral fractures upon discontinuation of denosumab (60.7%) compared with placebo (38.7%) (P = .049).[9,10] Bone turnover markers may remain elevated for 30 months after the last denosumab dose. This is responsible for an increased risk of multiple compression fractures between 7 and 18 months after the last denosumab dose.[10] It is important to consider the risk factors for rebound bone loss and vertebral fractures after denosumab discontinuation to individualize treatment approaches:

- Younger age
- Duration of denosumab therapy
- Greater improvement in hip BMD while on therapy
- Greater decline in hip BMD off therapy
- History of vertebral fractures
- Lower BMD at baseline
- High CTX at denosumab initiation

A history of bisphosphonate therapy prior to denosumab can decrease the degree of improvement in BMD with denosumab, which may be associated with less rebound bone loss upon cessation of denosumab. The authors' general recommendation is to consider denosumab as a second-line therapy for antiresorptive agents, particularly in younger patients, consistent with ACP guideline recommendations.

Additionally, DATA-SWITCH and romosozumab studies demonstrated that osteoanabolic therapy in patients with a high or very high fracture risk should be considered prior to or in addition to denosumab.[11-13] This is important to consider in young patients given the reversibility of the medication that would require lifelong therapy or transition to other therapy. The importance of sequences and risk of developing osteonecrosis of the jaw or atypical femoral fracture appear to be increased with cumulative exposure and length of therapy. Discontinuation of denosumab should be considered when adverse effects occur or if treatment goals are achieved but require bridge to alternative therapy to reduce the risk of rebound bone resorption and subsequent development of fractures. The optimal sequence for transition remains definitively unanswered, but existing data suggest some optimal approaches to reduce this risk. DATA-SWITCH demonstrates that the overlap of denosumab with an osteoanabolic agent likely is the most favorable approach in patients on denosumab who remain at very high fracture risk.[11] Bisphosphonates (oral and intravenous) can be effective options, especially if a course of denosumab is less than 2 years. However, in patients on long-term denosumab therapy, frequent monitoring of bone resorption markers is necessary to guide the dosing frequency of intravenous zoledronic acid.[14] Finally, low-dosage denosumab, 30 mg every 6 months over 24 months, resulted in modest improvement in spine BMD while maintaining hip BMD regardless of the therapy duration. Follow-up studies are ongoing to evaluate the efficacy of intravenous zoledronic acid following low-dosage denosumab.

Clinical Case Vignettes

Case 1

A 67-year-old woman with postmenopausal osteoporosis presents with a 6-month history of back and hip pain. The patient is concerned with preserving activities of daily living. She remains an active cigarette smoker (1 pack per day for the last 43 years). She had a myocardial infarction 10 months ago. Osteoporosis was diagnosed on her most recent DXA (*see Table*).

She previously delayed treatment with oral alendronate recommended by her primary care physician because she was concerned about adverse effects.

On physical examination, her blood pressure is 157/97 mm Hg and pulse rate is 84 beats/min. Her height is 65.7 in (167 cm), and weight is 107 lb (48.5 kg) (BMI = 17.4 kg/m^2). She has reportedly lost 2 in (5.08 cm) of height. She appears healthy and is in no apparent distress. She can easily rise from a seated position unassisted with good tandem gait with balance.

There is a history of low vitamin D and elevated alkaline phosphatase (documented 3 years ago) that normalized with vitamin D correction. Currently, calcium and vitamin D intake are adequate, and she exercises daily. She received a steroid injection for left hip pain 3 times in the last 3 years. There is no history of oral steroids, anticoagulation, thyroid medication, proton-pump inhibitors, or anticonvulsants. The secondary workup for osteoporosis and comorbid conditions was unrevealing.

X-ray reveals an L1:L2 compression fracture.

Which of the following is the most appropriate treatment recommendation for this patient?

A. PTH analogue

B. Denosumab

C. Romosozumab

D. Raloxifene

Answer: A) PTH analogue

Which of the following is the most compelling factor that supports the use of the recommended agent?

A. Compression fracture

B. Vegan diet

C. Age

D. BMD

Answer: A) Compression fracture

PTH analogues are preferred for this patient given the severity of her osteoporosis and history of compression fracture, which is the most compelling indication for therapy. The patient is treatment-naïve and as such, it is anticipated that she would get the greatest response from a PTH analogue as initial therapy. Bisphosphonates are often considered as initial therapy but would not be the preferred option due to the potential for blunting the benefits of teriparatide. In addition, this patient already experienced a compression fracture and is at very high risk for subsequent fractures. Thus, she needs optimization of treatment sequence with the most effective options. To optimally reduce her risk, it is recommended to start with the agent that would

Date/machine	Trabecular bone score (TBS)	Lumbar spine	Femoral neck	Total hip
Lunar	1.132	0.875 g/cm^2 T-score = −2.5 L1-L2 0.749 g/cm^2 T-score = −3.5 Degenerative disease L3-L4	Left 0.729 g/cm^2 T-score = −2.2 Right 0.673 g/cm^2 T-score = −2.6	Left 0.761 g/cm^2 T-score = −2.0 Right 0.704 g/cm^2 T-score = −2.4

most greatly impact BMD and with robust and timely fracture risk reduction. The VERO trial demonstrated greater fracture risk reduction and effectiveness with teriparatide compared with the oral bisphosphonate risedronate (24 months, new vertebral fractures 5.4% in teriparatide group vs 12.0% in the risedronate group (risk ratio 0.44; $P < .0001$).[15] Romosozumab could be considered; however, this patient has a contraindication to therapy given the cardiovascular event in the last 12 months. Denosumab may also be a referenced option, but it would not be the authors' preferred first-line therapy. First, DATA-SWITCH suggests that using denosumab prior to a PTH analogue will result in significant decreases in BMD. This limits the option for the next sequence of treatment. Second, the patient is young with a history of compression fractures, which places her at very high risk of rebound bone loss and development of further compression fractures with denosumab discontinuation. This is a significant concern with denosumab cessation, and hence duration of denosumab therapy would be unclear and create complications for transitions to alternative therapy.

Case 2

A 70-year-old woman with stress-induced cardiomyopathy and cardiac arrest 12 years ago presents for follow-up of postmenopausal osteoporosis. Osteoporosis was diagnosed by DXA with the lowest T-score of –2.9 at the lumbar spine and no history of fragility fractures. A PTH analogue was recommended twice, but the patient remains apprehensive of a daily self-administered injection. She also declines treatment with intravenous zoledronic acid due to concerns with intravenous infusions. Subsequently, the patient started denosumab 6 years ago. No adverse outcomes were reported, and she has been tolerating denosumab every 6 months except for a 2-month delay during the COVID pandemic and for dental work. Physical examination findings and laboratory evaluation are unremarkable. The most recent DXA (this year, after 9 doses of denosumab), demonstrates significant improvement with the lowest T-score of –2.3 at the spine, –2.2 at the left femoral neck, and –1.4 at the left total hip. She has heard about the adverse effects of osteonecrosis of the jaw and she would like to stop denosumab if possible.

How long should denosumab be continued for this patient?

A. Lifelong

B. 10 years

C. 5 years

D. Dependent on several factors

Answer: D) Dependent on several factors

The duration of denosumab therapy depends on several factors. Given results from the FREEDOM extension, there are efficacy data to suggest that treatment of 10 years (and potentially longer) is appropriate and safe. Consideration of cumulative exposure doses, as well as managing the need for invasive dental work and development of atypical femoral fracture is vital. Additionally, a system for ensuring appropriate administration and continuation of denosumab is an important aspect of management to prevent interruption or delay to avoid the risk of rebound fracture.[16] The patient is responding well to treatment overall as evidenced by no development of fractures and T-score improvement to greater than –2.5; thus, discontinuation of denosumab and transition to alternative therapy can be considered.

Which of the following would be the most appropriate pharmacological treatment option for transition?

A. Teriparatide

B. Romosozumab

C. Oral bisphosphonate

D. Intravenous zoledronic acid

Answer: D) Intravenous zoledronic acid

How often should intravenous zoledronic acid be administered?

A. Once

B. Every 12 months

C. Every 3 months

D. Dependent on monitored bone markers

Answer: D) Dependent on monitored bone markers

DATA-SWITCH demonstrates that transitioning to teriparatide is not the optimal treatment approach. Likewise, data from phase 2 and 3 studies of romosozumab suggest that after 2 doses of denosumab BMD did not decline with romosozumab, but there was a blunting in the degree of BMD improvement. No data are available regarding romosozumab after long-term therapy with denosumab. Oral bisphosphonates are a potential option, likely more effective after short-term denosumab therapy, but there is no option to adjust the frequency of bisphosphonate administration based on monitoring of bone turnover markers and subsequent elevations, which is a vital aspect of denosumab discontinuation and management. Hence, intravenous zoledronic acid is the optimal approach, as it can be given more frequently based on bone turnover markers.

Case 3

An 83-year-old woman presents for a follow-up visit for management of postmenopausal osteoporosis and low BMD. She was last seen in the office 12 months ago. She has received 2 doses of intravenous zoledronic acid over the last 2 years with reports of lower-extremity cramps 1 week after each infusion. She confirms this is tolerable and does not have concerns about continuing. The last infusion of intravenous zoledronic acid was given 11 months ago. Her lowest T-score at the time of diagnosis was –2.8 at the lumbar spine with no history of atraumatic fractures. She saw the dentist 2 months before the current visit and confirmed no plans for invasive dental work. The patient denies any concerning hip or pelvic pain

consistent with an atypical femur fracture. She has a history of atrial fibrillation and developed a stroke 6 months ago and is now treated with apixaban. She remains active with physical therapy and optimizing nonpharmacological treatment recommendations, including adequate supplementation of vitamin D and calcium. Follow-up DXA demonstrates a significant decline in BMD with the lowest T-score of –3.0 in femoral neck. The patient's CTX is 1269.1 pg/mL (reference range, 104-1008 pg/mL).

Which of the following is the most appropriate pharmacological treatment option?

A. Romosozumab

B. Denosumab

C. Continuation of intravenous zoledronic acid

D. PTH analogue

Answer: B) Denosumab

Which of the following statements best supports the need to transition to alternative therapy?

A. Significant decline in BMD suggests failure of current therapy

B. Bone turnover marker is elevated suggesting bisphosphonate is not optimally suppressing bone turnover

C. The patient has not had a fracture, so is responding to therapy and does not need to switch

D. The patient is having adverse effects from bisphosphonates

Answer: A) Significant decline in BMD suggests failure of current therapy

The patient has a history of cardiovascular disease with a stroke in the past 12 months, so romosozumab is contraindicated. The significant decline in BMD suggests the failure of antiresorptive therapy, and treatment escalation or transition is required. While CTX is elevated, these markers have not been validated to assess fracture risk and thus are not the primary reason for transition. PTH analogues will have less effect on BMD in the hip where the patient's BMD is lowest, so it would not be the optimal next step. Given her age and specific presentation, this is a scenario where denosumab is the preferred next treatment step.

Key Learning Points

- Risk stratification, future considerations, and treatment goals are important for deciding initial treatment.

- Risk factors, cost, insurance coverage, comorbidities, and patient preferences should be considered with all decisions.

- Long-term treatment goals should be considered to guide all treatment decisions.

References

1. Shoback D, Rosen CJ, Black DM, Cheung AM, Murad MH, Eastell R. Pharmacological management of osteoporosis in postmenopausal women: an Endocrine Society guideline update. *J Clin Endocrinol Metab.* 2020;105(3):587-594. PMID: 32068863

2. LeBoff MS, Greenspan SL, Insogna KL, et al. The clinician's guide to prevention and treatment of osteoporosis. *Osteoporos Int.* 2022;33(10):2049-2102. PMID: 35478046

3. Camacho PM, Petak SM, Binkley N, et al. American Association of Clinical endocrinologists/American College of Endocrinology clinical practice guidelines for the diagnosis and treatment of postmenopausal osteoporosis—2020 update. *Endocr Pract.* 2020;26(Suppl 1):1-46. PMID: 32427503

4. Qaseem A, Hicks LA, Etxeandia-Ikobaltzeta I, Shamliyan T, Cooney TG; Clinical Guidelines Committee of the American College of Physicians. Pharmacologic treatment of primary osteoporosis or low bone mass to prevent fractures in adults: a living clinical guideline from the American College of Physicians. *Ann Intern Med.* 2023;176(2):224-238. PMID: 36592456

5. Kanis JA, Cooper C, Rizzoli R, Reginster JY, on behalf of the Scientific Advisory Board of the European Society for Clinical and Economic Aspects of Osteoporosis (ESCEO) and the Committees of Scientific Advisors and National Societies of the International Osteoporosis Foundation (IOF). European guidance for the diagnosis and management of osteoporosis in postmenopausal women. *Osteoporos Int.* 2019;30(1):3-44. PMID: 30324412

6. Ahlborg HG, Johnell O, Turner CH, Rannevik G, Karlsson MK. Bone loss and bone size after menopause. *N Engl J Med.* 2003;349(4):327-334. PMID: 12878739

7. Saag KG, Petersen J, Brandi ML, et al. Romosozumab or alendronate for fracture prevention in women with osteoporosis. *N Engl J Med.* 2017;377(15):1417-1427. PMID: 28892457

8. Cummings SR, San Martin J, McClung MR, et al; FREEDOM Trial. Denosumab for prevention of fractures in postmenopausal women with osteoporosis. *N Engl J Med.* 2009;361(8):756-765. PMID: 19671655

9. Bone HG, Wagman RB, Brandi ML, et al. 10 years of denosumab treatment in postmenopausal women with osteoporosis: results from the phase 3 randomised FREEDOM trial and open-label extension. *Lancet Diabetes Endocrinol.* 2017;5(7):513-523. PMID: 28546097

10. Anastasilakis AD, Polyzos SA, Makras P, Aubry-Rozier B, Kaouri S, Lamy O. Clinical features of 24 patients with rebound-associated vertebral fractures after denosumab discontinuation: systematic review and additional cases. *J Bone Miner Res.* 2017;32(6):1291-1296. PMID: 28240371

11. Leder BZ, Tsai JN, Uihlein AV, et al. Denosumab and teriparatide transitions in postmenopausal osteoporosis (The data-switch study): extension of a randomised controlled trial. *Lancet.* 2015;386(9999):1147-1155. PMID: 26144908

12. McClung MR, Bolognese MA, Brown JP, et al. Skeletal responses to romosozumab after 12 months of denosumab. *JBMR Plus.* 2021;5(7):e10512. PMID: 34258507

13. Cosman F, Crittenden DB, Adachi JD, et al. Romosozumab treatment in postmenopausal women with osteoporosis. *N Engl J Med.* 2016;375(16):1532-1543. PMID: 27641143

14. Sølling AS, Harsløf T, Langdahl B. Treatment with zoledronate subsequent to denosumab in osteoporosis: a randomized trial. *J Bone Miner Res.* 2020;35(10):1858-1870. PMID: 32459005

15. Geusens P, Marin F, Kendler DL, et al. Effects of teriparatide compared with risedronate on the risk of fractures in subgroups of postmenopausal women with severe osteoporosis: the Vero Trial. *J Bone Miner Res.* 2018;33(5):783-794. PMID: 29329484

16. Lyu H, Yoshida K, Zhao SS, et al. Delayed denosumab injections and fracture risk among patients with osteoporosis: a population-based cohort study. *Ann Intern Med.* 2020;173(7):516-526. PMID: 3271670

Primary Hyperparathyroidism in Pregnancy

Dalal S. Ali, MD, MSc. Division of Endocrinology and Metabolism, McMaster University, Hamilton, ON, Canada; Email: dalal.ali@boneresearch.ca

Aliya A. Khan, MD. Division of Endocrinology and Metabolism, McMaster University, Hamilton, ON, Canada; Email: aliya@mcmaster.ca

Educational Objectives

After reviewing this chapter, learners should be able to:

- Explain the changes in calcium homeostasis during pregnancy.

- Evaluate and diagnose primary hyperparathyroidism (PHPT) during pregnancy.

- Manage PHPT during pregnancy, both medically and surgically.

- List the indications for genetic testing in women of childbearing age presenting with PHPT.

Figure 1. Calcium Homeostasis During Pregnancy

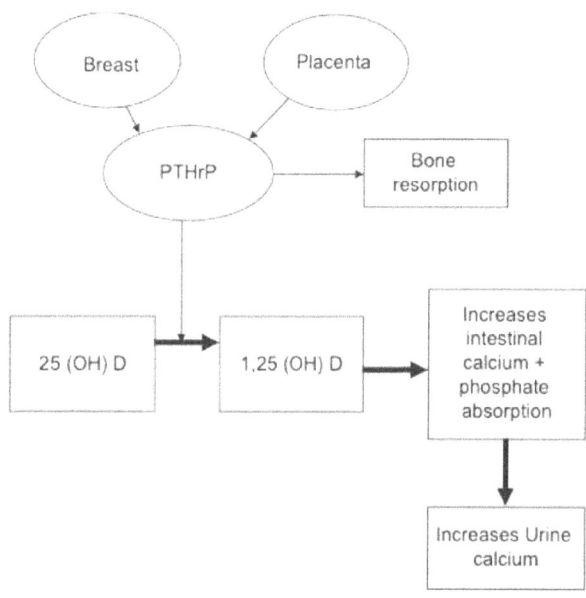

Reprinted with permission from Khan AA et al. *Eur J Endocrinol*, 2019; 180(2): R37-R44. © European Society of Endocrinology. Published by Oxford University Press on behalf of the Society.[1]

Significance of the Clinical Problem

Physiology

During pregnancy, PTH levels can decline in association with the physiological rise in PTHrP (*Figure 1*). The PTHrP level rises as early as 3 to 13 weeks' gestation and peaks in the third trimester. In pregnancies complicated by PHPT, the diagnosis is confirmed in the presence of hypercalcemia with elevated or (nonsuppressed) PTH.[1]

Epidemiology

PHPT is a leading cause of hypercalcemia in the nonpregnant population.[2] An increase in the incidence of PHPT in pregnancy was noted in a Canadian retrospective study evaluating 13,792,544 deliveries. Of these, 368 deliveries occurred in women with PHPT, representing an increase in the overall incidence of PHPT from 1.6 to 5.2 per 100,000 births ($P < .0001$) over the past 16 years.[3] Women with PHPT had a higher prevalence of comorbidities such as obesity, pregestational hypertension, and diabetes when compared with the control group. They also had a higher rate of preterm delivery (odds ratio, 1.69; 95% CI, 1.24-2.29), preeclampsia (odds ratio, 3.14; 95% CI, 2.30-4.28), and cesarean delivery (odds ratio, 1.69; 95% CI, 1.36-2.09). Another retrospective study that included 28 pregnancies showed a higher rate of preterm delivery and preeclampsia in women with PHPT treated medically during pregnancy.[4] Infants born to mothers with PHPT were more likely to experience growth restriction (odds ratio, 1.83 [95% CI, 1.08-3.07]) and be diagnosed with a congenital anomaly (odds ratio, 4.21 [95% CI, 2.09-8.48]) as noted in one retrospective study.[3]

Practice Gaps

- Diagnosing PHPT during pregnancy and excluding familial hypocalciuric hypercalcemia (FHH) types 1, 2, and 3 requires careful evaluation.

- Diagnosing and managing PHPT in pregnancy requires close follow-up.

- Medical management of PHPT in pregnancy is currently being further studied.

Discussion

Diagnosis

The diagnosis of PHPT in pregnancy is confirmed in the presence of hypercalcemia (elevated serum ionized calcium or calcium adjusted for albumin) with a nonsuppressed serum PTH.[5] PHPT results from a solitary parathyroid adenoma in approximately 85% of cases, with hyperplasia occurring in approximately 15% of patients. Fortunately, parathyroid cancer is extremely rare.[6] In those younger than 40 years, an underlying pathogenic variant resulting in the development of PHPT is present in approximately 10% of individuals.[7] These variants may result in the development of a syndromic or nonsyndromic form of PHPT. Syndromic forms include multiple endocrine neoplasia (MEN type 1, MEN type

2A, or MEN type 4) or hyperparathyroidism–jaw tumor syndrome. Nonsyndromic forms of PHPT or isolated PHPT also require further evaluation and in particular exclusion of familial hypocalciuric hypercalcemia (FHH). FHH is considered if the calcium-to-creatinine clearance ratio is less than 0.01 in the presence of hypercalcemia and a nonsuppressed PTH. If the calcium-to-creatinine clearance ratio is inconclusive (between 0.01 and 0.02), it is important to consider other causes of a low calcium-to-creatinine clearance ratio, including vitamin D inadequacy, kidney impairment, or inadequate calcium intake. Consideration may be given to completing DNA analysis of the *CASR*, *AP2S1*, and *GNA11* genes with exclusion of the 3 forms of FHH, namely FHH types 1, 2, and 3.

Maternal and Fetal Outcomes

Pregnancy in women with PHPT may be associated with several maternal complications, including hyperemesis gravidarum, nephrolithiasis, and/or pancreatitis,[5] as well as fetal complications, including neonatal hypocalcemia (in severe cases), tetany, intrauterine growth restriction, and fetal demise.[5] Early recognition of PHPT is associated with a reduced rate of complications compared with that observed in older literature. However, medically managed PHPT still seems to be linked to an increased risk of preeclampsia and miscarriage rates. The literature reports postpartum hypercalcemic crises as a potential complication of PHPT in pregnancy, likely occurring when the active transplacental transfer of calcium from the mother to the fetus is lost after placental delivery.[8]

Management

Medical

Mild cases of PHPT in pregnancy have been reported in the literature and have been successfully managed medically. Medical management includes ensuring adequate hydration, cessation of thiazide diuretics, calcium supplements and lithium if possible, and/or pharmacotherapy. Several pharmacological agents have been used in this context.[9] This includes calcitonin, a class B category drug that does not cross the placenta and can be used for a short duration to manage hypercalcemia.[9] Cinacalcet, a calcimimetic agent that reduces PTH secretion, has also been cautiously used in women with severe PHPT during pregnancy.[10] This is a class C category drug that crosses the placenta, and data on long-term safety in pregnancy are unfortunately lacking. Bisphosphonates (class C drug) are another category of medications used in hypercalcemia management. However, bisphosphonates carry a theoretical risk of affecting the fetal endochondral bone formation and should therefore be avoided.[9] Denosumab, a category D drug, should not be used during pregnancy due to its association with fetal skeletal adverse outcomes in animal studies.[9]

Surgical

Timely surgical intervention in the second trimester has been associated with favorable outcomes in patients with moderate to severe hypercalcemia during pregnancy (calcium adjusted for albumin greater than 11 mg/dL (>2.75 mmol/L) based on the Fifth International Workshop on the management of PHPT in pregnancy.[11] Other guidelines from Europe have a different threshold for recommending parathyroidectomy in pregnancy (calcium adjusted for albumin greater than 11.42 mg/dL (>2.85 mmol/L).[12] Surgery remains the only curative option for PHPT and is well-tolerated during pregnancy (ideally in the second trimester) with minimal adverse events. Parathyroid resection under local anesthesia may be possible to reduce risks of anesthesia-related complications during pregnancy.[13,14] Parathyroidectomy has also been reported in the third trimester in patients for whom medical therapy has failed and severe hypercalcemia is present. In such patients, surgery also appears to be safe in experienced hands with no negative maternal or fetal outcomes.[15] However, associated complications were reported in some cases, including preeclampsia, preterm labor, and severe neonatal hypocalcemia with third-trimester surgery.[15] These complications may be attributed to delayed presentation and prolonged exposure to maternal hypercalcemia.

Localization in Pregnancy

The diagnosis of PHPT is confirmed based on the biochemical profile, and imaging is only used to guide the surgical approach. Neck ultrasonography serves as the first-line imaging modality, with a sensitivity of 76% to 87% in identifying abnormal parathyroid tissue and a specificity of 94% to 96%.[5] If neck ultrasonography fails to identify a parathyroid adenoma, neck MRI[12] or CT with appropriate abdominal shielding would be appropriate.[16]

Clinical Case Vignettes

Case 1

A 30-year-old woman (G2A1L0) presents at 32 weeks' gestation with progressive leg pain of 2 months duration, and now requires wheelchair use. Her early pregnancy was complicated by nausea with intermittent vomiting. Two years ago, she presented with flank pain and a kidney stone was identified on kidney ultrasonography.

On physical examination, her blood pressure is 140/92 mm Hg and other vitals are stable. There is no cervical lymphadenopathy and there is a fullness in the left lower lobe of the thyroid. The left distal femur has a palpable, deep, soft-tissue mass that is mildly tender. The quadriceps tendon is intact. Motor examination documents 3/5 power in the left leg. The left quadriceps is tender. She has normal findings on sensory exam and musculoskeletal exam, including normal knee and hip function and intact reflexes. She has a gravid uterus.

Laboratory test results (sample drawn at admission):

Serum-corrected calcium = 16.83 mg/dL (8.62-10.4 mg/dL) (SI: 4.2 mmol/L [2.15-2.6 mmol/L])
PTH = 1394.6 pg/mL (15-65 pg/mL) (SI: 147.9 pmol/L [1.6-6.9 pmol/L])

Estimated glomerular filtration rate = 71 mL/min per
  1.73 m² (>60 mL/min per 1.73 m²)
Serum alkaline phosphatase = 183 U/L (50-136 U/L)
  (SI: 3.06 µkat/L [0.84-2.27 µkat/L])
Serum phosphate = 3.31 mg/dL (3-4.5 mg/dL)
  (SI: 1.07 mmol/L [0.81-1.45 mmol/L])
Magnesium = 1.14 mg/dL (1.7-2.2 mg/dL)
  (SI: 0.47 mmol/L [0.85-1.10 mmol/L])
25-Hydroxyvitamin D = 14.72 ng/mL (30-50 ng/mL)
  (SI: 36.8 nmol/L [75-125 nmol/L])
Serum AST, normal
Bilirubin, normal

Biochemical workup for MEN type 1 is unremarkable. Genetic test results are outstanding.

Femur x-ray demonstrated a large, aggressive bone lesion within the distal femoral diaphysis, with aggressive periosteal reaction and cortical thinning of approximately 7 cm (*Figure 2*). Histopathology identifies it as a brown tumor, with additional bone lesions found on a skeletal survey involving the right shoulder, right humerus, skull, and pelvis.

Figure 2. Femur X-ray

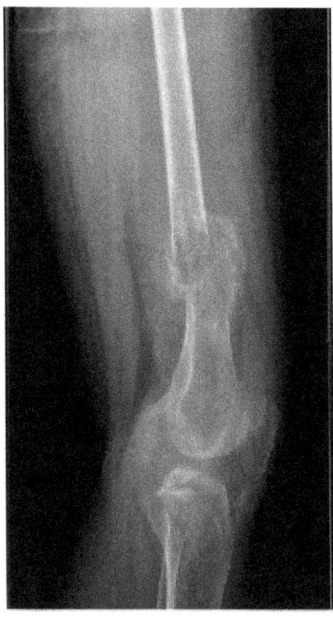

X-ray showing large, aggressive bone lesion in the distal femoral diaphysis (brown tumor). Courtesy of Dalal S. Ali and Aliya A. Khan, McMaster University, Ontario, Canada.

Neck ultrasonography shows a TR-4 right solid and cystic neck nodule favored to represent an exophytic thyroid nodule rather than a parathyroid adenoma, TR-2. Subsequent CT neck reveals a 4-cm parathyroid adenoma with no overt malignant features.

Which of the following is this patient's most likely diagnosis?

A. Severe PHPT

B. Solid-organ cancer with bone metastasis

C. Ectopic PTH-secreting tumour

D. Milk-alkali syndrome

Answer: A) Severe PHPT

This patient's biochemical profile is consistent with PTH-dependent hypercalcemia (thus, Answer A is correct).

Case 1 (continued)

In addition to intravenous fluid hydration and discontinuation of any drugs that may contribute to hypercalcemia, which of the following is the best course of action?

A. Start calcitonin

B. Start cinacalcet

C. Start a trial of calcitonin and normalize vitamin D

D. Start intravenous bisphosphonate therapy

Answer: C) Start a trial of calcitonin and normalize vitamin D

Calcitonin and vitamin D supplementation (Answer C) is safe during pregnancy. Correction of vitamin D inadequacy has been associated with reduced incidence of hungry bone syndrome following parathyroidectomy.

This patient had severe PTH-mediated hypercalcemia, confirmed to be PHPT. She was treated with intravenous fluids, and calcitonin was added. Cinacalcet was introduced after an inadequate response to previous measures, with a maximum dosage of 30 mg twice daily. Subtotal parathyroidectomy was performed at 33 weeks' gestation. PTH dropped to 44.3 pg/mL (4.7 pmol/L) postoperatively, signifying cure. The histopathologic report was consistent with an atypical parathyroid adenoma, and there was no evidence of malignancy. After parathyroidectomy, the patient experienced premature rupture of membranes and cesarean delivery was completed at 34 weeks' gestation. On day 8 post parathyroidectomy, the patient developed hungry bone syndrome requiring calcium and vitamin D supplementation. Unfortunately, she also experienced a mechanical fall, resulting in a pathological fracture of the femur at the site of the brown tumor (*Figure 3*). *Figures 4* and *5* represent the right humeral lesion before and 6 months after parathyroidectomy.

Figure 3. X-ray After Parathyroidectomy

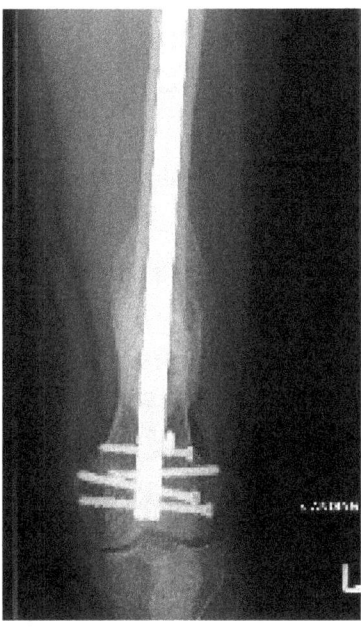

X-ray showing an intramedullary rod in the left femur. Exuberant bony callus formation in the distal diaphysis is noted with progressive bony healing. Courtesy of Dalal S. Ali and Aliya A. Khan, McMaster University, Ontario, Canada.

Figure 4. X-ray Before Parathyroidectomy

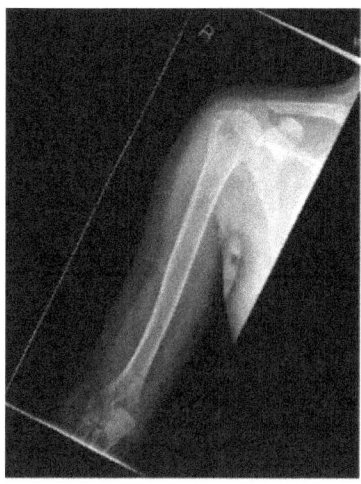

X-ray showing inhomogeneous increased density lesion in the proximal humerus, measuring approximately 5.3 × 2.2 cm. There is no obvious cortical involvement. Image courtesy of Dalal S. Ali and Aliya A. Khan, McMaster University, Ontario, Canada.

Figure 5. X-ray 6 Months After Parathyroidectomy

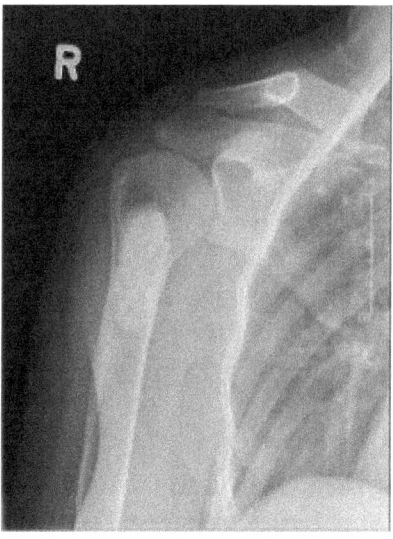

X-ray showing a densely sclerotic and elongated oval-shaped intramedullary focus at the level of the right humeral neck, measuring approximately 5.5 × 2 cm when compared with previous imaging, consistent with posttreatment changes with brown tumor. Image courtesy of Dalal S. Ali and Aliya A. Khan, McMaster University, Ontario, Canada.

Case 1 (continued)

Which of the following complications of maternal PHPT is a concern?

A. Post-term pregnancy

B. Neonatal hypocalcemia

C. Arrhythmias due to prolonged QT interval in the mother

D. Seizures

Answer: B) Neonatal hypocalcemia

Neonatal hypocalcemia (Answer B) can develop due to suppression of the fetal parathyroid glands in the presence of maternal hypercalcemia. The baby was admitted to neonatal intensive care with hypoparathyroidism, requiring pharmacological intervention with calcium and active vitamin D. Hypoparathyroidism resolved at 3 months of age.

Case 2

A 32-year-old woman (G1P0) presents at 27 weeks' gestation with incidental hypercalcemia and high PTH. Nausea and vomiting worsened at the 18th week of gestation. There is no end-organ involvement. Her corrected calcium is 12.18 mg/dL (3.04 mmol/L) and PTH concentration is 161.2 pg/mL (17.1 pmol/L). She is managed with intravenous fluids and remains symptomatic with no improvement in hypercalcemia.

Which additional investigations should be completed before surgery?

A. Exclusion of MEN and FHH by laboratory profile and DNA analysis

B. Sestamibi scan

C. Exclusion of MEN and FHH by laboratory profile

D. Family mapping

Answer: C) Exclusion of MEN and FHH by laboratory profile

Exclusion of familial causes of hypercalcemia is advised in young individuals.

Case 2 (continued)

Which of the following is the best next management step?

A. Surgery

B. Intravenous zoledronate

C. Cinacalcet

D. Calcitonin

Answer: A) Surgery

Parathyroidectomy (Answer A) in the second trimester is considered safe in pregnant women with severe PHPT. Parathyroidectomy was performed at 30 weeks' gestation with excellent maternal and fetal outcomes. Postoperatively, PTH dropped to 18.8 pg/mL (2.0 pmol/L), signifying cure (*Figure 6, following page*). Histopathologic findings were consistent with parathyroid adenoma. She had a spontaneous vaginal delivery at 39 weeks' gestation, and no neonatal hypocalcemia was noted. The baby was healthy and had normal APGAR scores. The biochemical workup for MEN was unremarkable, and DNA analysis is pending.

Case 2 (continued)

Which of the following complications is NOT a concern for the mother?

A. Kidney stones

B. Fractures

C. Preeclampsia

D. Basal ganglia calcifications

Answer: D) Basal ganglia calcifications

Basal ganglia calcifications (Answer D) are seen in hypoparathyroidism, not in PHPT.

Case 3

A 37-year-old pregnant woman (G2P1) is referred at 10 weeks' gestation for the evaluation and management of hypercalcemia in pregnancy. High serum calcium with high PTH were identified during the workup of dizziness. The

Figure 6. Patient's Laboratory Data Before and After Parathyroidectomy

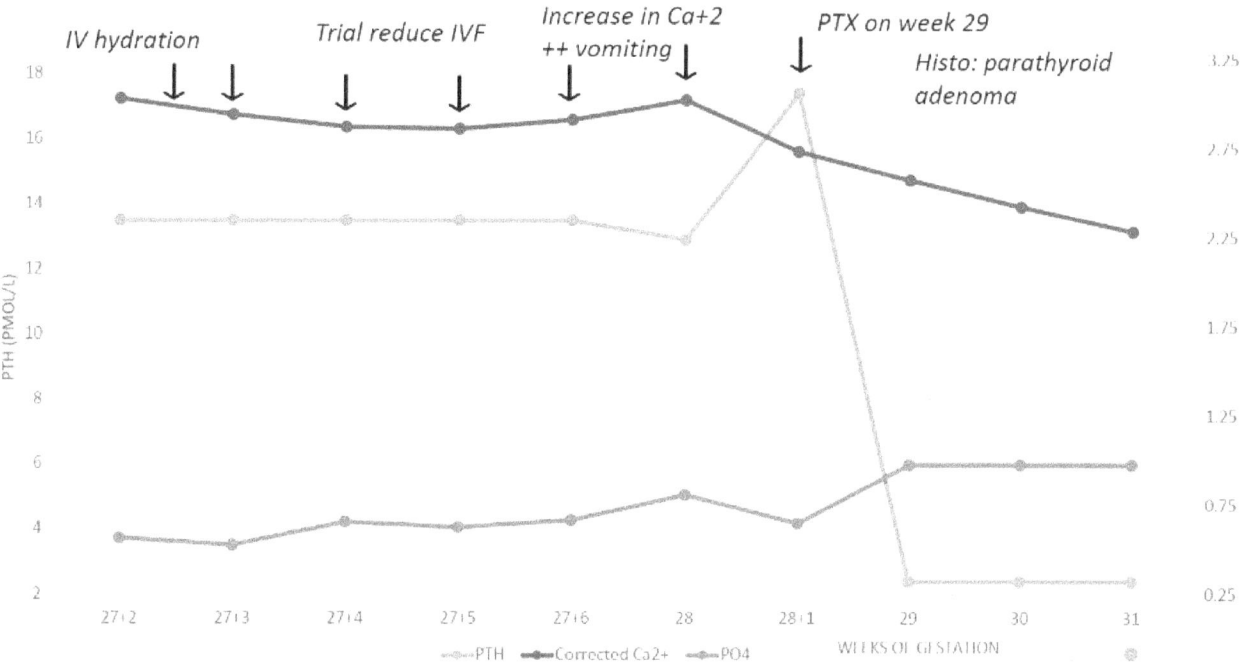

PTH, corrected Ca+2 and PO4 levels at presentation

[Color—Print (Color Gallery page CG7) or web & ePub editions]

25-hydroxyvitamin D concentration was low at presentation, and she was started on vitamin D$_3$, 1000 IU daily. The serum-corrected calcium fluctuated between normal and mildly elevated, while the serum ionized calcium was consistently mildly elevated. Nausea was present before pregnancy, and it significantly worsened during pregnancy, with no response to doxylamine. She currently has polyuria, excessive thirst, and nocturia. She drinks almost 3 L of fluids daily. She has mild abdominal pain and constipation. There is no history of kidney stones or fractures. She has had no changes in mental status. There is no history of lithium, thiazide, or calcium supplement use. She has no family history of hypercalcemia or parathyroid disorders and has never had an emergency department visit or hospital admission for hypercalcemia.

Laboratory test results:

> Serum ionized calcium = 6.2 mg/dL (4.6-5.4 mmol/L) (SI: 1.56 mmol/L [1.15-1.35 mmol/L])
> PTH = 78.2 pg/mL (SI: 8.3 pmol/L)
> 25-Hydroxyvitamin D = 24 pg/mL (SI: 60 nmol/L)
> Urinary calcium = 230 mg/24 h (SI: 5.76 mmol/d)
> Urinary creatinine = 1.1 g/24 h (SI: 9.7 mmol/d)
> Magnesium = 1.87 mg/dL (SI: 0.77 mmol/L)
> Phosphate = 2.2 mg/dL (SI: 0.71 mmol/L)
> Estimated glomerular filtration rate = 111 mL/min per 1.73 m²
> Creatinine = 0.7 mg/dL (SI: 62 μmol/L)
> Calcium-to-creatinine clearance ratio = 0.014

She is advised to increase her fluid intake and avoid dehydration. Genetic testing excludes FHH.

At 13 weeks' gestation, she starts experiencing increasing nausea and vomiting, the following laboratory values are documented:

> Serum ionized calcium = 6.2 mg/dL (SI: 1.56 mmol/L)
> Serum corrected calcium = 11.9 mg/dL (SI: 2.97 mmol/L)
> Calcium-to-creatinine clearance ratio = 0.019

At what serum calcium concentration (corrected for albumin) is parathyroidectomy considered during pregnancy?

A. 13 mg/dL (3.25 mmol/L)

B. >11 mg/dL (>2.75 mmol/L)

C. 10.8 mg/dL (2.7 mmol/L)

D. >13 mg/dL (>3.25 mmol/L)

Answer: B) >11 mg/dL (>2.75 mmol/L) based on the 5th International Workshop on PHPT management

Parathyroidectomy is recommended during pregnancy, preferably in the second trimester, if the serum-corrected calcium concentration exceeds 11 mg/dL (>2.75 mmol/L) (Answer B).

Case 3 (continued)

Which of the following is the first-line imaging modality for localizing parathyroid adenomas when considering parathyroidectomy during pregnancy?

A. Neck ultrasonography

B. 4D-CT with abdominal shielding

C. Neck MRI

D. ^{99m}Tc-MIBI

Answer: A) Neck ultrasonography

Neck ultrasonography (Answer A) is the safest imaging modality during pregnancy and should be used as the first-line imaging if parathyroidectomy is being considered. Neck ultrasonography revealed no clear parathyroid adenoma in this patient, but neck MRI identified the parathyroid adenoma.

Parathyroidectomy was completed at 15 weeks' gestation. Histopathology was consistent with right lower lipoadenoma. Postoperative PTH dropped to 22.6 pg/mL (2.4 pmol/L), signifying cure, and the following laboratory values were documented:

> Serum ionized calcium = 5.2 mg/dL (SI: 1.29 mmol/L)
> Serum corrected calcium = 9.42 mg/dL (SI: 2.35 mmol/L)
> Serum phosphate = 4.03 mg/dL (SI: 1.3 mmol/L)

Key Learning Points

- Medical management of PHPT in pregnancy is limited to hydration and calcitonin with close monitoring. There is limited evidence regarding the use of cinacalcet in pregnancy.

- Parathyroidectomy is well-tolerated in the second trimester of pregnancy in women with severe PHPT.

- Imaging options prior to surgical intervention for PHPT in pregnancy include neck ultrasonography, MRI, or CT with proper abdominal shielding.

References

1. Khan AA, Clarke B, Rejnmark L, Brandi ML. Management of endocrine disease: hypoparathyroidism in pregnancy: review and evidence-based recommendations for management. *Eur J Endocrinol.* 2019;180(2):R37-R44. PMID: 30444723

2. Khan AA, Hanley DA, Rizzoli R, et al. Primary hyperparathyroidism: review and recommendations on evaluation, diagnosis, and management. A Canadian and international consensus. *Osteoporosis International.* 2017;28(1):1-19. PMID: 27613721

3. Trahan M-J, Antinora C, Czuzoj-Shulman N, et al. Obstetrical and neonatal outcomes among pregnancies complicated by hyperparathyroidism. *J Matern Fetal Neonatal Med.* 2023;36(1):2170748. PMID: 36775282

4. Rigg J, Gilbertson E, Barrett HL, Britten FL, Lust K. Primary hyperparathyroidism in pregnancy: maternofetal outcomes at a quaternary referral obstetric hospital, 2000 through 2015. *J Clin Endocrinol Metab.* 2019;104(3):721-729. PMID: 30247615

5. Ali DS, Dandurand K, Khan AA. Primary hyperparathyroidism in pregnancy: literature review of the diagnosis and management. *J Clin Med.* 2021;10(13):2956. PMID: 34209340

6. Dematapitiya C, Perera C, Pathmanathan S, et al. Parathyroid carcinoma during pregnancy: a novel pathogenic CDC73 mutation – a case report. *BMC Endocr Disord.* 2022;22(1):259. PMID: 36284286

7. Marini F, Cianferotti L, Giusti F, Brandi ML. Molecular genetics in primary hyperparathyroidism: the role of genetic tests in differential diagnosis, disease prevention strategy, and therapeutic planning. A 2017 update. *Clin Cases Miner Bone Metab.* 2017;14(1):60-70. PMID: 28740527

8. Dandurand K, Ali DS, Khan AA. Hypercalcemia in pregnancy. *Endocrinol Metab Clin North Am.* 2021;50(4):753-768. PMID: 34774246

9. Bilezikian JP, Silverberg SJ, Bandeira F, et al. Management of primary hyperparathyroidism. *J Bone Miner Res.* 2022;37(11):2391-2403. PMID: 36245251

10. Vera L, Oddo S, Di Iorgi N, et al. Primary hyperparathyroidism in pregnancy treated with cinacalcet: a case report and review of the literature. *J Med Case Rep*. 2016;10(1):361. PMID: 27998296

11. Bilezikian JP, Khan AA, Silverberg SJ, et al. Evaluation and management of primary hyperparathyroidism: summary statement and guidelines from the Fifth International Workshop. *J Bone Miner Res*. 2022;37(11):2293-2314. PMID: 36245251

12. Bollerslev J, Rejnmark L, Zahn A, et al; 2021 PARAT Working Group. European Expert Consensus on practical management of specific aspects of parathyroid disorders in adults and in pregnancy: recommendations of the ESE Educational Program of Parathyroid Disorders. *Eur J Endocrinol*. 2022;186(2):R33-R63. PMID: 34863037

13. Mokrysheva NG, Eremkina AK, Mirnaya SS, et al. A case of pregnancy complicated by primary hyperparathyroidism due to a parathyroid adenoma. *Am J Case Rep*. 2019;20:53-59. PMID: 30636767

14. Sen S, Cherian AJ, Ramakant P, et al. Focused parathyroidectomy under local anesthesia - a feasibility study. *Indian J Endocrinol Metab*. 2019;23(1):67-71. PMID: 31016156

15. Nilsson IL, Adner N, Reihnér E, Plame-Kilander C, Edstrom G, Degerblad M. Primary hyperparathyroidism in pregnancy: a diagnostic and therapeutic challenge. *J Womens Health*. 2010;19(6):1117-1121. PMID: 20469964

16. McMullen TPW, Learoyd DL, Williams DC, Sywak MS, Sidhu SB, Delbridge LW. Hyperparathyroidism in pregnancy: options for localization and surgical therapy. *World J Surg*. 2010;34(8):1811-1816. PMID: 20386905

Osteoporosis in Underserved Populations

E. Michael Lewiecki, MD. University of New Mexico Health Sciences Center, Albuquerque, NM; Email: mlewiecki@gmail.com

Micol S. Rothman, MD. University of Colorado School of Medicine, Aurora, CO; Email: micol.rothman@cuanschutz.edu

Educational Objectives

After reviewing this chapter, learners should be able to:

- Identify disparities in the management of patients with osteoporosis.

- Recommend strategies for identifying and treating patients in underserved populations who are at high risk for fracture.

Significance of the Clinical Problem

Osteoporosis is a chronic systemic skeletal disorder characterized by low bone mineral density (BMD) and poor bone quality that results in loss of bone strength and increased risk of fractures. The consequences of fractures include chronic pain, impaired quality of life, loss of independence, and death. The global burden of osteoporosis and related fractures is vast and increasing, in large part due to aging of the population, with marked differences among world regions, countries, and population groups within countries. It is estimated that more than 200 million women have osteoporosis worldwide and that about 10 million adults in the United States have osteoporosis.

Despite the availability of excellent tools to assess fracture risk and many approved medications to reduce fracture risk, most patients at risk for fractures are not recognized and not treated. This large treatment gap constitutes a global crisis in the care of patients with osteoporosis.

Practice Gaps

- NonWhite women with osteoporosis are undertreated due to underuse of diagnostic services and potential bias in fracture risk assessment tools.

- Treatment of osteoporosis is low in populations with low income and low levels of education.

- Transgender and gender-diverse (TGD) individuals may be at risk for low BMD and may not receive appropriate skeletal health care screenings.

Discussion

Many factors contribute to the osteoporosis treatment gap, including fear of drug adverse effects, poor understanding of the balance of benefits and risks with treatment, poor appreciation of the potentially serious consequences of fractures, failure to recognize that a prior fracture is due to osteoporosis, conflicting clinical practice guidelines, limited available time for physician-patient encounters, and competing health care priorities. The gap in osteoporosis care is especially large in nonWhite women and in populations that are underserved due to factors such as race/ethnicity–adjustments in fracture risk algorithms, sexual orientation, socioeconomic status, age, geography, language, comorbidities, availability of diagnostic services, and expertise of local health care providers. Failure to address these issues represents many missed opportunities to prevent osteoporotic fractures and their consequences.

Since the prevalence of osteoporosis is lower in Black women than in White women, it would be expected that fewer Black women would have bone density testing; however, even when the indications are the same, fewer Black women than White women are tested.[1] There are racial and sex implications for the diagnosis of osteoporosis, with the International Society for Clinical Densitometry (ISCD) recommending that a White female reference database be used for hip T-score calculations in women and men of all race/ethnicities (https://iscd.org/official-positions-2023/). Adherence to these recommendations is not universal and may vary by DXA facility and by country. Z-score reference populations are matched for age, sex, race/ethnicity, and sometimes body weight, although there may be uncertainty regarding selection of sex in TGD patients and race/ethnicity in patients with mixed race/ethnicity. In the United States, the FRAX fracture risk calculator requires selection of 1 of 4 race/ethnicities, with controversy as to whether this results in discrimination and undertreatment of some patients.[2,3] The effect of transitioning to a single population-based FRAX calculator has been evaluated in a large registry-based study conducted on behalf of the American Society for Bone and Mineral Research Task Force on Clinical Algorithms for Fracture Risk (ASBMR Task Force). It was found that doing so would reduce differences in treatment qualification by race/ethnicity and may enhance equity and access of care for patients with osteoporosis.[4] These findings will be considered when developing recommendations for possible changes in FRAX USA.

Additional disparities exist in postfracture treatment rates and outcomes. Black women are less likely to be treated for osteoporosis than White women after adjustment for socioeconomic factors and clinical risk factors,[5] even after having a fracture.[6] Despite Black women having a lower risk of hip fracture than White women, Black women have higher morbidity and mortality following a hip fracture.[7] It is also notable that men have fewer hip fractures than women, yet have worse outcomes after having a hip fracture.[8]

TGD people have a gender identity that differs from their sex assigned at birth. Recent data from the Williams Institute found 0.5% of adults and 1.4% of youth aged 13 to 17 years in the United States identify as transgender.[9] Many transgender people may receive sex steroid–based gender-affirming hormone therapy (GAHT). This typically consists of estrogens and androgen blockers for those assigned male at birth/transgender women and testosterone for those assigned female at birth. Younger patients, as well as some adults, may receive GnRH agonists either at the time of puberty or in adulthood. These lead to suppression of endogenous gonadotropins and consequently testosterone and estradiol. It is well known that sex steroids, mainly estradiol, are a key factor in determination of peak bone mass in all people, regardless of assigned sex at birth.

Multiple studies have shown that transfeminine transgender youth and adults have lower BMD than their peers of the same sex assigned at birth even prior to initiating GAHT. The etiology is not completely understood, but may be related to decreased physical activity, low vitamin D, and other factors. Transgender youth who undergo treatment with GnRH agonists may have additional concerns for low peak bone mass. Although BMD initially improves with initiation of estrogen-based GAHT in adults, despite suppression of testosterone, this typically levels off after the first years of treatment.[10] Some long-term data also suggest that older transfeminine adults may have increased risk of fractures when compared with risk in cisgender men of similar age. Endocrine Society guidelines suggest consideration of DXA screening for transgender women at baseline prior to GAHT initiation, at age 60 years, and if GAHT is stopped after gonadectomy or with other risk factors.[11]

Transmasculine youth and adults tend to have BMD similar to that of their peers at the time GAHT is initiated. Testosterone-based GAHT leads to body-fat composition changes with increased muscle mass, but large alterations in BMD are not seen. Endocrine Society guidelines suggest screening only if GAHT is discontinued or other risk factors exist.[11] FRAX and other risk calculators are binary with respect to gender assessment and may need to be used with multiple inputs to gauge an individual's estimated fracture risk. The use of such calculators in the TGD population is not well studied.

The study of health care in underserved populations is confounded by ambiguous terminology. The concept of race itself has been called into question, since the genetic makeup of 2 individuals defined as having the same race may be very different, while 2 people of different races may be very similar genetically.[12] As far as reporting in the medical literature, race and ethnicity may be inappropriately used interchangeably and both are thought to be social constructs. Recent guidance from *JAMA* suggests, "these terms be unified into an aggregate, mutually exclusive set of categories as in 'race and ethnicity.'"[13] They stress that it is still important to report race and ethnicity to ensure health disparities that may occur in research are not overlooked but that race and ethnicity reporting be accompanied by reporting of other sociodemographic factors and determinants.[13] TGD individuals may or may not receive GAHT or surgeries of various types and may thus require different assessments with respect to BMD.

A distinction can be made between disparities and inequity in health care, although there may be overlap and ambiguity in how these terms are defined. Not all heath differences are disparities. There may be appropriate differences in health care in different populations because the prevalence or severity of disease is different. Equity often refers to social justice, meaning that no group is denied health care because of social or economic disadvantages. Disparity is unequal distribution of health care services based on such differences.

Clinical Case Vignettes
Case 1

A healthy 65-year-old woman of mixed race/ethnicity, with a White father and Black mother, identifies herself as Black. She has her first DXA according to standard guidelines. Her lowest relevant T-score, calculated with a White reference database, is −2.4 at the left femoral neck. Her White father died in a car accident at age 52 years. Her Black mother had a hip fracture from a fall at age 92 years. You use FRAX to estimate fracture risk and guide treatment decisions but are uncertain how to best use FRAX due to her mixed race/ethnicity and her mother's advanced age at time of her hip fracture. FRAX calculations using different race/ethnicities to estimate 10-year probabilities of major osteoporotic fracture and hip fracture are shown:

Race/ethnicity	Parental hip fracture	FRAX major osteoporotic fracture	FRAX hip fracture
White	Yes	20.0%	2.5%
Black	Yes	9.3%	1.1%

Which of the following is the most appropriate use of FRAX in this patient?

A. The ASBMR Task Force has stated that FRAX USA is invalid in patients of mixed ethnicity and therefore FRAX Canada should be used

B. FRAXplus is a recently updated version of FRAX that includes a race/ethnicity choice of Black/White for FRAX USA, which is most appropriate for this patient

C. Uncertainty and lack of evidence regarding the use of FRAX USA for different race/ethnicities should be discussed with the patient and considered when making treatment decisions

D. Since the patient self-identifies as Black, this is the race/ethnicity that should be used, and therefore she should not be treated according to current guidelines, because of low fracture risk with FRAX

E. FRAX USA with White race/ethnicity should be selected, since this results in the highest fracture risk and is therefore the most sensitive guide for making treatment decisions

Answer: C) Uncertainty and lack of evidence regarding the use of FRAX USA for different race/ethnicities should be discussed with the patient and considered when making treatment decisions

The ASBMR Task Force review of the best medical evidence in 2023 determined that there is "a paucity of evidence predicting incident fractures with and across race and ethnicity groups in US adults aged > 40 years" and "additional investigations should provide valuable information about whether inclusion of race and ethnicity in fracture risk assessment tools is warranted."[14] Recognition of the lack of evidence and uncertainty is reflected in Answer C.

There is no consensus recommending the use of FRAX Canada for any US patients (Answer A). There is no Black/White category for use with FRAXplus or FRAX (Answer B). There is no consensus on which ethnicity to use for FRAX USA in a patient of mixed race/ethnicity (Answers D and E).

Case 1 (continued)

In this patient, the femoral neck T-score was calculated using a White reference database, consistent with the ISCD Official Positions. However, these recommendations remain controversial, application may vary according to local requirements, and they are not universally applied. For Z-scores, reference databases should be matched for race/ethnicity.

Which of the following statements is applicable regarding reference databases for this patient?

A. Because of her mixed ethnicity and underestimation of fracture risk using a White reference database, AACE recommends using a Black database for T-scores

B. FRAX Canada, which is a single calculator for all Canadians, should be used for T-score calculations for Americans of mixed race/ethnicity

C. The use of an invalid reference database for T-score has confounding effects on FRAX calculations only when lumbar spine is used for FRAX input

D. FRAX calculation with input of femoral neck BMD rather than T-score is preferred because the reference database used with the DXA study may not be the same as that used with the FRAX calculator

E. Mixed race/ethnicity is not a concern with FRAX since the databases are updated annually

Answer: D) FRAX calculation with input of femoral neck BMD rather than T-score is preferred because the reference database used with the DXA study may not be the same as that used with the FRAX calculator

Using femoral neck BMD in g/cm^2 for FRAX input avoids the possibility of using a T-score that was calculated with a different reference database than what is used in the FRAX algorithm (Answer D). The recommendations of the ISCD for using a uniform reference database for men and women of all race/ethnicities are based on data showing fracture risk is similar in men and women of all race/ethnicities when BMD is similar.

There are no consensus recommendations for selecting race/ethnicity for FRAX USA in patients of mixed race/ethnicity (Answers A and B). Lumbar spine BMD/T-score is not validated for use with FRAX (Answer C). FRAX is not routinely updated on an annual basis (Answer E).

Case 2

A 26-year-old transgender woman presents for a clinic visit after a wrist fracture that occurred while playing soccer. She had undergone puberty blockade with a GnRH agonist followed by estradiol initiation at age 18 years, which she continues. DXA reveals the lowest relevant Z-score to be −2.1 using a female reference database.

Which of the following is true?

A. ISCD guidelines suggest her Z-scores be interpreted using a male database as her sex assigned at birth was male

B. Initiating estradiol likely led to low BMD due to suppression of testosterone

C. Data indicate that transgender girls and women frequently have low baseline BMD even prior to initiating GAHT

D. She should refrain from playing sports going forward due to her low BMD

E. Bisphosphonate therapy should be initiated

Answer: C) Data indicate that transgender girls and women frequently have low baseline BMD even prior to initiating GAHT

Transgender women often have low BMD at baseline, even prior to initiation of GAHT (Answer C). This has been documented in studies of both adults and youth; however, youth who have been treated with GnRH agonists may be at particular risk for low BMD, as sex steroids are suppressed during a time when velocity of BMD gains is typically accelerating. Although gains in BMD occur once estradiol is initiated (thus, Answer B is incorrect), transgender girls may not "catch up" to their expected peak BMD.[15] Some recent data are more reassuring,[16] but further study in this area is needed. Variations among countries and protocols as to timing of GnRH agonist initiation and duration of its use may be determining factors as well.

A fracture in a young patient would not be an indication to stop playing sports (Answer D), and physical activity should be encouraged in everyone, regardless of gender identity.

Pharmacologic treatment (Answer E) is rarely indicated in children and younger adults and certainly not before a more thorough assessment is undertaken.

The ISCD Official Positions suggest reporting Z-scores concordant with gender identity in transgender adults (thus, Answer A is incorrect).

Key Learning Points

- NonWhite women are undertreated due to underuse of diagnostic services and potential bias in fracture risk assessment tools.

- While risk calculators are helpful, they should be a springboard for discussion of risks, and their limitations must be recognized.

- TGD individuals, particularly transgender women, may be at risk for low BMD, and BMD screening should be considered prior to GAHT initiation.

References

1. Amarnath ALD, Franks P, Robbins JA, Xing G, Fenton JJ. Underuse and overuse of osteoporosis screening in a regional health system: a retrospective cohort study. *J Gen Intern Med.* 2015;30(12):1733-1740. PMID: 25986135

2. Vyas DA, Eisenstein LG, Jones DS. Hidden in plain sight - reconsidering the use of race correction in clinical algorithms. *N Engl J Med.* 2020;383(9):874-882. PMID: 32853499

3. Lewiecki EM, Wright NC, Singer AJ. Racial disparities, FRAX, and the care of patients with osteoporosis. *Osteoporos Int.* 2020;31(11):2069-2071. PMID: 32980922

4. Leslie WD, ASBMR Task Force on Clinical Algorithms for Fracture Risk. Effect of race/ethnicity on United States FRAX calculations and treatment qualification: a registry-based study. *J Bone Miner Res.* 2023;38(12):1742-1748. PMID: 37548387

5. Curtis JR, McClure LA, Delzell E, et al. Population-based fracture risk assessment and osteoporosis treatment disparities by race and gender. *J Gen Intern Med.* 2009;24(8):956-962. PMID: 19551449

6. Sattari M, Cauley JA, Garvan C, et al. Osteoporosis in the Women's Health Initiative: another treatment gap? *Am J Med.* 2017;130(8):937-948. PMID: 28366425

7. Cauley JA. Defining ethnic and racial differences in osteoporosis and fragility fractures. *Clin Orthop Relat Res.* 2011;469(7):1891-1899. PMID: 21431462

8. Bliuc D, Nguyen ND, Milch VE, Nguyen TV, Eisman JA, Center JR. Mortality risk associated with low-trauma osteoporotic fracture and subsequent fracture in men and women. *JAMA.* 2009;301(5):513-521. PMID: 19190316

9. Herman JL, Oneil KK, Flores A. *How Many Adults and Youth Identify as Transgender in the United States?* The Williams Institute, UCLA School of Law. 2022.

10. Wiepjes CM, de Jongh RT, de Blok CJ, et al. Bone safety during the first ten years of gender-affirming hormonal treatment in transwomen and transmen. *J Bone Miner Res.* 2019;34(3):447-454. PMID: 30537188

11. Hembree WC, Cohen-Kettenis PT, Gooren L, et al. Endocrine treatment of gender-dysphoric/gender-incongruent persons: an Endocrine Society clinical practice guideline. *J Clin Endocrinol Metab.* 2017;102(11):3869-3903. PMID: 28945902

12. Bamshad MJ, Olson SE. Does race exist? *Sci Am.* 2003;289(6):78-85. PMID: 14631734

13. Flanagin A, Frey T, Christiansen SL, Committee AMA Manual of Style Committee. Updated guidance on the reporting of race and ethnicity in medical and science journals. *JAMA.* 2021;326(7):621-627. PMID: 34402850

14. Fink HA, Butler ME, Claussen AM, et al. Performance of fracture risk assessment tools by race and ethnicity: a systematic review for the ASBMR Task Force on Clinical Algorithms for Fracture Risk. *J Bone Miner Res.* 2023;38(12):1731-1741. PMID: 37597237

15. Klink D, Caris M, Heijboer A, van Trotsenburg M, Rotteveel J. Bone mass in young adulthood following gonadotropin-releasing hormone analog treatment and cross-sex hormone treatment in adolescents with gender dysphoria. *J Clin Endocrinol Metab.* 2015;100(2):E270-E275. PMID: 25427144

16. van der Loos MATC, Vlot MC, Klink DT, Hannema SE, et al. Bone mineral density in transgender adolescents treated with puberty suppression and subsequent gender-affirming hormones. *JAMA Pediatr.* 2023;177(12):1332-1341. PMID: 37902760

Bone Health in the Orthopedic Surgery Population

Alexandra N. Krez, BA. Division of Endocrinology and Metabolic Bone Service, Hospital for Special Surgery, New York, NY; Email: kreza@hss.edu

Emily M. Stein, MD, MS. Division of Endocrinology and Metabolic Bone Service, Hospital for Special Surgery, New York, NY; Email: steine@hss.edu

Educational Objectives

After reviewing this chapter, learners should be able to:

- Explain the limitations of using dual x-ray absorptiometry (DXA) alone to evaluate bone health orthopedic surgery candidates.

- Illustrate the relationships between preoperative bone health and postoperative outcomes after orthopedic procedures.

- Consider potential strategies to optimize perioperative bone health.

Significance of the Clinical Problem

The prevalence of older individuals undergoing elective orthopedic surgery is burgeoning.[1,2] As a result, the number of surgical patients who have age-related osteoporosis is similarly rising. Osteoporosis is associated with several adverse orthopedic surgery outcomes.[3-6] Successful surgery requires early stability of hardware in bone and de novo bone formation. Osteoporotic bone can contribute to adverse outcomes following orthopedic procedures because of diminished efficacy of hardware fixation, increased risk of implant subsidence, and increased susceptibility to fractures during and after surgical instrumentation.[3-6] Although several studies have linked poor bone health to adverse outcomes after orthopedic surgery,[3,4,6] the evaluation and management of bone health have not been widely integrated into orthopedic clinical practice. This review will summarize the evidence linking bone health and outcomes after orthopedic surgery. We will focus on spine surgery, an increasingly prevalent procedure, which is associated with high rates of skeletal complications.

Spinal fusion surgery is one of the most commonly performed orthopedic procedures in the United States, with an annual incidence exceeding 400,000 cases. Related health care costs exceed $287 billion dollars per decade.[7] Skeletal complications occur in more than 30% of patients. Complications include fractures of vertebrae adjacent to the surgical hardware, screw loosening, rod breakage, and proximal junctional kyphosis (an abnormal kyphotic curvature that occurs directly proximal to the level of hardware).[4,5] These complications can lead to heightened levels of pain, increased disability, and reoperation, consequently amplifying both morbidity and health care expenses. Identifying those at highest risk for these skeletal complications is crucial for optimizing outcomes for patients who undergo spinal fusion surgery.

DXA remains the gold standard for assessing bone mineral density (BMD) and diagnosing osteoporosis. However, these scans are infrequently performed prior to spine and other elective orthopedic procedures. Further, when DXA is performed in patients with spinal disease, the presence of artifact poses a significant challenge to accurate assessment of BMD. Osteophytes, degenerative changes, and sclerosis are factors that can lead to falsely elevated readings. Scoliosis further contributes to the inaccuracy and imprecision of DXA. Thus, osteoporosis is frequently missed in this cohort when areal bone mineral density (aBMD) or trabecular bone score (TBS) measurements are used to screen patients.[5] As a result, there has been increased interest in using other modalities, including CT, for evaluation of bone health in patients who undergo spine surgery.

The fact that limited tools are available for accurate preoperative assessment of bone health contributes to missed or delayed diagnosis of osteoporosis and increased risk of postoperative complications in many patients. For those who are identified as having osteoporosis or abnormal bone quality, there is a lack of data regarding optimal treatment strategies. While anabolic agents may be beneficial in improving postoperative outcomes, few clinical trials have tested the efficacy or optimal duration of these agents for perioperative healing. Another challenge related to perioperative treatment of bone health in patients with skeletal deficits is the cost of medications. As none of the available osteoporosis treatments are approved for postoperative healing, they are not typically covered by insurance for this indication. Addressing the gaps in both identification and treatment of patients at high risk is crucial for developing strategies to optimize bone health and improve outcomes in those who undergo elective orthopedic surgery.

Practice Gaps

- Understanding the tools that can be used for evaluation of bone quality before elective orthopedic surgery.

- Determining which patients are at highest risk for complications after orthopedic surgery.

- Knowing whether osteoporosis therapies improve outcomes after orthopedic procedures.

- Assessing the optimal timing of perioperative treatment of bone health.

Discussion

This section reviews the literature investigating bone health in spine surgery candidates and treatment studies. We further present expert recommendations for the optimization of bone health in patients undergoing orthopedic surgery.

Preoperative Evaluation of Bone Quality

Most studies investigating the relationship between bone quality and outcomes following spinal fusion have been retrospective in nature and have relied solely on DXA for skeletal assessment. While some suggest that low BMD measured by DXA is a risk factor for complications such as adjacent fractures, proximal junctional kyphosis, screw loosening, and cage subsidence, these findings are not uniform in the literature. This discrepancy may relate to the fact that DXA is often artifactually normal in patients with spinal disease for the reasons previously outlined. CT images that have been obtained for diagnosis or surgical planning can be analyzed opportunistically for measurement of volumetric bone mineral density (vBMD). This alternative approach may help to capture patients with underlying skeletal deficits who are missed by standard DXA or never sent for evaluation. CT measurements of vBMD have been associated with postoperative outcomes. Our group performed a retrospective cohort study of 359 patients who underwent lumbar spine fusion surgery and found that low vBMD measured by quantitative CT was associated with an increased risk of skeletal complications (*Figure 1, following page*)[6]; each 10 g/cm³ decrease in baseline vBMD was associated with a 9% increase in likelihood of skeletal complications. Further, patients in the lowest tertile of vBMD experienced complications an average of 3 months earlier than those in the highest tertile.[6] Of note, cigarette smoking was also a risk factor for skeletal complications in this cohort. Similarly, another retrospective cohort study of 469 patients who underwent thoracic or lumbar fusion related CT measurements of vBMD and estimated bone strength to postoperative outcomes.[3] Patients with osteoporosis, defined as either low vBMD or low estimated bone strength, had a 4-fold increased risk of reoperation and 5-fold increased risk of vertebral fracture adjacent to the hardware compared with risks in those with normal BMD and strength.[3] These findings suggest that modalities beyond DXA may be valuable in assessing bone health in patients undergoing orthopedic procedures, particularly when artifact and structural abnormalities are prominent in the spine.

Figure 1. Complication-Free Survival Rates After Spine Fusion Surgery According to Tertile of Baseline Spine Volumetric BMD

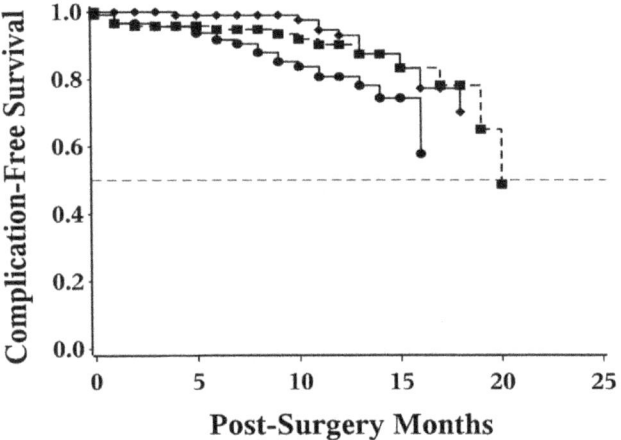

Lowest tertile indicated by circles and solid line, middle tertile indicated by diamonds and solid line, highest tertile indicated by squares and dashed line. Reprinted with permission from Liu Y et al. Osteoporos Int, 2020; 31(4): 647-654. © International Osteoporosis Foundation and National Osteoporosis Foundation. Published by Springer Nature.[6]

High-resolution peripheral quantitative CT (HR-pQCT) is a research tool that allows for direct measurement of vBMD, as well as assessment of trabecular and cortical bone microarchitecture at the radius and tibia. These measurements are associated with general skeletal health and fragility. We performed a prospective cohort study of 54 patients who underwent multilevel lumbar spine fusion and related skeletal health, using both DXA and HR-pQCT, to postoperative outcomes. In this cohort, DXA measurements of aBMD and TBS were normal in most patients and did not predict complications 6 months postoperatively.[4] In contrast, HR-pQCT measurements were markedly different between patients who did and did not go on to have skeletal complications, Specifically, those who had complications had lower preoperative trabecular vBMD, lower trabecular number and thickness, and thinner tibial cortices.[4] Further, in a recent prospective study of 50 postmenopausal women, most of whom were having multilevel fusion, we found that mean spine aBMD was normal and only 35% of women had osteoporosis by DXA at any site. However, 50% of the cohort developed skeletal complications. A higher risk of complications was found in women whose surgery was more complex (involved greater number of surgical levels, who had thinner cortices and smaller bones by HR-pQCT (*Figure 2, following page*).[5] These findings underscore the significance of bone quality, and microarchitecture in particular, in influencing the success of fusion procedures. However, as HR-pQCT is only available for research purposes at present, these measurements cannot be currently used to risk-stratify patients in clinical practice.

Use of Osteoporosis Medications to Improve Perioperative Bone Health

Most studies investigating the effects of treatment on postoperative outcomes are small, observational studies that have focused on anabolic agents, primarily teriparatide. These data suggest that patients who receive teriparatide have increased bone union and lower prevalence of screw loosening compared with untreated patients.[8,9] The literature is heterogenous regarding timing of treatment initiation, duration of treatment, and transition to antiresorptive agents after anabolics. In a prospective observational study of 29 postmenopausal women with osteoporosis, those who were treated with teriparatide for at least 1 month prior to surgery had higher insertional torque of pedicle screws, indicative of better bone strength, at the time of surgery. In a multicenter

Figure 2. Greater Cumulative Hazard of Complications Related to Greater Length of Fusion, Thinner Cortices, and Smaller Total Area of Bones at the Tibia

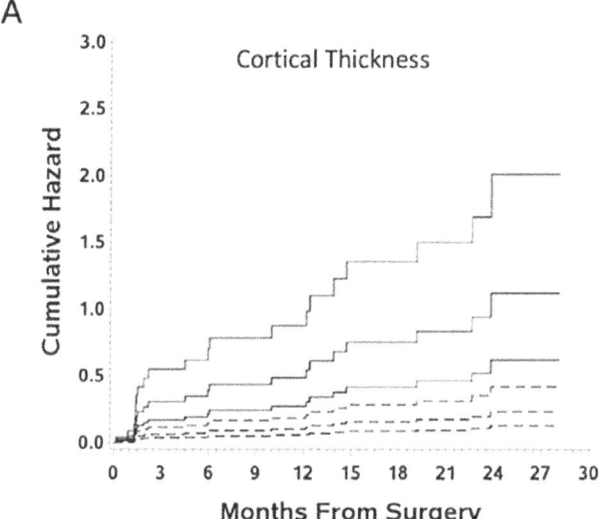

A

Cortical Thickness

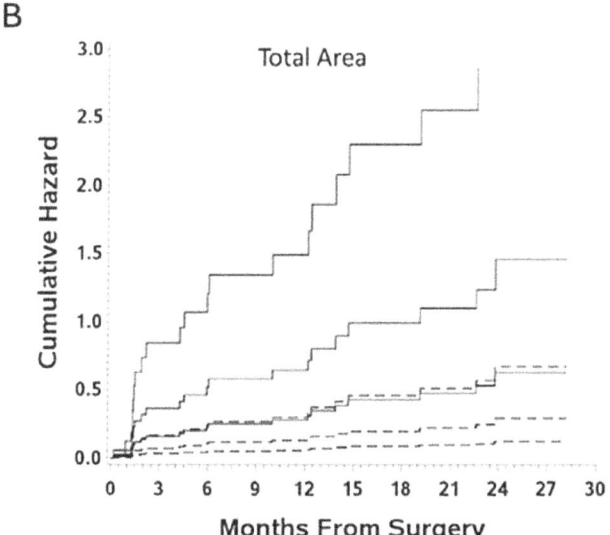

B

Total Area

Panel A, Participants grouped according to tertiles of cortical thickness with black line ≥1.7 mm, blue line 1.2-1.7 mm, and red line ≤1.2 mm. Panel B, Participants grouped according to tertile of total area with black line ≥712 mm, blue line 620-712 mm, and red line 430-620 mm. Solid line represents hazard for patients who had fusions involving ≥6 levels, and dashed lines represent hazard for patients who had fusions involving <6 levels. Reprinted with permission from Dash AS et al. Osteoporos Int, 2023; 35(3): 551–560. © International Osteoporosis Foundation and Bone Health and Osteoporosis Foundation. Published by Springer Nature.[5]

[Color—Print (Color Gallery page CG8) or web & ePub editions]

prospective randomized control trial, 75 women having interbody spine fusion were allocated to receive either weekly teriparatide for 6 months, beginning 1 week after surgery, or no treatment.[8] There was a 22% drop-out rate in the teriparatide group and few differences in the intention-to-treat analysis. However, in a per protocol analysis, patients who received teriparatide had greater fusion by CT at 6 months.[8] In a systematic review and meta-analysis of patients undergoing thoracolumbar spinal fusion, teriparatide use was associated with earlier fusion rates compared with fusion rates of bisphosphonates. However, it is important to note that there appeared to be beneficial effects of bisphosphonate use as well, which were associated with less cage subsidence and adjacent vertebral fractures compared with outcomes in control participants.[10]

Data from animal studies suggest that other anabolic agents such as abaloparatide and romosozumab may have beneficial effects promoting fusion.[11,12] Our group is currently conducting the FAST (Fusion with Anabolics after Spinal surgery Trial) Healing Study, a randomized, placebo-controlled, double-blind clinical trial investigating the effects of 6 months of abaloparatide on fusion in postmenopausal women (FDA IND # 143852, NCT03841058). Further, there may be a role for combination therapy (anabolic and antiresorptive) for the reduction of postoperative complications in the highest-risk patients who undergo spinal fusion surgery. A very small clinical trial found that combination therapy with denosumab and teriparatide resulted in an increase in fusion rates compared with teriparatide alone at 6 months, although there was no difference at 12 months.[13] Thus, additional data are needed to determine the efficacy of anabolic therapy, optimal agents to use, and timing of these medications.

Recommendations for Formal Bone Health Evaluation

There are few guidelines available to direct clinicians regarding the screening, evaluation, and treatment of orthopedic patients. This section highlights our clinical recommendations (*Figure 3, following page*), which align closely with those of a recent expert consensus, including orthopedic and neurological surgeons, endocrinologists, and rheumatologists, on preoperative management for elective spinal reconstruction surgery.[14]

Figure 3. Recommendations for Screening, Evaluation, and Management for Poor Bone Health in Patients Prior to Spinal Surgery

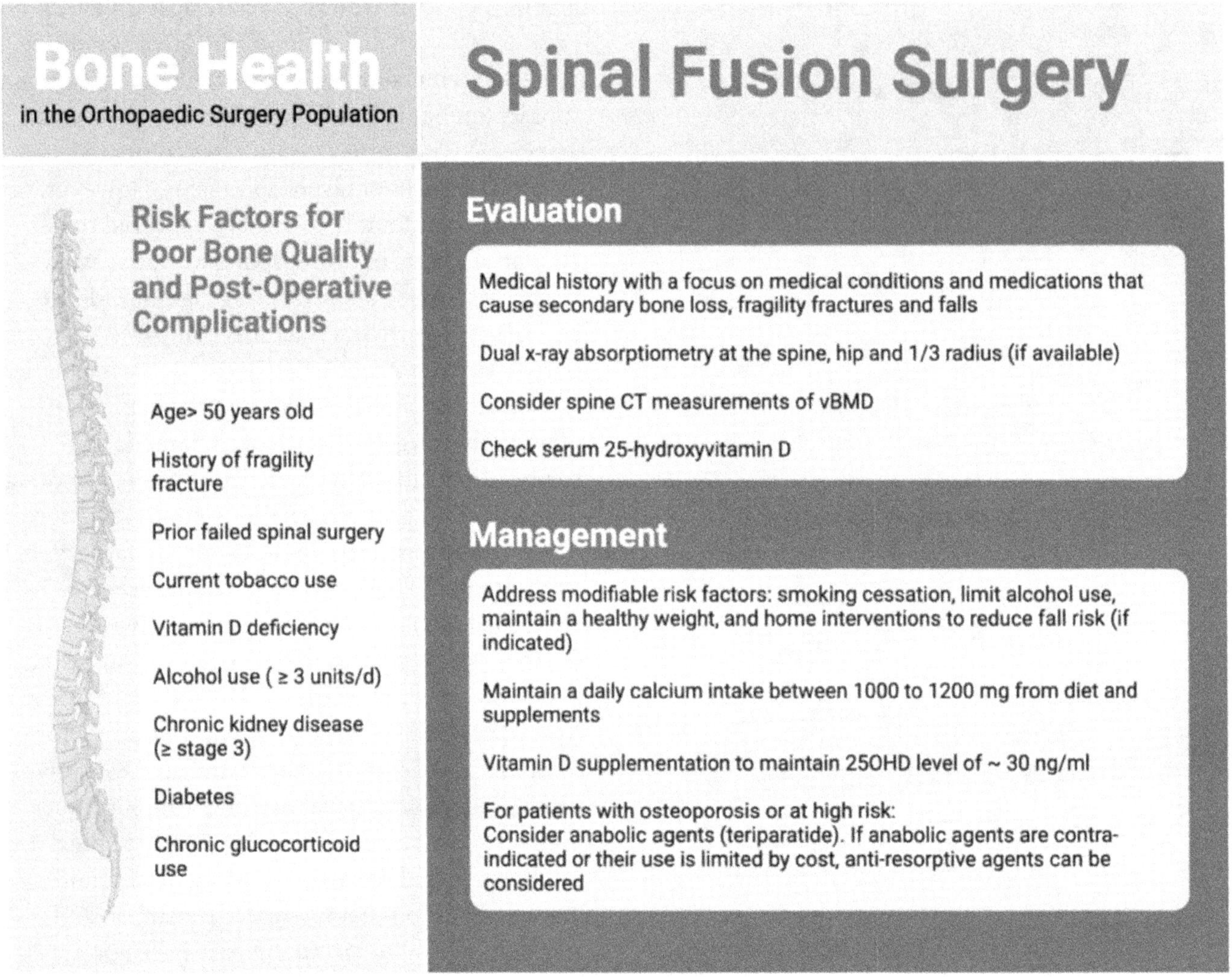

Bone Health
in the Orthopaedic Surgery Population

Spinal Fusion Surgery

Risk Factors for Poor Bone Quality and Post-Operative Complications

Age> 50 years old

History of fragility fracture

Prior failed spinal surgery

Current tobacco use

Vitamin D deficiency

Alcohol use (≥ 3 units/d)

Chronic kidney disease (≥ stage 3)

Diabetes

Chronic glucocorticoid use

Evaluation

Medical history with a focus on medical conditions and medications that cause secondary bone loss, fragility fractures and falls

Dual x-ray absorptiometry at the spine, hip and 1/3 radius (if available)

Consider spine CT measurements of vBMD

Check serum 25-hydroxyvitamin D

Management

Address modifiable risk factors: smoking cessation, limit alcohol use, maintain a healthy weight, and home interventions to reduce fall risk (if indicated)

Maintain a daily calcium intake between 1000 to 1200 mg from diet and supplements

Vitamin D supplementation to maintain 25OHD level of ~ 30 ng/ml

For patients with osteoporosis or at high risk:
Consider anabolic agents (teriparatide). If anabolic agents are contraindicated or their use is limited by cost, anti-resorptive agents can be considered

[Color—Print (Color Gallery page CG9) or web & ePub editions]

A bone health history should be obtained with focus on prior fragility fractures, falls, conditions, and medications associated with secondary osteoporosis in all patients prior to orthopedic surgery. Patients should be encouraged to maintain a daily calcium intake between 1000 to 1200 mg, depending on age and sex, from combined dietary sources and supplements. Serum 25-hydroxyvitamin D should be measured and moderate supplementation (1000-2000 IU daily) encouraged. In the absence of data that clearly identify a specific 25-hydroxyvitamin D threshold associated with outcomes, we advise targeting levels to approximately 30 ng/dL (75 nmol/L).

Modifiable risk factors for skeletal fragility should be addressed, including smoking cessation,[6] limiting alcohol, maintaining a healthy weight, and lowering fall risk. Use of medications that contribute to bone loss, including glucocorticoids, should be minimized as much as possible.

All patients older than 65 years should have a formal preoperative bone health evaluation with imaging.[14] Additionally, imaging assessment is suggested for patients between the ages of 50 and 64 years who have other risk factors for surgical failure. These risk factors include: history of previous fragility fracture, prior failed spine surgery, chronic glucocorticoid use, chronic kidney disease (≥stage 3), current tobacco use, alcohol use (≥3 units daily), vitamin D deficiency, and diabetes.[14] Screening is also recommended for patients younger than 50 years who take glucocorticoids on a long-term basis or have comorbidities associated with high fracture risk.[14] Although preoperative identification and evaluation of patients is preferred, those patients identified by their surgeon as having "soft bone" intraoperatively should also be referred for further evaluation. In recent work by our group, subjective assessment of soft bone intraoperatively directly related to low aBMD and vBMD.[5]

Although DXA measurements are often impacted by artifact in spine surgery and orthopedic populations, it remains the most widely accessible method for osteoporosis screening and should be used, particularly when other modalities are not available. The artifact may falsely elevate DXA readings, so that low values of aBMD should be considered as indicative of osteoporosis as they are in the general population. It may be valuable to obtain forearm DXA measurements, when possible, to have additional data for evaluation. CT measurements at the spine, if available, may be more sensitive for detecting patients with osteoporosis. There are commercially available tools for calculating vBMD, as well as simpler methods based on measurement of Hounsfield units.[14] Population-based reference data are available for diagnosis of osteoporosis based on quantitative CT measurements. Specifically, according to the American College of Radiology criteria for quantitative CT interpretation, osteoporosis is defined as a vBMD less than 80 mg/cc. Osteopenia is defined as vBMD of 80 to 120 mg/cc, and normal is defined as vBMD greater than 120 mg/cc.

For patients who are found to have osteoporosis by any imaging modality or clinical criteria, we recommend perioperative treatment to improve bone health. Although there are limited data directly comparing antiresorptive and anabolic therapy, we recommend using anabolic agents as first-line therapy given their ability to promote osteoanabolic activity, which may foster fusion, as well as the few studies showing faster rates of fusion in patients who receive anabolic agents. If anabolic agents are contraindicated or their use is limited by cost, antiresorptive agents should be considered. Given the potential for rebound bone loss and increased vertebral fragility with denosumab discontinuation, we discourage clinicians from discontinuing denosumab perioperatively. Some experts propose treatment with anabolic agents for 3 months prior to surgery, based on insights from studies on patients with osteoporosis that revealed positive changes in microarchitecture and fracture reduction in that period.[15] However, delaying surgery may not be an option for many patients. It is reasonable to begin treatment as soon as operative candidates with skeletal deficits are identified. It has been recommended that anabolic agents be continued for at least 8 months postoperatively.[14] The optimal treatment duration for operative healing is not known. In our practice, we aim to continue treating perioperative patients who have osteoporosis with a full 18- to 24-month course, so that they achieve the maximum medication benefit. Treatment should be considered for patients who do not meet densitometric criteria for osteoporosis but are otherwise at high-risk for skeletal complications based on age, complexity of surgery, reoperation, or other comorbidities.

Clinical Case Vignettes
Case 1

A 60-year-old woman with a medical history notable for gastroesophageal reflux disease treated with a proton-pump inhibitor presents to the metabolic bone practice for bone health optimization prior to T10-pelvis spinal fusion for spondylolisthesis and scoliosis. She has no history of fragility fractures or falls. She experienced menopause at age 48 years and did not use hormone therapy. DXA reveals a lumbar spine T-score of +1.8, total hip T-score of –2.2, femoral neck T-score of –1.9, and forearm T-score of –2.4. TBS is 1.504 (TBS reflective of normal microarchitecture ≥1.350). Laboratory workup is notable for a 25-hydroxyvitamin D concentration of 22 ng/mL (55 nmol/L).

Which of the following imaging modalities may provide additional information about this patient's underlying bone health as it relates to risk of postoperative complications?

A. Bone scan

B. PET

C. Ultrasonography

D. CT

E. DXA is sufficient to assess this patient's bone health

Answer: D) CT

While DXA (Answer E) remains the gold standard for diagnosing osteoporosis, it is not without limitations, including artifactually elevated BMD measurements in the setting of osteophytes, degenerative joint disease, sclerosis, and imprecision related to scoliosis. Measurements of vBMD from spine CT images (Answer D) can provide additional insights regarding underlying bone quality. Low vBMD measured by CT is associated with an increased risk of skeletal complications. In some cases, measurements can be performed opportunistically using CT imaging that has already been obtained clinically for surgical planning.

Bone scan (Answer A), PET (Answer B), ultrasonography (Answer C) measurements are not related to postoperative outcomes.

Case 1 (continued)

It was recommended that the patient start vitamin D supplementation and maintain a total calcium intake of 1200 mg daily from combined food and calcium citrate. Measurement of volumetric bone mineral density (vBMD) at L1-L2 from quantitative CT is 70 mg/cc.

According to the American College of Radiology, the patient's measurement falls within what range?

A. Osteoporosis

B. Osteopenia

C. Normal BMD

D. Partially degraded microarchitecture

E. Osteomalacia

Answer: A) Osteoporosis

According to the American College of Radiology criteria for quantitative CT interpretation, osteoporosis (Answer A) is defined as vBMD less than 80 mg/cc. Osteopenia (Answer B) is defined as vBMD 80 to 120 mg/cc, and normal (Answer C) is defined as vBMD greater than 120 mg/cc. Quantitative CT does not provide an assessment of the microarchitecture (Answer D) (partially degraded is a diagnostic category for DXA-based TBS), nor is it used to diagnose osteomalacia (Answer E).

Case 2

A 73-year-old woman presents to the metabolic bone practice for bone health optimization prior to revision T11-S1 spine fusion surgery. She has had 2 prior spine surgeries: a L2-4 fusion that was complicated by a broken surgical rod and a subsequent T12-L5 fusion complicated by continued pain and pseudarthrosis (failure to form new bone to stabilize the surgical construct). The patient's medical history is notable for multiple fragility fractures, including compression fractures of T12, L1, and ribs. Osteoporosis was diagnosed 2 decades earlier by DXA. HR-pQCT imaging was performed as part of a research protocol (*Figure 4*).

Figure 4. HR-pQCT Imaging

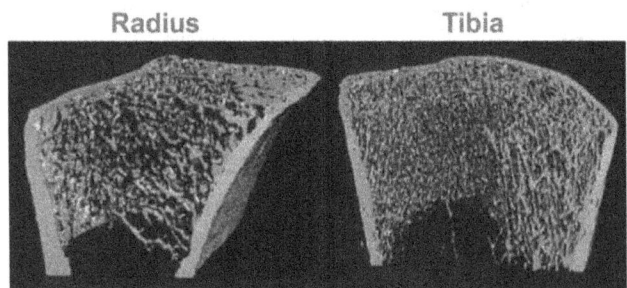

[Color—Print (Color Gallery page CG9) or web & ePub editions]

She took bisphosphonates for a cumulative period of 5 years and discontinued the treatment a decade prior to the current presentation. She has not taken any other osteoporosis treatment since. Her daily calcium intake includes 600 mg from diet and 500 mg of calcium carbonate. She also reported taking vitamin D_3 (cholecalciferol), 1200 international units daily.

Based on the available evidence, which pharmacologic agent is most likely to promote early, successful fusion in this patient?

A. Raloxifene

B. Ibandronate

C. Calcitonin

D. Teriparatide

E. Romosozumab

Answer: D) Teriparatide

Although there is limited evidence from randomized clinical trials of any agent for treatment of perioperative bone health in patients undergoing spine surgery, the pharmacologic agent for which there exists the largest amount of human data is teriparatide (Answer D). Teriparatide has been shown to increase fusion rates and lower the prevalence of screw loosening. Antiresorptive agents, including denosumab or bisphosphonates such as ibandronate (Answer B), may offer benefits in terms of lower rates of subsidence and adjacent fractures, but the few studies directly comparing treatments suggest that teriparatide is associated with faster rates of fusion. Abaloparatide or romosozumab (Answer E) have shown promise in animal studies but there are no published human data to date. Raloxifene (Answer A) and calcitonin (Answer C) have not been related to outcomes after spinal fusion surgery.

Teriparatide treatment was introduced prior to the patient's third spine surgery and continued for a 2-year duration. Notably, the patient had no complications during that time.

Key Learning Points

- Bone quality plays an important role in outcomes following orthopedic surgery. Poor bone quality can result in fractures during and after surgical fixation, diminished hardware stability, and decreased rates of fusion.

- While DXA remains the gold-standard for diagnosing osteoporosis, this modality may miss patients with osteoporosis because of artifact from underlying spinal pathology. Other modalities, including CT measurements of vBMD, may provide additional important insights regarding underlying bone.

- For patients known to have poor bone quality, or those who are at high risk for complications, pharmacologic therapy should be considered. At present, the literature favors the use of anabolic agents to promote fusion and reduce complications, but additional data from high-quality clinical trials are needed.

References

1. Mealy A, Sorensen J. Effects of an aging population on hospital costs related to elective hip replacements. *Public Health.* 2020;180:10-16. PMID: 31835140

2. O'Lynnger TM, Zuckerman SL, Morone PJ, Dewan MC, Vasquez-Castellanos RA, Cheng JS. Trends for spine surgery for the elderly: implications for access to healthcare in North America. *Neurosurgery.* 2015;77(Suppl 4):S136-S141. PMID: 26378351

3. Keaveny TM, Adams AL, Fischer H, et al. Increased risks of vertebral fracture and reoperation in primary spinal fusion patients who test positive for osteoporosis by biomechanical computed tomography analysis. *Spine J.* 2023;23(3):412-424. PMID: 36372353

4. Kim HJ, Dash A, Cunningham M, et al. Patients with abnormal microarchitecture have an increased risk of early complications after spinal fusion surgery. *Bone.* 2021;143:115731. PMID: 33157283

5. Dash AS, Billings E, Vlastaris K, et al. Pre-operative bone quality deficits and risk of complications following spine fusion surgery among postmenopausal women. *Osteoporos Int.* 2023 [Online ahead of print] PMID: 37932510

6. Liu Y, Dash A, Krez A, et al. Low volumetric bone density is a risk factor for early complications after spine fusion surgery. *Osteoporos Int.* 2020;31(4):647-654. PMID: 31919536

7. Goz V, Weinreb JH, McCarthy I, Schwab F, Lafage V, Errico TJ. Perioperative complications and mortality after spinal fusions: analysis of trends and risk factors. *Spine (Phila Pa 1976).* 2013;38(22):1970-1976. PMID: 23928714

8. Ebata S, Takahashi J, Hasegawa T, et al. Role of weekly teriparatide administration in osseous union enhancement within six months after posterior or transforaminal lumbar interbody fusion for osteoporosis-

associated lumbar degenerative disorders: a multicenter, prospective randomized study. *J Bone Joint Surg Am.* 2017;99(5):365-372. PMID: 28244906

9. Kaliya-Perumal AK, Lu ML, Luo CA, et al. Retrospective radiological outcome analysis following teriparatide use in elderly patients undergoing multilevel instrumented lumbar fusion surgery. *Medicine (Baltimore).* 2017;96(5):e5996. PMID: 28151894

10. Buerba RA, Sharma A, Ziino C, Arzeno A, Ajiboye RM. Bisphosphonate and teriparatide use in thoracolumbar spinal fusion: a systematic review and meta-analysis of comparative studies. *Spine (Phila Pa 1976).* 2018;43(17):E1014-E1023. PMID: 29462070

11. Morse KW, Moore H, Kumagai H, et al. Abaloparatide enhances fusion and bone formation in a rabbit spinal arthrodesis model. *Spine (Phila Pa 1976).* 2022;47(22):1607-1612. PMID: 35943233

12. Kim G, Inage K, Shiga Y, et al. Bone union-promoting effect of romosozumab in a rat posterolateral lumbar fusion model. *J Orthop Res.* 2022;40(11):2576-2585. PMID: 35088447

13. Ide M, Yamada K, Kaneko K, et al. Combined teriparatide and denosumab therapy accelerates spinal fusion following posterior lumbar interbody fusion. *Orthop Traumatol Surg Res.* 2018;104(7):1043-1048. PMID: 30179720

14. Sardar ZM, Coury JR, Cerpa M, et al. Best practice guidelines for assessment and management of osteoporosis in adult patients undergoing elective spinal reconstruction. *Spine (Phila Pa 1976).* 2022;47(2):128-135. PMID: 34690329

15. Anderson PA, Jeray KJ, Lane JM, Binkley NC. Bone health optimization: beyond own the bone: AOA critical issues. *J Bone Joint Surg Am.* 2019;101(15):1413-1419. PMID: 31393435

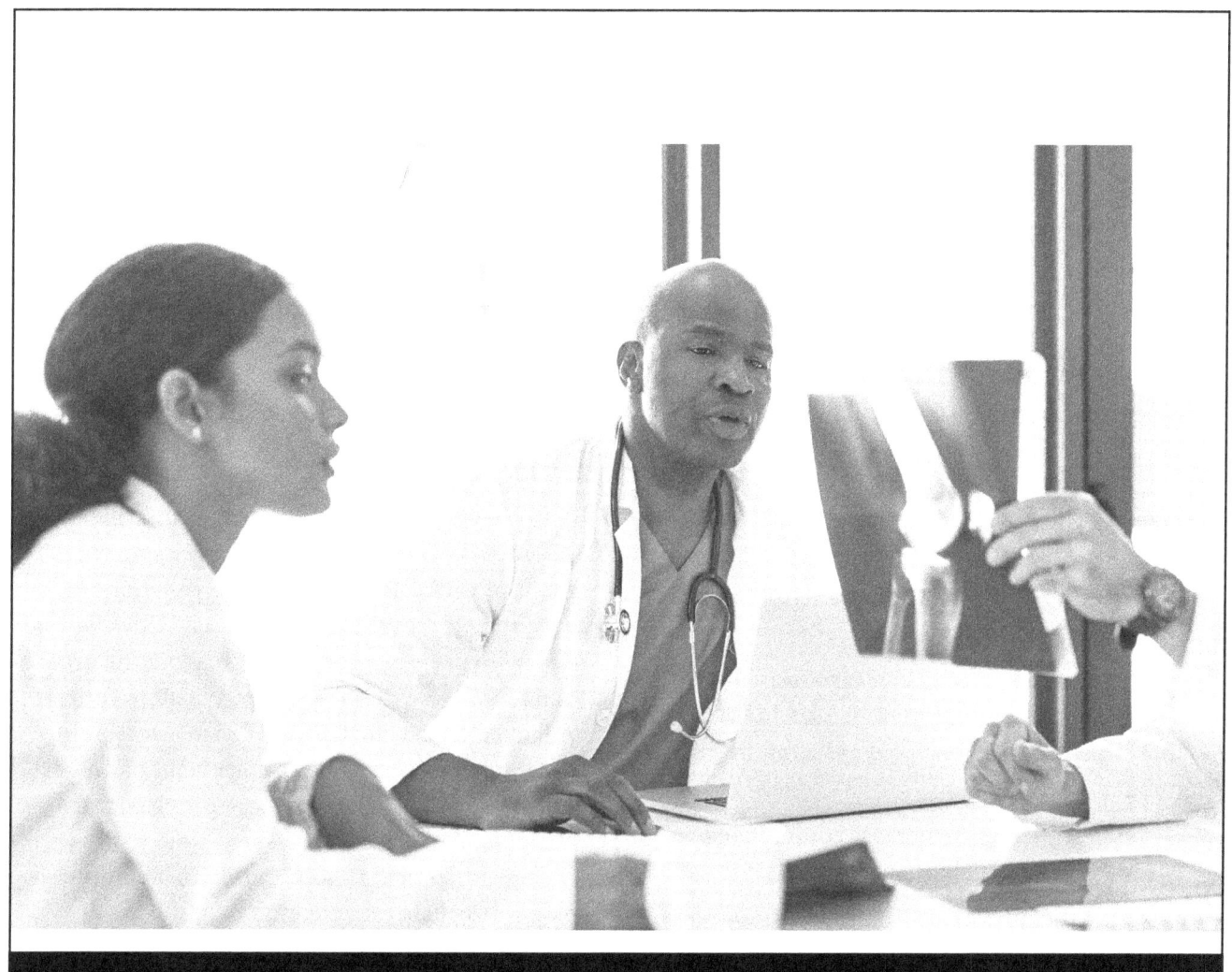

CARDIOVASCULAR
ENDOCRINOLOGY

Cardiovascular Outcomes With New Diabetes Medications

Jane E. B. Reusch, MD. Division of Endocrinology, Metabolism, and Diabetes and Ludeman Family Center for Women's Health Research University of Colorado, Anschutz Medical Campus, Aurora, CO; Email: Jane.reusch@cuanschutz.edu

Layla Abushamat, MD, MPH. Section of Cardiovascular Research, Baylor College of Medicine, Houston, TX; Email: Layla.abushamat@bcm.edu

Educational Objectives

- Describe the urgency of comprehensive care for people with diabetes.

- Summarize the outcomes of cardiovascular outcome trials over the past decade and explain their role in cardiorenal and heart failure risk mitigation.

- Develop strategies to increase comprehensive clinical care in the clinic setting.

- Describe the infrastructure needed to support preauthorization of the new cardiorenal protective agents and support for individuals safely initiating these agents.

Significance of the Clinical Problem

Diabetes affects 537 million people globally and 38.4 million people in the United States (11.6% of the US population). In the United States alone, the cost of diabetes was recently estimated to be 414 billion dollars, with most of that spent on treatment of complications. The leading cause of death and disability in people with diabetes is cardiovascular disease (CVD).[1] Thus, considering the use of agents to mitigate CVD risk in people with diabetes is a centerpiece of any discussion on diabetes management. The title of this Meet the Professor session is "Cardiovascular Outcomes With New Diabetes Medications." Data will be presented on agents approved in the last decade that have with cardiorenal protective actions in addition to glucose-lowering efficacy. However, it is seminal to place this conversation about the urgent need to incorporate these new agents into context with overall effective CVD risk management. In the United States, current management of drivers of CVD in people with diabetes—the classic ABCs (hemoglobin A_{1c}, blood pressure, cholesterol)—is inadequate, so this is a top priority to be addressed to optimize diabetes outcomes.

Practice Gaps

- In the United States and globally, we are failing to address comprehensive CVD risk factor management in people with diabetes.

- In the United States and globally, there is underuse of GLP-1 receptor agonists and SGLT-2 inhibitors in people at increased cardiorenal risk.

Discussion

CVD is leading cause of death and disability in the United States, and approximately one-third of CVD cases can be attributed to diabetes.[2] Goal-directed therapy for glucose lowering, blood pressure treatment, and cholesterol lowering in patients with diabetes in the United States ranges from 11% to 26%.[3,4] Classically, residual CVD risk is defined as the risk of CVD events that persists despite treatment for or achievement of goal-directed targets for risk factor reduction, and it is based on risk measured in prospective clinical trials. Thus, failure to mitigate risk by omission of goal-directed therapy leads to residual risk secondary to failure to control classic CVD risk factors. This excess risk is estimated to be increased by 62% of predicted CVD mortality. Risk of atherosclerotic cardiovascular disease (ASCVD) can be estimated using the American College of Cardiology risk engine (https://tools.acc.org/ASCVD-Risk-Estimator-Plus/#!/calculate/estimate/). All people with diabetes have increased CVD risk. However, not all people with diabetes have the same cardiovascular risk, so formal risk assessment is essential. An unmet health care priority for health span is lifespan without disability. CVD morbidity decreases healthy lifespan. As such, optimal evidence-based control of cholesterol, hypertension, and hyperglycemia will stem the health and financial cost of diabetes. Beyond this basic goal, in many cases, the addition of agents with proven cardiometabolic and kidney protection is warranted.

Diet, Physical Activity, and Sedentary Behavior

In all diabetes management guidelines, the foundation is enhancing diet quality, increasing physical activity, and decreasing sedentary time.[5] Behavior change, as outlined in this format, has a demonstrated a decrease in cardiovascular and all-cause mortality between 30% and 50% with a dose-response of single vs multiple changes in behavior. Behavior change is challenging; as clinicians, we need to explore opportunities to help patients increase their consumption of fruits and vegetables, incorporate sustainable physical activity, and interrupt sedentary time. Provider engagement around behavior change, similar to smoking cessation, has been demonstrated to positively benefit the likelihood of change for a patient.

Until recently, discussion of obesity was a bit of a clinical taboo because of stigma. This stigma has been partially overcome with the availability of agents that can meaningfully impart substantial (greater than 10% to 25%) and durable weight loss (up to 3 to 5 years). Still, providers must ask for permission to discuss weight issues and need to engage the same readiness-for-change models

Table 1. Crude Percentage of Adults Aged 18 Years or Older With Diagnosed Diabetes Meeting All ABCs Goals, United States, 2017-2020

Risk Factor	ABCs goals for many adults	Less stringent ABCs goals
A1C	<7.0%	<8.0%
Blood Pressure	<130/80 mmHg	<140/90 mmHg
Cholesterol, non-HDL	<130 mg/dL	<160 mg/dL
Smoking, current	Nonsmoker	Nonsmoker
Percentage meeting all ABCs goals	11.1 (8.1–14.9)	36.8 (31.8–42.1)

Notes: ABCs = A1C, blood pressure, cholesterol, and smoking. CI = confidence interval. Estimates are crude percentages and 95% confidence intervals. Data source: 2017–2020 National Health and Nutrition Examination Survey.

Centers for Disease Control and Prevention. National Diabetes Statistics Report website. https://www.cdc.gov/diabetes/data/statistics-report/index.html.[4]

[Color—Print (Color Gallery page CG10) or web & ePub editions]

that have been previously used for behavior modification. Most importantly, we need to consistently reinforce the importance of high nutritional–value food and physical activity. In many practice settings, we can further reinforce the importance of diet and physical activity by working with a dietician and a certified diabetes care and education specialist. If a patient has musculoskeletal issues that limit physical activity, it can be beneficial to make a referral to physical therapy to set up an exercise routine that decreases rather than exacerbates musculoskeletal pain. For both dietary changes and increases in physical activity, the greatest cardiovascular benefit comes with the initial modest changes. For example, adding fruits and vegetables, following the Mediterranean diet, or engaging in 5- to 10-minute bouts of physical activity confer an important and potentially durable benefit.[2,3]

Evidence-Based, Goal-Directed Therapy for Cardiorenal Risk Mitigation in the Post–Cardiovascular Outcomes Trials Era

In 2008, the FDA established a regulation that obliged formal cardiovascular outcome studies for all agents seeking FDA approval for glucose-lowering in diabetes. This legislation was prompted by agents that were providing signals for CVD excess after approval. The unintended consequence of this FDA guidance was the discovery that several newer agents, most notably the GLP-1 receptor agonists and SGLT-2 inhibitors, demonstrated cardiovascular safety compared with that of currently available agents AND superiority for prevention of CVD end points. With the data generated with more than 190,000 individuals with diabetes to date, a new evidence-based approach to mitigation of CVD risk in people with and without diabetes has emerged. Thus, in the American Diabetes Association Standards of Care for Medical Therapy of People with Diabetes in 2022, a new pillar for CVD risk reduction was endorsed (*Figure 1*).[6]

Figure 1. Overview of the Pillars of Comprehensive Risk Factor Modification for the Management of People With Diabetes

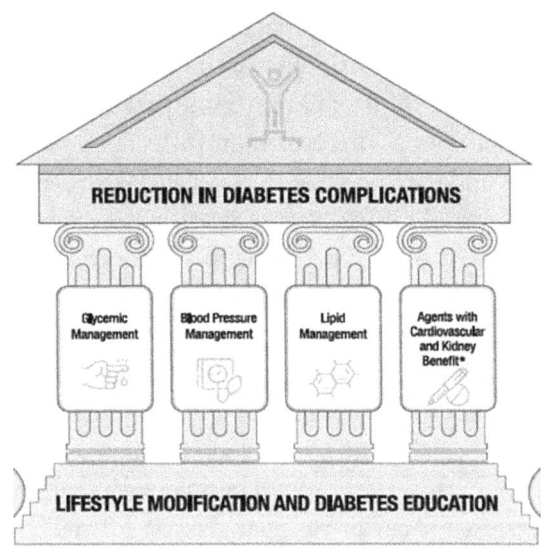

Reprinted from American Diabetes Association Professional Practice Committee. 10. Cardiovascular disease and risk management: Standards of Medical Care in Diabetes—2022. Diabetes Care, 2022; 45(Suppl. 1): S144–S174. © by the American Diabetes Association.[6]

[Color—Print (Color Gallery page CG10) or web & ePub editions]

Evidence for Cardiorenal Risk Mitigation With SGLT-2 Inhibitors

The initial release of the data from the empagliflozin clinical trial EMPA-REG was unexpected and demonstrated a decrease in 3-point Major Adverse Cardiovascular Events (MACE). Since that initial report, the data have been consistent and positive with some subtle differences in clinical trial outcomes between agents in the SGLT-2 inhibitor class. For the purpose of this chapter, I will use a recent review summarizing the cardiovascular outcomes with the SGLT-2 inhibitor class of antihyperglycemic and now cardiorenal protective agents.[7]

Figure 2 (following page) demonstrates the effect across the class of SGLT-2 inhibitors on 3-point MACE.[7] Empagliflozin and canagliflozin demonstrate significant lowering of CVD risk, whereas the confidence interval for dapagliflozin and ertugliflozin do not demonstrate superiority for cardiovascular lowering. Further analysis suggests that the effect on the MACE end point is

Figure 2. Effect Across Class of SGLT-2 Inhibitors on 3-Point MACE

A | Overall MACEs

	Treatment		Placebo					Weight, %
	No./total No.	Rate/1000 patient-years	No./total No.	Rate/1000 patient-years	Hazard ratio (95% CI)	Favors treatment	Favors placebo	
EMPA-REG OUTCOME	490/4687	37.4	282/2333	43.9	0.86 (0.74-0.99)			15.72
CANVAS program	NA/5795	26.9	NA/4347	31.5	0.86 (0.75-0.97)			20.12
DECLARE-TIMI 58	756/8582	22.6	803/8578	24.2	0.93 (0.84-1.03)			32.02
CREDENCE	217/2202	38.7	269/2199	48.7	0.80 (0.67-0.95)			10.92
VERTIS CV	735/5499	40.0	368/2747	40.3	0.99 (0.88-1.12)			21.23
Fixed-effects model (Q = 5.22; df = 4; P = .27; I² = 23.4%)					0.90 (0.85-0.95)			

0.2   1   2

HR (95% CI)

B | MACEs by ASCVD status

	Treatment		Placebo					Weight, %
	No./total No.	Rate/1000 patient-years	No./total No.	Rate/1000 patient-years	Hazard ratio (95% CI)	Favors treatment	Favors placebo	
Patients with ASCVD								
EMPA-REG OUTCOME	490/4687	37.4	282/2333	43.9	0.86 (0.74-0.99)			19.19
CANVAS program	NA/3756	34.1	NA/2900	41.3	0.82 (0.72-0.95)			21.16
DECLARE-TIMI 58	483/3474	36.8	537/3500	41.0	0.90 (0.79-1.02)			24.90
CREDENCE	155/1113	55.6	178/1107	65.0	0.85 (0.69-1.06)			8.82
VERTIS CV	735/5499	40.0	368/2747	40.3	0.99 (0.88-1.12)			25.93
Fixed-effects model (Q = 4.53; df = 4; P = .34; I² = 11.8%)					0.89 (0.84-0.95)			
Patients without ASCVD								
CANVAS program	NA/2039	15.8	NA/1447	15.5	0.98 (0.74-1.30)			21.70
DECLARE-TIMI 58	273/5108	13.4	266/5078	13.3	1.01 (0.86-1.20)			62.07
CREDENCE	62/1089	22.0	91/1092	32.7	0.68 (0.49-0.94)			16.23
Fixed-effects model (Q = 4.59; df = 2; P = .10; I² = 56.5%)					0.94 (0.83-1.07)			

0.2   1   2

HR (95% CI)

Reprinted from McGuire DK et al. *JAMA Cardiol*, 2021; 6(2):148–158.[7]

[Color—Print (Color Gallery page CG11) or web & ePub editions]

greatest for people with preexisting ASCVD. This is reflected in the American College of Cardiology and American Diabetes Association guidelines indicating the use of evidence-based agents in this class for people with preexisting ASCVD.

GLP-1 Receptor Agonists in Type 2 Diabetes: Effect on MACE

Prospective randomized cardiovascular outcomes trials examining cardiovascular safety and efficacy for the GLP-1 receptor agonist drug class demonstrate efficacy for liraglutide, semaglutide, albiglutide, and dulaglutide (*Figures 3* and *4*). Significant lowering of the 3-point MACE end point was consistent in people with preexisting ASCVD and nonsignificant in this review article in people without established CVD. Here again, these results are reflected in guidelines by the American

Diabetes Association, American Association of Clinical Endocrinology, American Heart Association, and American College of Cardiology on the indication of these specific GLP-1 receptor agonists in patients with preexisting ASCVD.[8]

Figure 3. Forest Plot of a Meta-Analysis of the 8 Cardiovascular Outcomes Trials With GLP-1 Receptor Agonists on MACE

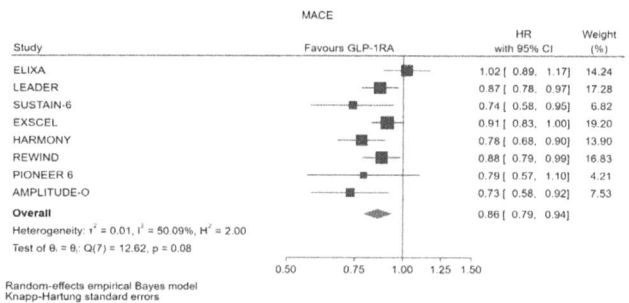

Reprinted from Giugliano D et al. *Cardiovasc Diabetol*, 2021; 20(1): 189.[8]

[Color—Print (Color Gallery page CG11) or web & ePub editions]

Figure 4. Forest Plot of a Meta-Analysis of the 6 Cardiovascular Outcomes Trials With GLP-1 Receptor Agonists on MACE in Patients With or Without CVD

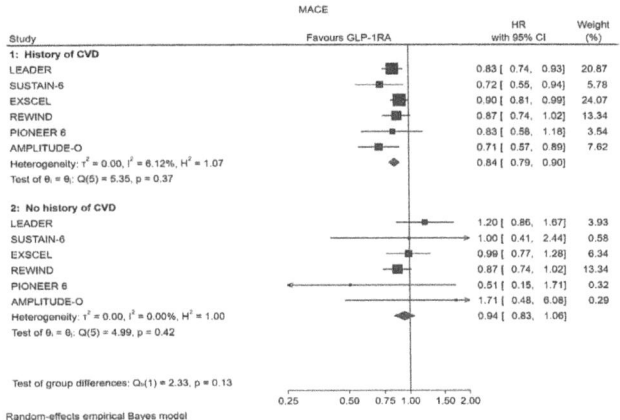

Patients with a history of CVD (top) and patients without such a history (bottom). Reprinted from Giugliano D et al. Cardiovasc Diabetol, 2021; 20(1): 189.[8]

[Color—Print (Color Gallery page CG12) or web & ePub editions]

Heart Failure Hospitalizations

The 2008 guidance by the FDA for evaluation of cardiovascular safety did not include heart failure as a primary end point. As such, in the earliest cardiovascular outcome studies, heart failure or heart failure hospitalization were not primary adjudicated end points. However, based on the data from EMPA-REG, heart failure and heart failure hospitalizations were formally embedded into the statistical analysis plan for all of the major cardiovascular outcome trials for diabetes agents. A consistent signal of about 30% decrease in heart failure hospitalizations has been observed across the class of SGLT-2 inhibitors. For GLP-1 receptor agonists in people with type 2 diabetes, there is a signal for safety but no signal for superiority in decreasing heart failure hospitalizations.[9] However, in recent studies using GLP-1 receptor agonists and combined GLP-1/GIP or other combinations agents with high weight-loss efficacy, there is a signal for decreased heart failure hospitalization. SGLT-2 inhibitors demonstrate the most consistent effect in heart failure and are thus indicated in all people with heart failure, unless there is a contraindication.

Beyond ASCVD and Heart Failure

Diabetes is associated with multiple comorbidities, including obesity, kidney disease, metabolic liver disease, and dyslipidemia. SGLT-2 inhibitors and GLP-1 receptor agonists (or GLP-1 plus other incretin combination agents) (especially in the high efficacy weight-loss dosing range) demonstrate benefits across the integrated physiology of diabetes. SGLT-2 inhibitors demonstrate consistent efficacy down to an estimated glomerular filtration rate of 25 mL/min per 1.73 m^2 of kidney protection in terms of slowing progressive kidney disease and slowing progressive albuminuria. GLP-1 receptor agonists slow progression of microalbuminuria without demonstrating a specific effect on progressive loss of estimated glomerular filtration rate. Metabolic liver disease improves with weight loss mediated by metabolic surgery, significant lifestyle change, GLP-1 receptor agonists, and GLP-1 combined agents. Metabolic liver disease is also responsive to pioglitazone.[10]

Placing the Newer Agents in Context

Tables 2 and *3* provide easy access to the primary data.

Table 2. Clinical ASCVD Risk-Benefit Profiles of Commonly Used Medications for Glucose Lowering

Medication	Risk-Benefit Profiles
Metformin	This is the standard to which all are compared; no evidence of increased CVD risk
Sulfonylureas	Recent head-to-head comparison with DPP-4 inhibitors demonstrated no excess cardiovascular risk; concerns exist for hypoglycemia (of high concern in patients with existing CVD)
Pioglitazone	Decrease stroke in the setting of insulin resistance and metabolic syndrome and 4-point MACE; negative cardiovascular outcome trials for 3-point MACE
DPP-4 inhibitors	Neutral
GLP-1 receptor agonists	Semaglutide, liraglutide, and dulaglutide decrease 3-point MACE
SGLT-2 inhibitors	All affect 3-point MACE except ertugliflozin
Bromocriptine	Small cardiovascular outcome trials favorable
Insulin	Neutral

Table 3. Clinical Heart Failure Benefit Profiles of Commonly Used Medications for Glucose Lowering

Medications	Clinical Heart Failure Benefits
Metformin	This is the standard to which all are compared; no evidence of increased heart failure risk
Sulfonylureas	Neutral
Pioglitazone	Fluid retention and increased heart failure hospitalization
DPP-4 inhibitors	Neutral except saxagliptin (increased heart failure hospitalization)
GLP-1 receptor agonists	Modest improvement in heart failure-class effect
SGLT-2 inhibitors	Significant decrease in heart failure hospitalization and benefit from use during hospitalization for heart failure (heart failure with reduced ejection fraction and heart failure with preserved ejection fraction)
Bromocriptine	No data
Insulin	Neutral

In the post–cardiovascular outcome trial era, we have strong evidence-based guidance to improve cardiovascular outcomes in people with diabetes. This evidence is in addition to the cardiovascular benefit of goal-directed management of glycemia, blood pressure, and dyslipidemia and effective lifestyle management. Of note for dyslipidemia, compelling data are available for the addition of ezetimibe to statins and for the use of icosapent ethyl in individuals with diabetes and hypertriglyceridemia on statin therapy. We have come a long way in harmonizing guidance for risk mitigation across leading experts (American Diabetes Association, Endocrine Society, American College of Cardiology, American Heart Association, American Association of Clinical Endocrinology, and international organizations). We are not currently meeting goal-directed therapy in diabetes for effective management of the diabetes ABCs or for timely adoption of newer agents with cardiorenal benefit.

Box. Evidence-Based Use of Glucose-Lowering Therapy for Cardiometabolic-Renal Benefit

GLP-1 receptor agonists
- All for diabetes type 2 management
- Liraglutide, dulaglutide, semaglutide for type 2 diabetes and **ASCVD/high CVD risk**
- Liraglutide, semaglutide, tirzepatide for **overweight with comorbidity or obesity**
- Semaglutide for obesity and **ASCVD/high CVD risk**
- Semaglutide for obesity and **heart failure with preserved ejection fraction**

SGLT-2 inhibitors
- All for type 2 diabetes management
- Canagliflozin, dapagliflozin, empagliflozin for **type 2 diabetes and ASCVD/high CVD risk**
- Canagliflozin, dapagliflozin for **chronic kidney disease with or without type 2 diabetes**
- Empagliflozin or dapagliflozin for **heart failure with reduced ejection fraction, heart failure with preserved ejection fraction with or without type 2 diabetes**

Table 4. Landmark Studies and Clinical Guidelines Informing CVD Risk Mitigation in Diabetes

General	
ADA SOC 2024	American Diabetes Association Professional Practice Committee. 10. Cardiovascular disease and risk management: standards of care in diabetes-2024. *Diabetes Care*. 2024;47(Suppl 1):S179-S218. PMID: 38078592
Data supporting the ABCs of diabetes CVD risk mitigation and current benefit	
Steno 2	Gaede P, Lund-Andersen H, Parving HH, Pedersen O. Effect of a multifactorial intervention on mortality in type 2 diabetes. *N Engl J Med*. 2008;358(6):580-591. PMID: 18256393
Therapeutic Inertia	Khunti K, Kosiborod M, Ray KK. Legacy benefits of blood glucose, blood pressure and lipid control in individuals with diabetes and cardiovascular disease: time to overcome multifactorial therapeutic inertia? *Diabetes Obes Metab*. 2018;20(6):1337-1341. PMID: 29405543

Landmark cardiovascular outcomes studies in diabetes	
EMPA-REG OUTCOME	Zinman B, Wanner C, Lachin JM, et al; EMPA-REF OUTCOME Investigators. Empagliflozin, cardiovascular outcomes, and mortality in type 2 diabetes. N Engl J Med. 2015;373(22):2117-2128. PMID: 26378978
	Palmer SC, Tendal B, Mustafa RA, et al. Sodium-glucose cotransporter protein-2 (SGLT-2) inhibitors and glucagon-like peptide-1 (GLP-1) receptor agonists for type 2 diabetes: systematic review and network meta-analysis of randomized controlled trials. BMJ. 2021;372:m4573. PMID: 33441402
CANVAS	Neal B, Perkovic V, Mahaffey KW, et al; CANVAS Program Collaborative Group. Canagliflozin and cardiovascular and renal events in type 2 diabetes. N Engl J Med. 2017;377(7):644-657. PMID: 28605608
CAROLINA	Marx N, Rosenstock J, Kahn SE, et al. Design and baseline characteristics of the CARdiovascular Outcome Trial of LINAgliptin Versus Glimepiride in Type 2 Diabetes (CAROLINA). Diab Vasc Dis Res. 2015;12(3):164-174. PMID: 25780262
DECLARE–TIMI 58	Wiviott SD, Raz I, Bonaca MP, et al; DECLARE–TIMI 58 Investigators. Dapagliflozin and cardiovascular outcomes in type 2 diabetes. N Engl J Med. 2019;380:347-357. PMID: 30415602
CREDENCE	Perkovic V, Jardine MJ, Neal B, et al; CREDENCE Trial Investigators. Canagliflozin and renal outcomes in type 2 diabetes and nephropathy. N Engl J Med. 2019;380(24):2295-2306. PMID: 30990260
DAPA-CKD	Heerspink HJL, Stefansson BV, Correa-Rotter R, et al; DAPA-CKD Trial Committees and Investigators. Dapagliflozin in patients with chronic kidney disease. N Engl J Med. 2020;383(15):1436-1446. PMID: 32970396
EMPEROR-Reduced	Packer M, Anker SD, Butler J, et al; EMPEROR-Reduced Trial Investigators. Cardiovascular and renal outcomes with empagliflozin in heart failure. N Engl J Med. 2020;383(15):1413-1424. PMID: 32865377
EMPEROR-Preserved	Anker SD, Butler J, Filippatos G, et al; EMPEROR-Preserved Trial Committees and Investigators. Baseline characteristics of patients with heart failure with preserved ejection fraction in the trial. Eur J Heart Fail. 2020;22(12):2383-2392. PMID: 33251670
VERTIS CV	Cannon CP, Pratley R, Dagogo-Jack S, et al; VERTIS CV Investigators. Cardiovascular outcomes with ertugliflozin in type 2 diabetes. N Engl J Med. 2020;383(15):1425-1435. PMID: 32966714
GLP-1 receptor agonist and combination	
LEADER	Marso SP, Daniels GH, Brown-Frandsen K, et al; LEADER Steering Committee; LEADER Trial Investigators. Liraglutide and cardiovascular outcomes in type 2 diabetes. N Engl J Med. 2016;375(4):311-322. PMID: 27295427
SUSTAIN-6	Marso SP, Bain SC, Consoli A, et a.; SUSTAIN-6 Investigators. Semaglutide and cardiovascular outcomes in patients with type 2 diabetes. N Engl J Med. 2016;375(19):1834-1844. PMID: 27633186
PIONEER 6	Husain M, Birkenfeld AL, Donsmark M, et al; PIONEER 6 Investigators. Oral semaglutide and cardiovascular outcomes in patients with type 2 diabetes. N Engl J Med. 2019;381(9):841-851. PMID: 31185157
HARMONY	Hernandez AF, Green JB, Janmohamed S, et al; Harmony Outcomes Committees and Investigators. Albiglutide and cardiovascular outcomes in patients with type 2 diabetes and cardiovascular disease (Harmony Outcomes): a double-blind, randomised placebo-controlled trial. Lancet. 2018;392(10157):1519-1529. PMID: 30291913
REWIND	Gerstein HC, Colhoun HM, Dagenais GR, et al.; REWIND Investigators. Dulaglutide and cardiovascular outcomes in type 2 diabetes (REWIND): a double-blind, randomised placebo-controlled trial. Lancet. 2019;394(10193):121-130. PMID: 31189511
ELIXA	Pfeffer MA, Claggett B, Diaz R, et al; ELIXA Investigators. Lixisenatide in patients with type 2 diabetes and acute coronary syndrome. N Engl J Med. 2015;373(23):2247-2257. PMID: 26630143
EXSCEL	Holman RR, Bethel MA, Mentz RJ, et al; EXSCEL Study Group. Effects of once-weekly exenatide on cardiovascular outcomes in type 2 diabetes. N Engl J Med. 2017;377(13):1228-1239. PMID: 28910237
AMPLITUDE-O	Gerstein HC, Sattar N, Rosenstock J, et al.; AMPLITUDE-O Trial Investigators. Cardiovascular and renal outcomes with efpeglenatide in type 2 diabetes. N Engl J Med. 2021;385(10):896-907. PMID: 34215025
GLP-1 plus SGLT-2	Lam CSP, Ramasundarahettige C, Branch KRH, et al. Efpeglenatide and clinical outcomes with and without concomitant sodium-glucose cotransporter-2 inhibition use in type 2 diabetes: exploratory analysis of the AMPLITUDE-O trial. Circulation. 2022;145(8):565-574. PMID: 34775781
SCORED	Bhatt DL, Szarek M, Pitt B, et al; SCORED Investigators. Sotagliflozin in patients with diabetes and chronic kidney disease. N Engl J Med. 2021;384(2):129-139. PMID: 33200891

Thiazolidinediones and bromocriptine	
PROactive	Dormandy JA, Charbonnel B, Eckland DJA, et al; PROactive Investigators. Secondary prevention of macrovascular events in patients with type 2 diabetes in the PROactive Study (PROspective pioglitAzone Clinical Trial In macroVascular Events): a randomised controlled trial. *Lancet.* 2005;366(9493):1279-1289. PMID: 16214598
Bromocriptine	Chamarthi B, Ezrokhi M, Rutty D, Cincotta AH. Impact of bromocriptine-QR therapy on cardiovascular outcomes in type 2 diabetes mellitus subjects on metformin. *Postgrad Med.* 2016;128(8):761-769. PMID: 27687032
Landmark heart failure outcomes studies	
EMPEROR-Reduced	Packer M, Anker SD, Butler J, et al; EMPEROR-Reduced Trial Investigators. Cardiovascular and renal outcomes with empagliflozin in heart failure. *N Engl J Med.* 2020;383(15):1413-1424. PMID: 32865377
EMPEROR-Preserved	Anker SD, Butler J, Filippatos G, et al; EMPEROR-Preserved Trial Investigators. Empagliflozin heart failure with a preserved ejection fraction. *N Engl J Med.* 2021;385(16):1451-1461. PMID: 34449189
DELIVER	Solomon SD, McMurray JJV, Claggett B, et al; DELIVER Trial Committees and Investigators. Dapagliflozin in heart failure with mildly reduced or preserved ejection fraction. *N Engl J Med.* 2022;387(12):1089-1098. PMID: 36027570
SGLT-2 inpatient	Voors AA, Angermann CE, Teerlink JR, et al. The SGLT2 inhibitor empagliflozin in patients hospitalized for acute heart failure: a multinational randomized trial. *Nat Med.* 2022;28(3):568-574. PMID: 35228754
REVERT	Colucci WS, Kolias TJ, Adams KF, et al; REVERT Study Group. Metoprolol reverses left ventricular remodeling in patients with asymptomatic systolic dysfunction: the REversal of VEntricular Remodeling with Toprol-XL (REVERT) trial. *Circulation.* 2007;116(1):49-56. PMID: 17576868
Metformin	Inzucchi SE, Masoudi FA, McGuire DK. Metformin in heart failure. *Diabetes Care.* 2007;30(12):e129. PMID: 18042738

Clinical Case Vignettes

Case 1

A 61-year-old man with an 8-year history of type 2 diabetes just moved to the area and presents for continuation of care. He also has hypertension and dyslipidemia. He has never smoked cigarettes. His family history is remarkable only for a brother with type 2 diabetes. He is unaware of any family members with CVD. His current medications include metformin, 1000 mg twice daily; lisinopril, 20 mg daily; hydrochlorothiazide, 25 mg daily; and atorvastatin, 10 mg daily. His diet is poor, he does not cook, and he entertains clients at lunchtime. He enjoys fruits and vegetables but has not figured out a way to incorporate them into his diet. He exercised regularly before he moved but has not gotten into the habit in his new home. He reports previous excellent glycemic control with hemoglobin A_{1c} values around 6.5% (48 mmol/mol) and is surprised that his hemoglobin A_{1c} is elevated today. He does not monitor blood glucose at home. He takes his medications regularly.

On physical examination, his height is 70 in (177.8 cm) and weight is 200 lb (90.7 kg) (BMI = 28.6 kg/m²). His blood pressure is 156/78 mm Hg (repeated measurement, 154/84 mm Hg), pulse rate is 80 beats/min, and respiratory rate is 20 breaths/min.

Preclinic laboratory test results:

Hemoglobin A_{1c} = 8.7% (72 mmol/mol)
Fasting plasma glucose = 180 mg/dL
    (SI: 10.0 mmol/L)
Total cholesterol = 140 mg/dL (SI: 3.63 mmol/L)
LDL cholesterol = 70 mg/dL (SI: 1.81 mmol/L)
HDL cholesterol = 35 mg/dL (SI: 0.91 mmol/L)
Triglycerides = 175 mg/dL (SI: 1.98 mmol/L)
Liver function test results, normal
Urinary albumin-to-creatinine ratio = 13 mg/g

Which of the following should be the priority in this patient's management?

A. Hemoglobin A_{1c}

B. Blood pressure

C. Cholesterol

D. BMI

E. All of the above

Answer: E) All of the above

In this case, the focus of the discussion with the patient will be on goal setting, using the information available to predict CVD to set the stage for a discussion of diabetes management and CVD risk mitigation and the use of SGLT-2 inhibitors and GLP-1 receptor agonists. This allows for a personalized approach to care, including identifying treatment barriers such as insurance coverage for and available supply of prescribed medications. He has what appears to be uncomplicated diabetes with poorly controlled hypertension and glycemia, LDL cholesterol at goal with a moderate-dosage statin, and, apparently, recent poor lifestyle changes. For this man with uncomplicated diabetes and a long lifespan ahead of him, his hemoglobin A_{1c} goal should be less than 7.0% (<53 mmol/mol) without hypoglycemia. Attaining this goal should not be delayed, so a combination of support from a certified diabetes care and education specialist/nutritionist and a GLP-1 receptor agonist could help him achieve his glycemic target. With 2 uncontrolled CVD risk factors (type 2 diabetes and hypertension), one can make the argument that he is at high risk for ASCVD, but it would probably be easier to get approval using the indication for glycemic lowering.

Case 2

A 50-year-old African American woman presents with a new diagnosis of type 2 diabetes. She was diagnosed in the hospital at the time of acute coronary syndrome (LAD PCIx2-without a myocardial infarction). She is G2P2 with a history of preeclampsia (P1) and gestational diabetes (P2). She is not interested in additional children. She was recently diagnosed with hypertension, which is still inadequately controlled.

Her current medications (started in the hospital) are metformin, 500 mg twice daily; lisinopril, 20 mg daily; metoprolol, 50 mg twice daily; and atorvastatin, 80 mg daily.

On physical examination, her BMI is 31.2 kg/m², blood pressure is 146/88 mm Hg (repeat measurement, 144/90 mm Hg), and pulse rate is 64 beats/min.

Laboratory test results from hospitalization:

> Random glucose = 243 mg/dL (SI: 13.5 mmol/L)
> Hemoglobin A_{1c} = 8.2% (66 mmol/mol)
> Total cholesterol = 239 mg/dL (SI: 6.19 mmol/L)
> Triglycerides = 260 mg/dL (SI: 2.94 mmol/L)
> HDL cholesterol = 32 mg/dL (SI: 0.83 mmol/L)
> LDL cholesterol = 155 mg/dL (SI: 4.01 mmol/L)
> Estimated glomerular filtration rate = 75 mL/min per 1.73 m²
> Urinary albumin-to-creatinine ratio = 38 mg/g

Which of the following glucose-lowering medications with high glycemic efficacy would be best?

A. SGLT-2 inhibitor

B. GLP-1 receptor agonist

C. SGLT-2 inhibitor or GLP-1 receptor agonist

D. Metformin

E. Insulin

Answer: C) SGLT-2 inhibitor or GLP-1 receptor agonist

This is a classic presentation of new-onset type 2 diabetes in the context of the new presentation of CVD. As such, treatment is warranted with either an SGLT-2 inhibitor and/or a GLP-1 receptor agonist (or both). Her glycemic goal should be a hemoglobin A_{1c} value less than 7.0% (<53 mmol/mol) without hyperglycemia. To achieve this goal, we would assess her lifestyle with the help of a certified diabetes care and education specialist/nutritionist and prescribe a glucose-lowering medication. A posthospitalization assessment of her overall glycemic status is essential, and it must be determined whether she needs monotherapy vs dual therapy for achieving glycemic targets while mitigating CVD risk. Her acute glucose elevation in the hospital may have been related to acute coronary syndrome; thus, she may need only a single agent for optimized glycemic control. In this setting, she could be on a background regimen of metformin, or medication management can be started with either an SGLT-2 inhibitor or a GLP-1 receptor agonist, both of which reduce CVD events. In this case, other cardiovascular risk factors should also be addressed, including a blood pressure goal of less than 130/80 mm Hg and an LDL-cholesterol goal of less than 55 mg/dL (<1.42 mmol/L).

Case 3

A 68-year-old Hispanic man has a 20-year history of type 2 diabetes complicated by myocardial infarction and diabetic kidney disease. He has recently noted decreased exercise tolerance due to dyspnea and weakness. He has not had accompanying chest pain.

Current medications include metformin, 500 mg twice daily; glipizide, 10 mg daily; atorvastatin, 80 mg daily; lisinopril, 20 mg daily; metoprolol, 50 mg twice daily; and aspirin, 81 mg daily.

On physical examination, her BMI is 33 kg/m², blood pressure is 138/84 mm Hg (repeat measurement, 136/78 mm Hg), and pulse rate is 64 beats/min. She has labored breathing walking into the clinic room and bilateral lower lung crackles cleared with cough. Liver span is 12 centimeters with a palpable edge at 2 cm (firm but not overly hard). She has lower-extremity edema, decreased sensation to 10 g monofilament, absent dorsalis pedis, and dependent rubor. She has no foot ulcers and mild dry skin on her feet without significant callus.

Laboratory test results:

Hemoglobin A$_{1c}$ = 7.3% (56 mmol/mol)
Total cholesterol = 124 mg/dL (SI: 3.21 mmol/L)
Triglycerides = 202 mg/dL (SI: 2.28 mmol/L)
HDL cholesterol = 34 mg/dL (SI: 0.88 mmol/L)
LDL cholesterol = 50 mg/dL (SI: 1.30 mmol/L)
Estimated glomerular filtration rate = 47 mL/min per 1.73 m²
Urinary albumin-to-creatinine ratio = 147 mg/g
Liver transaminases, twice the normal range

Which of the following glucose-lowering medications with high glycemic efficacy is the best choice?

A. SGLT-2 inhibitor

B. GLP-1 receptor agonist

C. SGLT-2 inhibitor or GLP-1 receptor agonist

D. Metformin

E. Insulin

Answer: A) SGLT-2 inhibitor

This patient has significant cardiorenal complications related to diabetes, previous ASCVD, and chronic kidney disease. His hemoglobin A$_{1c}$ goal is 7.0% to 8.0% (53-64 mmol/L) without hypoglycemia. He is currently a candidate for use of an SGLT-2 inhibitor or GLP-1 receptor agonist. In light of his comorbid kidney disease, an SGLT-2 inhibitor (Answer A) is the best choice. It is also probably a good idea to discontinue glipizide to prevent hypoglycemia and weight gain. His BMI is 33 kg/m², and, as such, decreasing the weight gain stimulus of glipizide and adding the modest weight loss associated with an SGLT-2 inhibitor could be beneficial. His need for glucose lowering does not currently demand use of 2 agents, so discontinuing glipizide and initiating the SGLT-2 inhibitor is a reasonable choice. If his glycemic control were to deteriorate further, the addition of a GLP-1 receptor agonist could be a reasonable choice or addition.

Case 4

A 24-year-old African American woman was diagnosed with type 2 diabetes at 19 years. She is new to this clinic and presents today for her initial intake exam and transition from pediatrics. She expresses interest in learning about new diabetes medications that are in the news, particularly the ones associated with weight loss.

She is feeling well, her weight is stable, she exercises for 20 to 30 minutes twice a week, her diet is varied, her intake of fruit and vegetables is low, and her job is desk based with few interruptions for movement during the day. She has met with a certified diabetes care and education specialist/nutritionist to work on increasing fruits and vegetables and decreasing sugary snacks. Retinopathy neuropathy and nephropathy screens are up-to-date and negative.

She is not currently anticipating pregnancy, but she does hope to have a child later in life. She is not currently sexually active, but when she is, she has used a barrier method (she does not like the adverse effects of oral contraceptives).

She was screened for the NIH RADIANT study and was told that she does not have "genetic diabetes" (records she brings with her suggest she has type 2 diabetes, not monogenic diabetes).

On physical examination, her pulse rate is 68 beats/min and respiratory rate is 17 breaths/min. Her height is 65 in (165.1 cm), and weight is 220 lb (98.8 kg) (BMI = 36.6 kg/m^2). Exam findings are otherwise unremarkable with no symptoms or signs of Cushing syndrome or acanthosis nigricans.

Laboratory test results:

Hemoglobin A$_{1c}$ = 7.3% (56 mmol/mol)
LDL cholesterol = 105 mg/dL (SI: 2.72 mmol/L)
HDL cholesterol = 53 mg/dL (SI: 1.37 mmol/L)
Triglycerides = 137 mg/dL (SI: 1.55 mmol/L)

Her only medication is metformin, 1000 mg twice daily.

Which of the following should be the biggest priority at today's appointment?

A. Educate her on weight-loss surgery

B. Start weight-loss medications today

C. Start insulin today

D. Educate her on weight-loss medications and provide preconception counseling

Answer: D) Educate her on weight-loss medications and provide preconception counseling

This is an increasingly common scenario. Individuals with adolescent-onset type 2 diabetes are at very high risk for progression to CVD and microvascular complications. The introduction of new agents such as SGLT-2 inhibitors and GLP-1 receptor agonists are revolutionizing our ability to optimize glycemic control in this population of people with younger-onset type 2 diabetes, To date, we do not have data to demonstrate the cardioprotective effects of these agents in this age group; however, we do not have any pathophysiological reason to suspect lack of efficacy. In addition, because of the potent weight loss efficacy of these agents, they are used more and more often in younger individuals of reproductive age, with or without diabetes. These agents are not approved for use during pregnancy, and preconception counseling is critical because weight loss may affect fertility (Answer D). In the setting of planned pregnancy in people taking these agents, strategies for prevention of profound pregnancy-related weight gain and timely discontinuation of these agents upon conception are critical.

References

1. Virani SS, Alonso A, Aparicio HJ, et al; American Heart Association Council on Epidemiology and Prevention Statistics Committee and Stroke Statistics Subcommittee. Heart disease and stroke statistics-2021 update: a report from the American Heart Association. *Circulation.* 2021;143(8):e254-e743. PMID: 33501848

2. Stokes A, Preston SH. Deaths attributable to diabetes in the United States: comparison of data sources estimation approaches. *PLoS One.* 2017;12(1):e0170219. PMID: 28121997

3. Wong ND, Zhao Y, Patel R, et al. Cardiovascular risk factor targets and cardiovascular disease event risk in diabetes: a pooling project of the atherosclerosis risk in communities study, multi-ethnic study of atherosclerosis, and Jackson Heart Study. *Diabetes Care.* 2016;39(5):668-676. PMID: 27208374

4. Centers for Disease Control. National Diabetes Statistics Report website. www.cdc.gov/diabetes/data/statistics-report/index.html. Accessed March 31, 2024.

5. American Diabetes Association Professional Practice Committee. 5. Facilitating positive health behaviors and well-being to improve health outcomes: standards of care in diabetes-2024. *Diabetes Care.* 2024;47(Suppl 1):S77-S110. PMID: 38078584

6. American Diabetes Association Professional Practice Committee. 10. Cardiovascular disease and risk management: standards of care in diabetes-2024. *Diabetes Care.* 2024;47(Suppl 1):S179-S218. PMID: 38078592

7. McGuire DK, Shih WJ, Cosentino F, et al. Association of SGLT2 inhibitors with cardiovascular and kidney outcomes in patients with type 2 diabetes: a meta-analysis. *JAMA Cardiol.* 2021;6(2):148-158. PMID: 33031522

8. Giugliano D, Scappaticcio L, Longo M, et al. GLP-1 receptor agonists and cardiorenal outcomes in type 2 diabetes: an updated meta-analysis of eight CVOTs. *Cardiovasc Diabetol.* 2021;20(1):189. PMID: 34526024

9. Zelniker TA, Wiviott SD, Raz I, et al. Comparison of the effects of glucagon-like peptide receptor agonists and sodium-glucose cotransporter 2 inhibitors for prevention of major adverse cardiovascular and renal outcomes in type 2 diabetes mellitus. *Circulation.* 2019;139(17):2022-2031. PMID: 30786725

10. Belfort-DeAguiar R, Lomonaco R, Cusi K. Approach to the patient with nonalcoholic fatty liver disease. *J Clin Endocrinol Metab.* 2023;108(2):483-495. PMID: 36305273

Treatment of Primary Aldosteronism

Anand Vaidya, MD, MMSc. Center for Adrenal Disorders, Division of Endocrinology, Diabetes, and Hypertension, Brigham and Women's Hospital, Harvard Medical School, Boston, MA; Email: anandvaidya@bwh.harvard.edu

Educational Objectives

After reviewing this chapter, learners should be able to:

- Identify the treatment objectives for primary aldosteronism.
- Optimize medical therapy for patients with primary aldosteronism.

Significance of the Clinical Problem

Primary aldosteronism is an endocrinopathy characterized by dysregulated aldosterone production that occurs despite suppression of renin and angiotensin II and that cannot be suppressed by volume and sodium-loading maneuvers. Primary aldosteronism pathophysiology causes increased activation of the mineralocorticoid receptor (MR) in the kidney, resulting in volume expansion and hypertension but also increased MR activation in extra-renal tissues, which leads to increased inflammation, fibrosis, and development of adverse cardiometabolic and kidney outcomes (*Figure 1, following page*). Importantly, the pathophysiology of primary aldosteronism contributes to adverse outcomes beyond the effects of hypertension alone. For these reasons, it is imperative that patients with primary aldosteronism be treated with targeted therapy to abolish or neutralize the deleterious effects of aldosterone excess.

The main treatment modalities for primary aldosteronism include surgical adrenalectomy and MR antagonist therapy. Other nonsurgical therapies that can be effective include dietary sodium restriction and the use of epithelial sodium channel (ENaC) inhibitors. Radiofrequency ablation is effective in selected cases of lateralizing primary aldosteronism, and new evidence suggests that aldosterone synthase inhibitors may be an effective treatment in the future; however, these modalities will not be discussed in this chapter. This chapter will highlight 3 clinical vignettes demonstrating the implementation of treatment of primary aldosteronism and how to gauge therapeutic success.

Practice Gaps

- Surgical adrenalectomy effectively treats lateralizing primary aldosteronism; however, many clinicians are not comfortable interpreting adrenal venous sampling results and/or assessing efficacy of therapy postoperatively.
- Most patients with primary aldosteronism are ultimately be treated medically rather than surgically, yet there is a lack of guidance on how to optimize medical therapy and the key metrics of success.

Discussion

The effectiveness of surgical adrenalectomy for patients with lateralizing primary aldosteronism is characterized by the attenuation of excess aldosterone production to induce reductions in

Figure 1. Pathophysiology of Primary Aldosteronism

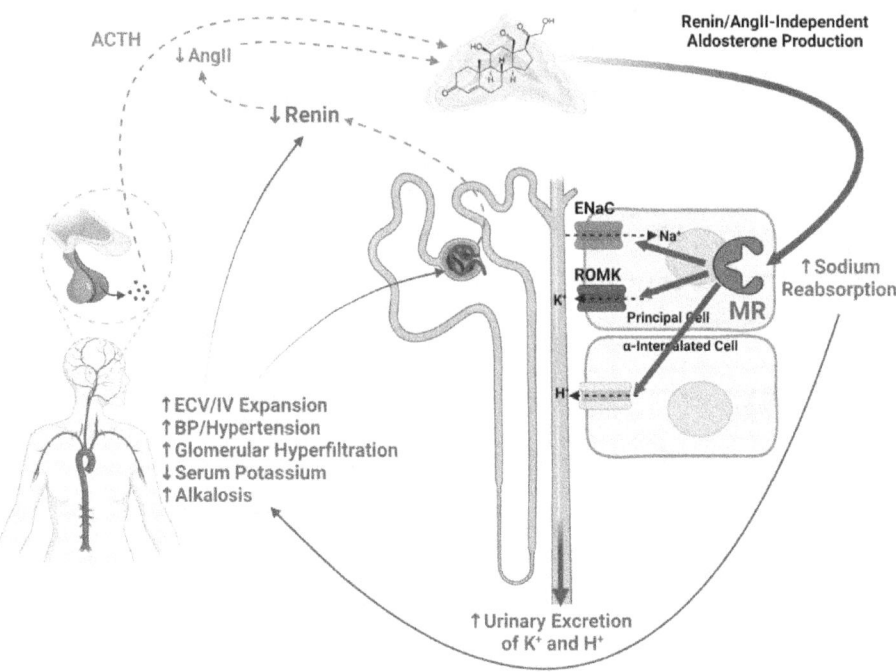

Abbreviations: ACTH, adrenocorticotropic hormone; Ang II, angiotensin II; BP, blood pressure; ECV, extracellular volume; ENaC, epithelial sodium channel; H+, hydrogen; IV, intravascular; K+, potassium; MR, mineralocorticoid receptor; Na+, sodium; ROMK, renal outer medullary potassium channel. Aldosterone is physiologically regulated by the renin-angiotensin system, adrenocorticotropic hormone, and potassium. In primary aldosteronism, one or both adrenal glands contain foci of dysregulated aldosterone synthase capable of producing aldosterone independent of stimuli by angiotensin II and/or adrenocorticotropic hormone. This excess aldosterone production activates the MR in principal cells even in volume-expanded states wherein renin and angiotensin II are suppressed, resulting in inappropriate sodium reabsorption via ENaC along with a commensurate excretion of potassium and hydrogen ions. This vicious cycle can induce the clinical manifestations of elevated blood pressure and hypertension, glomerular hyperfiltration, hypokalemia, and metabolic alkalosis. Created with biorender.com. Reprinted from Hundemer GL et al, Endocrine Reviews, 2024; 45(1): 69–94. © The Endocrine Society.[1]

[Color—Print (Color Gallery page CG12) or web & ePub editions]

blood pressure, normalization of serum potassium, and increases in renin. These biomarkers collectively indicate a reversal of primary aldosteronism pathophysiology and restoration of normal physiology. When surgical adrenalectomy is pursued in patients with lateralizing primary aldosteronism, it offers the potential to cure the aldosteronism and hypokalemia while substantially improving blood pressure (and in some cases, curing hypertension).[1,2] Postoperatively, there is a risk for transient hypoaldosteronism, as the ability of the contralateral zona glomerulosa to produce aldosterone may be diminished, and the ability to secrete renin may be suppressed. The more severe the lateralizing primary aldosteronism, the more likely there is to be postoperative hypoaldosteronism. The main risks of hypoaldosteronism are hyperkalemia, hypotension, and acute kidney injury. For these reasons, patients

should have their serum potassium, kidney function, blood pressure, renin, and aldosterone followed every 7 to 10 days after the surgery until there is reassurance of homeostatic physiology. If needed, low-dosage fludrocortisone can be used transiently. Preoperative treatment with MR antagonists can reduce the risk of postoperative hypoaldosteronism.[3] Surgical adrenalectomy can also be pursued in patients with nonlateralizing primary aldosteronism who have asymmetric disease and/or who have severe disease that is not amenable to medical therapy. In these cases, the objective of surgical adrenalectomy is not to cure primary aldosteronism, but rather to attenuate its severity such that subsequent medical therapy is more likely to succeed (*Table, following page*).[1,4,5]

Most patients with primary aldosteronism will ultimately be treated medically rather than surgically, owing to the fact that most cases are

Table. Expected Biochemical and Clinical Sequelae of Therapies for Primary Aldosteronism

Parameters	Curative adrenalectomy for lateralizing disease	Noncurative unilateral adrenalectomy for nonlateralizing disease	MR antagonist therapy	ENaC inhibitors	Dietary sodium restriction
Aldosterone	↓↓	↓	↑	↑	↑
Renin	↑↑	↑↑	↑↑	↑↑	↑
Aldosterone-to-renin ratio	↓↓	↓	↔/↓	↔/↓	↓
Serum potassium	↑	↑	↑	↑	↑
Base excess/alkalosis	↓	↓	↓	↓	↓
Estimated glomerular filtration rate	↓	↓	↓	↓	↓
Blood pressure	↓↓	↓	↓	↓	↓
Risk for incident cardiovascular and kidney disease	↓*	Unknown	↓*	Unknown	↓#

* Observations from longitudinal cohort studies comparing curative adrenalectomy with MR antagonist therapy.

Observations from population-based studies evaluating dietary sodium restriction in essential hypertension.

Reprinted from Hundemer GL et al, *Endocrine Reviews*, 2024; 45(1): 69–94. © The Endocrine Society.[1]

nonlateralizing, and/or due to the lack of availability of adrenal venous sampling, and/or due to patient preference for medical therapy. Medical therapy can be effective if titrated and monitored appropriately. Medical treatment options include dietary sodium restriction to decrease the substrate that fuels primary aldosteronism, MR antagonists to block the effects of aldosterone, ENaC inhibitors to block the effects of MR activation, and potentially in the future, aldosterone synthase inhibitors to decrease aldosterone production (*Figure 2, following page*). The objectives of medical therapy in primary aldosteronism should aspire to restore normal physiology and attenuate excess cardiometabolic and kidney disease risk (*Table*).[1] Ideally, dietary sodium restriction should be combined with MR antagonist therapy to afford the greatest synergy. In cases of MR antagonist intolerance, ENaC inhibitors can also be used to effectively improve blood pressure and hypokalemia; however, it should be noted that this medication class does not block extrarenal MR, and therefore ENaC inhibitors may not address deleterious aldosterone-MR interactions that contribute to cardiovascular injury.

Accruing evidence indicates that the key biomarkers reflective of optimized medical therapy mirror the physiologic expectations following surgical adrenalectomy: control of blood pressure with the fewest number of antihypertensive agents, normalization of serum potassium without supplementation, and a rise in renin.[1] Adequate up-titration of MR antagonist dosing should result in a reversal of volume expansion, which in turn should manifest with a rise in renin (*Figure 3, following page*).

Multiple studies have now shown that a rise in renin, from a suppressed to an unsuppressed state, is associated with improved cardiovascular and kidney outcomes.[1,6,7] This approach requires active titration of MR antagonists, usually in intervals of every few months. In some patients, it may not be possible to raise renin due to the effects of high-dosage β-adrenergic blockers and/or chronic kidney disease. In these instances, renin may not be a useful biomarker, but blood pressure and potassium levels can still serve as proxies for optimized therapy. In patients with chronic kidney disease, increased MR antagonist dosing can increase the risk for hyperkalemia. In these instances, diuretics, SGLT-2 inhibitors, and novel

Figure 2. Medical Treatments for Primary Aldosteronism

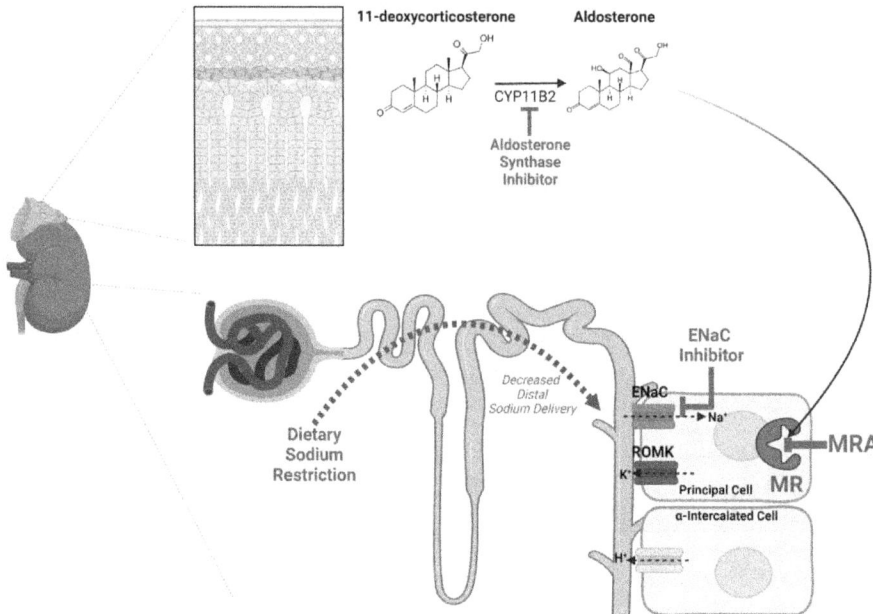

Abbreviations: ENaC, epithelial sodium channel; H+, hydrogen; K+, potassium; MR, mineralocorticoid receptor; MRA, mineralocorticoid receptor antagonist; Na+, sodium; ROMK, renal outer medullary potassium channel. Dietary sodium restriction leads to volume contraction, decreased glomerular filtration, and decreased sodium delivery to the distal nephron thereby limiting aldosterone-MR-ENaC-mediated sodium reabsorption. MR antagonists prevent the interaction between aldosterone and the MR in the principal cell, thereby preventing ENaC-mediated sodium reabsorption. ENaC inhibitors directly block ENaC-mediated sodium reabsorption. Aldosterone synthase inhibitors block CYP11B2-mediated conversion of 11-deoxycorticosterone to aldosterone in the adrenal cortex. Created with biorender.com. Reprinted from Hundemer GL et al, *Endocrine Reviews*, 2024; 45(1): 69–94. © The Endocrine Society.[1]

[Color—Print (Color Gallery page CG13) or web & ePub editions]

Figure 3. Biomarkers of Optimal Medical Therapy in Primary Aldosteronism

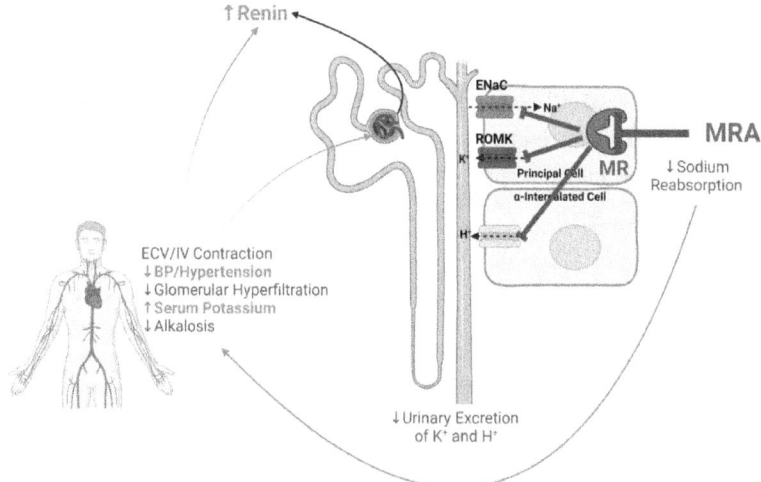

Abbreviations: BP, blood pressure; ECV, extracellular volume; ENaC, epithelial sodium channel; H+, hydrogen; IV, intravascular; K+, potassium; MR, mineralocorticoid receptor; MRA, mineralocorticoid receptor antagonist; Na+, sodium; ROMK, renal outer medullary potassium channel. Through blockade of the interaction between aldosterone and the MR in the principal cell of the distal nephron, MR antagonists decrease ENaC-mediated sodium reabsorption. This, in turn, results in decreased volume expansion along with decreased potassium and hydrogen ion urinary excretion. If the degree of MR blockade is sufficient to cause intravascular volume contraction and relative kidney hypoperfusion, renin will rise due to secretion from the juxtaglomerular cells. Thus, a rise in renin along with a lowering of blood pressure and normalization of serum potassium serve as biomarkers of adequate MR blockade in primary aldosteronism. In bold are the key biomarkers that reflect optimized medical therapy in primary aldosteronism: normalization of blood pressure, normalization of serum potassium, and a rise in renin. Created with biorender.com. Adapted from Hundemer GL et al, *Endocrine Reviews*, 2024; 45(1): 69–94. © The Endocrine Society.[1]

[Color—Print (Color Gallery page CG13) or web & ePub editions]

Figure 4. Approaches to Address MR Antagonist–Associated Hyperkalemia

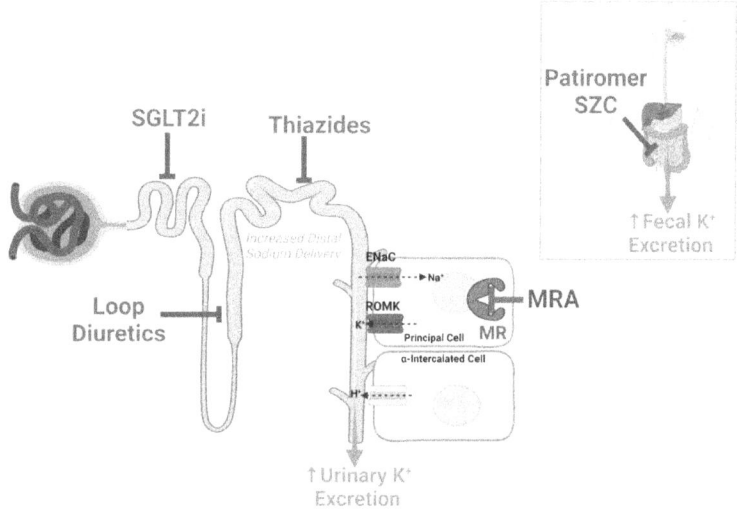

Abbreviations: ENaC, epithelial sodium channel; H+, hydrogen; K+, potassium; MR, mineralocorticoid receptor; MRA, mineralocorticoid receptor antagonist; Na+, sodium; ROMK, renal outer medullary potassium channel; SGLT2i, sodium-glucose cotransporter-2 inhibitor; SZC, sodium zirconium cyclosilicate. SGLT-2 inhibitors (via blockade of SGLT-2 in the proximal tubule), loop diuretics (via blockade of the Na+-K+-Cl- cotransporter along the thick ascending loop of Henle), and thiazide diuretics (via blockade of the sodium-chloride symporter in the distal convoluted tubule) all cause increased urinary distal sodium delivery and reabsorption, which enhances the electronegative charge in the tubular lumen thereby driving urinary potassium excretion in the collecting duct. Patiromer and sodium zirconium cyclosilicate serve to bind potassium in the gastrointestinal tract, thereby increasing fecal potassium excretion. Created with biorender.com. Reprinted from Hundemer GL et al, Endocrine Reviews, 2024; 45(1): 69–94. © The Endocrine Society.[1]

[Color—Print (Color Gallery page CG14) or web & ePub editions]

potassium binders can all be used to mitigate the risk for hyperkalemia and permit the continued use of MR antagonists (*Figure 4*). A treatment algorithm summarizing the approaches to primary aldosteronism therapy is shown in *Figure 5* (*following page*).[1]

Clinical Case Vignettes

Case 1

A 62-year-old man with a history of hypertension, obesity, and diabetes is referred for evaluation of difficult-to-control hypertension. Hypertension was diagnosed at age 40 years. Records indicate multiple episodes of hypokalemia, with the lowest recorded value of serum potassium at 2.8 mEq/L (2.8 mmol/L). In the last 10 years, his blood pressure has been very difficult to control, and he currently takes 7 antihypertensive medications: hydrochlorothiazide, amlodipine, olmesartan, doxazosin, hydralazine, atenolol, and spironolactone. On this regimen, his blood pressure is 130-140/80-90 mm Hg, plasma

aldosterone is markedly elevated at 61 ng/dL (1692 pmol/L), plasma renin activity is suppressed at 0.19 ng/mL per h, and the aldosterone-to-renin ratio is markedly elevated at 321 ng/dL per ng/mL/h (8900 pmol/L per ng/mL/h). Primary aldosteronism is diagnosed. Abdominal CT shows 2 subcentimeter left adrenocortical adenomas and a normal-appearing right adrenal gland. Results of a dexamethasone-suppression test are normal. Adrenal venous sampling demonstrates overt lateralization to the left side (lateralization index >40) and simultaneous contralateral suppression of right-sided aldosterone production (demonstrated as an aldosterone-to-cortisol ratio from the right adrenal vein that is less than that of the inferior vena cava, and an absolute aldosterone concentration from the right adrenal vein that is less than that of the inferior vena cava). The patient is scheduled to undergo retroperitoneoscopic left adrenalectomy.

Figure 5. Recommended Approach to Primary Aldosteronism Treatment

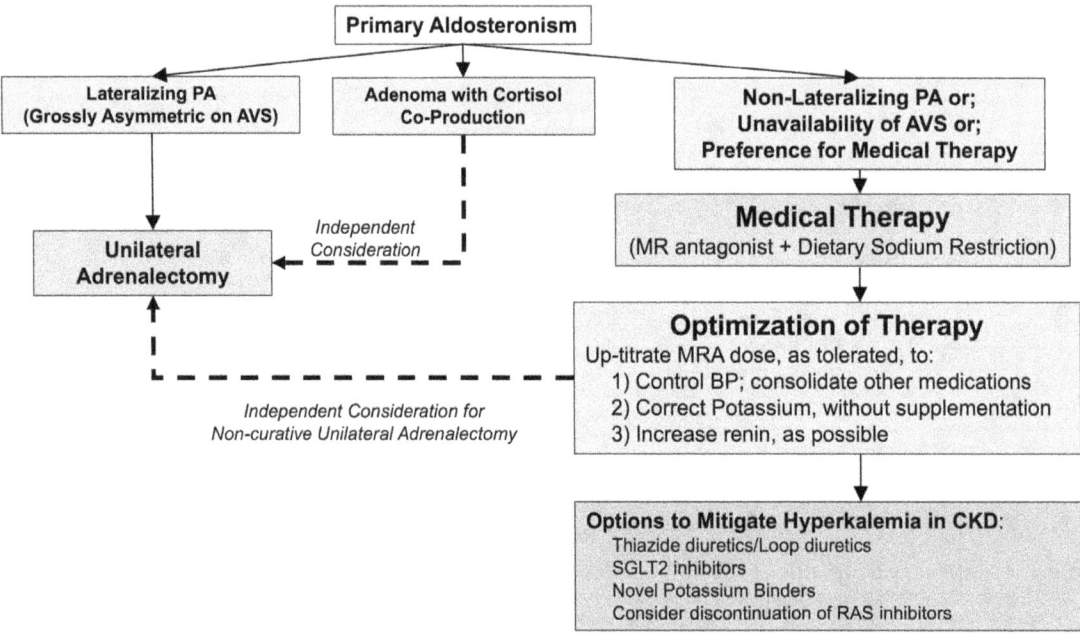

Abbreviations: AVS, adrenal vein sampling; BP, blood pressure; HTN, hypertension; K+, potassium; MRA, mineralocorticoid receptor antagonist; PA, primary aldosteronism; RAS, renin-angiotensin system; SGLT2, sodium-glucose cotransporter-2. For patients with lateralizing PA, unilateral adrenalectomy is the standard recommendation. Unilateral adrenalectomy should also be considered for patients with an adenoma with cortisol co-production. For patients with nonlateralizing PA, those for whom AVS is not available, or those with lateralizing PA who have declined surgical treatment, we suggest treating with MR antagonist therapy and dietary sodium restriction. To optimize MR antagonist therapy, we recommend up-titrating the dose as tolerated with the goals of normalizing blood pressure (and ideally reducing other antihypertensive medications in the process), normalizing serum potassium without the use of potassium supplementation (if applicable), and achieving a rise in renin as a biomarker of restoration of normal renin-angiotensin system activity. If hyperkalemia becomes a barrier to MR antagonist up-titration, addition of a potassium-wasting diuretic (thiazide or loop), an SGLT-2 inhibitor, a novel potassium binder (patiromer or sodium zirconium cyclosilicate), and/or discontinuing renin-angiotensin system inhibitors should be considered. If a case of PA is severe enough and refractory to maximal medical therapy, unilateral adrenalectomy may be considered for disease attenuation (rather than disease cure). Reprinted from Hundemer GL et al, Endocrine Reviews, 2024; 45(1): 69–94. © The Endocrine Society.[1]

[Color—Print (Color Gallery page CG14) or web & ePub editions]

The patient should be counseled to expect which of the following postoperative outcomes?

A. Adrenal insufficiency

B. Cure of hypertension

C. Hyperkalemia

D. Hypokalemia

E. Persistent primary aldosteronism

Answer: C) Hyperkalemia

This patient has lateralizing primary aldosteronism that has been clearly demonstrated on adrenal venous sampling. In addition, adrenal venous sampling demonstrates complete suppression of right-sided aldosterone production. As a result, it is very likely that this patient will achieve postoperative cure of his primary aldosteronism and hypokalemia; however, this also means that he has a high likelihood of developing postoperative hypoaldosteronism, which can manifest as hyperkalemia (Answer C), volume depletion, a decline in glomerular filtration rate owing to the decrease in glomerular hyperfiltration, and in some instances, hypotension. Indeed, for several weeks after the operation, this patient had undetectable renin and aldosterone values, and his serum potassium concentration rose to 5.6 mEq/L (5.6 mmol/L). At that point he was treated with low-dosage fludrocortisone for 3 weeks, and this was then tapered with normalization of renin and aldosterone. This case highlights the importance of close monitoring in the postoperative period. Preoperative treatment with MR antagonists can reduce the risk of postoperative hypoaldosteronism, especially when they induce a rise in renin.[3] Patients with severe and longstanding hypertension are unlikely to achieve normalization of their blood pressure even after curing primary aldosteronism because of the irreversible vascular damage that has occurred. However, improvement in blood pressure should be anticipated. This patient ultimately required only 2 blood pressure medications after his surgery: hydrochlorothiazide and amlodipine. Adrenal insufficiency, or cortisol insufficiency, should not be expected unless there was preoperative evidence of hypercortisolism.

Case 2

A 68-year-old woman with nonlateralizing primary aldosteronism is treated with spironolactone. Hypertension was diagnosed in her 40s, and she had had multiple episodes of hypokalemia and chronic metabolic alkalosis. Her diagnostic plasma aldosterone concentration was 15 ng/dL (416 pmol/L) with a plasma renin activity less than 0.6 ng/mL per h while on hydrochlorothiazide, 25 mg daily, amlodipine, 10 mg daily, and atenolol, 50 mg daily. Abdominal CT at the time revealed no adrenal nodules. Adrenal venous sampling did not demonstrate lateralizing aldosterone production amenable to surgical adrenalectomy. Therefore, spironolactone, 12.5 mg daily, was added to her antihypertensive medication regimen and she was counseled to decrease dietary sodium intake, as best as possible, with a goal of less than 2 g per day. One month later, her blood pressure has declined from 160-170 mm Hg systolic to 130-140 mm Hg. Her serum potassium is now 3.7 mEq/L (3.7 mmol/L) without potassium supplementation, and her plasma renin activity remains less than 0.6 ng/mL per h.

Which of the following should be recommended?

A. Continue treatment with the current regimen

B. Increase the spironolactone dosage to 25 mg daily

C. Prescribe ACE inhibitor or angiotensin receptor blocker

D. Prescribe potassium supplementation to target a serum potassium ≥4.0 mEq/L

Answer: B) Increase the spironolactone dosage to 25 mg daily

The goals of medical therapy for primary aldosteronism should aspire to achieve the same objectives as surgical adrenalectomy: improvement/normalization of blood pressure with the fewest medications, normalization of serum potassium without the aid of supplementation, and normalization of renin as a proxy for reversal of primary aldosteronism pathophysiology (*Figure 3, Table*). These objectives can be achieved in most patients by gradually up-titrating the dosage of the MR antagonist. The critical importance of normalizing blood pressure has been validated in numerous prospective studies and remains a foundation of primary aldosteronism therapy. Multiple studies have also demonstrated that an increase in renin, from a suppressed to unsuppressed state, serves as a proxy for decreased risk for incidence of adverse cardiovascular and kidney outcomes.[1,6,7] Achieving a rise in renin can take several medication titrations spanning the course of several months and up to 1 year.[8,9] In some patients, particularly those who have advanced kidney disease or are on high dosages of β-adrenergic antagonists, it may not be possible to see substantial rises in renin. Therefore, in these patients, MR antagonists can be titrated to the highest dosage permitted by blood pressure and serum potassium objectives. In patients with chronic kidney disease, hyperkalemia can be an issue with higher MR antagonist dosing. When encountered, hyperkalemia induced by MR antagonists can be mitigated with diuretics, SGLT-2 inhibitors (which are also indicated in many patients with kidney disease), and novel potassium binders (such as patiromer) (*Figure 4*).[1,10] Because this patient's blood pressure is still above the target range and renin is suppressed, increasing the spironolactone dosage (Answer B) is the best next step. In the subsequent 3 to 6 months after increasing the spironolactone dosage to 25 mg daily, this patient's systolic blood pressure ranged from 118 to 130 mm Hg, her serum potassium concentration ranged from 3.9 to 4.3 mEq/L, and her plasma renin activity ranged from 0.9 to 3.3 ng/mL per h.

Case 3

A 48-year-old man is referred for further evaluation regarding treatment of primary aldosteronism. Hypertension was diagnosed at age 31 years, and he had multiple episodes of hypokalemia with a serum potassium concentration as low as 2.9 mEq/L (2.9 mmol/L). After primary aldosteronism was diagnosed, CT showed 3 right-sided adrenal nodules (ranging in size from 0.4 to 2.2 cm) and 1 subcentimeter left-sided adrenal nodule, all with attenuation characteristics of benign adenomas. Adrenal venous sampling revealed a lateralization ratio of 2, favoring the right side, and lack of contralateral suppression, suggesting bilateral primary aldosteronism. He was treated with eplerenone in addition to amlodipine and atenolol. Over the next few years, his eplerenone was titrated to a dosage of 500 mg daily (300 mg in the morning and 200 mg in the evening), in addition to amlodipine, 10 mg daily, and atenolol, 50 mg daily. Despite this high dosage of eplerenone, his plasma renin activity remained suppressed (<0.6 ng/mL per h), and his plasma aldosterone concentration was greater than 200 ng/dL (>5540 pmol/L). He required potassium chloride supplementation for persistent hypokalemia, his blood pressure remained in the range of 150-160/90-100 mm Hg, and he developed new-onset atrial fibrillation and an occipital stroke.

Which of the following is most likely to improve this patient's cardiovascular risk profile?

A. Add amiloride, 5 mg daily

B. Add hydrochlorothiazide, 25 mg daily

C. Add lisinopril, 40 mg daily

D. Increase the eplerenone dosage to 600 mg daily

E. Perform right-sided laparoscopic adrenalectomy

Answer: E) Perform right-sided laparoscopic adrenalectomy

Despite aggressive medical therapy, this patient has persistent primary aldosteronism pathophysiology, as evidenced by uncontrolled high blood pressure, hypokalemia, and suppressed renin. Increasing his current medication dosages, or adding more medications, is likely to provide only diminishing gains that are not sustainable in a 48-year-old patient. His risk for adverse cardiovascular outcomes is very high, especially because he has already developed a stroke and atrial fibrillation. Noncurative right-sided surgical adrenalectomy can attenuate the magnitude of aldosterone production to facilitate improved medical therapy outcomes.[1,4]

In this case, the patient underwent uncomplicated adrenalectomy. Postoperatively, his plasma aldosterone concentration declined to 30 ng/dL (832 pmol/L) and his blood pressure normalized to less than 130/80 mm Hg with eplerenone, 50 mg daily, amlodipine, 10 mg daily, and atenolol, 25 mg daily. His pathology revealed multiple adrenocortical adenomas harboring pathogenic somatic variants known to cause primary aldosteronism.[11] This pathogenesis of primary aldosteronism is suspected to occur in a bilateral and diffuse manner, suggesting a similar process is likely ongoing in his contralateral left adrenal cortex.[12] In subsequent years, his eplerenone dosage was gradually increased to 50 mg twice daily, and his renin activity rose to 0.8 to 1.4 ng/mL per h. This case highlights that surgical therapy for primary aldosteronism can be very effective, even when it is not used to induce cure (*Table, Figure 5*).

Key Learning Points

Adapted from Hundemer GL et al, *Endocrine Reviews*, 2024; 45(1): 69–94. © The Endocrine Society.[1]

- Primary aldosteronism is an endocrinopathy characterized by dysregulated aldosterone production that occurs despite suppression of renin and angiotensin II, and that cannot be suppressed by volume and sodium-loading maneuvers. This underlying pathophysiology of primary aldosteronism increases the risk for adverse cardiometabolic and kidney outcomes.

- The effectiveness of surgical adrenalectomy for patients with lateralizing primary aldosteronism is characterized by the attenuation of excess aldosterone production to induce reductions in blood pressure, normalization of serum potassium, and increases in renin, which are biomarkers that collectively indicate a reversal of pathophysiology and restoration of normal physiology.

- Most patients with primary aldosteronism are ultimately treated medically rather than surgically; the objectives of medical therapy in primary aldosteronism should aspire to restore normal physiology and attenuate excess cardiometabolic and kidney disease risk.

- Accruing evidence indicates that the key biomarkers reflective of optimized medical therapy mirror the physiologic expectations following surgical adrenalectomy: control of blood pressure with the fewest number of antihypertensive agents, normalization of serum potassium without supplementation, and a rise in renin.

References

1. Hundemer GL, Leung AA, Kline GA, Brown JM, Turcu AF, Vaidya A. Biomarkers to guide medical therapy in primary aldosteronism. *Endocr Rev.* 2024;45(1):69-94. PMID: 37439256

2. Williams TA, Lenders JWM, Mulatero P, et al; Primary Aldosteronism Surgery Outcome (PASO) Investigators. Outcomes after adrenalectomy for unilateral primary aldosteronism: an international consensus on outcome measures and analysis of remission rates in an international cohort. *Lancet Diabetes Endocrinol.* 2017;5(9):689-699. PMID: 28576687

3. Zhang J, Libianto R, Lee JC, et al. Preoperative mineralocorticoid receptor antagonist reduces postoperative hyperkalaemia in patients with Conn syndrome. *Clin Endocrinol (Oxf).* 2022;96(1):40-46. PMID: 34743353

4. Williams TA, Gong S, Tsurutani Y, et al. Adrenal surgery for bilateral primary aldosteronism: an international retrospective cohort study. *Lancet Diabetes Endocrinol.* 2022;10(11):769-771. PMID: 36137555

5. Hundemer GL, Vaidya A. Management of endocrine disease: the role of surgical adrenalectomy in primary aldosteronism. *Eur J Endocrinol.* 2020;183(6):R185-R196. PMID: 33077688

6. Hundemer G, Curhan G, Yozamp N, Wang M, Vaidya A. Incidence of atrial fibrillation and mineralocorticoid receptor activity in patients with medically and surgically treated primary aldosteronism. *JAMA Cardiology.* 2018;3(8):768-774. PMID: 30027227

7. Hundemer GL, Curhan GC, Yozamp N, Wang M, Vaidya A. Cardiometabolic outcomes and mortality in medically treated primary aldosteronism: a retrospective cohort study. *Lancet Diabetes Endocrinol.* 2018;6(1):51-59. PMID: 29129576

8. Mansur A, Vaidya A, Turchin A. Using renin activity to guide mineralocorticoid receptor antagonist therapy in patients with low renin and hypertension. *Am J Hypertens.* 2023;36(8):455-461. PMID: 37013957

9. Tezuka Y, Turcu AF. Mineralocorticoid receptor antagonists decrease the rates of positive screening for primary aldosteronism. *Endocr Pract.* 2020;26(12):1416-1424. PMID: 33471733

10. Agarwal R, Rossignol P, Budden J, et al. Patiromer and spironolactone in resistant hypertension and advanced CKD: analysis of the randomized AMBER Trial. Kidney360. 2021;2(3):425-434. PMID: 35369022

11. Omata K, Yamazaki Y, Nakamura Y, et al. Genetic and histopathologic intertumor heterogeneity in primary aldosteronism. *J Clin Endocrinol Metab.* 2017;102(6):1792-1796. PMID: 28368480

12. van de Wiel E, Chaman Baz AH, Kusters B, et al. Changes of the CYP11B2 expressing zona glomerulosa in human adrenals from birth to 40 years of age. *Hypertension.* 2022;79(11):2565-2572. PMID: 36036158

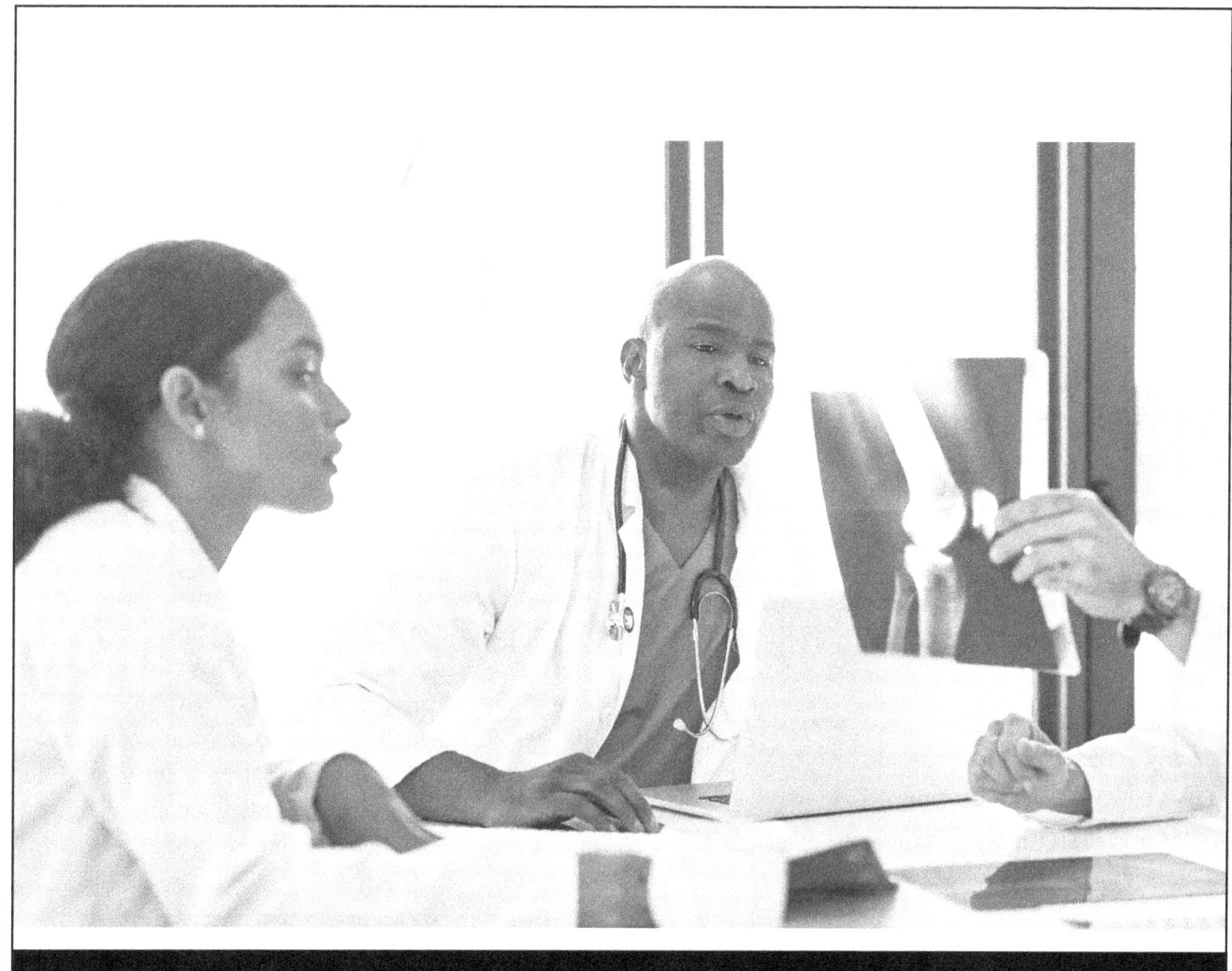

DIABETES MELLITUS AND GLUCOSE METABOLISM

What's New in Diabetes Technology?

Grazia Aleppo, MD. Division of Endocrinology, Metabolism and Molecular Medicine, Feinberg School of Medicine, Northwestern University, Chicago, IL; Email: aleppo@northwestern.edu

Educational Objectives

After reviewing this chapter, learners should be able to:

- Identify discrepancies in continuous glucose monitoring (CGM), connected pens, and automated insulin delivery (AID) reports and glucometrics due to the patient's behavior.

- Diagnose algorithm-induced hypoglycemia and recommend strategies to reduce its prevalence by optimizing system features.

- Manage AID setting changes according to the specific system.

Significance of the Clinical Problem

Numerous CGM systems, AID systems, and connected pens are commercially available for persons with type 1 and type 2 diabetes mellitus. Since late 2019, advances have been made regarding each aspect of diabetes technology, and the vast and growing literature supports the clinical benefits of CGM and AID systems.[1,2] With this plethora of available devices and systems for diabetes management, clinicians must learn the many features of multiple devices and AID systems to best advise patients on a personalized care plan.

Data suggest that preparedness to adopt advanced diabetes technology is still somewhat lacking. Therapeutic inertia in diabetes technology is partially due to the provider's or care team's unfamiliarity and discomfort with these systems.[3]

With the rapidly evolving integration of diabetes technology in clinical practice and diabetes self-management, health care professionals must stay current not only with practice guidelines, but also with knowledge about the technological aspects of diabetes care. Certified diabetes education care and specialists (CDCESs) are well positioned to support clinicians, but the reality is that not every clinical practice has a CDCES. Often the burden of unraveling the information about these systems and trying to assist patients during the limited time of an office visit falls on clinicians. In such circumstances, it is crucial that the entire care team, whether small or large, engages in the necessary steps to enable technology-driven diabetes care. Historically, health care professionals' attitude toward CGM was found to be a barrier to CGM expansion.[4] Readiness charts for clinicians (MD and CDCES) describe which type of provider is expected to prescribe diabetes technology tools. Tannenbaum et al described 3 "clinician personas" based on readiness to promote diabetes technology and comfort in keeping up with technology advances.[5] In this report, only 20% were "ready," 41% were "cautious," and 40% were "not yet ready."

While the uptake of CGM has increased since 2018, there is still much work to be done to enhance providers' comfort with and knowledge about prescribing diabetes technology devices and successfully implementing these systems in clinical practice. In particular, AID systems require not only the knowledge of each system, but also the ability to interpret each report and what can be gleaned to optimize patient care.

Practice Gaps

- Detailed management of each AID system is often delegated to the CDCES in clinical practice. However, in many clinical practices, a CDCES are not readily available, and clinicians require expanded knowledge of each type of algorithm and the settings that can be modified and those that cannot. Setting patient expectations for various systems (eg, CGM, connected pens, or AID systems), and understanding the impact of the end-user's behaviors on optimal technology adoption are crucial to enhance patient satisfaction and outcomes.

- Multiple types of software are necessary to review specific AID systems, and some agnostic data aggregators are also available. However, software/data review proficiency for each commercially available AID system can be challenging and time consuming. Providers may not have readily available resources to efficiently and correctly navigate the many available reports to design a care plan during office visits.

Discussion

Several CGM systems have been FDA cleared and are commercially available, and all of them are now approved for nonadjunctive use (ie, without the need for confirmatory blood glucose measurement by fingerstick to make insulin dosing decisions). Furthermore, all FDA-cleared CGM systems have seen substantially increased accuracy with lower median absolute relative difference, between 7.9% and 10.4%. Among these, the long-wear, implantable Senseonic Eversense E3 CGM (Senseonics, Germantown, MA, USA) was cleared in February 2022 for persons 18 years and older, with 24-hour warm-up time and up to 180 days duration. This system has an external rechargeable transmitter placed over the implanted sensor, which in turn charges the sensor and transmits data to a smartphone app. In mid-2022, the Abbott FreeStyle Libre 3 (Abbott Laboratories, Alameda, CA, USA) also received FDA clearance for persons

4 years and older. The sensor/transmitter unit has 1 hour warm-up time and 14 days wear. Libre 3, which has optional alerts and alarms, can be used with a reader or a smartphone app. In December 2022, the FDA cleared Dexcom G7 (Dexcom, San Diego, CA, USA), a class II iCGM, for persons 2 years and older. This is an all-in-one sensor/transmitter unit, with a 30-minute warm-up time, 10-day sensor wear, and a 12-hour grace period that allows users to replace the sensors up to 12 hours after the sensor's 10-day life has expired without losing CGM signal or data. Dexcom G7 can be used with a receiver or via a smartphone app and has no restriction for use in pregnancy. This system has predictive alerts and alarms, an urgent "low soon" alert, and the options to delay the first alert or turn off all alerts up to 6 hours. Similar to Dexcom G6, this newer, much smaller system can be integrated with the Tandem t:slim X2 with Control IQ and the Tandem Mobi (with Control IQ) AID systems (Tandem Diabetes Care, San Diego, CA, USA). In March 2023, a modified version of the Abbott Libre 2 CGM and the Libre 3 CGM (Abbott Laboratories, Alameda, CA, USA) received FDA clearance for integration with AID systems, and their use was expanded to pregnant patients as well. Lastly, in April 2023, the Medtronic Guardian 4 CGM, a 7-day sensor requiring no calibrations, was FDA cleared for the use with the Medtronic MiniMed 780G (Medtronic Diabetes, Northridge, CA, USA) AID system.

Several AID systems have received FDA clearance since late 2019, substantially expanding insulin delivery options for persons with diabetes. In December 2019, the Tandem t:slim X2 with Control IQ AID system (Tandem Diabetes Care, San Diego, CA, USA) was cleared by the FDA. At that time, it was the first advanced AID system that offered automated correction boluses based on a glucose concentration threshold and the first alternate controller enabled interoperable pump. The Tandem t:slim X2 with Control IQ algorithm uses and maintains preset basal rates while the sensor glucose levels are stable between 112.5 and 160 mg/dL (6.2-8.8 mmol/L). When the sensor glucose levels are predicted to increase in the following 30 minutes to greater than 160 mg/dL (>8.8 mmol/L) the system modulates basal delivery by increasing the infusion. Similarly, when the sensor glucose levels are predicted to decrease below 112.5 mg/dL (<6.2 mmol/L) insulin delivery is decreased, and it is stopped if the sensor glucose levels are predicted to be below 70 mg/dL (<3.9 mmol/L). The system delivers an automated correction if the sensor glucose levels reach greater than 180 mg/dL (>10 mmol/L). Additional features include exercise activity that modulates insulin delivery to a target of 140 to 160 mg/dL (7.8-8.8 mmol/L) to reduce hypoglycemia risk and the sleep activity where the algorithm maintains the sensor glucose concentration between 112.5 and 120 mg/dL (6.2-6.7 mmol/L) without any additional automated correction boluses.

After a hiatus of 2 years, in February 2022, the Insulet OmniPod 5 (Insulet Corporation, Acton, MA, USA), a tubeless, advanced AID system, received FDA clearance for persons older than 2 years. This first in its class, all-on-body AID system with the algorithm on the pod is connected with the Dexcom G6 CGM through a controller or a smartphone app, and it offers adjustable glucose targets from 110 to 150 mg/dL (6.1- 8.3 mmol/L). These targets, which can be adjusted in 10 mg/dL (0.55 mmol/L) increments, can be used for a full 24 hours or combined in multiple segments (up to 8) per day. The system delivers insulin via the SmartAdjust technology every 5 minutes, modulating insulin doses based on the current sensor glucose values and their projected direction in the following 60 minutes to the preset glucose target. In addition, the system offers the SmartBolus Calculator, which combines CGM trend arrows and insulin on board to the carbohydrate grams entered to calculate insulin dose for mealtimes. The Activity Mode, with a glucose target of 150 mg/dL (8.3 mmol/L) that can be programmed up to 24 hours, allows the users to reduce hypoglycemia risk with a higher sensor glucose target and a more conservative insulin delivery mode.

In 2023, FDA clearance of AID systems accelerated. In April 2023, the Medtronic MiniMed 780G system with Guardian 4 was cleared for patients older than 7 years. The system's innovative 3 separate glucose targets allow users the options of setting sensor glucose targets at either 100 mg/dL, 110 mg/dL, or 120 mg/dL (5.55 mmol/L, 6.1 mmol/L, 6.7 mmol/L, respectively). In addition, the 780G SmartGuard technology in Auto Mode automatically adjusts basal insulin delivery based on sensor glucose values every 5 minutes, including automatically suspending and resuming delivery based on directional sensor glucose values and preset low sensor glucose limits. Finally, the advanced feature Meal Detection technology automatically delivers correction boluses up to every 5 minutes when it detects rapid rises in sensor glucose levels (eg, a missed meal bolus). Shortly thereafter, in May 2023, the Beta Bionics iLet (Beta Bionics, Irvine, CA, USA) advanced AID system (ACE pump) connected with Dexcom G6 and G7 received FDA clearance for individuals 6 years and older. This system is substantially different from other AID systems in that the algorithm requires only the person's weight to initialize. It does not include nor allow preset manual settings or manual basal rates/manual bolus settings. It is based on a semiqualitative way to deliver insulin for meals and does not require carbohydrate counting. The user enters the information for the meal type (breakfast, lunch, dinner) and bases it on "usual for me," "more," or "less."

The iLet has adjustable glucose targets, with the default glucose target being 120 mg/dL (6.7 mmol/L). The glucose targets can be shifted by 10 mg/dL (5.5 mmol/L) "lower" or "higher" (110-130 mg/dL [6.1-7.2 mmol/L]). Lastly, the most recent AID system of 2023, the Tandem Mobi advanced AID system, was approved in July, for patients older than 6 years (Tandem Diabetes Care, San Diego, CA, USA). This is the smallest (to date) AID system and consists of a screenless, 200 units reservoir (with a bolus button), controlled solely by a smart phone app that connects with either Dexcom G6, G7, or a modified version of FreeStyle Libre 2 CGM using the Control IQ technology. It includes a 5-inch tubing option or regular tubing, as well as an on-body option with a lightweight adhesive sleeve.

In addition to the numerous CGM and AID systems, connected pens (InPen, Medtronic, Northridge, CA, USA) and pen caps (Tempo Pen and Cap, Eli Lilly, Indianapolis, IN, USA) have been brought to market to aid patients with diabetes with bolus calculators, insulin dose reminders, and integration with CGM. The Medtronic InPen (Northridge, CA, USA) is a reusable insulin pen (with half-unit increments) compatible with short-acting insulin lispro and aspart and fast-acting aspart 3-mL cartridges. It has a 1-year battery life and is connected with a smartphone app. The smartphone app features a bolus calculator for insulin dose recommendations. The bolus calculator can be programmed (by the health care provider) for carbohydrate counting with insulin-to-carbohydrate ratio(s), insulin sensitivity factor, blood glucose target, and active insulin time. In the carbohydrate-counting mode, the bolus calculator also shows the insulin-on-board from previous insulin doses and advises the user of the presence of active insulin when calculating correction doses or premeal bolus doses in the setting of premeal hyperglycemia. The bolus calculator can also be programmed for fixed mealtime insulin doses or doses based on meal estimates (ie, small, medium, large), where the insulin-on-board is also calculated but not shown. The app provides reminders for missed doses (for both long- and short-acting insulin as long as long-acting insulin is recorded), provides alerts, and tracks insulin temperature. The InPen integrates with several CGM systems, including the Medtronic Guardian and Dexcom G6 CGM. Reports are available either through Medtronic CareLink, via Dexcom Clarity, or through the smartphone app.

The Lilly Tempo personalized diabetes management platform (Eli Lilly, Indianapolis, IN, USA) includes multiple components to allow users to track insulin doses, receive dose reminders, enter blood glucose readings, be integrated with CGM (Dexcom), and monitor carbohydrate intake and fitness activities. The components of this platform include the Tempo Smart Button and the Tempo Pen (available for glargine and lispro),

as well as the TempoSmart App and the Tempo Blood Glucose Meter. The adoption of CGM use among persons with diabetes has increased substantially in the last year, particularly since the Centers for Medicare and Medicaid Services have expanded CGM coverage to patients on basal insulin (or any insulin) and increased risk for or evidence of hypoglycemia.[6] Coverage for CGM in less-intensively treated people with diabetes has also been implemented by main commercial insurance payors. Therefore, in daily practice, there could theoretically be several patients using CGM whose data need to be reviewed to create a care plan during the short time of an office visit.

In addition, currently available AID systems have a variety of features with differences specific to each system that may be complex for both the provider and patient without proper training and understanding of their nuances. Education and training are essential for patients using these systems. It is increasingly necessary that health care providers and support staff are proficient in their knowledge of all aspects of technology, including prior authorizations, onboarding, downloading and interpreting data, and supporting ongoing use of these devices.[7] In 2021, the Association for Diabetes Care Education Specialists formed a working group to determine the core competencies required for the entire care team, from support staff to technology experts. In their report, the authors identified several domains of diabetes technology competencies, from fundamental (ie, schedulers), to intermediate (ie, RN, PharmD, RD, etc), to advanced (MD, DO, PA, NP, CDCES) based on the specific staff roles.

Without a systematic approach to the data, providers, who are often expected to have advanced proficiency with this technology, may be unsuccessful in their tasks, and this in turn can perpetuate therapeutic inertia. Stepwise, systematic approaches to data interpretation of CGM and AID systems must be available to clinicians. A systematic approach to CGM interpretation published in 2022 offers a stepwise review of the data to assist providers in making a care plan (*Table, following page*).[8]

Table. Stepwise Approach to CGM Interpretation[8]

Before starting, assess whether CGM data are sufficient for analysis	Look at percentage of time CGM is active (must be >70%)
Questions	**Answers**
1. What is the problem?	Look at CGM metrics
2. Where is the problem?	Look at the ambulatory glucose profile
3. How should therapy be adjusted?	Look at the daily glucose data

Reprinted from Szmuilowicz ED & Aleppo G. Postgrad Med, 2022; 134(8): 743-751. © Taylor & Francis.

Similarly, when reviewing AID systems, a structured approach to interpreting the data is necessary.

In March 2023, the first consensus recommendations for the use of AID technologies in clinical practice were published.[9] This first of its kind consensus addressed multiple points, from the evolution of AID systems to their clinical evidence, to target populations. The consensus also reviewed essentials of initiation and education, training, and support. In addition to establishing the first clinical recommendations for AID use to date, this consensus emphasized the need to standardize AID reports. These reports should provide valuable information, so clinicians can quickly ascertain the overall degree of glucose management. There are 3 recommended portions: an upper panel, middle panel, and lower panel.

The upper panel should have 4 components:

1. Time-in-range (time-in-range, time-below-range, and time-above-range)

2. Description of how the patient is using the device, indicating percentage of active AID and CGM, as well as information on frequency of changing the infusion set and sensor

3. Glucose metrics: average glucose, glucose management indicator, glucose variability

4. Insulin metrics, divided into AID- and user-initiated insulin delivery, including the amount of bolus for food, correction, or overrides per day

The middle panel should include the ambulatory glucose profile with the AID settings (including insulin-to-carbohydrate ratios, correction factor, and algorithm setpoints).

The lower panel should include the mealtime glucose metrics starting 1 hour before meals and ending 4 hours after the start of the meal.

With these new recommendations and visualization standards, providers should be able to identify how the system is used by the patient and identify concerns (hypoglycemia or hyperglycemia), as well as ways to improve use the AID system to allow for optimal results.

Clinical Case Vignettes
Case 1

A 42-year-old man with history of type 1 diabetes since age 10 years has a hemoglobin A_{1c} value of 7.0% (53 mmol/mol). In the last 12 months, he has self-updated his pump to the Tandem with Control IQ AID. He has not attended his postupdate training or follow-up visits. He is concerned that the system is not working well and does not think there is a great advantage over his previous system (Basal IQ). His report is shown (*Figure 1, following page*).

Which of the following is the most likely cause of this patient's hyperglycemia?

A. Incorrect insulin-to-carbohydrate ratio

B. He is overriding the system

C. Insufficient basal rates

D. Glucose target is too high

E. Active insulin time is too long

Answer: B) He is overriding the system

This patient is overriding the system (Answer B) and is using overrides (ie, manually entering boluses without using the bolus calculator) 93% of the time. This is easily recognized on the dashboard where there are 17 boluses per day, 6 g of total carbohydrates consumed per day.

Figure 1A. Data Derived From Tandem Device

CGM summary

Average reading	152 mg/dL
Time in range	78 %
Time CGM in use	99 %
Standard deviation	48 mg/dL
Coefficient of variation	32 %
GMI	6.9 %

Time in range comparison

Current 2 Weeks		Previous 2 Weeks
4%	> 250	6%
17%	181 - 250	19%
78%	In Range 70 - 180	74%
0%	54 - 69	1%
0%	< 54	0%

Control-IQ summary

Time active	98 %	13 d 8 hrs
Control-IQ off	0 %	0 hrs
CGM inactive	2 %	6 hrs
Pump inactive	0 %	2 hrs

Average sleep		Average exercise	
Duration	8 hrs	Duration	0 hrs
Weekly	6 times	Weekly	0 times

Insulin summary

Average daily dose		82.78 u
Basal	44 %	36.08 u
Bolus	56 %	46.70 u
Average daily boluses		17 boluses
Manual	86 %	14 boluses
Control-IQ	14 %	2 boluses
Average daily carbs		6 g

Bolus review (daily average)

Type		
Food	1 %	0.67 u
Correction	1 %	0.37 u
Override	93 %	43.26 u
Control-IQ	5 %	2.40 u

Delivery Method		
Standard	95 %	44.29 u
Extended	0 %	0.00 u
Quick	0 %	0.00 u
Control-IQ	5 %	2.40 u

Load activity

Cartridge change	every	2.0 d
Tubing fill	every	2.0 d
Cannula fill	every	2.0 d

Dashboard shows average glucose levels, GMI, time-in-range, and use of Control IQ in the upper panels. Lower panels show the insulin summary with basal insulin delivered by the algorithm, bolus doses, number of boluses per day, and average daily grams of carbohydrate entered. Bolus review shows how the user has used the bolus (whether by bolus calculator or otherwise) and the average cartridge change (number of days).

[Color—Print (Color Gallery page CG15) or web & ePub editions]

Figure 1B. Data Derived From Tandem Device

Pump Profile Settings - Base

Time	Basal Rate (u/hr)	Correction Factor	Carb Ratio	Target BG (mg/dL)
12:00am	1.400	1:30	1:8	110
3:00am	1.500	1:30	1:6	105
8:00am	1.700	1:30	1:6	100
9:30am	1.650	1:30	1:8	100
10:40am	1.450	1:30	1:8	100
2:00pm	1.450	1:30	1:8	100
8:00pm	1.350	1:30	1:8	115

Total Daily Basal: 35.108 u   Insulin Duration: 3:15 hrs

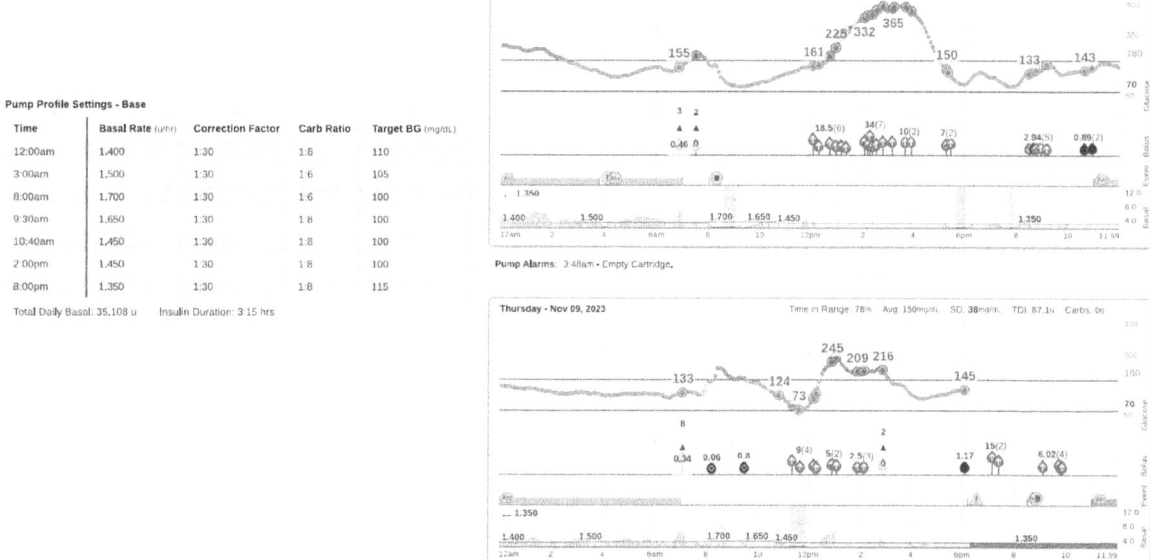

The left panel shows the pump profile settings, with basal rates, correction factor, carbohydrate ratio, and target blood glucose. The right panel shows the daily views with information on the CGM data, the boluses entered by the user, and the basal insulin delivery information.

[Color—Print (Color Gallery page CG16) or web & ePub editions]

The patient is not using the bolus calculator at all, so the hyperglycemia cannot be attributed to an incorrect insulin-to-carbohydrate ratio (Answer A).

He has overall good time-in-range, and the preprogrammed basal rates are very similar to the delivered automated basal insulin doses. Thus, insufficient basal rates (Answer C) is not the explanation.

The Tandem t:slim X2 with Control IQ has a nonmodifiable glucose target of 110 mg/dL (6.1 mmol/L). Even though the patient has set the target at various values between 100 and 115 mg/dL (5.6-6.4 mmol/L), these targets are not relevant while the Control IQ is on (thus, Answer D is incorrect).

The active insulin time (Answer E) cannot be modified in this AID system; it is automatically set at 5 hours.

After implementing recommended changes, the patient contacted the clinic 10 days later and was very happy about his glycemic control. He started using the bolus calculator, and his time-in-range had already improved. The number of overrides decreased from 93% to 12% with most boluses entered via the bolus calculator for either meals or corrections (*Figure 2*, *following page*).

Case 2

A 58-year-old man was diagnosed with type 1 diabetes at age 9 years. His hemoglobin A_{1c} value is 6.7% (50 mmol/mol). He has used various AID systems in the past. He currently uses the Insulet Omnipod 5 with a glucose target between 110 and 120 mg/dL (6.1-6.7 mmol/L), insulin-to-carbohydrate ratio of 1:7, correction factor of 35 mg/dL (1.9 mmol/L), and insulin-on-board 2.5 hours. He reports challenges with hyperglycemia in the late evening and overnight (blood glucose target = 110 mg/dL [6.1 mmol/L]). He follows a low–glycemic index meal plan with high protein and low carbohydrate intake. He reports that a few nights ago, he developed hypoglycemia in the early hours of the morning (*Figure 3, following pages*), and he is seeking advice.

Which of the following is the most likely cause of this patient's hyperglycemia in the evening into the overnight hours?

A. Insulin-to-carbohydrate ratio is too strong because of the low–glycemic index meal plan

B. Correction factor is too strong given the high-protein meal plan

C. Blood glucose target is too high

D. Bolus should be split in 2 halves to accommodate high-protein and low–glycemic index meal plan

E. Active insulin time is too long

Answer: D) Bolus should be split in 2 halves to accommodate high-protein and low–glycemic index meal plan

In view of this patient's low–glycemic index and high-protein meal plan, there may be a mismatch between food absorption and insulin action. Therefore, the patient would benefit from taking 2 boluses (Answer D) to accommodate for protein and fiber in the low–glycemic index carbohydrates.

If the insulin-to-carbohydrate ratio were too strong (Answer A) he would be experiencing postprandial hypoglycemia instead of hyperglycemia.

An inappropriately strong correction factor (Answer B) would reduce postprandial hyperglycemia and likely cause hypoglycemia at bedtime.

The patient is using the lowest glucose target (thus, Answer C is incorrect), which usually helps achieve the best time-in-range.

At 2.5 hours, the active insulin time (Answer E) sets the system to allow correction factors very frequently and would help achieve more optimal postprandial glucose levels with reduced overnight hyperglycemia.

The patient was experiencing hypoglycemia in the early-morning hours because of fake carbohydrate bolus entries. With guidance, the patient started taking premeal and postmeal boluses and overnight hyperglycemia resolved (*Figure 4*, *following pages*).

Figure 2A. Data Derived From the Tandem Device

Pre=152 mg/dL

Pre= 48

Pre=32%

Pre=6.9%

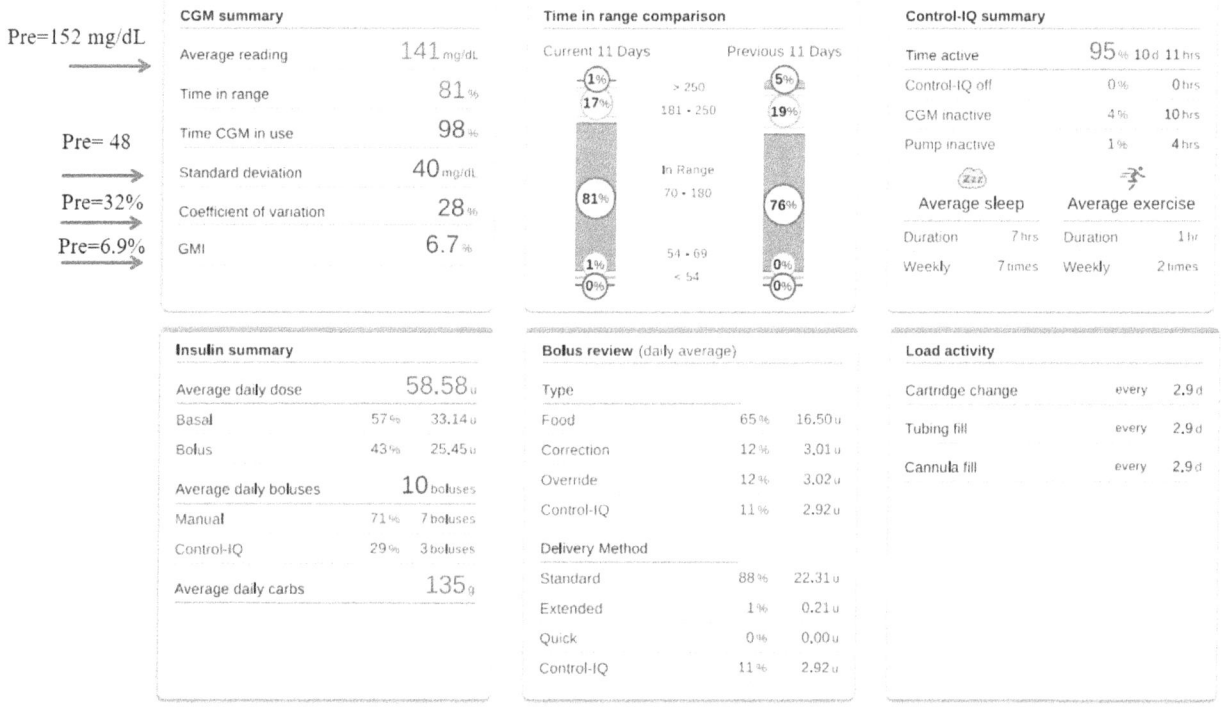

[Color—Print (Color Gallery page CG16) or web & ePub editions]

Figure 2B. Data Derived From the Tandem Device

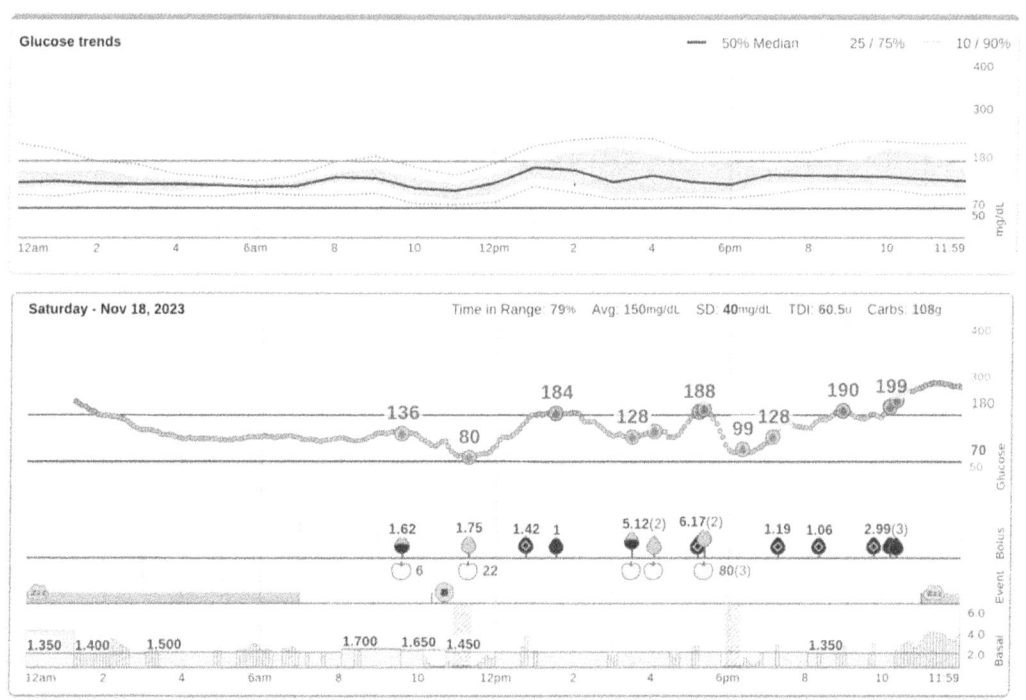

[Color—Print (Color Gallery page CG17) or web & ePub editions]

Figure 3A. Data Derived From the Glooko Device

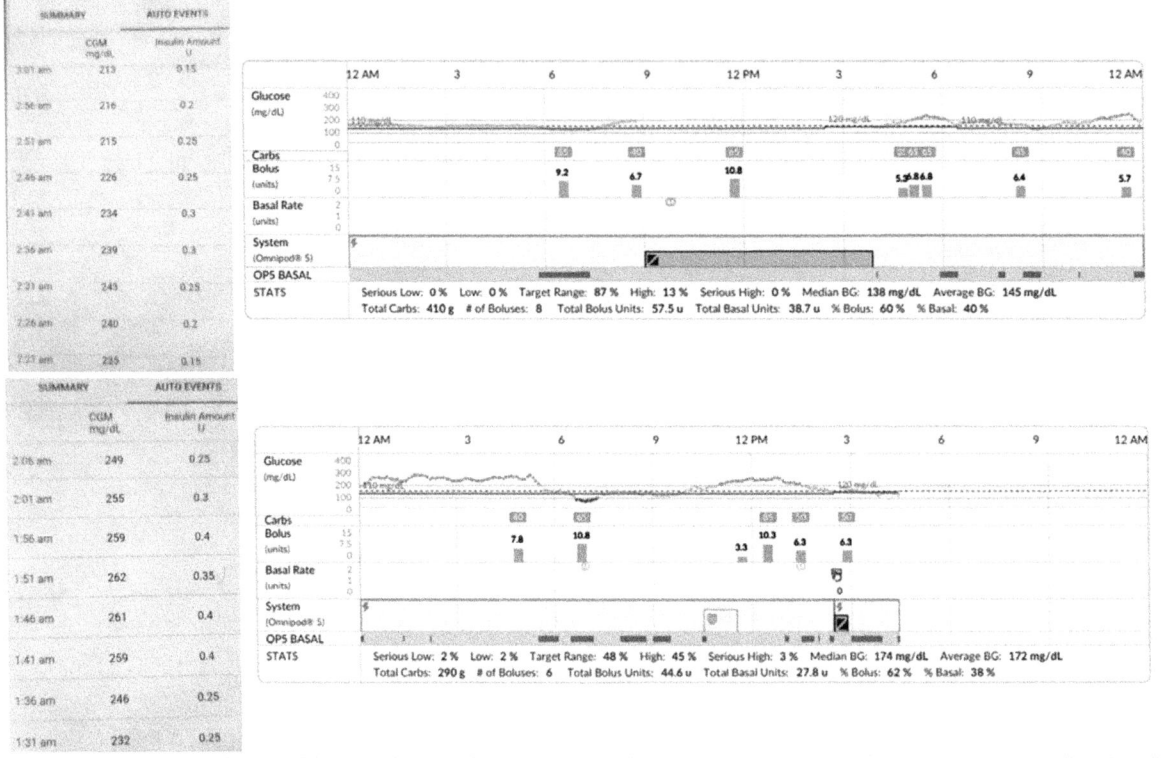

[Color—Print (Color Gallery page CG17) or web & ePub editions]

Figure 3B. Data Derived From the Glooko Device

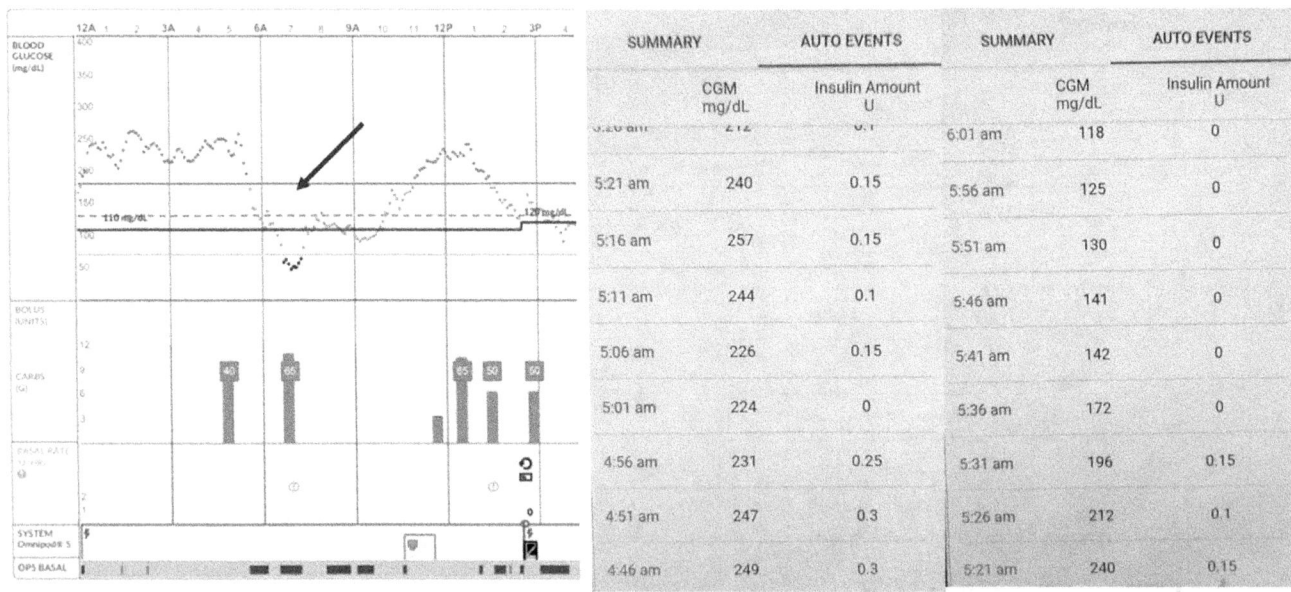

[Color—Print (Color Gallery page CG18) or web & ePub editions]

Figure 4. Data Derived From the Glooko Device

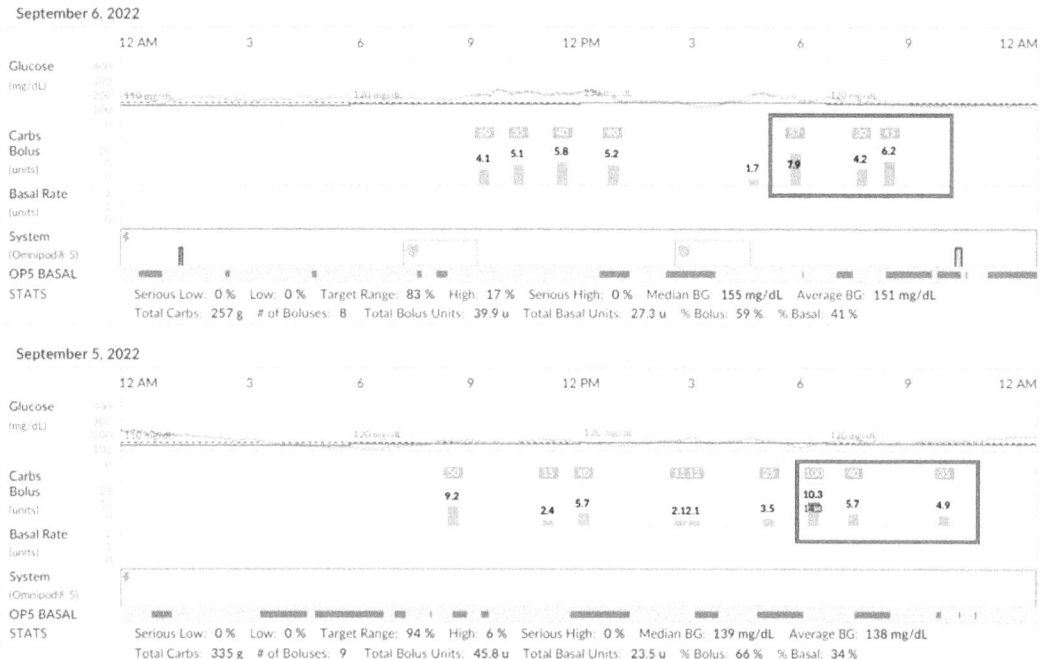

September 6, 2022

STATS	Serious Low: 0%	Low: 0%	Target Range: 83%	High: 17%	Serious High: 0%	Median BG: 155 mg/dL	Average BG: 151 mg/dL

Total Carbs: 257 g # of Boluses: 8 Total Bolus Units: 39.9 u Total Basal Units: 27.3 u % Bolus: 59% % Basal: 41%

September 5, 2022

STATS	Serious Low: 0%	Low: 0%	Target Range: 94%	High: 6%	Serious High: 0%	Median BG: 139 mg/dL	Average BG: 138 mg/dL

Total Carbs: 335 g # of Boluses: 9 Total Bolus Units: 45.8 u Total Basal Units: 23.5 u % Bolus: 66% % Basal: 34%

[Color—Print (Color Gallery page CG18) or web & ePub editions]

Case 3

A 45-year-old man presents for a routine follow-up appointment. Type 1 diabetes was diagnosed at age 30 years. He current treatment regimen consists of multiple daily insulin injections with insulin detemir, 9 units twice daily, and insulin aspart via an InPen connected pen for his meal via carbohydrate counting. He also uses Dexcom G6 CGM. He would like to improve his hemoglobin A_{1c} level (current value = 7.5% [58 mmol/mol]). His CGM tracing and InPen data are shown (*Figure 5, following page*).

Which of the following is the most likely cause of this patient's wide glycemic variability?

A. Insulin-to-carbohydrate ratio is too strong, and the patient reduces doses of mealtime insulin

B. Basal insulin dose is excessive and causes hypoglycemia between meals

C. Patient is overriding boluses and rarely using the bolus calculator

D. Correction factor is not strong enough and does not reduce hyperglycemia when the patient uses the correction dose via the bolus calculator

E. Active insulin time is too long, and the bolus calculator does not allow the patient to take frequent correction doses

Answer: C) Patient is overriding boluses and rarely using the bolus calculator

If one uses the stepped approach to interpreting the CGM data in *Figure 5*, it becomes clear that there are sufficient data to analyze with 97.8% active CGM time.

Question: What is the problem?
Answer: Low time-in-range at 52% with a high coefficient of variability at 41.6%, and above target time-above-range.

Question: Where is the problem?
Answer: The ambulatory glucose profile clearly shows midday hyperglycemia.

Figure 5A. Data Derived From Dexcom Clarity Device

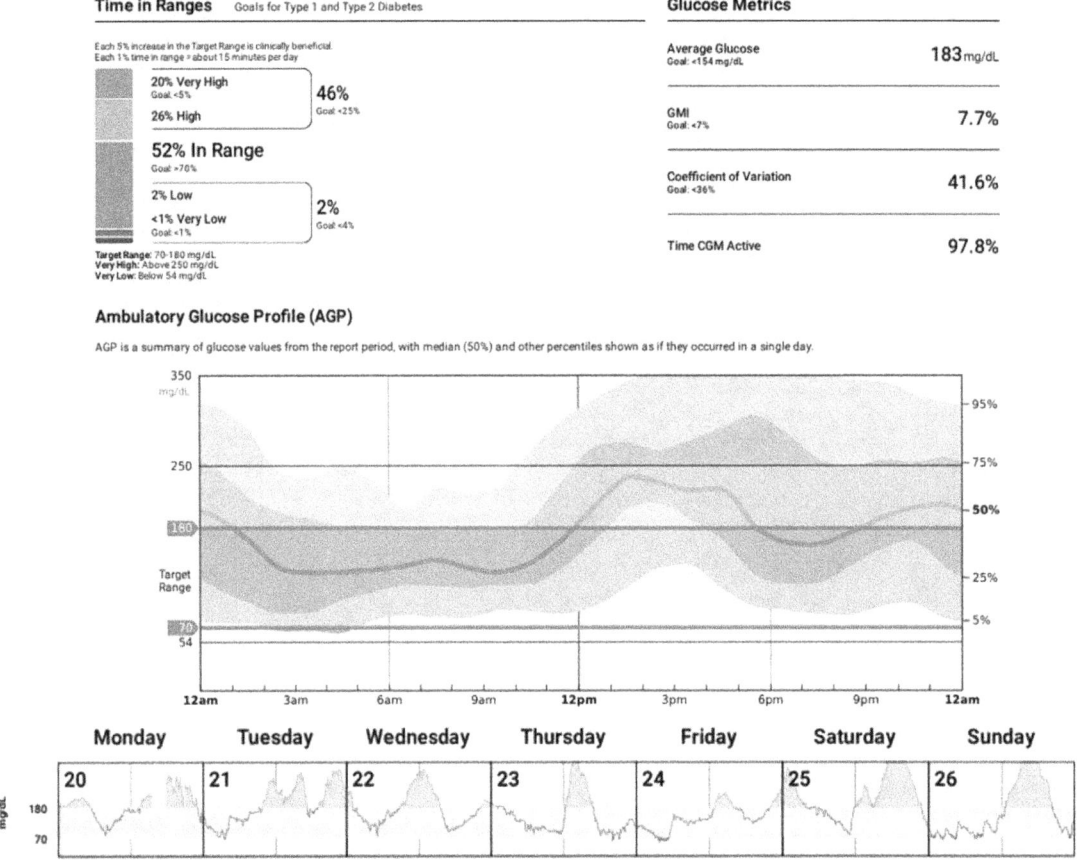

[Color—Print (Color Gallery page CG19) or web & ePub editions]

Figure 5B. Data Derived From InPen Device

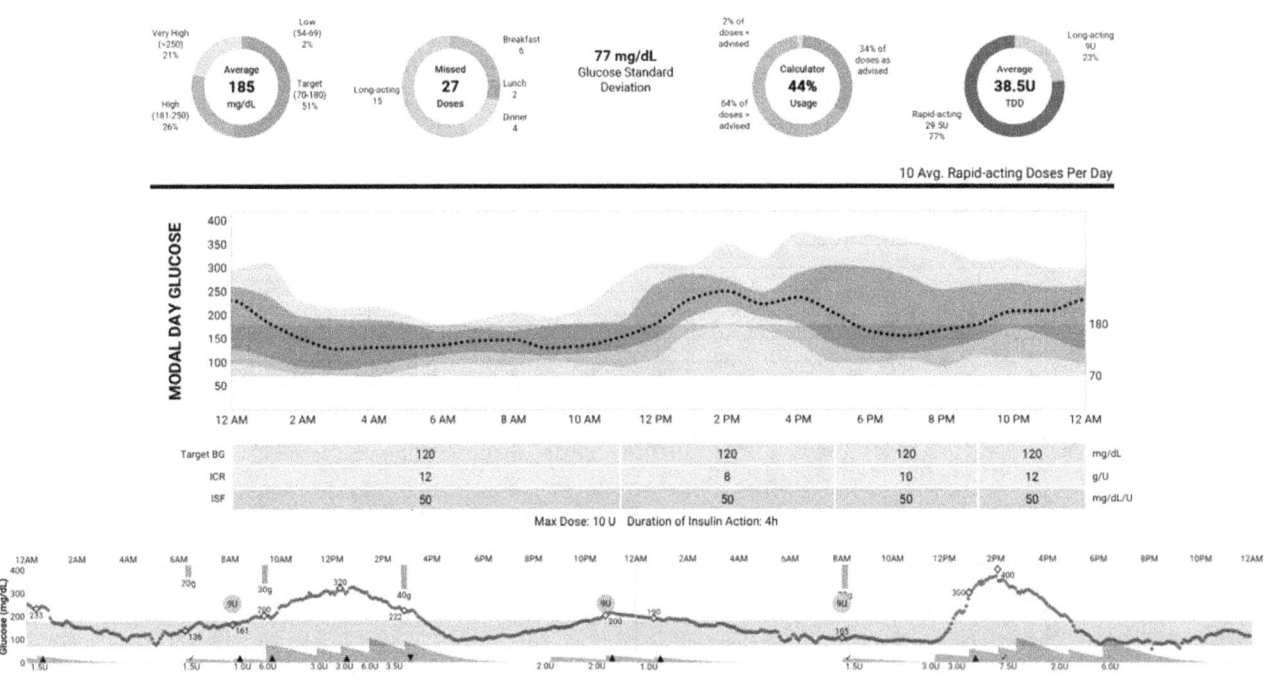

[Color—Print (Color Gallery page CG19) or web & ePub editions]

Question: How should therapy be adjusted?

Answer: The InPen report shows that the patient uses the bolus calculator only 44% of the time and overrides the bolus calculator many times during the day (Answer C), taking 4 to 6 boluses for the midday meal on more than 1 day. Therefore, the patient must be counseled on how to use the bolus calculator and adjust the insulin-to-carbohydrate ratio. Meal planning should be discussed to optimize postprandial glucose concentrations.

The patient takes many boluses at lunchtime, whereas the breakfast boluses are adequate. This suggests that the insulin-to-carbohydrate ratio at lunch may not be aggressive enough (thus, Answer A is incorrect).

There is no hypoglycemia between meals or overnight, the glucose concentrations are stable overnight, and patient wakes up with glucose values between 105 and 110 mg/dL (5.8-6.1 mmol/L) (thus, Answer B is incorrect).

The patient is not using the correction, so the correction factor cannot be evaluated until patient uses the bolus calculator more often and data are generated for review (thus, Answer D is incorrect).

The duration of insulin does not seem to affect postprandial hyperglycemia (thus, Answer E is incorrect). Generally, a duration of insulin set at 4 hours is accepted as ideal for adults who are taking multiple daily injections. This is expected to limit the occurrence of insulin stacking that could take place with a shorter active insulin time, allowing correction doses too close to each other.

Key Learning Points

- There are multiple CGM systems with different features, and providers must be knowledgeable on the nuances of these systems and be proficient in interpreting the reports with a systematic, stepped approach.

- There are multiple AID systems, and providers should be familiar with the details of each system's specific features, so that they can best advise patients and set realistic expectations for each system.

- AID reports contain valuable information that can guide providers in understanding the patient's behavior and deciding how to best adjust settings to optimize outcomes.

References

1. Galindo RJ, Aleppo G. Continuous glucose monitoring: the achievement of 100 years of innovation in diabetes technology. *Diabetes Res Clin Pract.* 2020;170:108502. PMID: 33065179

2. Sherr JL, Heinemann L, Fleming GA, et al. Automated insulin delivery: benefits, challenges, and recommendations. A consensus report of the Joint Diabetes Technology Working Group of the European Association for the Study of Diabetes and the American Diabetes Association. *Diabetologia.* 2023;66(1):3-22. PMID: 36198829

3. ElSayed NA, Aleppo G, Aroda VR, et al; American Diabetes Association. 1. Improving care and promoting health in populations: standards of care in diabetes-2023. *Diabetes Care.* 2023;46(Suppl 1):S10-S18. PMID: 36507639

4. Pickup JC, Ford Holloway M, Samsi K. Real-time continuous glucose monitoring in type 1 diabetes: a qualitative framework analysis of patient narratives. *Diabetes Care.* 2015;38(4):544-550. PMID: 25552422

5. Tanenbaum ML, Adams RN, Lanning MS, et al. Using cluster analysis to understand clinician readiness to promote continuous glucose monitoring adoption. *J Diabetes Sci Technol.* 2018;12(6):1108-1115. PMID: 29991281

6. AAFP. Medicare expands coverage of continuous glucose monitoring. https://www.aafp.org/pubs/fpm/blogs/gettingpaid/entry/medicare-cgm-expansion.html. Accessed December 11, 2023.

7. Patil SP, Albanese-O'Neill A, Yehl K, Seley JJ, Hughes AS. Professional competencies for diabetes technology use in the care setting. *Sci Diabetes Self Manag Care.* 2022;48(5):437-445. PMID: 36048025

8. Szmuilowicz ED, Aleppo G. Stepwise approach to continuous glucose monitoring interpretation for internists and family physicians. *Postgrad Med.* 2022;134(8):743-751. PMID: 35930313

9. Phillip M, Nimri R, Bergenstal RM, et al. Consensus recommendations for the use of automated insulin delivery technologies in clinical practice. *Endocr Rev.* 2023;44(2):254-280. PMID: 36066457

Addressing Social Determinants of Health in Routine Diabetes Care

A. Enrique Caballero, MD. Latino Diabetes Health, Division of Endocrinology, Diabetes, and Hypertension; Division of Global Health Equity, Brigham and Women's Hospital; International Innovation Programs, Harvard Medical School, Boston, Massachusetts; Email: enrique_caballero@hms.harvard.edu

Educational Objectives

- Evaluate social determinants of health (SDOH) in routine diabetes care.

- Describe how medical, psychological, social, financial, and cultural factors influence patients' diabetes self-care behaviors.

- Identify the widespread presence of unconscious biases among health care professionals that may affect clinical outcomes of people living with diabetes.

Significance of the Clinical Problem

Important scientific and technological advances have been made in the field of diabetes over the last few decades. However, most people living with diabetes across the world are not achieving common treatment targets. In the United States, only 1 in 4 people with diabetes have achieved hemoglobin A_{1c}, blood pressure, and non–HDL-cholesterol targets and nonsmoking status.[1] Many individuals who do not achieve basic treatment goals are likely to develop diabetes-related chronic complications, which often shorten their lifespan and negatively affect their quality of life. In addition to the huge burden diabetes can impose on people living with the disease, as well as on

their families, health care systems are constantly facing enormous challenges in providing optimal diabetes care at a reasonable cost. A significant proportion of health care dollars is spent on patients who are often hospitalized due to severe acute and chronic diabetes-related complications.[2]

Why is it that despite all the great scientific advances in diabetes care, we are not yet able to help the majority of individuals achieve treatment goals? Although multiple complex factors related to patients, health care providers, health care systems, and political and social structures certainly contribute to suboptimal health care, the lack of solid efforts across the board to address SDOH in routine diabetes care has a major role.[3]

According to the World Health Organization, SDOH are the conditions in which people are born, grow, live, work, and age. These circumstances are shaped by the distribution of money, power, and resources at global, national, and local levels. The SDOH are mostly responsible for health inequities—the unfair and avoidable differences in health status seen within and between countries.[4]

Practice Gaps

- Clinicians often underestimate the effect that SDOH have on patients' diabetes self-care behaviors.

- The limited time available to interact with patients in routine clinical practice, as well as the common lack of multidisciplinary diabetes care teams, makes health care professionals particularly address the traditional "biomedical" factors, paying very little attention to SDOH.

- Health care professionals may not be fully aware of specific strategies to incorporate the evaluation of SDOH into routine diabetes care.

- Clinicians are often not familiar with local, regional, and national programs that may be beneficial for people living with diabetes who struggle financially to implement expected diabetes self-care behaviors.

- Health care professionals need to enhance their knowledge, competence, and performance skills to effectively address social, financial, emotional, and cultural challenges in diverse patient populations.

Discussion

The impact of SDOH on the development and course of diabetes has been well demonstrated, and it is highly recommended that health care professionals address patients' social and cultural factors in routine clinical activities.[3,5,6] Multiple social factors routinely affect patients' health status. Five general categories are shown in *Box 1*[3]:

Box 1. Social Determinants of Health in Patients With Diabetes

---

1. Socioeconomic status (education, income, occupation)

2. Neighborhood and physical environment (housing, built environment, toxic environmental exposures)

3. Food environment (food insecurity, food access, food availability, food affordability)

4. Health care (access, affordability, quality)

5. Social context (social cohesion, social capital, social support)

Adapted from Hill-Briggs F et al. Diabetes Care, 2020; 44(1): 258–79. © by the American Diabetes Association.[3]

Socioeconomic Status

Socioeconomic status is a multidimensional construct that includes educational, economic, and occupational status. Lower socioeconomic status has been clearly associated with higher prevalence rates of type 2 diabetes and its complications, as well as higher mortality rates.[7] Engaging in adequate diabetes self-care behaviors is an expensive task. We often recommend that patients improve their meal plans and physical activity; these behaviors usually require proper financial means to be achieved. In addition, the cost of regular glucose monitoring and multiple medications to help them control their diabetes and related disorders can be quite challenging. People living with diabetes are expected to take 8 to 10 different medications on a regular basis; some are for diabetes management and others are for conditions frequently present such as hypertension, dyslipidemia, obesity, cardiovascular disease, kidney disease, etc. Even if patients have health insurance coverage, the "copay" (obligatory out-of-pocket expense for obtaining most medications) is often prohibitive.

Socioeconomic status can be assessed through information related to education level, income, and occupation.[3]

Neighborhood and Physical Environment

Housing instability among individuals with diabetes has been associated with increased use of outpatient services.[8] Not having a stable home influences diabetes self-care behavior. Patients with diabetes may not have access to homemade foods or safe and proper places to store their medications.

The built environment, as defined by the US Centers for Disease Control and Prevention, includes the physical parts of where people live and work, such as infrastructure, buildings, streets, and open spaces. Walkability is the ability to safely walk to services and amenities within a reasonable distance, and it has been associated with diabetes-related outcomes. In general, more walkable neighborhoods are associated with lower prevalence and incidence rates of type 2 diabetes.[8] Toxic environmental exposures are also becoming highly relevant in diabetes care and should be assessed in routine clinical practice.[3]

Food Environment

The Centers for Disease Control define food environment as the physical presence of food that affects a person's diet; a person's proximity to food store locations; the distribution of food stores, food service, and any physical entity by which food may be obtained; or a connected system that allows access to food. Key dimensions of the food environment include accessibility, availability, affordability, and quality. It is clear that in some geographical areas around the country and the world, access to healthy and affordable foods is quite challenging. People living with diabetes are often affected by not having access to the foods that are generally recommend to them. Patient and family education about how to improve eating habits within their budget is of paramount importance. An open discussion about how the food environment is affecting patients' diabetes self-care behaviors should routinely take place in health care.[3,5,6]

Health Care

Having health insurance is the strongest predictor of whether adults with diabetes have access to diabetes screenings and care.[9] Furthermore, having both insurance and a usual source of care, rather than one or the other, confers the greatest odds of receiving at least minimum diabetes health care.

Affordability of current health care systems is quite challenging for many people living with diabetes. On average, health care costs of people with diabetes are 2.3 times those of people without diabetes. Approximately 14% to 20% of adults with diabetes report reducing or delaying medications due to their high cost. In fact, many patients are often left with the difficult decision of not taking their medications consistently to reduce costs. This phenomenon, known as cost-related or

cost-reducing nonadherence, is associated with income, insured status, and type of insurance.[3]

Regarding quality of diabetes care, having insurance is the strongest single predictor of whether adults with diabetes are likely to meet individual quality measures of diabetes care. Therefore, discussing with patients their health insurance coverage and its practical implications is not out of our scope of important factors to regularly incorporate into routine diabetes care.[3,5,6]

Social Context

Social capital is defined as the features of social structures that serve as resources for collective action (eg, interpersonal trust, reciprocity norms, and mutual aid). Social cohesion refers to the extent of connectedness and solidarity among groups in a community. Social support describes experiences in individuals' formal and informal personal relationships, as well as their perceptions of those relationships.[3] Interestingly, higher neighborhood social cohesion is associated with lower incidence of diabetes.[10] Not surprisingly, increased social support is often associated with improved glycemic control and better quality of life among people living with diabetes.

Therefore, discussing patients' social network is extremely important in routine diabetes care. People who are lonely in their fight against diabetes often struggle more than those who have a strong support system.[3,5,6]

Ultimately, it is important to remember that multiple medical, social, financial, psychological, and cultural factors influence the development and course of diabetes. Addressing these factors in routine diabetes care is crucial. The "A-to-Z" list of factors to consider when providing diabetes care is shown in *Box 2* (*following page*).

Box 2. A-to-Z Factors to Consider
When Providing Diabetes Care

Acculturation	Nutrition and Food Availability
Biology	Other Forms of Medicine
Clinicians' Cultural Awareness	Perception of Body Image
Depression and Emotional Distress	Quality of Life
Educational Level	Religion and Faith
Fears	Socioeconomic Status
Group Engagement/Family/ Community Support	Technology
Health Literacy	Unconscious Bias
Intimacy/Sexual Dysfunction	Vulnerable Groups
Judging	Why? (Always get the patient's perspective)
Knowledge of the Disease	Xercise!
Language	You Are in Charge. (Patient-Centered Approach)
Medical Adherence	Zip it! (Let the Patient Talk!)

Caballero AE. Front Endocrinol (Lausanne), 2018; 9(479): 1-15. © by the Author. Published by Frontiers Media S.A.[6]

[Color—Print (Color Gallery page CG20) or web & ePub editions]

Clinical Case Vignettes

Case 1

A 59-year-old Hispanic/Latina woman with type 2 diabetes has obesity, hypertension, dyslipidemia, and a history of coronary artery disease. She is asymptomatic. Her BMI is 33 kg/m^2 and blood pressure is 140/90 mm Hg.

Most recent laboratory test results:

Hemoglobin A$_{1c}$ = 8.6% (70 mmol/mol)
LDL cholesterol = 100 mg/dL (SI: 2.59 mmol/L)
Triglycerides = 180 mg/dL (SI: 2.03 mmol/L)
HDL cholesterol = 45 mg/dL (SI: 1.17 mmol/L)

Her kidney and liver function is normal. She lives in a small city with a high population of immigrants. She does not work outside the home; she is separated and has 3 children and 2 grandchildren. She does not speak English well, has low health literacy, and requires assistance to follow her treatment recommendations. Her health care coverage is limited. She lives with her oldest daughter and her family. She often misses her appointments because of transportation issues

and lives in an unsafe neighborhood. She has not been able to implement significant changes in her meal plan and has not engaged in regular physical activity. She has been prescribed oral antidiabetes agents, as well as medications for blood pressure and dyslipidemia.

What additional issue is the most important to address with the patient during this visit?

A. Fear of starting insulin injections due to specific cultural issues in the Latino/Hispanic population

B. The need to monitor blood glucose levels routinely to assess her glucose patterns more effectively

C. Referral to the cardiology department for further testing due to her high cardiovascular risk

D. Evaluation of food insecurity through the validated 2-item screening tool

E. Referral to a program to improve her English language skills to better engage in her visits with the diabetes care team

Answer: D) Evaluation of food insecurity through the validated 2-item screening tool

Evaluation of SDOH in all patients with diabetes is important.[3] This patient has provided information that allows you to have a better sense of the 5 major areas to explore in routine care.[3] You have an idea about her socioeconomic status, education, health literacy level, neighborhood and physical environment, food environment, and social context.

Health beliefs are influenced by race/ethnicity and culture. The fear to inject insulin (Answer A) due to the negative connotation it carries is common in many populations. The belief that insulin can cause complications such as blindness, in particular, is highly prevalent among many members of the Latino/Hispanic community.[11,12] It is always important to assess health beliefs in diabetes care.[3,6] However, it is uncertain whether insulin therapy is strictly necessary at this point in this patient's case.

Evaluation of glucose patterns (Answer B) is always important. However, unless this patient is taking a sulfonylurea, it is unlikely that she is having hypoglycemic episodes. Based on her hemoglobin A_{1c} value, she is likely experiencing both fasting and postprandial hyperglycemia.

Referral to cardiology (Answer C) does not seem to be warranted at this time. Certainly, addressing all cardiovascular risk factors and implementing strategies to reduce cardiovascular risk is paramount.

Referral to a program to improve her English language skills (Answer E) is certainly not adequate. She has low education and low health literacy levels. If desired by the patient, improving her English skills would be important. However, our commitment as health care professionals is to provide optimal diabetes care to everyone regardless of their preferred language. Ensuring we have well-trained interpreters in our health care systems and adequate culturally and socially oriented patient education materials and programs is crucial.[3,5,6]

The best answer is to evaluate food insecurity through the validated 2-item screening tool (Answer D) Food insecurity is defined as limited or uncertain access to adequate, nutritious food for an active and healthy lifestyle. It is estimated that up to 14% of people living with diabetes have food insecurity. In this particular patient, assessing whether food insecurity is an issue is of paramount importance. A validated 2-item screening tool has been widely recommended:

1. Within past 12 months, we worried whether our food would run out before we got money to buy more.

2. Within past 12 months, the food we bought just didn't last and we didn't have money to get more.

Affirmative response to either item has a sensitivity of 97% and specificity of 83%.

Openly discussing with patients whether food insecurity is a problem should be incorporated in routine diabetes care.

Case 1 (continued)

The patient reports she has food insecurity. In fact, she lives in an area of the country that is considered a food desert. Access to adequate foods is challenging.

Which of the following is the best course of action regarding her food insecurity?

A. Include this important piece of information in her medical record, so that other health care professionals are aware of the situation

B. Refer her to the department in the clinic or hospital where other health care professionals can provide guidance on how to face this challenge

C. Refer her to local, regional, or national programs for which she may qualify to help her obtain healthier foods at a lower or no cost

D. Discuss specific changes in her meal plan she can start implementing that consider her limited budget and limited access to nutritious foods

E. All the above

Answer: E) All the above

All these strategies are likely to help the patient in this challenging situation (Answer E). It is important for health care professionals to become familiar with how to evaluate food insecurity, discuss this sensitive issue with patients, and, most importantly, identify programs and activities that can help patients and families with this crucial situation. Clinics and hospitals across the country may have local programs that can be offered to patients. For instance, our group developed a program in which we were able to guide patients and families on how to obtain healthier foods within their budget. This particular program involved visits to the supermarket with patients and their families along with culturally and socially oriented education activities.[13] Peer-to-peer education programs can also be helpful in guiding members of communities at high risk in improving their diabetes self-care behaviors.[14]

Case 2

A 45-year-old woman with a 10-year history of type 2 diabetes presents as a new patient. She has obesity, hypertension, and dyslipidemia. She is asymptomatic. Her BMI is 33 kg/m², and blood pressure is 140/90 mm Hg.

> Most recent laboratory test results:
> Hemoglobin A$_{1c}$ = 8.6% (70 mmol/mol)
> LDL cholesterol = 100 mg/dL (SI: 2.59 mmol/L)
> Triglycerides = 180 mg/dL (SI: 2.03 mmol/L)
> HDL cholesterol = 45 mg/dL (SI: 1.17 mmol/L)

Her kidney and liver function is normal. Both her primary care physician and the endocrinologist who last saw her have provided specific recommendations on how to improve her meal plan and physical activity. However, the patient has not been able to implement many changes in her meal plan and does not exercise routinely. She takes metformin and a sulfonylurea to control her diabetes, lisinopril for blood pressure, and a statin for LDL cholesterol.

Which of the following actions is the most appropriate now?

A. Review the meal plan and physical activity recommendations in more detail to ensure she understands what she needs to do to improve her metabolic status

B. Inquire about her medications and specifically address adherence to her current pharmacological regimen before considering the addition of and/or a change to a new medication

C. Ask her about specific challenges she is currently facing to implement recommended diabetes self-care behaviors

D. Obtain more information about her glucose patterns, ideally through continuous glucose monitoring, to ensure accurate data are available to gauge next steps in her treatment plan

E. A and B

Answer: C) Ask her about specific challenges she is currently facing to implement recommended diabetes self-care behaviors

Although all the above strategies could make sense in her case, the one that may prove to be the most useful now is asking her about particular challenges she is currently facing to implement recommended diabetes self-care behaviors (Answer C). Dedicating time during this initial visit to better understand the challenges she is facing in modifying her lifestyle and with her overall treatment plan is of paramount importance. A guided, respectful, and open conversation about her experience with living with diabetes is likely to uncover important information. Inquiring about the 5 areas of SDOH would be very helpful.

She has received information on how to improve her meal plan and physical activity multiple times. It is possible she has a general sense of what to do and reviewing again (Answer A) may be helpful. However, it is likely she is facing particular barriers in modifying her current lifestyle.

Evaluating adherence to pharmacological therapies (Answer B) is always important. However, it is uncertain whether just taking her medications more regularly would be enough to improve her glycemic control and that of other comorbidities.

Although continuous glucose monitoring (Answer D) may be very helpful for most people living with diabetes, this does not seem to be the best time to introduce a new strategy in her treatment plan when we do not know what barriers she may be facing in implementing diabetes treatment recommendations.

Case 2 (continued)

Additional information is learned about this patient. She is Hispanic/Latina, works full time as an accountant, is divorced, and has one son. She lives in a modest but safe neighborhood. She owns the apartment where she lives. She is fully bilingual and bicultural and explains that she is under constant stress due to her work and being a single mother. She has no difficulty in obtaining recommended foods but states she lacks the time and motivation to cook healthy meals at home. She has full health insurance and has been able to obtain all recommended medications. However, she is really frustrated by trying to improve her diabetes control without success. She feels lonely and says that she spends most of her time working and caring for her son.

After learning all this information, which of the following is the best next step?

A. Ask her to fill out the depression in diabetes 10-item survey

B. Apply the Patient Health Questionnaire-2 (PHQ-2)

C. Prescribe a third pharmacological agent to improve her diabetes control

D. Ask her to meet with a nutritionist to review her meal plan in more detail

E. None of the above

Answer: B) Apply the Patient Health Questionnaire-2 (PHQ-2)

There is no 10-item survey on depression in diabetes (Answer A).

Prescribing a third pharmacological agent to improve her diabetes control (Answer C) may not be sufficient since she is clearly struggling with implementing current recommendations.

Although meeting with a nutritionist (Answer D) is always important and helpful, this patient is going through particular challenges that underpin her overall lack of motivation to effectively engage in diabetes self-care behaviors.

A general assessment of 5 key areas of SDOH has taken place in this patient's case: her socioeconomic status, neighborhood and physical environment, food environment, health care access, and social context. The fact that she reports feeling lonely and is frustrated with her diabetes outcomes requires further evaluation of her emotional and psychological well-being. An important step would be to determine whether she is depressed. Asking her the 2 questions on the Patient Health Questionnaire-2 (PHQ-2) (Answer B) would be important: over the last 2 weeks, how often have you been bothered by the following problems: (a) little interest or pleasure in doing things and (b) feeling down, depressed, or hopeless.[15]

Certainly, this patient is one of many people living with diabetes who have diabetes-related emotional distress or depression. Proper evaluation of these conditions is important in routine diabetes care. Referral to experts in behavioral health would be the optimal strategy upon which all other recommendations can be further discussed and addressed.[6]

Case 3

A 70-year-old Black man comes for follow-up on his diabetes and related comorbidities. He has had type 2 diabetes for more than 20 years and has hypertension, obesity, and dyslipidemia. He reports shortness of breath when walking short distances. Congestive heart failure was diagnosed several years ago and he takes multiple medications to control all his medical problems. He has struggled over the years to implement self-care behaviors. He does not follow a good meal plan, exercise regularly, measure his blood glucose levels at home often, or take his medications regularly. His wife recently died of cancer, and he lives in an assisted living facility. He missed his last 2 appointments in the endocrinology department.

It is apparent that he has an exacerbation of congestive heart failure and is therefore referred him to the emergency department. This hospital is well known for having a great inpatient cardiology department. When you later check on his status, you learn that he was admitted to the general medicine department.

Which of the following is the most likely explanation for why this patient was admitted to the general medicine department instead of cardiology department?

A. The cardiology department is often so crowded with patients that there was simply no room for anyone else

B. The patient did not know there was an option as to where he should have been admitted and did not ask for any particular department

C. The health care professional in charge decided to admit the patient to the general medicine department instead of the cardiology department because she usually reserves the cardiology department for only particular cases

D. A and B

E. A, B, and C

Answer: E) A, B, and C

There is no doubt that this patient is one of many who need to be admitted to the hospital, and there is a lack of available rooms in many hospitals. It is also possible that patients do not have a good idea regarding the specific department where they should be hospitalized and rarely advocate for themselves in this type of situation.

The main point to raise in this case is that related to unconscious biases. "Implicit bias," also called "unconscious bias," refers to associations outside of conscious awareness that adversely affect one's perception of a person or group.[16] It is extremely common for health care professionals to have biases that influence decisions and behavior. Within the well-intended care provided to patients, health care professionals may favor special diagnostic and treatment strategies in some individuals and not in others. Could it be that the health care professional in charge of admitting this patient to the general medicine ward instead of the cardiology service has biases that favor some patients over others? A recent analysis of this particular situation at the Brigham and Women's Hospital, a large academic center considered one of the best in the country and the world (and where I have the privilege of working), showed that during a period it was more likely for Black and Hispanic patients with heart failure seen in the emergency department to be admitted to the general medicine department than to the cardiology department. White patients with the same condition were more likely to be admitted to the cardiology service. Clinical outcomes and hospitalization rates are usually better when patients are managed in the cardiology department.[17]

A careful analysis of the data related to patients' quality of care is of the upmost importance.

Identifying biases based on race/ethnicity, gender, age, sexual preference, disabilities, and other characteristics should be routinely performed in health care systems. It is an activity in which we all need to engage to correct underlying conditions that favor some patients. Ultimately, optimal health care for everyone is the goal. Optimal diabetes care is achievable if we combine the latest scientific advances with routine evaluation of SDOH and the implementation of fair and equitable measures across health care systems.

We should continue to be inspired by Sir William Osler, who once said, "The good physician treats the disease; the great physician treats the patient that has the disease."

Key Learning Points

- SDOH are the conditions in which people are born, grow, live, work, and age. They influence the development and progression of diabetes and related conditions.

- Addressing SDOH in routine diabetes care is warranted.

- Socioeconomic status, neighborhood and physical environment, food environment, health care, and social context are the 5 general categories that should be routinely evaluated in patients with diabetes.

- Multiple medical, psychological, social, financial, and cultural factors influence patients' diabetes self-care behaviors and must also be routinely assessed in clinical practice (the A-to-Z list).

- Referring patients to existing programs in health care institutions and/or the communities where patients live is extremely important.

- Identifying unconscious biases among health care professionals, administrators, and everyone who may participate in health care decisions is crucial. Implementing effective strategies to eliminate these biases is necessary in our common task of achieving optimal health care for all.

References

1. Chen Y, Rolka D, Xie H, Saydah S. Imputed state-level prevalence of achieving goals to prevent complications of diabetes in adults with self-reported diabetes - United States, 2017-2018. *MMWR Morb Mortal Wkly Rep.* 2020;69(45):1665-1670. PMID: 33180755

2. Caballero AE, Davidson J, Elmi A, et al. Previously unrecognized trends in diabetes consumption clusters in medicare. *Am J Manag Care.* 2013;19(7):541-548. PMID: 23919418

3. Hill-Briggs F, Adler NE, Berkowitz SA, et al. Social determinants of health and diabetes: a scientific review. *Diabetes Care.* 2020;44(1):258-279. PMID: 33139407

4. World Health Organization. Social determinants of health. www.who.int/social_determinants/sdh_definition/en/. Accessed Dec 27, 2023.

5. Caballero AE. Transcultural diabetes care: a call for addressing the patient as a whole. Invited commentary. *Endocr Pract.* 2019;25(7):766-768. PMID: 31298951

6. Caballero AE. The "A to Z" of managing type 2 diabetes in culturally diverse populations. *Front Endocrinol (Lausanne).* 2018;9:479. PMID: 30233490

7. Agardh E, Allebeck P, Hallqvist J, Moradi T, Sidorchuk A. Type 2 diabetes incidence and socio-economic position: a systematic review and meta-analysis. *Int J Epidemiol.* 2011;40(3):804-818. PMID: 21335614

8. Berkowitz SA, Meigs JB, DeWalt D, et al. Material need insecurities, control of diabetes mellitus, and use of health care resources: results of the Measuring Economic Insecurity in Diabetes study. *JAMA Intern Med.* 2015;175(2):257-265. PMID: 25545780

9. Kazemian P, Shebl FM, McCann N, Walensky RP, Wexler DJ. Evaluation of the cascade of diabetes care in the United States, 2005-2016. *JAMA Intern Med.* 2019;179(10):1376-1385. PMID: 31403657

10. Gebreab SY, Hickson DA, Sims M, et al. Neighborhood social and physical environments and type 2 diabetes mellitus in African Americans: the Jackson Heart Study. *Health Place.* 2017;43:128-137. PMID: 280

11. Aguayo-Mazzucato C, Diaque P, Hernandez S, Rosas S, Kostic A, Caballero AE. Understanding the growing epidemic of type 2 diabetes in the Hispanic population living in the United States. *Diabetes Metab Res Rev.* 2019;35(2):e3097. PMID: 30445663

12. Gutierrez RR, Ferro AM, Caballero AE. Myths and misconceptions about insulin therapy among Latinos/Hispanics with diabetes: a fresh look at an old problem. *J Diabetes Metab.* 2015;6:482.

13. Cortés DE, Millán-Ferro A, Schneider K, Vega RR, Caballero AE. Food purchasing selection among low-income, Spanish-speaking Latinos. *Am J Prev Med.* 2013;44(3 Suppl 3):S267-S273. PMID: 23415192

14. Castillo-Hernandez KG, Laviada-Molina H, Hernandez-Escalante VM, Molina-Segui F, Mena-Macossay L, Caballero AE. Peer support added to diabetes education improves metabolic control and quality of life in Mayan adults living with type 2 diabetes: a randomized controlled trial. *Can J Diabetes.* 2021;45(3):206-213. PMID: 33129754

15. Kroenke K, Spitzer RL, Williams JB. The Patient Health Questionnaire-2: validity of a two-item depression screener. *Medical Care.* 2003;41(11):1284-1292. PMID: 14583691

16. Caballero AE, ElSayed NA, Golden SH, Bannuru RR, Gregg B. Implicit or unconscious bias in diabetes care. *Clin Diabetes.* 2023.

17. Eberly LA, Wispelwey B, Richterman A, et al.Identification of racial inequities in access to specialized inpatient heart failure care at an academic medical center. *Circ Heart Fail.* 2019;12(11):e006214. PMID: 31658831

When to Consider Testing for Monogenic Diabetes

Kevin Colclough, DClinSci. Exeter Genomics Laboratory, Royal Devon University Healthcare NHS Foundation Trust, Exeter, United Kingdom; Email: kevin.colclough@nhs.net

Kashyap A. Patel, PhD. Exeter Genomics Laboratory, Royal Devon University Healthcare NHS Foundation Trust and University of Exeter Medical School, College of Biomedical Science, Exeter, United Kingdom; Email: k.a.patel@exeter.ac.uk

Educational Objectives

After reviewing this chapter, learners should be able to:

- Identify the clinical features that can trigger genetic testing for monogenic diabetes.

- Effectively use existing or novel biomarkers and tools to identify patients with a higher probability of having monogenic diabetes who should be offered genetic testing.

- Request the appropriate gene panel for patients being evaluated for monogenic diabetes.

Significance of the Clinical Problem

Monogenic diabetes is a rare familial form of diabetes caused by monoallelic or biallelic pathogenic variants in 1 of more than 60 different genes. Pathogenic variants typically cause diabetes due to β-cell dysfunction or destruction leading to reduced insulin secretion. Some pathogenic variants cause severe insulin resistance through dysfunction of the insulin receptor or dyslipidemia secondary to lipodystrophy. Monogenic diabetes can be inherited in an autosomal dominant or recessive manner, or a pathogenic variant can arise spontaneously (de novo). Some subtypes are associated with isolated diabetes and others with a multisystem disorder with additional extrapancreatic syndromic features. Monogenic diabetes is typically diagnosed in the neonatal period (before the age of 6 months; neonatal diabetes can be permanent or transient) or in adolescence and early adulthood. Maturity-onset diabetes of the young (MODY) is the most common subtype of monogenic diabetes and is responsible for 2% to 4% of all patients with diabetes diagnosed between the ages of 1 and 30 years.[1] MODY has an autosomal dominant mode of inheritance, and affected patients typically presents with nonsyndromic, non–insulin-dependent diabetes in adolescence or early adulthood (median age of diagnosis, 17 years).[2] Affected individuals typically do not have obesity and may have a parent with diabetes. Neonatal diabetes is a rare subtype of monogenic diabetes that presents in the first 6 months of life. In the transient form, diabetes typically remits within 3 months of diagnosis and may relapse in adolescence/adult life. The prevalence of neonatal diabetes is approximately 1 in 100,000. Syndromic forms of monogenic diabetes may be diagnosed at any age from the neonatal period to early adulthood and exhibit a wide range of additional characteristic features with variable clinical expressivity and penetrance.

The genetic diagnosis of monogenic diabetes is important since the specific genetic subtype determines the most effective treatment. Patients with GCK-MODY have mild, stable fasting hyperglycemia from birth that does not increase the risk of microvascular and macrovascular complications. Hyperglycemia in *GCK*-MODY cannot be changed by treatment, and therefore does not require therapy.[3] Conversely, the *HNF1A*- and *HNF4A*-MODY subtypes can be well controlled with low-dosage sulfonylurea therapy.[4] The permanent neonatal diabetes caused by pathogenic variants in the potassium channel genes *KCNJ11* and *ABCC8* also responds to sulfonylurea therapy but requires a significantly higher dosage.[5] The transient form of *KCNJ11* and *ABCC8* neonatal diabetes requires a lower dosage of sulfonylurea, and if there is a relapse of diabetes in later life, this will also respond well to low-dosage sulfonylurea therapy.[6] Syndromic forms of monogenic diabetes are typically managed with insulin. A diagnosis of monogenic diabetes also has implications for clinical management during pregnancy and the risk of the fetus being large-for-gestational-age. *HNF4A* pathogenic variants cause fetal hyperinsulinism in utero resulting in an average birth weight increase of 700 g and risk of neonatal hyperinsulinemic hypoglycemia.[7] A fetus that does not inherit a MODY-causing *GCK* variant from their hyperglycemic mother is also at increased risk of being large-for-gestational-age due to the fetal pancreas sensing the maternal hyperglycemia and increasing insulin secretion, leading to increased fetal growth and birth weight.[3] In addition to informing the management of hyperglycemia, the diagnosis can provide important prognostic information, opportunities for testing family members, and counseling on the risk of diabetes to healthy at-risk relatives or to future offspring. For example, finding the mitochondrial DNA pathogenic variant m.3243A>G in a patient with isolated diabetes can inform the risk of developing additional symptoms associated with mitochondrial disease (eg, myopathy and hearing loss) and help counsel the family that the variant will only be transmitted when the affected parent is female (due to maternal inheritance of mitochondrial DNA). Noninvasive prenatal genetic testing of cell-free fetal DNA in maternal blood is available in the United Kingdom to assist in the management of pregnancies affected by *GCK*- and *HNF4A*-MODY.[8]

Identifying individuals with suspected monogenic diabetes in routine clinical practice is challenging due to the high background prevalence of young-onset polygenic type 1 and type 2 diabetes. Despite important clinical implications and advances in sequencing technology that enable rapid testing of all monogenic diabetes subtypes in a single assay, currently in the United Kingdom there is a median 3-year delay from diabetes diagnosis to the correct diagnosis of monogenic diabetes (based on unpublished data from 255 individuals with monogenic diabetes diagnosed by the Exeter Genomics Laboratory from January 1, 2021, to November 12, 2023, and an estimated 70% of cases in the United Kingdom have not yet been diagnosed.[9] There are 5 main reasons for this: (1) monogenic diabetes is rare; therefore, these cases are lost among the much higher background prevalence of young-onset polygenic type 1 and type 2 diabetes; (2) no simple clinical criteria accurately identify all patients with monogenic diabetes; (3) patients with monogenic diabetes have clinical features that overlap with the more common types of diabetes (eg, the traditional clinical diagnostic criteria for MODY; diagnosed <25 years, not–insulin-treated, and a parent affected with diabetes]), resulting in a genetic diagnosis in less than half of cases[9]; (4) a lack of genetics training and awareness of monogenic diabetes among endocrinologists; and (5) limited access to monogenic diabetes genetic testing globally.

Practice Gaps

- Lack of awareness of the clinical features that characterize patients with monogenic diabetes and the ability to differentiate from those with common polygenic disease.

- Suboptimal knowledge of the current tools/investigations/biomarkers/biochemical tests that can help identify patients with a higher probability of having monogenic diabetes who should be offered genetic testing.

Discussion

Clinical Features of Monogenic Diabetes

Although there is significant phenotypic overlap between monogenic and common types of diabetes, there are certain features that either individually, or in combination, can identify patients with suspected monogenic diabetes who should be offered genetic testing. Neonatal onset of diabetes (diagnosed before age 6 months) is a stand-alone criterion for genetic testing, regardless of any other clinical features. This is because more than 90% of these patients have a monogenic cause and nearly half have a pathogenic variant in a potassium channel gene (*KCNJ11* or *ABCC8*) and can be treated with sulfonylurea.[10] The presence of additional nonautoimmune syndromic features (eg, kidney cysts, deafness, neurologic disease, intellectual disability/developmental delay) in a patient with nonautoimmune diabetes (ie, negative islet autoantibodies and a low polygenic risk for type 1 diabetes) is also a strong indication for genetic testing with nearly 20% having monogenic diabetes.[11]

However, there is no single clinical feature that is suggestive of a MODY diagnosis, and affected patients have overlapping features with type 1 and type 2 diabetes. Combining some key discriminatory features using a statistical model (the MODY probability calculator) is a very powerful tool to identify patients who are most likely to have MODY. The MODY calculator is freely accessible at https://www.diabetesgenes.org/exeter-diabetes-app/ModyCalculator. It combines the patient's age, age at diabetes diagnosis, sex, BMI, current hemoglobin A_{1c} value, current treatment, time to insulin treatment, and parental diabetes status to provide a probability.[12] This is not a tool that returns a yes or no answer for selecting patients, but rather provides a percentage likelihood of a diagnosis. Health care providers can determine their own thresholds for testing depending on resources available and the number of patients they have the capacity to test. Some MODY subtypes are associated with additional characteristic features that can increase likelihood of a genetic diagnosis. *HNF4A* pathogenic variants causing MODY also result in hyperinsulinism in utero that results in an average birth weight increase of 700 g for a fetus that inherits the variant from either parent, and the newborn will be at risk of hyperinsulinemic hypoglycemia.[7] *GCK*-MODY has a very characteristic blood glucose profile (fasting blood glucose in range of 99-145 mg/dL [5.5-8.0 mmol/L], 2-hour increment <54 mg/dL [<3 mmol/L]) in 70% of patients and a hemoglobin A_{1c} value in the range of 5.5% to 7.5% [40-60 mmol/mol]) that is stable, persistent from birth, asymptomatic, and not changed by treatment.[3] *GCK*-MODY is typically incidentally diagnosed and accounts for approximately 40% of cases of asymptomatic pediatric hyperglycemia[13] and 30% of gestational diabetes cases in women with fasting blood glucose values greater than 99 mg/dL (>5.5 mmol/L) and a BMI less than 25 kg/m². [14]

Biomarkers

There are no generalized biomarkers for all subtypes of monogenic diabetes. Therefore, the aim of these biochemical tests is to exclude patients with likely type 1 and type 2 diabetes from having genetic testing. Islet autoantibody positivity (GAD, IA2A, IAA, and ZnT8) can be used as an exclusionary test because the probability of having a single positive antibody and MODY is less than 1 in 8000.[15] Antibody testing has the highest sensitivity when performed at diagnosis but can be undertaken at any time after diagnosis (acknowledging that a decline in antibody titers over time can lead to a negative result that may have been positive at diagnosis) and should be performed in all patients with insulin-treated diabetes. Persistent endogenous secretion is a strong feature of the most common subtypes of MODY (*GCK, HNF1A, HNF4A*) but can also be seen in other rarer subtypes such as *WFS1*-related diabetes. In contrast, more than 95% of patients with type 1 diabetes have severe endogenous insulin deficiency. Therefore, the presence of C-peptide (nonfasting blood C-peptide >0.6 ng/mL [>200 pmol/L]) 3 years after diagnosis in a patient with clinically diagnosed type 1 diabetes and negative islet autoantibodies is a strong indication for genetic testing. In other words, severe insulin deficiency (C-peptide <0.6 ng/mL [<200 pmol/L]) in a patient with clinically suspected type 1 diabetes effectively rules out the most common subtypes of MODY. However, it is important to be aware that C-peptide is a marker of endogenous insulin secretion and not a marker of all monogenic diabetes subtypes. There are rare subtypes in which C-peptide can be very low, including diabetes due to pathogenic variants in the *HNF1B* and *INS* genes, K-ATP channel gene variants causing permanent neonatal diabetes mellitus, and the mitochondrial DNA pathogenic variant m.3243A>G.

The identification of monogenic diabetes within a large population of polygenic type 2 diabetes with negative islet autoantibodies and normal C-peptide is more challenging. Continuous variables (age of diagnosis, BMI) are more discriminatory but are best combined with other features using a validated probability model such as the MODY calculator to help select patients for genetic testing. However, additional markers such as low HDL cholesterol and high triglycerides and other features of insulin resistance with obesity (acanthosis nigricans, hyperandrogenism, hypertension) point towards type 2 diabetes. Identifying good candidates for genetic testing is especially difficult in nonWhite populations such as patients from South Asia and the Middle East where there is a significantly higher background prevalence of young-onset type 2 diabetes at a lower BMI threshold for increased risk of insulin resistance.[16]

Clinical Case Vignettes

Case 1

A 23-year-old woman is newly diagnosed with diabetes. Her hemoglobin A_{1c} value at diagnosis was 9.3% (78 mmol/mol). She has no family history of diabetes, and her BMI is 24 kg/m². Type 1 diabetes is suspected, and she is started on a basal-bolus regimen (10 units of long-acting insulin and 1 to 5 units of short-acting insulin with meals). She mentions she was acutely unwell at birth and required insulin for a few months as a neonate. Her birth weight was 2.7 kg at full term. Her islet autoantibodies are negative and MODY probability is 4.9%.

Which of the following is the most appropriate recommendation regarding genetic testing for this patient?

A. Genetic testing is not indicated because the MODY probability is very low

B. Genetic testing for MODY should be performed despite low prior probability of MODY

C. Genetic testing should be performed for all monogenic diabetes subtypes that includes neonatal diabetes genes

D. Genetic testing should be performed for monogenic diabetes only after a positive C-peptide measurement

Answer: C) Genetic testing should be performed for all monogenic diabetes subtypes that includes neonatal diabetes genes

This patient had transient neonatal diabetes diagnosed when she was younger than 6 months. Therefore, genetic testing is recommended regardless of any other clinical features or biomarker test results. A test that includes all subtypes of neonatal diabetes is essential (Answer C). Sequencing methodologies will not detect methylation defects at the 6q24 locus, which account for 70% of cases of transient neonatal diabetes, and this must be assessed using a methylation- and dosage-sensitive assay when there is a clinical suspicion of transient neonatal diabetes.

Case 1 (continued)

Genetic testing documents a pathogenic variant in the *ABCC8* gene.

Which of the following is the best management of this patient's diabetes?

A. Recommend no treatment change because her diabetes will remit

B. Add a sulfonylurea to her insulin regimen

C. Stop insulin treatment and start a low-dosage sulfonylurea

D. Stop insulin treatment and start a sulfonylurea after C-peptide testing to confirm endogenous insulin secretion

E. Increase the insulin dosage

Answer: D) Stop insulin treatment and start a sulfonylurea after C-peptide testing to confirm endogenous insulin secretion

Patients in the relapsing diabetes stage of transient neonatal diabetes should respond well to sulfonylurea therapy and insulin can be discontinued. The safe practice in all scenarios where a patient is being transitioned from insulin to low-dosage sulfonylurea is to establish the level of endogenous insulin production prior to changing the regimen (Answer D).

Case 2

A 24-year-old South Asian woman (BMI = 21 kg/m^2) is referred for gestational diabetes screening at 28 weeks' gestation. Gestational diabetes is diagnosed based on a 75-g 2-hour oral glucose tolerance test: fasting blood glucose/0 hour = 111 mg/dL (6.2 mmol/L) and 2-hour value = 160 mg/dL (8.9 mmol/L). She is treated with insulin during pregnancy (30 units long-acting insulin overnight and 5 to 10 units of short-acting insulin with meals). Her slim mother also had gestational diabetes in her 2 pregnancies and was treated with metformin for type 2 diabetes after her second pregnancy.

Which of the following is the most appropriate recommendation regarding genetic testing for this patient?

A. Do not test because she has gestational diabetes

B. Use the results of the MODY probability calculator to decide whether to test

C. Test for pathogenic variants in all known monogenic diabetes genes

D. Test for pathogenic variants in the *GCK* gene only

Answer: D) Test for pathogenic variants in the GCK gene only

This patient has gestational diabetes but does not have a formal diagnosis of diabetes, so testing for other monogenic diabetes subtypes is not indicated now. Approximately 1 in 3 patients with gestational diabetes diagnosed with a fasting glucose value greater than 99 mg/dL (>5.5 mmol/L) and a BMI less than 25 kg/m^2 have *GCK*-MODY. Although *GCK*-MODY can be diagnosed through sequencing of all known monogenic diabetes genes by next-generation sequencing, a more rapid and cheaper Sanger sequencing method can be used to sequence *GCK* only (Answer D). This is a better first-line test option when the clinical suspicion and prior probability of a diagnosis of *GCK*-MODY is high. This applies to atypical gestational diabetes cases or children with mild hyperglycemia. A rapid diagnosis of *GCK*-MODY is particularly useful in patients with gestational diabetes because subsequent noninvasive prenatal testing can be undertaken to help guide clinical management of the pregnancy.

Case 3

A 37-year-old White man who developed diabetes at age 27 years undergoes medical review. His BMI is 28 kg/m^2. He has been treated with insulin from the time of diagnosis (basal-bolus regimen with a total daily dose of 0.8 units/kg per day) with a hemoglobin A$_{1c}$ value of 7.8% (62 mmol/mol). All islet autoantibodies were tested recently and are negative. His mother and maternal aunt have diabetes; they are both slim and treated with metformin and insulin. His 15-year-old daughter was diagnosed with diabetes at age 12 years and is treated with an insulin pump. She tested positive for GAD and IA2 autoantibodies. The

MODY probability calculator score for this man is low (8%).

Which of the following is the most appropriate recommendation regarding genetic testing for this patient?

A. Do not test because the most likely diagnosis is type 1 diabetes

B. Perform genetic testing now

C. Transition his treatment regimen from insulin to a sulfonylurea and consider genetic testing if glycemic control improves and there is no diabetic ketoacidosis

D. Measure C-peptide first and proceed with genetic testing only if C-peptide is greater than 0.6 ng/mL (>200 pmol/L)

Answer: D) Measure C-peptide first and proceed with genetic testing only if C-peptide is greater than 0.6 ng/mL (>200 pmol/L)

Given this patient's long duration of diabetes (>5 years), C-peptide is very likely to be negative if the diagnosis is type 1 diabetes. C-peptide measurement is a quick, inexpensive, and widely available first-line test (compared with genetic testing), and it significantly increases the likelihood of a diagnosis of monogenic diabetes if positive (Answer D). Treatment changes should not be undertaken without first confirming the genetic diagnosis of the monogenic diabetes subtype that would lead to the change.

Case 3 (continued)

The patient's random nonfasting C-peptide measurement is 1057 ng/mL (350 pmol/L).

Which of the following genetic testing options is most appropriate?

A. Testing for MODY only for the father

B. Testing for all forms of monogenic diabetes, including syndromic and mitochondrial diabetes, for the father

C. Testing for *GCK*-MODY only for the daughter

D. Testing for neonatal diabetes only for the daughter

E. Recommend no genetic testing since the lab results are consistent with polygenic type 1 diabetes mellitus

Answer: B) Testing for all forms of monogenic diabetes, including syndromic and mitochondrial diabetes, for the father

Approximately 20% of individuals referred for MODY testing have a pathogenic variant in a syndromic monogenic diabetes gene, and a genetic diagnosis might be missed if comprehensive testing of both MODY and syndromic genes (Answer B) is not undertaken. In this vignette, the daughter has confirmed type 1 diabetes and should not be tested as the proband in this family.

Case 3 (continued)

Genetic testing for all known subtypes of monogenic diabetes is undertaken in the father, and the mitochondrial DNA pathogenic variant m.3243A>G is identified, thus confirming a diagnosis of mitochondrial diabetes.

Which of the following is an appropriate action based on this result?

A. Transition the patient's regimen from insulin to metformin

B. Assess for other clinical features associated with the m.3243A>G variant

C. Advise the patient that his daughter with diabetes should be tested to confirm she also has mitochondrial diabetes

D. Transition the patient's regimen from insulin to high-dosage sulfonylurea

Answer: B) Assess for other clinical features associated with the m.3243A>G variant

This particular variant is associated with other extrapancreatic clinical features (Answer B), and in individuals with diabetes this is most likely to be bilateral sensorineural hearing loss as part of the maternally inherited diabetes and deafness

(MIDD) syndrome. Other less common features include myopathy (including skeletal and cardiac muscle), kidney disease (specifically focal and segmental glomerulosclerosis), short stature, retinal changes, and gastrointestinal problems. The clinical expressivity of these features is highly variable even among individuals in the same family, and patients commonly have isolated diabetes without deafness. This is likely related to the level of heteroplasmy in specific tissues, and this makes predicting disease progression challenging.

Insulin is the most appropriate treatment for mitochondrial diabetes and should be continued (thus, Answers A and D are incorrect).

Because mitochondrial DNA is maternally inherited, he was never at risk for transmitting the variant to his daughter and genetic testing of his offspring (Answer C) is not required.

Key Learning Points

- All patients younger than 6 months who are diagnosed with diabetes should be referred for genetic testing regardless of their current age and diabetes status, and regardless of antibody and C-peptide results.

- Pathogenic variants in the *GCK* gene are a common cause of gestational diabetes in slim women and have important implications for clinical management of the pregnancy.

GCK genetic testing should be offered to all women with gestational diabetes and a fasting blood glucose value greater than 99 mg/dL (>5.5 mmol/L) and BMI less than 25 kg/m^2.

- Islet autoantibodies and C-peptide are highly sensitive and specific biomarkers for discriminating MODY from type 1 diabetes. Islet autoantibodies help at diagnosis, whereas C-peptide is more informative with longer diabetes duration (3-5 years after diagnosis).

- Distinguishing MODY from common type 2 diabetes is more challenging due to a lack of biomarkers. Using multiple clinical features and family history within a statistical probability model is the best approach here and allows thresholds for probability of a diagnosis to be considered when deciding who should be tested.

- A genetic test that screens for pathogenic variants in all known monogenic diabetes genes should be offered, including genes causing syndromic forms of diabetes and the mitochondrial DNA variant m.3243A>G. Syndromic subtypes can be diagnosed unexpectedly due to clinical variability and should not be excluded from testing on the basis of an absence of associated extrapancreatic clinical features.

References

1. Shields BM, Shepherd M, Hudson M, et al; UNITED study team. Population-based assessment of a biomarker-based screening pathway to aid diagnosis of monogenic diabetes in young-onset patients. *Diabetes Care*. 2017;40(8):1017-1025. PMID: 28701371

2. Colclough K, Patel K. How do I diagnose maturity onset diabetes of the young in my patients? *Clin Endocrinol (Oxf)*. 2022;97(4):436-447. PMID: 35445424

3. Chakera AJ, Steele AM, Gloyn AL, et al. Recognition and management of individuals with hyperglycemia because of a heterozygous glucokinase mutation. *Diabetes Care*. 2015;38(7):1383-1392. PMID: 26106223

4. Shepherd M, Pearson ER, Houghton J, Salt G, Ellard S, Hattersley AT. No deterioration in glycemic control in HNF-1alpha maturity-onset diabetes of the young following transfer from long-term insulin to sulphonylureas. *Diabetes Care*. 2003;26(11):3191-3192. PMID: 14578267

5. Pearson ER, Flechtner I, Njolstad PR, et al; Neonatal Diabetes International Collaborative Group. Switching from insulin to oral sulfonylureas in patients

with diabetes due to Kir6.2 mutations. *N Engl J Med*. 2006;355(5):467-477. PMID: 16885550

6. Flanagan SE, Patch AM, Mackay DJ, et al. Mutations in ATP-sensitive K+ channel genes cause transient neonatal diabetes and permanent diabetes in childhood or adulthood. *Diabetes*. 2007;56(7):1930-1937. PMID: 17446535

7. Pearson ER, Boj SF, Steele AM, et al. Macrosomia and hyperinsulinaemic hypoglycaemia in patients with heterozygous mutations in the HNF4A gene. *PLoS Med*. 2007;4(4):e118. PMID: 17407387

8. Caswell RC, Snowsill T, Houghton JAL, et al. Noninvasive fetal genotyping by droplet digital PCR to identify maternally inherited monogenic diabetes variants. *Clin Chem*. 2020;66(7):958-965. PMID: 32533152

9. Shields BM, Hicks S, Shepherd MH, Colclough K, Hattersley AT, Ellard S. Maturity-onset diabetes of the young (MODY): how many cases are we missing? *Diabetologia*. 2010;53(12):2504-2508. PMID: 20499044

10. De Franco E, Flanagan SE, Houghton JA, et al. The effect of early, comprehensive genomic testing on clinical care in neonatal diabetes: an international cohort study. *Lancet.* 2015;386(9997):957-963. PMID: 26231457

11. Colclough K, Ellard S, Hattersley A, Patel K: Syndromic monogenic diabetes genes should be tested in patients with a clinical suspicion of maturity-onset diabetes of the young. *Diabetes.* 2022;71(3):530-537. PMID: 34789499

12. Shields BM, McDonald TJ, Ellard S, Campbell MJ, Hyde C, Hattersley AT. The development and validation of a clinical prediction model to determine the probability of MODY in patients with young-onset diabetes. *Diabetologia.* 2012;55(5):1265-1272. PMID: 22218698

13. Feigerlova E, Pruhova S, Dittertova L, et al. Aetiological heterogeneity of asymptomatic hyperglycaemia in children and adolescents. *Eur J Pediatr.* 2006;165(7):446-452. PMID: 16602010

14. Chakera AJ, Spyer G, Vincent N, Ellard S, Hattersley AT, Dunne FP. The 0.1% of the population with glucokinase monogenic diabetes can be recognized by clinical characteristics in pregnancy: the Atlantic Diabetes in Pregnancy cohort. *Diabetes Care.* 2014;37(5):1230-1236. PMID: 24550216

15. McDonald TJ, Colclough K, Brown R, et al. Islet autoantibodies can discriminate maturity-onset diabetes of the young (MODY) from type 1 diabetes. *Diabet Med.* 2011;28(9):1028-1033. PMID: 21395678

16. Misra S, Shields B, Colclough K, et al. South Asian individuals with diabetes who are referred for MODY testing in the UK have a lower mutation pick-up rate than white European people. *Diabetologia.* 2016;59(10):2262-2265. PMID: 27435864

Diabetes and Varied Diets: Intermittent Fasting, Ketogenic Diets, and Holiday Fasting

Nancy Samir Elbarbary, MBBCh, MSc, MD, PhD. Diabetes Unit, Department of Pediatrics, Ain shams University, Cairo, Egypt; Email: nancy_elbarbary@yahoo.com and nancy_elbarbary@med.asu.edu.eg

Educational Objectives

After reviewing this chapter, learners should be able to:

- Identify different ways of fasting and alternative dietary approaches in people living with diabetes.

- Explain the risks and benefits of ketogenic diets in people with type 1 diabetes mellitus (T1DM).

- Determine strategies to conduct safe fasting using multiple daily injection (MDI) insulin therapy.

- Illustrate the optimal approach to effective fasting using advanced hybrid closed-loop (AHCL) systems.

Significance of the Clinical Problem

While the use of technology and newer drugs (insulin or add-ons) help patients reach their glycemic targets, nutrition therapy is still the main cornerstone of diabetes management. Lowering the carbohydrate ratio is reportedly a successful strategy in the management of obesity, type 2 diabetes (T2DM), and T1DM.[1] Despite modern advancements in glucose monitoring, many individuals with T1DM experience marked variability in blood glucose concentrations and have difficulty achieving glycemic targets,[2] which increases the risk for several acute and chronic health complications such as cardiovascular disease. Consequently, effective treatment strategies are needed that achieve hemoglobin A_{1c} targets while minimizing the frequency and severity of hyperglycemia and hypoglycemia.[3]

The term *intermittent fasting* connotes reduced caloric intake on an intermittent basis. This can vary from several hours during the day to a complete 24-hour period. Intermittent fasting refers to either nonreligious fasting for health reasons, including weight loss, or religious fasting, such as Yom Kippur or during the holy month of Ramadan (practiced by Muslims worldwide [involves abstaining from all oral intakes between sunrise and sunset]).[4]

This chapter addresses appropriate changes that should be made in the therapeutic regimens of people living with T1DM who engage in alternative dietary approaches.

Practice Gaps

- Lack of knowledge of appropriate changes in the insulin regimen that would promote weight loss or be weight neutral, particularly in people living with T1DM.

- Nonexistent medical guidelines on how to manage therapeutic intermittent fasting in people living with diabetes.

- Most endocrinologists have not been formally trained in the evaluation and management of religious fasting in patients using AHCL systems.

- Adequately powered randomized clinical trials comparing different treatment regimens and algorithms for dosage adjustments in people living with T1DM who seek to engage in fasting are lacking. The guidance and recommendations have predominantly been targeted toward adults.

- A few small prospective studies in adults and observational studies in children exist regarding low-carbohydrate diets in people with T1DM, but controlled studies are deficient, especially in pediatric and adolescent patients.

Discussion

Background: Fasting and Alternative Dietary Approaches in People Living With Diabetes

Intermittent fasting has increased in popularity in recent years because of accumulating evidence regarding its favorable metabolic effect on various aspects of human health. this chapter addresses nonreligious and religious intermittent fasting and reviews the benefits, therapeutic adjustments, and safety concerns in patients with T1DM.[4] Intermittent fasting is also the term used when a patient withholds caloric intake for several consecutive hours during the day (time-restricted feeding often 16 hours, with all energy intake during the other 8 hours of the day). Other approaches to intermittent fasting focus on capping calories at 500 for 2 days per week (5:2 diet) or on an alternate-day protocol. Some protocols allow protein intake but no carbohydrates and still label it intermittent fasting. In all instances, noncaloric fluid intake is permitted (which is one of the main differences when compared with religious fasting), which significantly reduces the risk of dehydration and hypotension, an important concern in religious fasting.[5]

Adjusting Diabetes Therapies

In clinical practice, the total bolus dosage is lower in patients with T1DM on a low-carbohydrate diet than in patients with T2DM on a high-carbohydrate diet, with the total daily insulin dose reduced by 44.3% with similar basal insulin requirements.[6] If the hemoglobin A_{1c} value is near target, the daily dosage of basal insulin may need to be decreased by 10% to 20%.[7] This is similar to that observed in clinical trials of patients with T2DM who are starting a low-carbohydrate diet, in which insulin dosages are typically decreased by 50%.[8] It is reasonable that low carbohydrate intake and resulting lower prandial insulin bolus requirements may lead to better glycemic control, less blood glucose variability, and improved quality of life. Further, patients can be instructed to take additional correction doses of short-acting insulin to address hyperglycemia and to closely follow adjusted insulin doses on a weekly basis in the initial stages of weight loss.[7]

Adjusting Boluses Based on Fat and Protein Intake

T1DM guidelines recommend that fat and protein be considered in the meal insulin strategy. For carbohydrate meals containing more than 30 g of fat or more than 15 g fat with more than 25 g protein, findings support an insulin dose increase of 30% of the insulin-to-carbohydrate ratio, and a split insulin strategy could be applied.[9] In open-pump therapy, extended or dual boluses can be used, with 60% or more of the insulin calculated for carbohydrate given 15 minutes before eating.[10]

Other Diabetes Medications

With the aim of weight loss, many patients with T1DM also take off-label medications that are approved by the US FDA for T2DM, including metformin, SGLT-2 inhibitors, and GLP-1 receptor agonists. SGLT-2 inhibitors are associated with an increased risk of euglycemic diabetic ketoacidosis (DKA), particularly in T1DM. Accordingly, SGLT-2 inhibitors should be stopped before starting a ketogenic diet because of the risk of DKA, which often presents as euglycemic, making it difficult to recognize.[11] GLP-1 receptor agonists, when used in T1DM, may increase the risk of hypoglycemia and DKA. They can be continued with close monitoring in patients following a ketogenic diet, although some providers prefer to stop them. Metformin is generally considered safe to continue.[12]

Fasting in Ramadan

Management of T1DM During Ramadan for Patients on MDI Therapy

The period of fasting, which can exceed more than 20 hours in some countries, imposes a high risk of dehydration to all people living with T1DM. An individualized approach is important, and suggested guidelines to adjust insulin therapy are illustrated in *Figures 1* and *2*.[13-16]

Management of T1DM During Ramadan in Patients Using Open-Loop Insulin Pump Therapy

Most studies of open-loop insulin pump therapy in young individuals and adolescents during Ramadan reduced the dose of basal insulin by 20% to 35% during fasting hours and increased the basal rate during nonfasting hours (10%-30%) (*Figure 3, following page*).[17]

Management of T1DM During Ramadan in Patients Using AHCL Systems

A recent study compared satisfactory glycemic control without significant change in time-in-range and without influencing the percentage of time spent with low glucose values during Ramadan and before Ramadan.[18] The optimal approach for AHCL is illustrated in *Figure 4* (*following pages*).

Figure 1. Recommended Use of MDI Therapy in Adolescents With T1DM Who Are Fasting During Ramadan

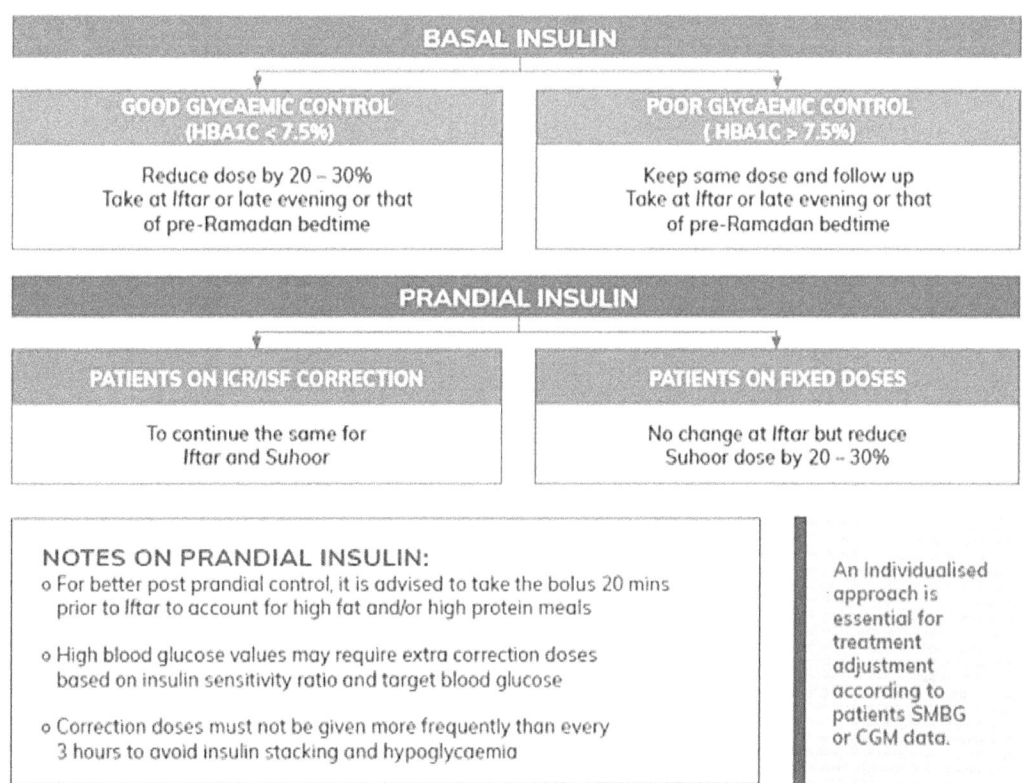

Adapted from Hassanein M et al. *Diabetes Res Clin Pract*, 2022; 185: 109185. © Elsevier B.V.

[Color—Print (Color Gallery page CG20) or web & ePub editions]

Figure 2. Schematic Adjustments of Insulin and/or Food Considerations During Fasting and Nonfasting Hours

ONCE DAILY LONG ACTING BASAL ANALOGUE
TWICE DAILY BASAL INSULIN ANALOGUE
MEASURE BG IN FASTING HOURS (morning, mid-day and before Iftar)
• No adjustments in BG between 90-160 mg/dL
• If BG between 160-250 mg/dL, consider increasing basal insulin by 10-15%
• If BG > 250 mg/dL, consider increasing basal insulin by 20-30%
• If BG < 90 mg/dL, consider decreasing basal insulin by 15-20%
• No adjustments of late evening dose if BG between 90-160 mg/dL
• If BG between 160-250 mg/dL, consider increasing late evening dose by 10-15%
• If BG > 250 mg/dL, consider increasing late evening dose by 20-30%
• If BG < 90 mg/dL, consider decreasing late evening basal insulin by 15-20%
MEASURE BG IN NON-FASTING HOURS (post-Iftar, midnight, predawn)
• Dose adjustment depends on short acting insulin at Iftar, Suhoor and snack in between
• Apply ICR calculation of meal contents for dose changes
• Avoid high carbohydrate and fat contents in meals as that will reflect on BG levels through night and early morning
• No adjustments of Iftar basal dose if BG between 90-150 mg/dL
• If BG between 160-250 mg/dL, consider increasing Iftar basal insulin by 10-15%
• If BG >250 mg/dL, consider increasing Iftar basal insulin by 20-30%
• If BG < 90 mg/dL, consider decreasing Iftar basal insulin by 15-20%
• ICR changes apply according to BG 2 hours after Iftar or Suhoor

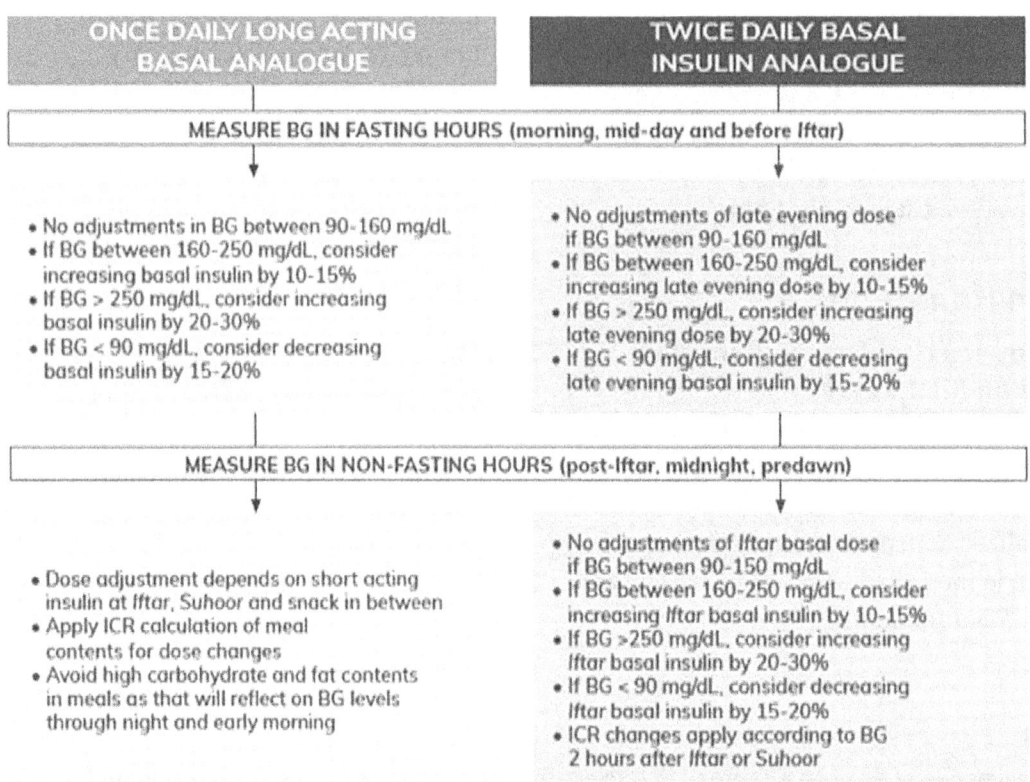

Reprinted from International Diabetes Federation & Diabetes and Ramadan, *Diabetes and Ramadan: Practical Guidelines 2021*, Chapter 9, "Management of Type 1 diabetes when fasting during Ramadan."

[Color—Print (Color Gallery page CG21) or web & ePub editions]

Figure 3. Basal and Bolus Insulin During Ramadan

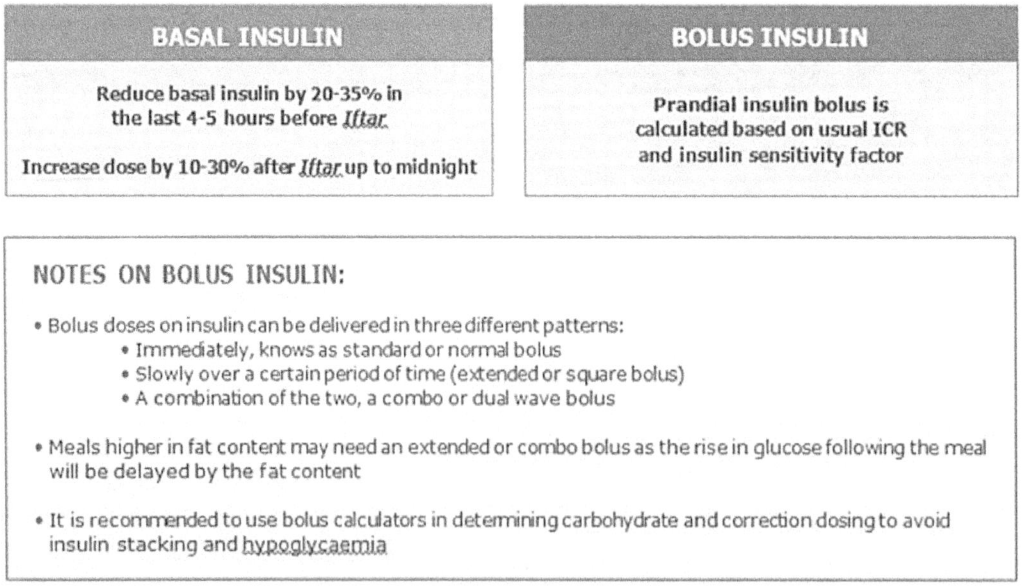

BASAL INSULIN
Reduce basal insulin by 20-35% in the last 4-5 hours before Iftar
Increase dose by 10-30% after Iftar up to midnight
BOLUS INSULIN
Prandial insulin bolus is calculated based on usual ICR and insulin sensitivity factor
NOTES ON BOLUS INSULIN:
• Bolus doses on insulin can be delivered in three different patterns:
• Immediately, knows as standard or normal bolus
• Slowly over a certain period of time (extended or square bolus)
• A combination of the two, a combo or dual wave bolus
• Meals higher in fat content may need an extended or combo bolus as the rise in glucose following the meal will be delayed by the fat content
• It is recommended to use bolus calculators in determining carbohydrate and correction dosing to avoid insulin stacking and hypoglycaemia

Adapted from Hassanein M et al. *Diabetes Res Clin Pract*, 2022; 185: 109185. © Elsevier B.V.

[Color—Print (Color Gallery page CG21) or web & ePub editions]

Figure 4. Management of Glycemic Control During Ramadan in Patients Using AHCL Systems

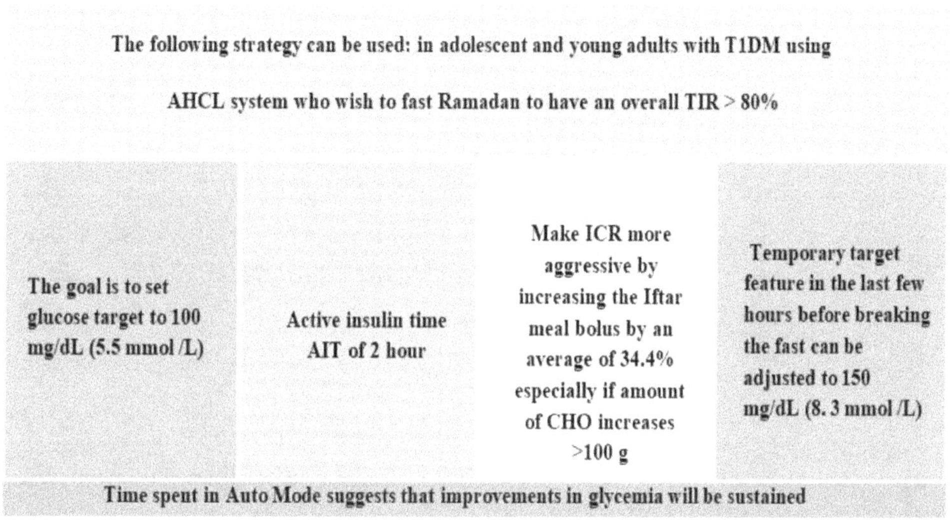

The following strategy can be used: in adolescent and young adults with T1DM using AHCL system who wish to fast Ramadan to have an overall TIR > 80%

| The goal is to set glucose target to 100 mg/dL (5.5 mmol /L) | Active insulin time AIT of 2 hour | Make ICR more aggressive by increasing the Iftar meal bolus by an average of 34.4% especially if amount of CHO increases >100 g | Temporary target feature in the last few hours before breaking the fast can be adjusted to 150 mg/dL (8.3 mmol /L) |

Time spent in Auto Mode suggests that improvements in glycemia will be sustained

Reprinted from Elbarbary NS, Ismail EAR. Glycemic control during Ramadan fasting in adolescents and young adults with type 1 diabetes on MiniMed™ 780G advanced hybrid closedloop system: a randomized controlled trial. *Diabetes Res Clin Pract.* 2022;191:110045.[18]

[Color—Print (Color Gallery page CG22) or web & ePub editions]

Yom Kippur and Other Fasts in Jewish Law

Yom Kippur fasting is the most solemn religious fast of the Jewish year and the holiest day in the Jewish religion and calendar. It is the last of the 10 days of penitence that begin with Rosh Hashana (the Jewish New Year); also called Day of Atonement. Various approaches for diabetes management during fasting have been used. Before the era of glucose meters and continuous glucose monitoring, people with diabetes were exempt from fasting. In the last 2 decades, several studies showed that insulin dose adjustments and close monitoring may enable safe fasting for individuals with T1DM.[19]

Christian Orthodox Fasting

Christian Orthodox fasting is a kind of periodical diet that recommends abstaining from meat, dairy products, and eggs for 180 days annually and from fish for 155 days annually. The diet during periods of fasting is characterized by increased consumption of cereals, legumes, fruits, vegetables, nuts, and seafood. It is characterized by low total energy intake, low-fat intake (total, saturated, and trans), low-animal and high-vegetable protein intake, and high complex carbohydrate and fiber intake. Thus, it is advisable for people with T1DM to choose carbohydrates with a low glycemic index and to consume them in combination with fiber, proteins (legumes, seafood), or fats (olive oil).[20]

Clinical Case Vignettes

Case 1

A 23-year-old woman with a 3-year history of T1DM uses an AHCL system (MiniMed 780G) and is fasting 17 hours per day for the month of Ramadan. When she was previously on an MDI regimen, she had hemoglobin A_{1c} values between 7.2% and 8.8% (55-73 mmol/mol). The AHCL system was initiated 9 months ago, and a hemoglobin A_{1c} value of 6.7% (50 mmol/mol) and time-in-range (70-180 mg/dL [3.9-10.0 mmol/L]) of 79% were achieved. She is fasting from 4:00 AM until 6:30 PM. She broke the fast twice in the afternoons during the first week of Ramadan because of mild hypoglycemic events between 5:00 and 6:30 PM. Her pump and sensor data are shown (*Figure 5, following page*).

Figure 5. Patient's Pump and Sensor Data

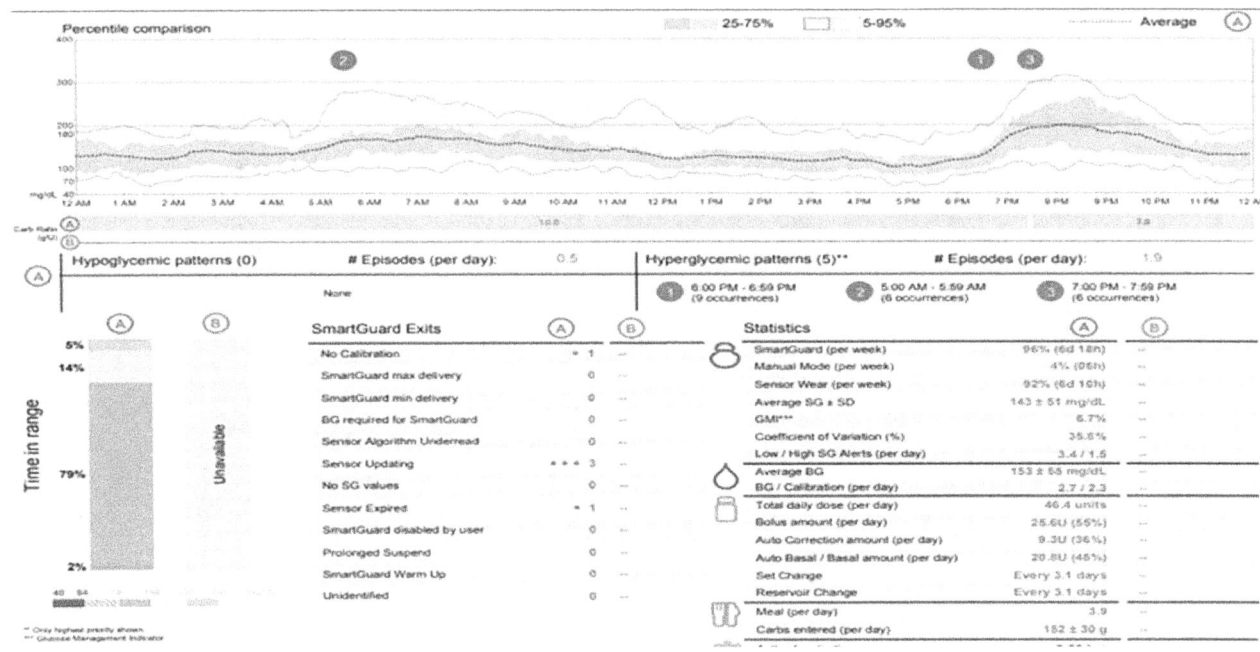

[Color—Print (Color Gallery page CG22) or web & ePub editions]

Which of the following is the best advice to help her avoid hypoglycemia in the late afternoons during fasting hours?

A. Change active insulin time

B. Change insulin-to-carbohydrate ratio for meals

C. Change blood glucose target

D. Set Temp Target of SmartGuard

E. Exit Auto Mode and go to manual mode

Answer: D) Set Temp Target of SmartGuard

Setting a Temp Target in SmartGuard technology (Answer D) of 150 mg/dL (8.3 mmol/L) is a safe approach to mitigate glycemic excursions and avoid hypoglycemia during fasting hours. The use of a temporary target for 2 to 4 hours if the glucose concentration reaches 80 mg/dL (4.4 mmol/L) is always advised to be used during fasting hours to avoid further glucose decrease. Optimal settings including an active insulin time of 2 hours, glucose target of 100 mg/dL (5.5 mmol/L), intensified insulin-to-carbohydrate ratio, and being on Auto Mode allow maintaining time-in-range greater than 80% as described (*Figure 4*). An AHCL system with automatic adjustments of basal insulin delivery in response to sensor readings, temporary target feature, and good collaboration between health providers and the patient allows satisfactory glucose control during 17 hours of fasting per day during the month of Ramadan. Of note, average autobasal/basal insulin amount per day is significantly lower in the period of 4:00 AM to 6:30 PM in the fasting hours during Ramadan compared with amounts during the same period in the nonfasting hours before Ramadan. This is different than open-loop continuous subcutaneous insulin infusion where there is a reduction in the basal rate by 20% to 35% during fasting hours and even up to a 35% to 40% reduction in the last few hours of breaking the fast. Weekly reassessment for further adjustments is recommended.

Case 1 (continued)

Despite correct carbohydrate counting, an increase in glucose values (7:00 PM-11:00 PM) is noted due to the evening sunset fast-breaking meal for Muslims during the month of Ramadan (known as Iftar) (*Figure 6, following page*).

Figure 6. Patient's Glucose Tracing

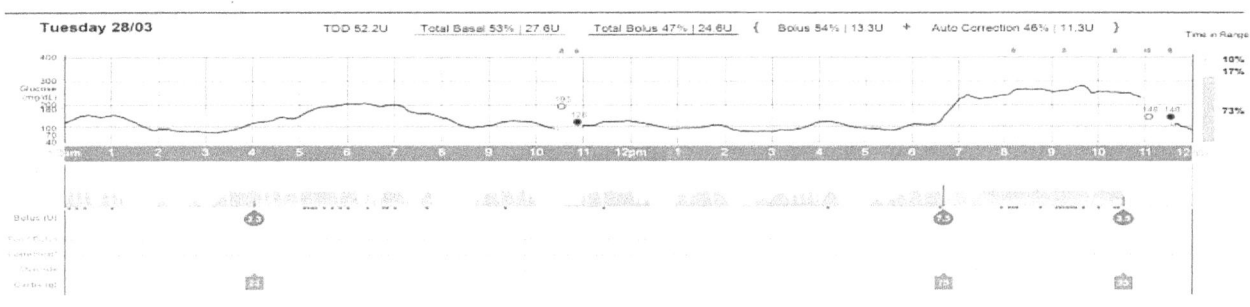

[Color—Print (Color Gallery page CG23) or web & ePub editions]

Which of the following is the best recommendation to avoid this postmeal hyperglycemia?

A. Use dual bolus

B. Use square bolus

C. Change the insulin-to-carbohydrate ratio

D. Change the type of insulin

E. Increase the meal bolus by 10% to 20%

Answer: E) Increase the meal bolus by 10% to 20%

The meal bolus should be increased by 10% to 20% (Answer E) if the meal contains more than 100 g of carbohydrates (eg, increase the bolus by 20% when 130 g of carbohydrates are eaten, so 156 g of carbohydrates would be entered into the bolus wizard calculator) and bolus insulin should be 40% to 50% before and 50% to 60% after the meal, as the "dual-wave" and "square" boluses are disabled in the MiniMed 780G AHCL system. AHCL demonstrated simple management in T1DM during Ramadan fasting. The patient in this vignette had satisfactory glucose control without changing the active insulin time, glucose target, insulin-to-carbohydrate ratio, and time-in-range, without influencing the percentage of time spent with low glucose values during Ramadan.

AHCL requires minimal adjustment of the system before and during Ramadan with use of a temporary target in the afternoon and increasing the meal bolus by 10% to 20% for huge meals in the evening (Answer E), without any change in basal and bolus insulin settings.

Case 2

A 19-year-old college student with a 6-year history of T1DM presents for routine follow-up. He has been on an AHCL system for 2 years. Before using AHCL, he used an MDI regimen, and hemoglobin A_{1c} values ranged from 7.5% to 8.3% (58-67 mmol/mol). Glycemic control improved on insulin pump therapy, but he had high glycemic variability and was very keen to maintain a healthy body weight. He self-initiated a low-carbohydrate diet with a gradual decrease in the amount of carbohydrate consumed on a weekly basis (he aimed to reach approximately 50 g of carbohydrates per day). He did not adjust his insulin pump settings and kept the same active insulin time, glucose target, and insulin-to-carbohydrate ratio. He reports that his glycemic control has improved with minimal hypoglycemia. His glucose management indicator (estimated hemoglobin A_{1c}) is 6.2% (44 mmol/mol), and he has lost 11 lb (5 kg). Glucose concentrations are reported to be within the desired range (70-180 mg/dL [3.9-10.0 mmol/L]) 90% to 98% of the time, with very few insulin boluses required. The patient inquires whether this dieting program is safe for him. His pump and sensor data are shown (*Figure 7, following page*).

According to sensor download, his bolus insulin requirements have decreased. His blood glucose level remains within the goal range of 70 to 180 mg/dL (3.9-10.0 mmol/L) 94% of the time. No episodes of hypoglycemia or DKA are reported.

Figure 7. Patient's Pump and Sensor Data

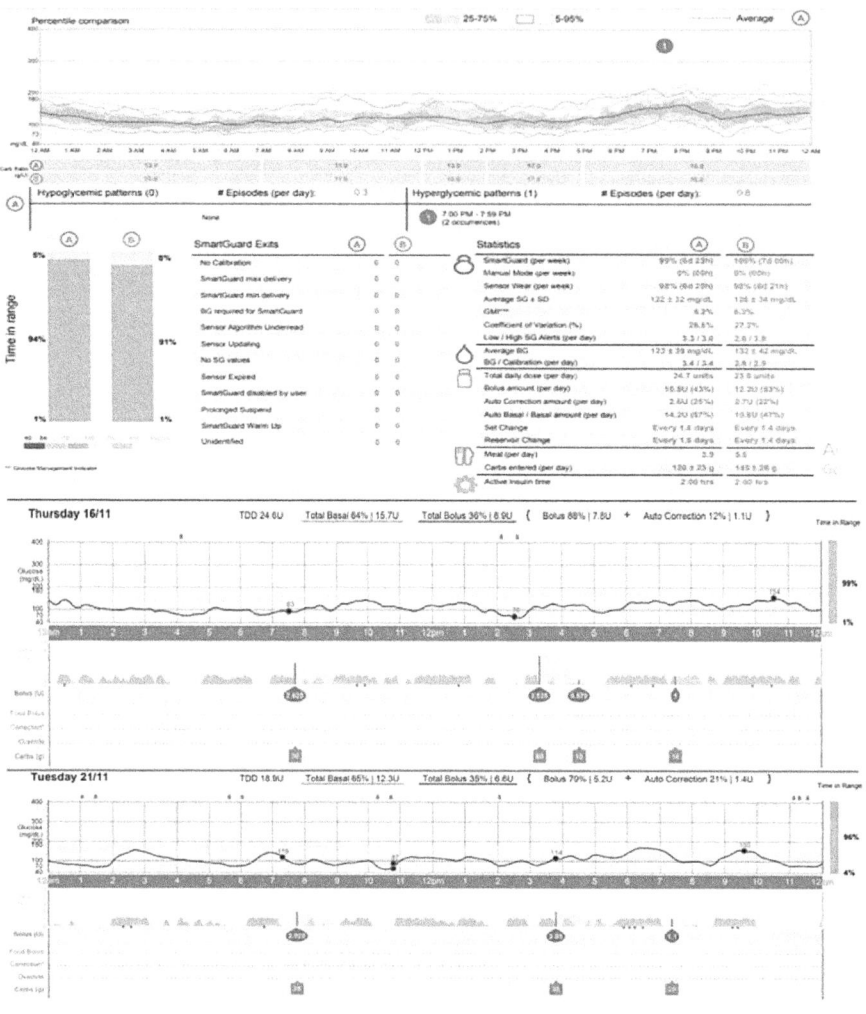

[Color—Print (Color Gallery page CG23) or web & ePub editions]

He wants to use add-on therapy to lose more weight. His friend advised him to take a medication that is off-label use for T1DM but is approved by the US FDA for T2DM.

Which of the following medications should he avoid using?

A. Metformin

B. SGLT-2 inhibitors

C. GLP-1 receptor agonists

D. DPP-4 inhibitors

E. Thiazolidinedione

Answer: B) SGLT-2 inhibitors

SGLT-2 inhibitors (Answer B) are associated with an increased risk of euglycemic DKA, particularly in T1DM. SGLT-2 inhibitors should be discontinued when following a ketosis-inducing diet, but metformin is considered safe. GLP-1 receptor agonists can be continued with close monitoring.

This may occur through multiple mechanisms, including reduction in insulin-mediated suppression of lipolysis and ketogenesis, volume contraction, promotion of glucagon secretion, and decreased kidney clearance of ketone bodies. Accordingly, SGLT-2 inhibitors should be stopped before starting a ketogenic diet because DKA often presents as euglycemic, making it difficult to recognize. For patients with T1DM, monitoring ketones is important to identify and prevent DKA.

Under normal physiologic circumstances, glucose is the main substrate for glycolysis, resulting in the production of adenosine triphosphate, the body's main energy source. Most glycogen is stored in the liver, which has the greatest role in the maintenance of blood glucose during the first 24 hours of a fast. After fasting for 24 hours, glycogen stores are depleted, causing the body to use energy stores from adipose tissue and protein stores.[21] Without glucose as a substrate for adenosine triphosphate production, the liver breaks down triglycerides to make ketone bodies that travel to target tissues (eg, brain, muscles) and ultimately generates adenosine triphosphate. This process of ketogenesis is regulated by insulin; low carbohydrate intake leads to low insulin levels, promoting ketosis.

Case 2 (continued)

Which of the following is the most important follow-up assessment for this patient on a ketogenic diet?

A. Time-in-range

B. Estimated hemoglobin A_{1c} level (by glucose management indicator)

C. Lipid profile

D. Patient weight (kg)

E. Patient waist circumference (cm)

Answer: C) Lipid profile

Concerns have been raised regarding ketogenic diets and adverse lipid profile changes (Answer C), but the literature is inconsistent and few publications have assessed the issue specifically in T1DM.[7,22-25] Effects of ketogenic diets include dyslipidemia (triglycerides >130 mg/dL [>1.47 mmol/L], LDL cholesterol >130 mg/dL [>3.37 mmol/L], or HDL cholesterol <35 mg/dL [<0.91 mmol/L]). Dyslipidemia in this setting may be due to a high proportion of saturated animal fat in ketogenic diets.

Case 3

A 15-year-old girl has T1DM that was diagnosed at age 9 years. Over the last 2 years, her hemoglobin A_{1c} values have ranged between 6.9% and 8.2%

(52-66 mmol/mol). For the last year, she has been using a continuous glucose monitor for better glycemic control. Her current diabetes therapy consists of insulin degludec and insulin aspart with meals. She has no microvascular disease, no hypoglycemia unawareness, and no associated diseases.

On physical examination, her height is 61.4 in (156 cm) and weight is 142.9 (64.8 kg) (BMI = 26.6 kg/m²).

She eats 3 meals per day with 3 to 4 carbohydrate exchanges. She swims twice per week.

Her daily pattern profile is shown (*Figure 8, following page*).

She would like to lose weight and wants to try intermittent fasting for 16 hours per day. Data from the first week of fasting are shown (*Figure 9, following page*).

She administers 20 units of insulin degludec at 7 AM and insulin aspart with meals according to insulin carbohydrate counting and average insulin-to-carbohydrate ratio of 1:10 g carbohydrate.

Which of the following is the best recommendation for basal insulin dosage adjustment?

A. Reduce basal dosage by 20%

B. Reduce insulin dosage by 50%

C. Move administration of her insulin degludec dose to the evening

D. Change basal insulin to intermediate-acting insulin (neutral protamine Hagedorn)

E. Continue the same regimen, as her time-in-range is 71%

Answer: A) Reduce basal dosage by 20%

The usual starting basal insulin dose reduction in first week is 20% (Answer A), especially in those with good glycemic control, and then follow-up is recommended. Patients should be educated about when breaking the fast is necessary, which includes symptomatic hypoglycemia and asymptomatic hypoglycemia with glucose values below 70 mg/dL (<3.9 mmol/L). Patients with hypoglycemia unawareness should not fast because of a high

Figure 8. Patient's Glucose Tracing

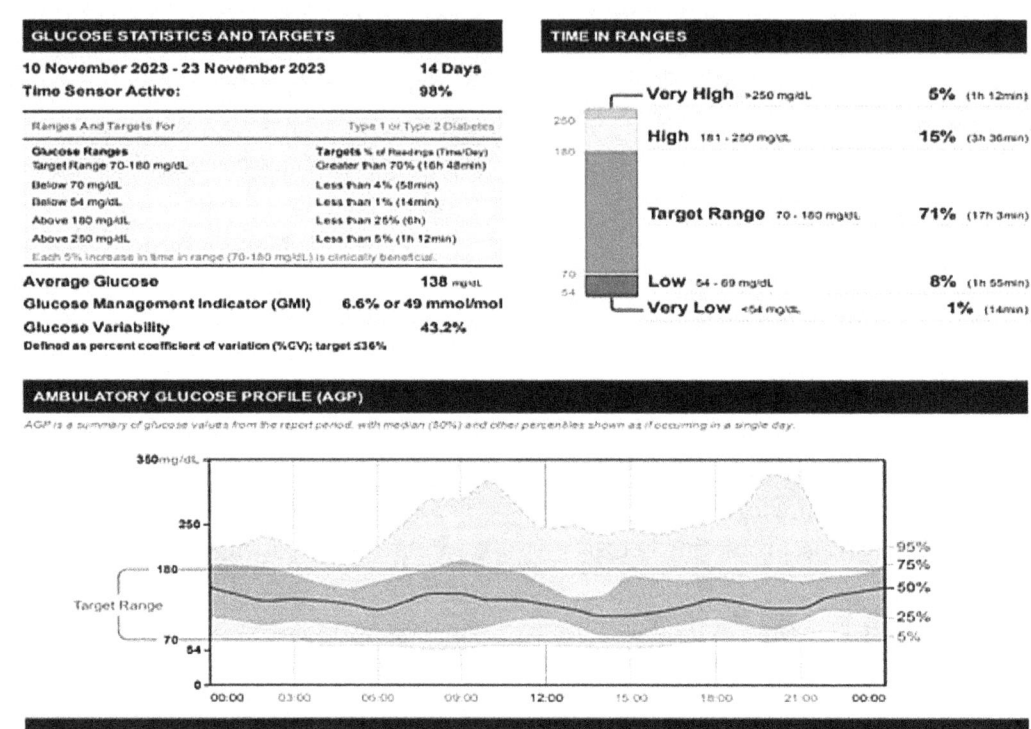

[Color—Print (Color Gallery page CG24) or web & ePub editions]

Figure 9. Patient's Glucose Tracing

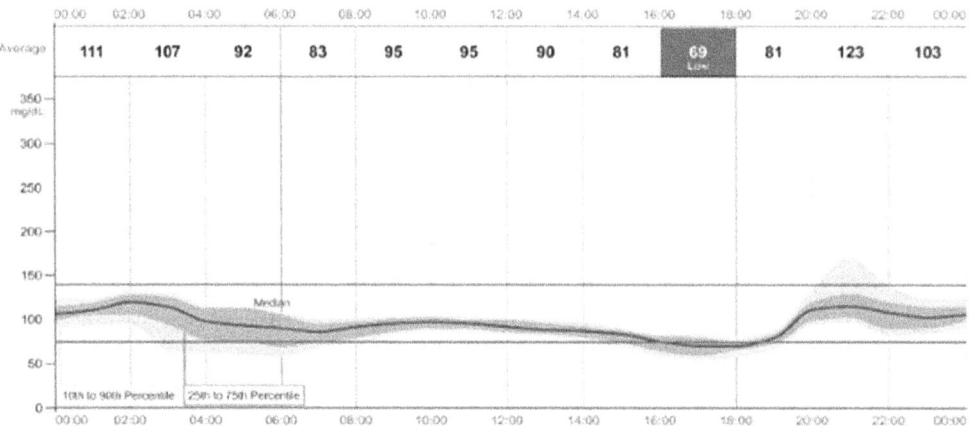

[Color—Print (Color Gallery page CG24) or web & ePub editions]

risk of hypoglycemia. Although glycogenolysis, gluconeogenesis, and negative feedback of insulin secretion are protective against fasting-induced hypoglycemia in normal physiology, they may not have the same effect in individuals with T1DM. Persons with T1DM have an inherently higher risk of hypoglycemia due to the hypoglycemic effect of unregulated exogenous insulin therapy. Other potentially predisposing risks for hypoglycemia include impaired or loss of glucagon response to hypoglycemia in longstanding T1DM, increased risk of celiac disease, and increased risk of hypoadrenalism due to the predisposition of a shared autoimmune background.

Case 3 (continued)

The next download (*Figure 10*) after the first week shows a better glucose profile.

The meal pattern at 7:00 PM indicates which of the following?

A. Improper type of insulin was used

B. The meal contained high fat and high protein

C. The insulin-to-carbohydrate ratio should be readjusted

D. The patient needs to be re-educated about accurately count carbohydrates

E. Late-meal bolus injection due to high–glycemic index food

Answer: E) Late-meal bolus injection due to high–glycemic index food

High–glycemic index carbohydrates should not be the basis of foods consumed at the breaking-fast meal and should be discouraged because dietary carbohydrate is absorbed and rapidly increases the blood glucose concentration, leading to postprandial hyperglycemic spikes. Preferred meals have a low glycemic index and limit the consumption of high– and moderate–glycemic index carbohydrates.

Carbohydrates with a low glycemic index are associated with a slower and more constant glycemic response, so it has been proposed that a low–glycemic index diet could promote better glycemic control and be an important adjuvant strategy together with insulin therapy for achieving glycemic balance in patients with T1DM.

Preprandial bolus insulin is preferable to insulin administered to avoid an early postprandial surge. Patients should be properly educated about how to count carbohydrates in special foods and adjust the insulin-to-carbohydrate ratio. Meals should be based on low–glycemic index carbohydrates, and monounsaturated and polyunsaturated fats should be used instead of saturated fat.

Hydration should be maintained by drinking water during nonfasting hours. Adjusting the insulin strategy for fat and protein meal content should always be discussed in the context of a healthful diet with individualized guidance regarding appropriate energy intake and physical activity.

Studies in people with T1DM have clearly shown that the amount of fat and protein in a meal affects postmeal blood glucose. Specifically, fat is known to blunt the blood glucose rise in the first 2 to 3 hours and to delay the peak glucose level due to delayed gastric emptying. While eating significant amounts of protein without carbohydrates will not affect blood glucose, protein eaten with carbohydrates will result in higher peak blood glucose than that same amount of carbohydrates without protein. Bolus calculators use in insulin pump therapy are important to prevent insulin "stacking."[9]

Figure 10. Patient's Glucose Tracing

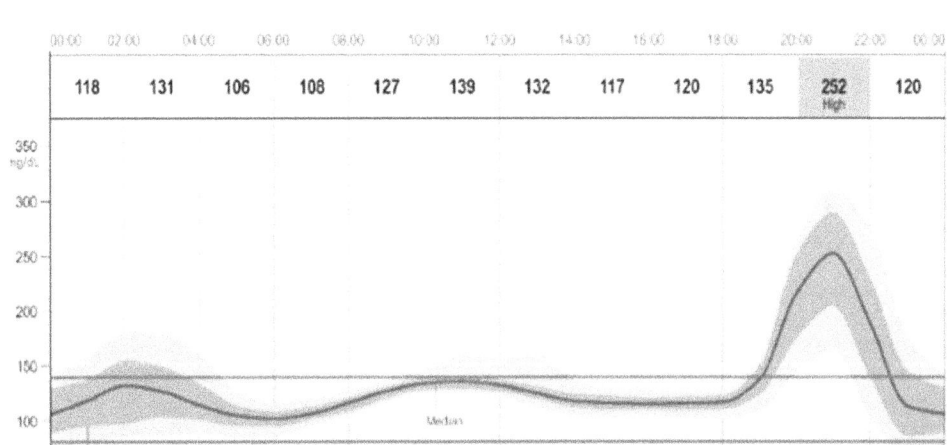

[Color—Print (Color Gallery page CG25) or web & ePub editions]

Key Learning Points

- Fasting is a practical dietary strategy. Therapeutic fasting is an underused dietary intervention that can provide superior blood glucose reduction compared with standard pharmacological agents. Optimal insulin dose adjustments are needed for different types of fasting and regimens.

- Patient with T1DM who use an AHCL system and wish to fast and have an overall time-in-range greater than 80% can set their devices accordingly:

  - Glucose target of 100 mg/dL (5.6 mmol/L)

  - Active insulin time of 2 hours

  - More aggressive insulin-to-carbohydrate ratio; increase the meal bolus with Iftar by an average of 20% to 30%, especially if the amount of carbohydrate is greater than 100 g

  - Adjust the temporary target feature in the last few hours before breaking to 150 mg/dL (8.3 mmol/L)

  - Sustain using Auto Mode

- The simultaneous growth of interest in ketogenic diets and knowledge development in this field have contributed to the increasingly frequent application of ketogenic diets in diabetes treatment. This type of diet is becoming more common among patients with T1DM, but its clinical impact remains unclear, as much of the literature consists of retrospective case reports and series. It has not been well investigated, and long-term data of its risks and complications are lacking.[23,26-28] Hence, close follow-up and adjustment of insulin doses is required to monitor patients' lipid profile, risk of DKA, hypoglycemia, growth, and psychosocial status.

- A ketogenic diet may be appropriate for select patients, but only after a thorough discussion between patient and care team about the risks and benefits. A registered dietitian and specialists in diabetes care, education, endocrinology, and pharmacy should be part of any discussion. For patients on a ketogenic diet, extra monitoring is critical, preferably with a continuous glucose monitor.

- Ketogenic diets have the potential to reduce hemoglobin A_{1c} levels, blood glucose variability, and insulin dosage and to improve time-in-range and cardiovascular risk factors.

- SGLT-2 inhibitors should be discontinued when following a ketogenic diet, but metformin is considered safe. GLP-1 receptor agonists can be continued with close monitoring.

- Taking protein and fat into consideration in the calculation of insulin boluses could potentially improve postmeal glucose control in T1DM, but this would increase the complexity of management of prandial insulin doses. Adjustments should also be considered in the context of AHCL for high-fat or high-protein meals.

References

1. Zhou Z, Sun B, Huang S, Zhu C, Bian M. Glycemic variability: adverse clinical outcomes and how to improve it? *Cardiovasc Diabetol.* 2020;19(1):102. PMID: 32622354

2. Monnier L, Colette C, Wojtusciszyn A, et al. Toward defining the threshold between low and high glucose variability in diabetes. *Diabetes Care.* 2017;40(7):832-838. PMID: 28039172

3. Harding JL, Pavkov ME, Magliano DJ, Shaw JE, Gregg EW. Global trends in diabetes complications: a review of current evidence. *Diabetologia.* 2019;62(1):3-16. PMID: 30171279

4. Grajower MM, Horne BD. Clinical management of intermittent fasting in patients with diabetes mellitus. *Nutrients.* 2019;11(4):873. PMID: 31003482

5. Furmli S, Elmasry R, Ramos M, Fung J. Therapeutic use of intermittent fasting for people with type 2 diabetes as an alternative to insulin. *BMJ Case Rep.* 2018;2018:bcr2017221854. PMID: 30301822

6. Ranjan A, Schmidt S, Damm-Frydenberg C, Holst JJ, Madsbad S, Nørgaard K. Short-term effects of a low carbohydrate diet on glycaemic variables and cardiovascular risk markers in patients with type 1 diabetes: a randomized open-label crossover trial. *Diabetes Obes Metab.* 2017;19(10):1479-1484. doi: 10.1111/dom.12953. Epub 2017 Jul 10. PMID: 28345762

7. Buehler LA, Noe D, Knapp S, Isaacs D, Pantalone KM. Ketogenic diets in the management of type 1 diabetes: Safe or safety concern? *Cleve Clin J Med.* 2021;88(10):547-555. PMID: 34598919

8. Saslow LR, Daubenmier JJ, Moskowitz JT, et al. Twelve-month outcomes of a randomized trial of a moderate-carbohydrate versus very low-carbohydrate diet in overweight adults with type 2 diabetes mellitus or prediabetes. *Nutr Diabetes*. 2017;7(12):304. PMID: 29269731

9. Smith TA, Marlow AA, King BR, Smart CE. Insulin strategies for dietary fat and protein in type 1 diabetes: A systematic review. *Diabet Med*. 2021;38(11):e14641. PMID: 34251692

10. Bell KJ, Smart CE, Steil GM, Brand-Miller JC, King B, Wolpert HA. Impact of fat, protein, and glycemic index on postprandial glucose control in type 1 diabetes: implications for intensive diabetes management in the continuous glucose monitoring era. *Diabetes Care*. 2015;38(6):1008-1015. PMID: 25998293

11. Handelsman Y, Henry RR, Bloomgarden ZT, Dagogo-Jack S, DeFronzo RA, Einhorn D, Ferrannini E, Fonseca VA, Garber AJ, Grunberger G, LeRoith D, Umpierrez GE, Weir MR. American Association of Clinical Endocrinologists and American College of Endocrinology position statement on the association of SGLT-2 inhibitors and diabetic ketoacidosis. *Endocr Pract*. 2016;22(6):753-762. PMID: 27082665

12. Mathieu C, Zinman B, Hemmingsson JU, et al; ADJUNCT ONE Investigators. Efficacy and safety of liraglutide added to insulin treatment in type 1 diabetes: The ADJUNCT ONE Treat-To-Target Randomized Trial. *Diabetes Care*. 2016;39(10):1702-1710. PMID: 27506222

13. Hassanein M, Afandi B, Yakoob Ahmedani M, et al. Diabetes and Ramadan: practical guidelines 2021. *Diabetes Res Clin Pract*. 2022;185:109185. PMID: 35016991

14. Deeb A, Elbarbary N, Smart CE, et al. ISPAD clinical practice consensus guidelines: fasting during Ramadan by young people with diabetes. *Pediatr Diabetes*. 2020;21(1):5-17. PMID: 31659852

15. Ibrahim M, Davies MJ, Ahmad E, et al. Recommendations for management of diabetes during Ramadan: update 2020, applying the principles of the ADA/EASD consensus. *BMJ Open Diabetes Res Care*. 2020;8(1):e001248. PMID: 32366501

16. Deeb A, Babiker A, Sedaghat S, et al. ISPAD Clinical Practice Consensus Guidelines 2022: Ramadan and other religious fasting by young people with diabetes. *Pediatr Diabetes*. 2022;23(8):1512-1528. PMID: 36537522

17. Elbarbary NS. Effectiveness of the low-glucose suspend feature of insulin pump during fasting during Ramadan in type 1 diabetes mellitus. *Diabetes Metab Res Rev*. 2016;32(6):623-633. PMID: 26789012

18. Elbarbary NS, Ismail EAR. Glycemic control during Ramadan fasting in adolescents and young adults with type 1 diabetes on MiniMed™ 780G advanced hybrid closedloop system: a randomized controlled trial. *Diabetes Res Clin Pract*. 2022;191:110045. PMID: 35987309

19. Grajower MM, Zangen D. Expert opinion and clinical experience regarding patients with type 1 diabetes mellitus fasting on Yom Kippur. *Pediatr Diabetes*. 2011;12(5):473-477. PMID: 21794045

20. Tromba V, Silvestri F. Vegetarianism and type 1 diabetes in children. *Metabolism Open*. 2021;11:100099. PMID: 34159308

21. Sanvictores T, Casale J, Huecker MR. Physiology, Fasting. In: StatPearls [Internet]. Treasure Island, FL: StatPearls Publishing; 2024 Jan. PMID: 30521298

22. Lennerz BS, Barton A, Bernstein RK, et al. Management of type 1 diabetes with a very low-carbohydrate diet. *Pediatrics*. 2018;141(6):e20173349. PMID: 29735574

23. de Bock M, Lobley K, Anderson D, et al. Endocrine and metabolic consequences due to restrictive carbohydrate diets in children with type 1 diabetes: an illustrative case series. *Pediatr Diabetes*. 2018;19(1):129-137. PMID: 28397413

24. Krebs JD, Parry Strong A, Cresswell P, Reynolds AN, Hanna A, Haeusler S. A randomised trial of the feasibility of a low carbohydrate diet vs standard carbohydrate counting in adults with type 1 diabetes taking body weight into account. *Asia Pac J Clin Nutr*. 2016;25(1):78-84. PMID: 26965765

25. O'Neill BJ. Effect of low-carbohydrate diets on cardiometabolic risk, insulin resistance, and metabolic syndrome. *Curr Opin Endocrinol Diabetes Obes*. 2020;27(5):301-307. PMID: 32773574

26. Leow ZZX, Guelfi KJ, Davis EA, Jones TW, Fournier PA. The glycaemic benefits of a very-low-carbohydrate ketogenic diet in adults with type 1 diabetes mellitus may be opposed by increased hypoglycaemia risk and dyslipidaemia. *Diabet Med*. 2018 [Online ahead of print] PMID: 29737587

27. McClean A-M, Montorio L, McLaughlin D, McGovern S, Flanagan N. Can a ketogenic diet be safely used to improve glycaemic control in a child with type 1 diabetes? *Arch Dis Child*. 2019;104(5):501-504. PMID: 30470684

28. Cogen FR. Incorporation of the ketogenic diet in a youth with type 1 diabetes. *Clin Diabetes*. 2020;38(4):412-415. PMID: 33132514

Managing Type 1 Diabetes and Exercise

Joseph Henske, MD. Department of Medicine, Division of Endocrinology, Diabetes, and Metabolism, University of Arkansas for Medical Sciences, Little Rock, AR; Email: jahenske@uams.edu

Educational Objectives

After reviewing this chapter, learners should be able to:

- Explain the effects of various forms of exercise on blood glucose levels in type 1 diabetes (T1D).

- Describe practical solutions to common problems faced by individuals with T1D undertaking an exercise regimen.

- Compare and contrast the features of commonly used automated insulin delivery (AID) systems with respect to exercise.

Significance of the Clinical Problem

Regular exercise is recommended for cardiovascular health and well-being for those living with T1D. According to recommendations, adults in the United States should perform 150 minutes of moderate physical activity divided into 3 to 5 days per week and 2 additional strength training sessions per week. However, most are falling well short of these goals, particularly those living with T1DM.[1] Beyond a lack of time or resources for exercise, individuals with T1D face additional barriers such as fear of hypoglycemia and a lack of knowledge and confidence as to how to exercise safely while managing their disease.

Nearly 100 years ago, it was shown that increases in contraction-mediated muscle glucose uptake and insulin sensitivity commonly lead to hypoglycemia during physical activity for individuals with T1D.[2] Despite the advent of modern rapid- and ultra-rapid–acting insulins, the duration of insulin action in subcutaneous tissue is prolonged and its actions cannot be stopped quickly in the event of unplanned exercise. Therefore, individuals with T1D who adopt a regular exercise regimen require careful advanced planning to avoid hypoglycemia. While carbohydrate intake can mitigate the risks of low blood glucose, rebound hyperglycemia often occurs. Adjustments to insulin delivery may require planning, sometimes 12 to 24 hours in advance of activity (in the case of injected basal insulin) or up to 4 hours prior to activity in the case of mealtime and corrective rapid-acting insulin. When starting an exercise regimen, it is common to see increased glucose variability—ranging from the intentional mild hyperglycemia leading up to exercise, to frequent hypoglycemia during exercise, to rebound hyperglycemia immediately post exercise, to spontaneous hypoglycemia overnight—all of which can be quickly discouraging to individuals with T1D and dissuade them from making the effort to participate in exercise at all.

Thankfully, recent advances in diabetes technology, including insulin pumps, continuous glucose monitors, and more recently AID systems, have been shown to improve time-in-range and reduce hypoglycemia with physical activity.[3] Challenges persist, however, with practical use of AID systems during exercise. Commercial AID algorithms are optimized at baseline to react quickly to avoid sustained hyperglycemia by automating basal and corrective insulin and generally recommend using aggressive insulin-to-carbohydrate ratios surrounding meals. These algorithms function well to increase insulin delivery and minimize hyperglycemia during relatively sedentary periods; however, the same algorithms may lead to rapid occurrence of hypoglycemia during exercise unless the user modifies the delivery settings to prepare for heightened insulin sensitivity as a result of physical activity. The astute clinician should be aware that each available AID system (*Table*) has unique settings that can be customized and adjusted by the user to reduce but not prevent all hypoglycemia without additional carbohydrate intake, particularly in the setting of unplanned exercise.[4]

Practice Gaps

- Addressing common key scenarios faced by individuals with T1D regarding glycemic management during exercise.

- Assisting patients with T1D to understand key features of insulin delivery and AID systems to optimize performance and glycemia during exercise.

Discussion

There are several key elements in an initial clinical encounter to discuss exercise and T1D. The first step in discussing a new exercise regimen with an individual with T1D is understanding their goals and motivation. Is the primary goal to achieve a cardiovascular benefit, to lose weight, or to exercise in a competitive way? Understanding a

Table. Exercise Targets for Available Commercial AID Systems[a]

System	Exercise terminology	Exercise glucose target	Effects of using exercise mode	Practical considerations
CamAPS Fx (CamDiab)	Ease-Off Planned Ease-Off	Customizable	- Reduces basal insulin delivery - Raises glucose target	- Can pre set a time for exercise adjustment and duration of activity
Control IQ (Tandem)	Exercise Activity	140-160 mg/dL (SI: 7.8-8.9 mmol/L)	- Decreases insulin delivery when predicted blood glucose below target, raises insulin delivery when above target range - Continues to auto-bolus	- Consider making alternative "exercise profile" to reduce insulin delivery - Consider a "phantom bolus" - Can pre set duration of activity 30 minutes to 8 hours
iLet (Beta Bionics)	None	130 mg/dL (SI: 7.2 mmol/L)	- Can raise target glucose modestly - No reduction in insulin delivery during exercise; continues to bolus to achieve target	- Disconnection from pump may be helpful during exercise
Omnipod 5 (Insulet)	Activity Mode	150 mg/dL (SI: 8.3 mmol/L)	- Raises target glucose - Decreases insulin delivery 50%	- Can set a duration of exercise from 1-24 hours - OP5 does not have automatic boluses
MiniMed 780g (Medtronic)	Temp Target	150 mg/dL (SI: 8.3 mmol/L)	- Raises target decreases insulin delivery - Disables automated boluses	- Can set a duration of exercise up to 24 hours

[a] Not listed: open-source AID systems (Loop, FreeAPS, OpenAPS, Android APS, FreeAPS X) that offer freely customizable targets, scalable delivery parameters, and programming options.

Adapted from Zaharieva DP et al. *Diabetes Spectr*, 2023; 36(2): 127-136. © by the American Diabetes Association.[4]

patient's motivations and goals helps the provider ensure that the clinical discussion is time-efficient and focused. For example, someone exercising to lose weight will need to first reduce insulin and take in carbohydrate only when necessary to avoid hypoglycemia. In contrast, a competitive athlete may prioritize a need for higher carbohydrate intake for fuel to muscles to achieve the best performance outcomes.

Second, one must determine the type, duration, and intensity of the planned exercise, as this will dictate the anticipated glycemic effects.[5] Broadly, exercise can be classified into 3 major subtypes: aerobic/endurance (running, cycling, walking), anaerobic/resistance (sprinting, weightlifting, high-intensity interval training), or interval/mixed (soccer, basketball). Aerobic/endurance activities cause a drop in blood glucose due to increased glucose disposal via both insulin-mediated and muscle contraction–mediated mechanisms, as well as suppression of hepatic glucose production by hyperinsulinemia. Anaerobic activities cause blood glucose levels to rise, sometimes sharply, due to high levels of counterregulatory hormones and lactate formation. These factors are unopposed in individuals with T1D, given their inability to produce endogenous insulin. Knowing what type of glycemic effect to expect allows the individual living with T1D to prepare for exercise by reducing insulin levels (ie, insulin-on-board) for aerobic exercise or maintain or increase insulin levels for anaerobic exercise. Longer durations of exercise require additional foresight and planning for both insulin adjustment and carbohydrate replacement. Increased intensity of aerobic activity causes a more rapid decline in glucose levels until the anaerobic threshold is reached—around 80% of the VO_2 max.[6] Once the body's glycogen stores are depleted, carbohydrate intake is necessary to avoid hypoglycemia if glucose levels continue to drop.

After understanding the exercise goals, it is essential to determine how the individual with T1D is going to monitor their blood glucose with regard to exercise. Given the risks of dysglycemia, the need for insulin adjustment and carbohydrate

intake in response to rapid changes in glucose, the use of a continuous glucose monitor (CGM) is strongly recommended during exercise.[7] The value of CGM lies not only in the absolute determination of blood glucose but in the trend arrows and described rate of change. The absolute accuracy of CGM may be reduced (% or mean absolute relative difference [MARD]), and the lag time between interstitial fluid vs blood glucose may be increased during exercise.[8] Accounting for these factors, it is recommended to self-treat with rapid-acting carbohydrates when blood glucose levels are trending down below 90 mg/dL (<5 mmol/L) during exercise.

Finally, it is necessary to assess the current insulin management strategy, whether the individual is using MDI or an insulin pump. For the latter, one must further consider whether the insulin pump is operating in an "open-loop" with blood glucose monitoring/CGM for assistance or in a "closed-loop" AID system. The strategies for adjusting insulin before, during, and after exercise vary with each of these insulin strategies.

For MDI users, the key is managing insulin-on-board in advance of planned activity. Adjusting basal insulin often requires adjustment the night before the next day's activity. The downside of this adjustment, however, is that it can also lead to hyperglycemia if exercise does not occur as planned and it does not limit the insulin reduction to only the period of exercise. For MDI users, adjusting mealtime bolus insulin is therefore a more useful strategy. The most effective intervention is to reduce mealtime insulin boluses by 25% to 75% (depending on duration and intensity of exercise) if the meal is within 2 hours of planned activity.[9] For those just starting out, the simplest recommendation is to reduce premeal insulin by 50% in anticipation of exercise for the first attempt and make further adjustments based on individualized response. Exercise in the fasting state, particularly in the morning, can be also useful to avoid hypoglycemia although carbohydrate replacement still may be needed due to the ongoing action of basal insulin and contraction-mediated muscle glucose uptake.

For insulin pump users, the strategies vary widely depending on the nature of the system. For those who use an "open loop" (ie, not an AID system), the key recommendations are to reduce basal insulin by 50% to 80% approximately 60 to 90 minutes prior to activity and to reduce bolus insulin for a meal occurring within 2 hours of activity (as noted above for MDI users).[5] For those using AID systems, the ways to reduce risk of hypoglycemia are to reduce basal insulin delivery, adjust the "exercise blood glucose target," and to reduce the premeal insulin bolus. As a special caveat for these systems, it is critical to avoid hyperglycemia leading up to exercise as this will lead to increases in AID and increase insulin-on-board. Also note that the insulin-on-board reported by the device screen may underestimate the "true" insulin-on-board, which would include increases in basal delivery. To avoid preexercise hyperglycemia and inadvertent increases in insulin delivery, one should try to consume carbohydrate snacks only within 15 minutes of exercise if needed based on blood glucose. The target glucose concentration to begin aerobic exercise should be approximately 125 mg/dL (6.9 mmol/L). The exercise target mode should be started 90 minutes prior to exercise.[5]

The system features of commercially available AID systems are summarized in the *Table*. Each system has a unique terminology for its exercise mode, and each varies in ability to customize the exercise target glucose. The user must understand what happens when the system is placed in exercise mode: whether the basal is adjusted right away, whether the target is a specific number or a range, whether you can preset the start and stop times for activity, and whether the system will continue to automatically bolus during activity.

After exercise, careful consideration should be given to avoid overnight hypoglycemia. This more commonly occurs with afternoon exercise than with morning exercise. If wearing an open-loop insulin pump, one could set a 20% reduction in basal insulin for 4 to 6 hours in the early overnight period (or up to 12 hours after exercise). If wearing an AID system, one could use an extended

period of using a higher exercise target glucose level to cover the same interval.

Both preceding episodes of hypoglycemia and exercise itself have been demonstrated to increase risk of future hypoglycemia due to loss of counterregulatory responses.[10] This can result in a dangerous cycle of hypoglycemia, especially in those with hypoglycemia unawareness. If a severe hypoglycemic event occurs, it is recommended to wait 24 hours before resuming exercise to allow for some restoration of counterregulatory responses.[5]

Many individuals struggle to avoid hypoglycemia despite insulin reductions, so a carbohydrate intake strategy is important. Carbohydrate needs vary but are increased for aerobic vs anaerobic exercise, longer vs shorter duration of activity, and higher levels of active insulin-on-board. Most aerobic activities lasting greater than 30 minutes require 30 to 60 g of carbohydrates per hour during exercise to prevent hypoglycemia, with some elite endurance athletes requiring up to 90 g per hour or more to maintain optimal performance. Refueling with 1 g carbohydrate per kg body weight and 20 to 25 g of protein within 1 hour of exercise can assist with muscle recovery and replenishment of glycogen stores, as well as avoiding postexercise hypoglycemia.[5]

Clinical Case Vignettes
Case 1

A 25-year-old woman with well-controlled T1D (most recent hemoglobin A_{1c} = 6.5% [48 mmol/mol]) presents to your clinic. She has started to exercise with a goal of losing weight and improving her overall health and well-being. She is discouraged, however, by frequent hypoglycemic events occurring during exercise. To manage her diabetes, she injects 25 units of insulin glargine once daily in the morning, 1 unit of insulin lispro for every 10 g of carbohydrates eaten, and 1 unit of insulin lispro for every 40 mg/dL (2.2 mmol/L) of corrective insulin above a glucose target of 120 mg/dL (6.6 mmol/L). She usually engages in 45 minutes of moderate-intensity jogging on a treadmill 5 days per week in the morning after breakfast. She tries to keep her blood glucose concentrations greater than 200 mg/dL (>11.1 mmol/L) prior to exercise, yet she still has recurrent low blood glucose after only about 30 minutes of activity.

Which of the following is the best recommendation now?

A. Take additional carbohydrates prior to exercise to maintain blood glucose higher from the outset

B. Move the timing of exercise to after dinner

C. Reduce long-acting insulin dose in the morning prior to exercise

D. Try to exercise in the fasted state

E. Change to high-intensity exercise in the morning

Answer: D) Try to exercise in the fasted state

Hypoglycemia during aerobic exercise is one of the most common challenges faced by individuals with T1D. The first key learning point in this vignette is to consider the patient's primary motivation for exercise. Her goal is to lose weight; therefore, the correct solution in line with her goals would not be one of consuming more carbohydrates, but rather reducing the insulin requirement. The best recommendation for her would be to try to exercise in the fasted state (Answer D). Exercising in the morning in a fasted state, when insulin-on-board is low, reduces the need for carbohydrate intake and is associated with less risk of exercise-associated hypoglycemia.[11]

Consuming additional carbohydrates prior to exercise (Answer A) would be incorrect, as consuming additional calories may lead to additional weight gain, and unless she reduces her insulin adequately for these carbohydrates, this could still lead to hypoglycemia.

Moving her exercise to after dinner instead of after breakfast (Answer B) would not help. Postmeal exercise would increase risk of hypoglycemia as discussed above, and exercise in the evening can be associated with increased risk of hypoglycemia, especially overnight.

A reduction in the dose of long-acting insulin on the morning of exercise (Answer C) would likely be insufficient to prevent hypoglycemia during exercise, especially in the face of increased insulin-on-board from a recent meal bolus.

High-intensity exercise in the morning (Answer E) may help her to avoid hypoglycemia. However, this leads to further hyperglycemia, which can then cause rebound hypoglycemia if insulin is given.[12]

One reasonable alternative not provided as an option would be for her to perform mixed-intensity exercise instead of pure aerobic exercise, which may result in more stable glucose levels.

Case 1 (continued)

The patient notices that with adjustment of her exercise timing in relation to meals and manipulating her insulin dosing, she has been able to successfully avoid hypoglycemia during exercise with minimal extra carbohydrate intake. Now she notices, however, that her blood glucose concentration tends to sharply spike *after* exercise, especially after higher-intensity workouts. She usually eats a small protein and carbohydrate snack after exercise for "refueling," but the spike occurs even before this.

Which of the following is the best recommendation?

A. Take a full correction bolus of insulin as blood glucose is peaking

B. Give an insulin bolus 15 minutes prior to stopping activity

C. Perform a 15-minute low-intensity cool-down after exercise

D. Avoid the protein and carbohydrate snack after exercise

Answer: C) Perform a 15-minute low-intensity cool-down after exercise

Hyperglycemia can occur shortly after aerobic, anaerobic, and mixed types of exercise related to increases in adrenaline and lactate formation. Liver metabolism causes excess lactate to be converted to glucose and high adrenaline levels cause release of stored glycogen and further worsening of hyperglycemia.[13] The most effective solution, especially in this patient who is concerned about avoiding hypoglycemia and excessive carbohydrate intake, would be to engage in a low-intensity cool-down activity (Answer C) such as walking to reduce postexercise lactate levels.

Administering additional insulin boluses, particularly full corrective insulin boluses (Answers A and B) may prevent hyperglycemia, but this could lead to significant rebound hypoglycemia given her increased postexercise muscle insulin sensitivity. Giving insulin boluses during activity should be done with extreme caution as the response can be unpredictable and dangerous. Insulin absorption kinetics are more rapid due to increased blood flow to the injection site.

Having a protein and carbohydrate snack after exercise is beneficial for muscle and liver glycogen replacement and is indeed recommended with a bolus of 50% of usual insulin requirements to avoid hypoglycemia. While this patient is trying to avoid taking in extra calories, this refueling step (Answer D) is important to restore glycogen stores, reduce risk of future hypoglycemia, and prepare for subsequent exercise sessions.[14]

Case 2

A 30-year-old man with a 16-year history of T1D is using an AID system (Tandem T-slim X2 with Control IQ), but he struggles with hypoglycemia during exercise. He is a cyclist who rides for 2 hours on weekends, usually in the middle of the day. He has frequent hypoglycemia near the beginning of his rides but also sometimes in the middle. He tries to eat a small snack 15 to 30 minutes prior to his ride to keep his blood glucose elevated (>180 mg/dL [>10 mmol/L]) at the start, knowing that his blood glucose will drop shortly thereafter. He has started enabling the "exercise" activity mode on the pump approximately 60 minutes prior to exercise but finds that this has not prevented hypoglycemia from occurring.

Which of the following is the best solution?

A. Switch to MDI

B. Eat a larger snack prior to exercise

C. Start exercise activity mode 2 hours prior to exercise

D. Discontinue Control IQ and use manual (open-loop) mode with 50% basal rate reductions starting 60 to 90 minutes prior to exercise

E. Switch from current pump to Beta Bionics iLet pump

Answer: D) Discontinue Control IQ and use manual (open-loop) mode with 50% basal rate reductions starting 60 to 90 minutes prior to exercise

This patient may be having trouble with hypoglycemia during exercise for several specific reasons. First, AID systems increase basal insulin delivery to achieve a target glucose, either a range (in the case of T-slim X2 with Control IQ) or to target a specific number (100-150 mg/dL [5.6-8.3 mmol/L] depending on the system). By attempting to begin exercise with glucose elevated, his pump is automatically increasing insulin-on-board, which is counterproductive in avoiding hypoglycemia. His goal should be to minimize insulin-on-board during aerobic exercise by reducing basal insulin and reducing any prandial insulin or corrective insulin given in the last 2 to 3 hours.

Eating a larger snack prior to exercise (Answer B) would lead to higher preexercise glucose levels and would only serve to increase insulin-on-board when using an AID system.

Starting exercise activity mode earlier (Answer C) would be of some benefit but is not likely sufficient to reduce insulin-on-board, as this adjustment alone may often be insufficient to avoid hypoglycemia during aerobic activity. Notably, the Control IQ algorithm does not reduce basal insulin delivery while in exercise activity mode when the blood glucose levels are greater than 140 mg/dL (>7.8 mmol/L), as is the case for this individual who is keeping his glucose levels elevated at the outset. This is contrast to the function of the

Minimed 780g, Omnipod 5, and CamAPS Fx algorithms, which do reduce basal insulin delivery immediately when the exercise function is activated regardless of blood glucose levels.

The best choice to reduce hypoglycemia is this case is stopping Control IQ mode, reverting to "open-loop" with a 50% basal rate reduction 60 to 90 minutes prior to exercise (Answer D). This also avoids the possibility of getting a Control-IQ automated bolus, which would be too aggressive for exercise. Another option to achieve a similar effect with this system would be to use a second "exercise" profile that could be preprogramed for a 50% basal rate reduction and a 200% increase in correction factor (eg, from 40 mg/dL [2.2 mmol/L] to 80 mg/dL [4.4 mmol/L]), so that there is less insulin delivery at baseline and any automated corrections are reduced. One way of temporarily suspending automated corrections with this pump is to give a 0.05 unit bolus after disconnecting the pump and then reconnecting as this will prevent any automated boluses for 1 hour.

Using MDI instead of a pump (Answer A) would be an option in some circumstances if appropriate adjustments are made; however, this would be likely too extreme of a change given that there are solutions with his current system as described above.

Switching to the iLet pump (Answer E) would not reduce his risk of hypoglycemia, as this pump does not provide a way to announce exercise or reduce basal insulin delivery in anticipation of exercise. Additionally, the maximum target glucose for the iLet is approximately 130 mg/dL (7.2 mmol/L), which is still lower than the 140 to 160mg/dL (7.8-8.9 mmol/L) exercise activity target with his current system. With the iLet pump, disconnection prior to exercise, as well as increased carbohydrate intake during exercise, would be recommended.

Case 2 (continued)

After further education and instruction, the patient is able to successfully complete his training bike rides without excessive hypoglycemia. He feels increasingly fit and confident and starts to exercise more frequently. He sometimes spontaneously bikes with friends or rides his bike to meet them for another activity, occasionally without a planned strategy for insulin management.

Which of the following spontaneous situations would cause the greatest immediate risk of hypoglycemia?

A. Jumping on his bike 30 minutes after lunch to squeeze in a 30-minute ride before his break-time is over

B. Waking up and riding 8 miles before breakfast

C. Going for a 30-minute ride after work at 5 PM, heading to dinner and a night out with friends

D. Challenging his friend to a brief but all-out intensity sprint competition

Answer: A) Jumping on his bike 30 minutes after lunch to squeeze in a 30-minute ride before his break-time is over

The key element here is understanding the importance of insulin-on-board and what situations tend to increase or decrease it. If the patient just ate lunch and he spontaneously decides to for a 30-minute ride (Answer A), more than likely he administered a full carbohydrate bolus for his meal. This is the highest-risk situation for hypoglycemia: exercise less than 2 hours after a meal when a full bolus has been given. A meal bolus should be reduced by 25% to 75% when exercise occurs within 2 hours of a meal. The only option for him at this point if he has already given the full meal bolus would be to consume additional carbohydrates (which may be difficult to tolerate from a gastrointestinal standpoint) or to delay or omit the exercise.

Exercise in the fasting state (Answer B) would not put him at the greatest risk of hypoglycemia, even if it were spontaneous. Often in the morning, due to increased cortisol, GH, and counterregulatory hormones such as norepinephrine, insulin resistance is greatest and there is the least likelihood of hypoglycemia compared with other times of day. Additionally, in patients using AID systems, often by the morning the blood glucose has been in the low target range for several hours and the system has kept insulin-on-board to an absolute minimum. Therefore, additional requirement for carbohydrates during exercise is negligible.

Going for a 30-minute ride after work at 5 PM and heading to dinner and a night out with friends (Answer C) implies that the exercise is being done in the fasting state (before dinner). Although he may later be at increased risk of overnight hypoglycemia due to performing evening exercise (as glycogen stores are replenished 7 to 11 hours after exercise), he would not currently be at the highest risk of hypoglycemia in the moment due to minimal insulin-on-board.

Brief bursts of maximal intensity aerobic activity (Answer D) would be expected to increase blood glucose levels, not decrease them, even in the context of high levels of insulin-on-board.

Case 3

A 45-year-old woman with a 35-year history of T1D has been recently struggling with recurrent hypoglycemic events during exercise. Her hemoglobin A_{1c} values run between 7.0% and 7.5% (53-58 mmol/mol), which she prefers to maintain due to some mild hypoglycemia unawareness (score of 4 on the Gold questionnaire). She has been increasing her weekly mileage in training for a half-marathon, and she feels overall that her fitness is improving. She exercises 5 out of 7 days per week, always in the mornings in the fasted state. She has had level 3 hypoglycemia (<55 mg/dL [<3 mmol/L]) twice in the last week. She uses an MDI regimen and has been gradually reducing her insulin doses in the last few weeks to try to decrease the number of hypoglycemic episodes.

Which of the following is a significant adverse risk factor for this individual who is having recurrent hypoglycemia during exercise?

A. Female sex
B. Hemoglobin A_{1c} ≥7.5% (≥58 mmol/mol)
C. Morning exercise
D. Exercise in the fasted state
E. Hypoglycemia in the last 24 hours before exercise

Answer: E) Hypoglycemia in the last 24 hours before exercise

A number of participant-related and exercise event-related characteristics can predict the degree of glucose changes and therefore the hypoglycemia risk during exercise. According to the T1DEXI study,[15] a recent comparison of 3 types of structured at-home exercise, several characteristics influence glucose decline during exercise: exercise type, participant sex, baseline A_{1c}, blood glucose levels at the start of exercise, rate of change at the start of exercise, percentage of time with glucose levels less than 70 mg/dL (<3.9 mmol/L) in the 24 hours prior to exercise, heart rate prior to exercise, time of day of exercise, and insulin-on-board prior to exercise. In this study, all 3 types of exercise (aerobic, resistance, and interval) caused a drop in blood glucose levels, although the drop was greatest for aerobic exercise. Male sex, not female sex (Answer A), was associated with a greater decline in blood glucose, although this finding was not significant after post hoc adjustment for confounders of insulin-on-board (male patients tended to be higher) and heart rate (male patients tended to be lower). The risk of hypoglycemia during exercise was greater for those with lower hemoglobin A_{1c} values, not higher values (Answer B). Morning exercise (Answer C) is associated with a smaller decline in blood glucose than the decline with afternoon, evening, or nighttime exercise. Higher levels of insulin-on-board are associated with a larger decline in glucose; therefore, exercise in the fasted state (Answer D) is not associated with increased risk of recurrent hypoglycemia.

Spending more time with blood glucose values less than 70 mg/dL (<3.9 mmol/L) (Answer E) is associated with increased risk of recurrent hypoglycemia. The act of exercise itself reduces the counterregulatory response to hypoglycemia, and sustained (>15 minutes) hypoglycemic events can lead to increased risk of subsequent events in the next 24 hours.[10] As fitness increases, as in this vignette, it is common to see an increase in hypoglycemic events due to higher glucose use rates, increased insulin sensitivity, and overall increase in exercise volume. To stop this cycle of recurrent hypoglycemia, the best recommendation for this patient would be to further reduce insulin doses and avoid exercise and hypoglycemic events for at least 24 to 48 hours to allow for restoration of her counterregulatory responses.

Key Learning Points

- Exercise can induce both hypoglycemia and hyperglycemia in individuals with T1D based on the type, duration, and intensity of activity.

- Managing T1D and exercise requires a customized plan for insulin adjustment and carbohydrate intake while understanding the individual's goals and motivations.

- AID systems are helpful but require active management and user-initiated changes to avoid glycemic disturbances during and after exercise.

References

1. American Diabetes Association Professional Practice Committee 5. Facilitating positive health behaviors and well-being to improve health outcomes: standards of care in diabetes-2024. *Diabetes Care.* 2024;46(Suppl 1):S77-S110. PMID: 38078584

2. Lawrence RD. The effect of exercise on insulin action in diabetes. *Br Med J.* 1926;1(3406):648-650. PMID: 20772477

3. Eckstein ML, Weilguni B, Tauschmann M, et al. Time in range for closed-loop systems versus standard of care during physical exercise in people with type 1 diabetes: a systematic review and meta-analysis. *J Clin Med.* 2021;10(11):2445. PMID: 34072900

4. Zaharieva DP, Morrison D, Paldus B, Lal RA, Buckingham BA, O'Neal DN. Practical aspects and exercise safety benefits of automated insulin delivery systems in type 1 diabetes. *Diabetes Spectr.* 2023;36(2):127-136. PMID: 37193203

5. Riddell MC, Gallen IW, Smart CE, et al. Exercise management in type 1 diabetes: a consensus statement. *Lancet Diabetes Endocrinol.* 2017;5(5):377-390. PMID: 28126459

6. Shetty VB, Fournier PA, Davey RJ, et al. Effect of exercise intensity on glucose requirements to maintain euglycemia during exercise in type 1 diabetes. *J Clin Endocrinol Metab.* 2016;101(3):972-980. PMID: 26765581

7. Moser O, Riddell MC, Eckstein ML, et al. Glucose management for exercise using continuous glucose monitoring (CGM) and intermittently scanned CGM (isCGM) systems in type 1 diabetes: position statement of the European Association for the Study of Diabetes (EASD) and of the International Society for Pediatric and Adolescent Diabetes (ISPAD) endorsed by JDRF and supported by the American Diabetes Association (ADA). *Diabetologia.* 2020;63(12):2501-2520. PMID: 33047169

8. Da Prato G, Pasquini S, Rinaldi E, et al. Accuracy of CGM systems during continuous and interval exercise in adults with type 1 diabetes. *J Diabetes Sci Technol.* 2022;16(6):1436-1443. PMID: 34111989

9. Rabasa-Lhoret R, Bourque J, Ducros F, Chiasson JL. Guidelines for premeal insulin dose reduction for postprandial exercise of different intensities and durations in type 1 diabetic subjects treated intensively with a basal-bolus insulin regimen (ultralente-lispro). *Diabetes Care.* 2001;24(4):625-630. PMID: 11315820

10. Sandoval DA, Aftab Guy DL, Richardson MA, Ertl AC, Davis SN. Effects of low and moderate antecedent exercise on counterregulatory responses to subsequent hypoglycemia in type 1 diabetes. *Diabetes.* 2004;53(7):1798-1806. PMID: 15220204

11. Gomez AM, Gomez C, Aschner P, et al. Effects of performing morning versus afternoon exercise on glycemic control and hypoglycemia frequency in type 1 diabetes patients on sensor-augmented insulin pump therapy. *J Diabetes Sci Technol.* 2015;9(3):619-624. PMID: 25555390

12. Riddell MC, Pooni R, Yavelberg L, et al. Reproducibility in the cardiometabolic responses to high-intensity interval exercise in adults with type 1 diabetes. *Diabetes Res Clin Pract.* 2019;148:137-143. PMID: 30641168

13. Yardley JE, Kenny GP, Perkins BA, et al. Resistance versus aerobic exercise: acute effects on glycemia in type 1 diabetes. *Diabetes Care.* 2013;36(3):537-542. PMID: 23172972

14. Campbell MD, Walker M, Bracken RM, et al. Insulin therapy and dietary adjustments to normalize glycemia and prevent nocturnal hypoglycemia after evening exercise in type 1 diabetes: a randomized controlled trial. *BMJ Open Diabetes Res Care.* 2015;3(1):e000085. PMID: 26019878

15. Riddell MC, Li Z, Gal RL, et al; T1DEXI Study Group. Examining the acute glycemic effects of different types of structured exercise sessions in type 1 diabetes in a real-world setting: the Type 1 Diabetes and Exercise Initiative (T1DEXI). *Diabetes Care.* 2023;46(4):704-713. PMID: 36795053

Diabetes and Pregnancy

Alon Y. Mazori, MD. The Icahn School of Medicine at Mount Sinai, New York, NY;
Email: alon.mazori@mssm.edu

Carol J. Levy, MD, CDCES. The Icahn School of Medicine at Mount Sinai, New York, NY;
Email:carol.levy@mssm.edu

Educational Objectives

After reviewing this chapter, learners should be able to:

- Explain the effect of maternal dysglycemia on maternal and neonatal outcomes and the important elements of preconception counseling for persons with diabetes mellitus.

- Describe the pattern of gestational changes in insulin sensitivity and identify pregnancy-specific glycemic targets for blood glucose and continuous glucose monitoring (CGM).

- Explain different treatment strategies to achieve glycemic goals for pregnancy.

Significance of the Clinical Problem

Optimal glycemic control throughout pregnancy complicated by diabetes mellitus is crucial for maternal and neonatal health. Pregnancies complicated by diabetes display an increased maternal risk of severe hypoglycemia, preeclampsia, and cesarean delivery.[1] Simultaneously, these pregnancies exhibit a higher risk of intrauterine fetal demise and perinatal mortality, congenital malformations, and large-for-gestational-age (LGA), and neonatal hypoglycemia requiring neonatal intensive care unit (NICU) admission.[1] The impact of these adverse events is tremendous not only for the individual, but also for society at large. One study[2] estimated that the total annual cost savings

afforded by CGM in pregnancy neared £10 million for England's National Health Service, the primary drivers of which were the number and duration of NICU admissions.

While maternal dysglycemia plays a central role in maternal and fetal health, multiple obstacles hinder glycemic control in pregnancy. Health care disparities worsen outcomes (eg, hemoglobin A_{1c}, frequency of diabetic ketoacidosis) by influencing the use of diabetes technology and measures of glycemic control across multiple social determinants of health, including race/ethnicity, socioeconomic status, and insurance status.[3] Fewer than 40% of women with type 1 diabetes mellitus (T1DM) receive formal prepregnancy care, which is known to improve gestational glycemic management and is cost saving.[1,4] Limited dietary guidance exists for pregnancies complicated by diabetes,[1,4] and current recommendations are difficult to consistently implement. Blood glucose monitoring is burdensome at the recommended frequency of 4 times daily outside of pregnancy, but a frequency of 7 times daily or more is often needed throughout pregnancy for those with preexisting diabetes.[4] Women and their health care teams use real-time continuous glucose monitoring (rtCGM) during pregnancy to provide a broader overview of glucose data for patients and providers. Yet, the US FDA first approved rtCGM for use in pregnancy in 2022.

The chief obstacle to maternal glycemic control is achieving optimal pregnancy-specific glycemic control prior to and throughout pregnancy, while balancing the risks of hypoglycemia and hyperglycemia and self-care burden. Insulin sensitivity changes with advancing gestation,[5,6] and the response to insulin therapy is modulated by maternal nutritional status and delayed insulin absorption.[7] These gestational metabolic alterations combine with the need for strict glycemic control and impaired hypoglycemia awareness to raise the risk of severe hypoglycemia by as much as 5-fold during pregnancy.[8] Continuous subcutaneous insulin infusion (CSII) therapy, including sensor-augmented pump therapy and hybrid closed-loop (HCL) systems, reduces the risk of hypoglycemia; however, studies on CSII use during pregnancy have been conflicting. HCL systems offer the potential to improve glycemic control and maternal and fetal outcomes, but most commercially available systems cannot be customized to pregnancy-specific targets.

Practice Gaps

- Variable implementation of preconception counseling.

- Challenges associated with preconception optimization of nutritional intake and glycemic control.

- Elevated risk of first-trimester hypoglycemia due to tighter glycemic targets.

- Need to preemptively transition prepregnancy medications to those without teratogenic potential.

- Unstandardized core CGM metrics for people with T1DM, T2DM, and gestational diabetes mellitus (GDM).

- Absence of formal treatment strategies to optimize glycemic control.

- Systemic barriers to use of diabetes technology impacted by social determinants of health.

- Absence of commercial HCL systems with pregnancy-specific glycemic targets.

Discussion

Preconception Counseling and Optimization

Preconception counseling has become central to the management of diabetes in pregnancy within the past decade. One meta-analysis and systematic review found that preconception counseling reduced the risk of congenital malformations by 71%, perinatal mortality by 54%, NICU admission by 25%, and preterm delivery by 15%.[1,4] Such counseling is a multidisciplinary endeavor that integrates subspecialists in endocrinology, maternal-fetal medicine, nutrition, and diabetes care and education.[4]

A key element of preconception counseling is to ensure all individuals of childbearing potential are aware of the ideal glycemic and health goals prior to pregnancy. To this end, preconception counseling should be introduced by pediatric diabetes specialists, include detailed counseling on contraceptive options, and emphasize the risks and benefits of prepregnancy planning. Such counseling should be continued for individuals seeing adult specialists. If available, referrals can be offered for classes on the management of diabetes during major life transitions (eg, adolescence to adulthood).

Ideally, the timing of the desire for future pregnancies is established, and the medical team coordinates the optimization of glycemic control for pregnancy 3 to 6 months prior to conception attempts. Pregestational glycemic goals are strict and specify a target hemoglobin A_{1c} of 6.5% (47 mmol/mol)[4]; a lower value of 6.0% (42 mmol/mol) is encouraged if attainable without hypoglycemia. Prospective parents should receive education on the maternal and fetal risks of hypoglycemia and hyperglycemia. Accordingly, the preconception visit is a crucial opportunity to review diabetes self-management techniques such as carbohydrate counting, to examine dietary and exercise patterns, and to introduce medical nutrition therapy. Clinicians should also inform patients about pregnancy-specific glycemic targets and provide anticipatory guidance about gestational changes in insulin sensitivity and absorption.[5-7]

Preconception preparation also centers on screening for and management of diabetes-related complications. Retinopathy can worsen in pregnancy; accordingly, dilated eye exams are recommended prior to pregnancy and during each trimester.[1,4] Nephropathy screening is also recommended due to a higher risk of preeclampsia during pregnancy,[1,4] and the potential risk of nephropathy progression if renoprotective medications are withheld due to teratogenicity. Other preconception topics such as folate supplementation, thyroid and hypertensive disorders, and genetic counseling should also be addressed.

Many persons with pregestational T2DM use antihyperglycemic medications with an understudied safety profile in pregnancy; examples include GLP-1 receptor agonists and SGLT-2 inhibitors. Accordingly, planning is needed to replace these medications with safer ones prior to conception. Similar attention should be given to the medical treatment of hypertension. Medications such as ACE inhibitors are first-line outside of pregnancy, but they are teratogenic and only a few antihypertensive medications have well-established safety in pregnancy. Careful review and monitoring are required to transition antihypertensive and antihyperglycemic medications to those with established safety in pregnancy.

Glucose Monitoring

Blood Glucose Monitoring

Historically, frequent fingerstick glucose testing was the method of choice for glucose monitoring. Blood glucose monitoring accurately and rapidly reports glucose levels. While glycemic targets should always be tailored to individual risk of hypoglycemia, the target ranges listed[4] are commonly used in pregnancy for individuals with preexisting diabetes or diabetes diagnosed during pregnancy. During a given day, blood glucose monitoring should be completed while fasting in the morning, before and after each meal, and ideally at least once overnight. In contrast to pregnancies complicated by T1DM, there

is a lower risk of hypoglycemia in pregnancies complicated by T2DM and GDM. As a result, pregnant individuals with T2DM or GDM are typically asked to perform fasting and postprandial measurements.

- Fasting: 70-95 mg/dL (3.9-5.3 mmol/L)
- One-hour postprandial: 110-140 mg/dL (6.1-7.8 mmol/L)
- Two-hour postprandial: 100-120 mg/dL (5.6-6.7 mmol/L)

Hemoglobin A$_{1c}$

Hemoglobin A$_{1c}$ is a macroscopic measure of glycemic control and has historically been used to estimate maternal and fetal risks associated with pregnancies complicated by diabetes. Hemoglobin A$_{1c}$ cannot elucidate the patterns or severity of hypoglycemia and hyperglycemia. While modest hemoglobin A$_{1c}$ decrements with advancing gestation are associated with improved neonatal outcomes,[9] other glucose-monitoring techniques such as CGM offer more precise and detailed information that can be incorporated into treatment strategies in real time.

Continuous Glucose Monitoring

CGM, particularly rtCGM, is a useful technology for managing diabetes in pregnancy. Measuring interstitial glucose levels every 1 to 5 minutes, rtCGM transmits these measurements to a compatible receiver, insulin pump, or smartphone application, and displays glycemic data in real time to the pregnant individual and others if a sharing option is enabled.[10] CGM enables providers to better examine glycemic patterns and tailor insulin therapy, and empowers patients to better understand the relationship between glycemic targets and patterns in diet, insulin dosing, and exercise. The most recent devices also reduce self-care burden because calibration is not required. Given CGM's temporally dynamic nature, consensus guidelines based on earlier data[11] led to the establishment of CGM-based glycemic goals to support clinicians and patients in pregnancies complicated by T1DM (*Figure 1*).[4,11] While similar criteria have not been established for T2DM and GDM, the lower risk of hypoglycemia in pregnancies complicated by these types of diabetes would ideally permit a narrower target range to optimize maternal and neonatal outcomes.

Figure 1. Glycemic Targets for Diabetes in Pregnancy Described in CGM-Based Measures

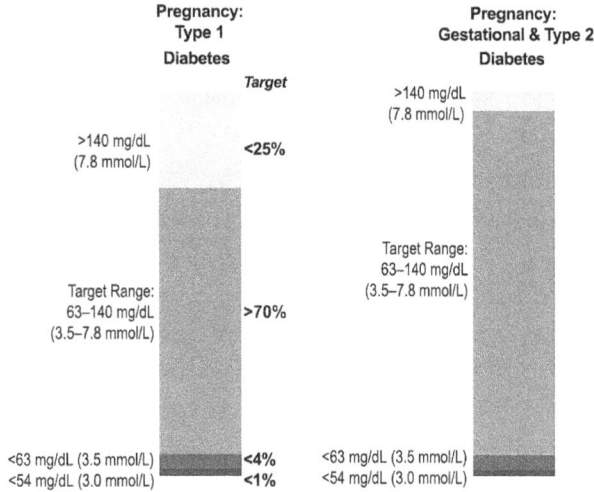

Reprinted from Battelino T et al. *Diabetes Care*, 2019; 42(8): 1593-1603. © by the American Diabetes Association.[11]

[Color—Print (Color Gallery page CG25) or web & ePub editions]

CGM Use in T1DM

Prior investigations into CGM use in pregnancies complicated by T1DM illustrate multiple advantages. CONCEPTT,[9] the largest randomized controlled trial, found that CGM use was associated with higher time-in-range, lower time-above-range, and reduced glycemic variability. CGM use was also linked to a lower incidence of adverse neonatal outcomes such as NICU admission, LGA, and hypoglycemia requiring intravenous dextrose. A smaller observational study[6] supported that higher time-in-range and lower time-above-range were associated with fewer maternal complications such as preeclampsia and preterm labor. A secondary analysis[2] of CONCEPTT further demonstrated that CGM use would afford cost savings close to £10 million while balancing the risk of adverse maternal and fetal outcomes.

CGM Use in GDM

Many of the benefits associated with CGM use in pregnancies complicated by T1DM have also been observed in those complicated by GDM. Yu et al[12] prospectively assigned a population of 340 Chinese women with GDM to either intermittently scanned CGM or blood glucose monitoring, and noted that women with intermittently scanned CGM exhibited a lower risk of preeclampsia, cesarean delivery, and preterm delivery. The study also demonstrated reduced risk of macrosomia, LGA, and neonatal hypoglycemia. FLAMINGO,[13] a more recent randomized controlled trial based in Poland, assigned 100 individuals with GDM to intermittently scanned CGM or blood glucose monitoring and found that intermittently scanned CGM conferred a lower risk of macrosomia.

Medication Strategies

T2DM and GDM

While lifestyle modifications and medical nutrition therapy are first-line interventions for T2DM and GDM, insulin is first-line pharmacologic therapy for GDM, T1DM, and T2DM. Both metformin and sulfonylureas cross the placenta and are associated with neonatal hypoglycemia, and long-term safety data are unclear. Moreover, metformin should be avoided in pregnancies with risk factors for an ischemic environment such as placental insufficiency, hypertension, preeclampsia, or growth restriction.

T1DM

Optimal glycemic control is challenging with insulin therapy because gestational changes in insulin sensitivity and absorption vary throughout pregnancy.[5,6] Prior work has documented that insulin requirements typically rise modestly early in the first trimester[5,6] and significantly decrease in the later first trimester with an increased risk of hypoglycemia (up to 5-fold in early pregnancy) (*Figure 2, following page*).[5,6,8] Nausea can further modulate the risk of hypoglycemia through sporadic meal intake; strategies include frequent smaller meals, extended mealtime boluses, and less aggressive basal-insulin dosing. The second and third trimesters, in contrast, are characterized by monotonically worsening insulin resistance and resultant hyperglycemia primarily driven by daytime postprandial hyperglycemia.[5,6]

Recent work on HCL systems with pregnancy-specific glycemic targets has demonstrated improvements in glycemic outcomes; however, further studies are needed to confirm reductions in maternal and neonatal complications. The largest trial to date occurred in the United Kingdom and was an open-label, multicenter, randomized controlled trial[14] of 124 patients using the Cambridge model predictive control algorithm targeting 100 mg/dL (5.6 mmol/L) in early pregnancy and lower values thereafter (*Figure 3, following page*). Significant improvements were seen in both time-in-range and time-above-range without an increase in hypoglycemia. A small observational study[15] in the United States of 10 pregnant individuals who used a noncommercial HCL system at home with zone model predictive control with pregnancy-tailored glycemic targets (daytime: 80-110 mg/dL [4.4-6.1 mmol/L]; nighttime: 80-100 mg/dL [4.4-5.6 mmol/L]) demonstrated that the HCL

system achieved significantly higher time-in-range with lower time-above-range and time-below-range compared with run-in data (*Figure 4, following page*).

Intrapartum Care

To reduce the risk of maternal and neonatal hypoglycemia, the target blood glucose range during delivery for persons with T1DM is 70 to 126 mg/dL (3.9-7.0 mmol/L). Continuous insulin infusion with hourly fingerstick glucose monitoring is a safe and effective approach; continuation of insulin pump therapy can be considered in select individuals whose on-site clinical teams possess expertise in using these systems.

Postpartum Care

Insulin requirements fall dramatically in the immediate postpartum period following delivery of the placenta, and reduction of antepartum insulin regimen dosing by 50% or more is often necessary. The choice of agents included in the postpartum antihyperglycemic regimen depends on the mother's lactation status. Metformin is

Figure 2. Mean Insulin Requirements and Self-Monitored Blood Glucose in Pregnant Women With T1DM

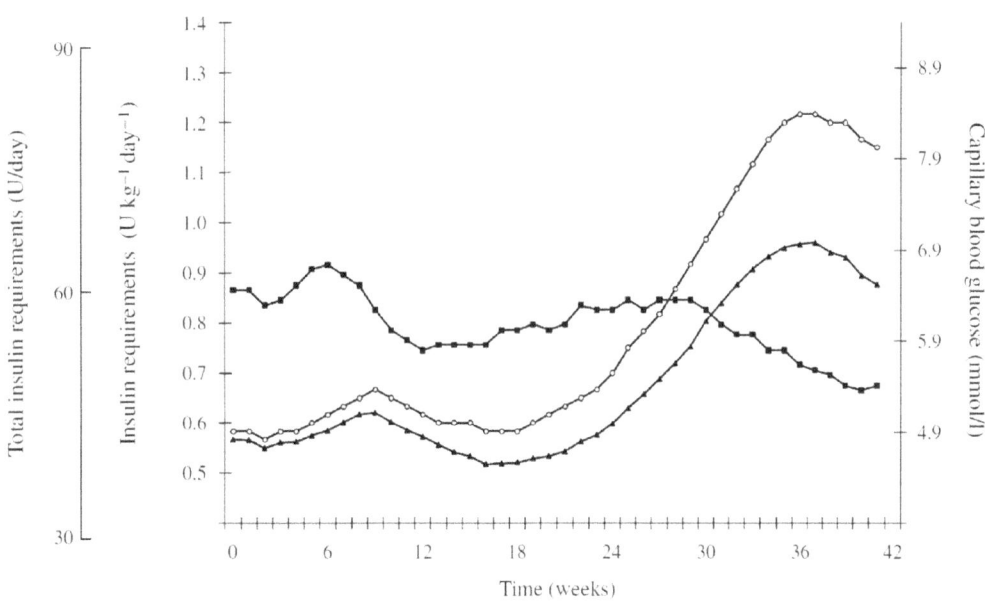

Squares represent capillary blood glucose. Circles show daily insulin requirements (units/day), and triangles depict weight-based daily insulin requirements (units kg⁻¹ day⁻¹). Reprinted with permission from García-Patterson A et al. *Diabetologia*, 2010; 53(3): 446-51. © Springer-Verlag.[5]

Figure 3. Pregnancy-Specific Target Glucose Range

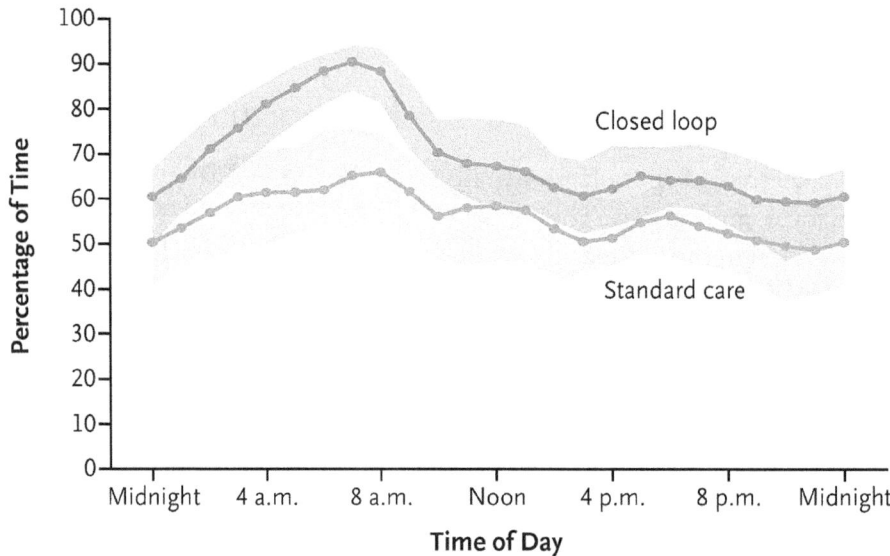

B Time in Target Glucose Range According to Time of Day

Panel B shows an envelope plot of time in the pregnancy-specific target glucose range, as measured by CGM, for each treatment group, according to the time of day, from 16 weeks' gestation until delivery. Shaded areas indicate the interquartile range. Reprinted with permission from Lee TTM et al. *N Engl J Med*, 2023; 389(17): 1566-78. © Massachusetts Medical Society.[14]

[Color—Print (Color Gallery page CG26) or web & ePub editions]

Figure 4. Median Continuous Glucose Monitoring Glucose Values During Run-In vs CLC-P Use

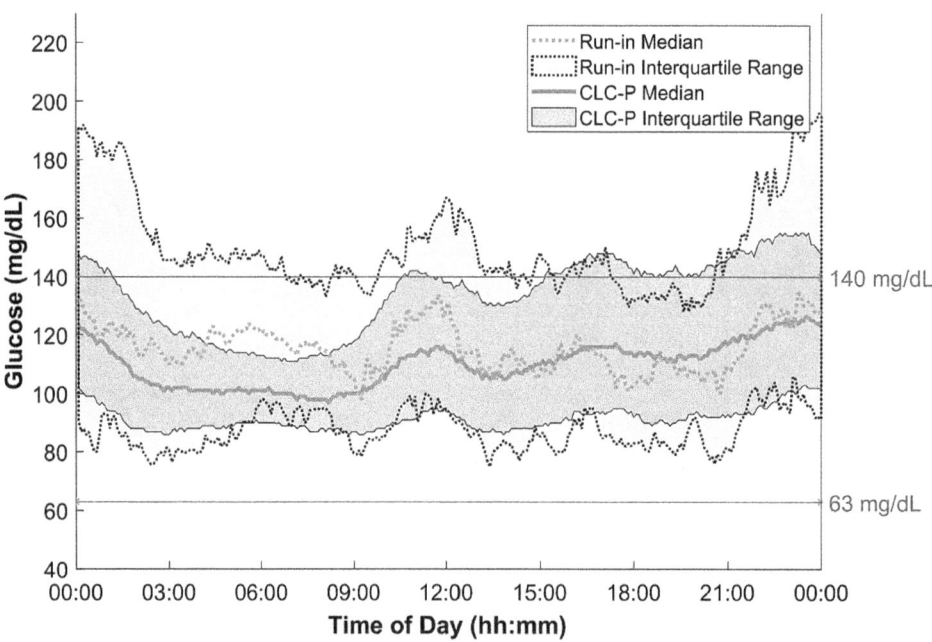

Comparison of glucose levels based on continuous glucose monitoring data between CLC-P (solid lines indicating median, and green shading indicating interquartile range) and run-in (dashed lines indicating median, and yellow shading indicating interquartile range). To convert values for glucose to millimoles per liter, multiply by 0.05551. Reprinted from Levy CJ et al. Diabetes Care, 2023; 46(7): 1425-1431. © by the American Diabetes Association.[15]

[Color—Print (Color Gallery page CG26) or web & ePub editions]

excreted into breastmilk and carries an unclear safety profile in the postnatal period and beyond. In addition, breastfeeding can increase the risk of hypoglycemia. If the mother breastfeeds, an antihyperglycemic regimen comprising only insulin confers no medication exposure to the neonate, but potentially increases the risk of maternal hypoglycemia.

GDM typically diminishes after delivery without the need for continued medication in many persons. However, the risk of developing T2DM is dramatically greater in those with prior GDM.[4] As hemoglobin A_{1c} exhibits a suboptimal detection rate during the postpartum period, all individuals should undergo oral glucose tolerance testing with 75 g of dextrose between 4 and 12 weeks after delivery. If the results are normal, testing with hemoglobin A_{1c} measurement or oral glucose tolerance testing should be repeated every 1 to 3 years.

Disparities in Diabetes Care

Prior work has shown that multiple social determinants of health (eg, race/ethnicity, socioeconomic status, insurance status) are linked to worse glycemic control, as evidenced by higher hemoglobin A_{1c} values and frequency of diabetic ketoacidosis and severe hypoglycemia.[3] Use of diabetes technology such as CGM and insulin pumps is also lower in these groups.[3] While the administrative burden of insurance documentation and requirements has fallen recently, a multifaceted approach is required to improve rates of technology adoption and health outcomes. Strategies include leveraging telemedicine to increase access to care by endocrinologists, lowering barriers to the prescription of diabetes technology by primary care providers, and systematizing the prescription of diabetes technology to mitigate implicit bias.

Clinical Case Vignettes

Case 1

A 26-year-old primigravid woman with T1DM presents to establish care for diabetes in pregnancy. She had a positive pregnancy test a week ago, and her obstetrician estimates that she is at 6 weeks' gestation. She had not received preconception counseling.

T1DM was diagnosed at age 14 years, and her treatment regimen was transitioned to an insulin pump at age 23 years; she currently uses sensor-augmented pump therapy. Hemoglobin A_{1c} values were less than 7.0% (<53 mmol/mol) for years, and her hemoglobin A_{1c} value last week was 6.0% (42 mmol/mol). She describes frequent symptomatic hypoglycemia and has noted recent episodes of hypoglycemia while at work, as well as one episode overnight; her husband gave her glucose tablets because she was confused. She has been self-administering more correction boluses, both after meals and overnight, because she is worried about the fetal consequences of hyperglycemia. She has also been experiencing nausea and is inconsistently eating meals. Her last episode of diabetic ketoacidosis was 1 year after T1DM was diagnosed.

She uses an rtCGM approved for use during pregnancy with supplemental blood glucose monitoring on occasion when feasible. Her CGM data over the past 2 weeks are shown (*Figure 5, following page*).

Retinopathy screening was negative last month, and her urinary albumin-to-creatinine ratio was 16 mg/g 6 months ago. She takes a prenatal multivitamin, and her only medication is rapid-acting insulin in her pump.

Today, her blood pressure is 108/70 mm Hg and pulse rate is 65 beats/min. Her weight is 169.8 lb (77 kg) (BMI = 24 kg/m²).

Which of the following statements is most accurate?

A. Her preconception A_{1c} goal was ≤6.0% (≤42 mmol/mol); recommend no dose changes

B. The recent hypoglycemia is to be expected in the first trimester; recommend no dose changes

C. Dysglycemia is limited to fasting hypoglycemia

Figure 5. The Patient's CGM Tracing for the Past 2 Weeks (Currently 6 Weeks' Gestation)

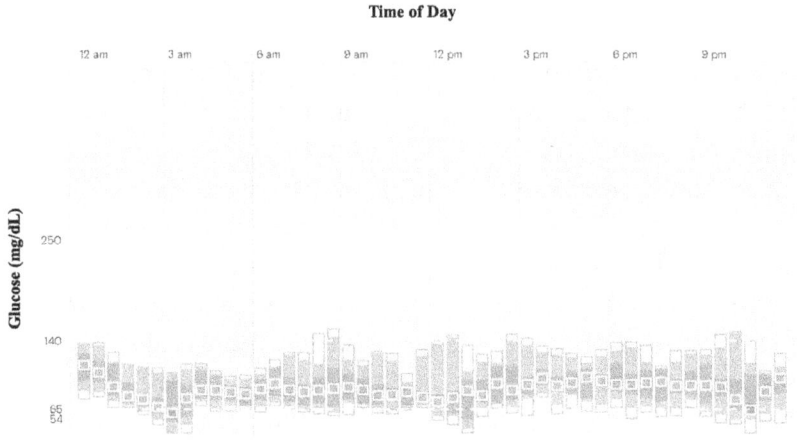

[Color—Print (Color Gallery page CG27) or web & ePub editions]

D. She should avoid exercise to reduce the risk of hypoglycemia

E. She has both nocturnal and postprandial hypoglycemia; pump settings should be adjusted with concurrent counseling to avoid overcorrection of hyperglycemia and hypoglycemia

Answer: E) She has both nocturnal and postprandial hypoglycemia; pump settings should be adjusted with concurrent counseling to avoid overcorrection of hyperglycemia and hypoglycemia

Multiple factors contribute to this patient's postprandial and nocturnal hypoglycemia. Nocturnal hypoglycemia is related to her increased reliance on correction boluses and likely supratherapeutic basal rates, as well as the expected increase in insulin sensitivity in the first trimester. These factors yield a higher proclivity for hypoglycemia that can be 5-fold for persons with T1DM in early pregnancy.[8] In addition, she exhibits postprandial hypoglycemia related to 3 key factors: (1) sporadic meal intake due to nausea, which is common in the first trimester; (2) potentially delayed gastric emptying; and (3) supratherapeutic correction doses. Fasting hyperglycemia is likely related to corrective measures to remedy nocturnal hypoglycemia (eg, glucose tablets). Adjustment in insulin delivery settings with close follow-up will reduce these risks.

While a preconception hemoglobin A_{1c} value of 6.0% or below (≤42 mmol/mol) is ideal, this strict target is reserved for individuals who can safely achieve this degree of glycemic control without hypoglycemia. A target of 6.5% or below (≤47 mmol/mol) is better suited for this patient. Glycemic targets in pregnancy are: fasting, 70-95 mg/dL (3.9-5.3 mmol/L); 1-hour postprandial, 110-140 mg/dL (6.1-7.8 mmol/L); and 2-hour postprandial, 100-120 mg/dL (5.6-6.7 mmol/L). Over the course of a given day, blood glucose monitoring should be completed while fasting in the morning, before and after each meal, and ideally at least once overnight. Hemoglobin A_{1c} underestimates hyperglycemia in pregnancy because of increased erythrocyte turnover; values above 7.0% (>53 mmol/mol) translate to maternal hyperglycemia during pregnancy and raise the risk of complications.

Case 1 (continued)

The patient's insulin pump settings are adjusted, and she returns for follow-up 1 week later. During a detailed diet and medication review, she shares that she occasionally delivers a bolus a few minutes after she has started eating because her workday can have unpredictable lunch times. When this happens, glucose as measured by her sensor often reaches 200 mg/dL (11.1 mmol/L) 1 hour after eating. The pump does not offer a correction bolus during these situations, so she overrides and develops hypoglycemia later in the afternoon.

How should this patient's insulin regimen be adjusted and why?

A. Increase the daytime basal rate to combat daytime hyperglycemia

B. Make the lunchtime insulin-to-carbohydrate ratio more aggressive to prevent postprandial hyperglycemia

C. Encourage her to dose 15 to 20 minutes before meals and make no other changes until re-evaluation

D. Make the daytime correction factor more aggressive so she will not need to override the pump

E. Recommend that she skip lunch to avoid postprandial hyperglycemia

Answer: C) Encourage her to dose 15 to 20 minutes before meals and make no other changes until re-evaluation

Postprandial hyperglycemia should first be targeted by better synchronizing bolus delivery with mealtimes (Answer C), and the insulin-to-carbohydrate ratio adjusted if such hyperglycemia persists.

Case 1 (continued)

In pregnancies complicated by T1DM, CGM use does which of the following?

A. Raises time-below-range and lowers time-above-range; no neonatal benefit

B. Raises time-in-range and lowers time-above-range; both maternal and neonatal benefit

C. Raises time-in-range and raises time-above-range; only maternal benefit

D. Lowers time-below-range and lowers time-above-range; both maternal and neonatal benefit

E. Raises time-below-range and time-in-range; only neonatal benefit

Answer: B) Raises time-in-range and lowers time-above-range; both maternal and neonatal benefit

Prior investigations into CGM use in pregnancies complicated by T1DM illustrate multiple advantages. CONCEPTT,[9] the largest randomized controlled trial to date, found that CGM use conferred higher time-in-range and lower time-above-range and reduced glycemic variability. CGM use was also linked to a lower risk of neonatal complications such as NICU admission, LGA, and hypoglycemia requiring intravenous dextrose. LOIS-P[6] noted that higher time-in-range and lower time-above-range were associated with fewer maternal complications such as preeclampsia and preterm labor.

Case 1 (continued)

The patient incorporates the recommendations for timing of bolus delivery. After several weeks without contact, she returns at 27 weeks' gestation. She reports that during the time between visits, her glucose values have been stable and hypoglycemia has fallen markedly. She also shares that it is still difficult to optimize premeal-bolus timing. She has gained 22 lb (10 kg) since conception and has not developed obstetric complications. Her CGM tracing for the last 2 weeks is shown (*Figure 6, following page*).

Which of the following is the best next step and/or anticipatory guidance?

A. Nighttime basal rate should be lowered to prevent nocturnal hypoglycemia

B. Observed hyperglycemia is unlikely to be related to advancing gestation

C. Careful review is needed to assess dietary patterns, insulin-administration timing, and basal-rate changes with potential adjustments in bolus settings

D. Glycemic control will improve with advancing gestation as insulin resistance decreases

E. Daytime basal rate should be raised to counter daytime hyperglycemia

Answer: C) Careful review is needed to assess dietary patterns, insulin administration timing, and basal-rate changes with potential adjustments in bolus settings

Figure 6. The Patient's CGM Tracing for the Past 2 Weeks (Currently 27 Weeks' Gestation)

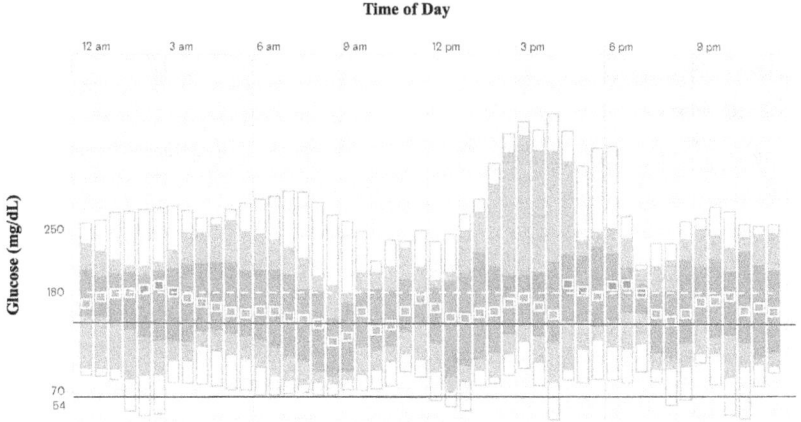

[Color—Print (Color Gallery page CG27) or web & ePub editions]

Sensor data show that pregnancy-specific time-in-range is below the goal of 70%, time-above-range is above the goal of 25%, and most hyperglycemic excursions appear to be postprandial and overnight. Premeal boluses should be administered 15 to 20 minutes before carbohydrate consumption earlier in gestation, while 30 to 45 minutes is often required in the third trimester to reduce postprandial hyperglycemia. Thus, careful review is needed to assess dietary patterns, insulin administration timing, and basal-rate changes with potential adjustments in bolus settings (Answer C).

Case 1 (continued)

Two years after delivery, the patient returns to clinic for preconception counseling. Over the past 3 months, time-in-range (70-180 mg/dL [3.9-10.0 mmol/L]) has been 51%, time-above-range has been 45%, and time-below-range has been 4%. Her hemoglobin A_{1c} value is 8.3% (67 mmol/mol). Her job continues to be demanding and stressful, and the unpredictable schedule impacts her ability to optimize prandial-insulin timing and administer correction boluses. She shares that her glycemic control would be worse if she could not use her HCL system, as she relies on the predictive low-glucose suspend feature and automated correction boluses. She also reports trouble sleeping related to frequent CGM

alerts. She asks whether she could use her HCL system during her next pregnancy.

Which recommendation should be made regarding the use of an HCL system in pregnancy?

A. Discourage use; no HCL system has been approved by the US FDA for use in pregnancy

B. Review the benefits and risks of off-label HCL system use in pregnancy and strategize with the patient on how her specific insulin pump and rtCGM could best be used

C. Discontinue rtCGM and insulin pump; transition to blood glucose monitoring and insulin injections

D. Always recommend only daytime HCL-system use with nighttime senor-augmented pump therapy

E. Always recommend only nighttime HCL-system use with daytime senor-augmented pump therapy

Answer: B) Review the benefits and risks of off-label HCL system use in pregnancy and strategize with the patient on how her specific insulin pump and rtCGM could best be used

While providers should seek to first use FDA-approved treatments, no HCL system has received approval for use in pregnancy complicated by diabetes. This patient's CGM-based measures of glycemic control are concerning for frequent hypoglycemia and marked hyperglycemia and glycemic variability.

HCL systems are useful tools to improve glycemic control in nonpregnant individuals. While glycemic targets in commercially available HCL systems exceed gestational targets (eg, nighttime target of 110 mg/dL [6.1 mmol/L]), such systems offer automated correction boluses to curb hyperglycemia and the predictive low-glucose suspend feature to prevent hypoglycemia. Simultaneously, off-label HCL system use in pregnancy can be complicated for pregnant individuals and their providers. Effective use requires a detailed understanding of which insulin pump parameters can be adjusted, as well as how the pump algorithm will respond to CGM-measured glucose. Mealtimes represent challenging situations. Insulin-to-carbohydrate ratios are made more aggressive to counter postprandial hyperglycemia; if the HCL system permits, basal rates after mealtimes may need to be reduced to prevent postprandial hypoglycemia. The opposite situation is also relevant: the doses of late premeal boluses may need to be lowered to reduce the risk of delayed postprandial hypoglycemia. Some pregnant individuals with T1DM achieve euglycemia by applying different modes of insulin delivery in different trimesters in response to pregnancy-mediated metabolic changes.

Case 2

A 33-year-old primigravid woman with T2DM presents for preconception counseling. T2DM was diagnosed 3 years ago on routine screening; both of her parents were diagnosed with T2DM after the age of 60 years. Retinopathy, nephropathy, and neuropathy screening were all negative 6 months ago. She has never experienced a hyperglycemic crisis. Her hemoglobin A_{1c} value was 6.8% (51 mmol/mol) 1 month ago. She does not engage in blood glucose monitoring. Her current antihyperglycemic regimen consists of dulaglutide, 4.5 mg weekly, and empagliflozin, 25 mg daily. She trialed metformin shortly after diabetes was

diagnosed, but she discontinued the medication within 5 days because of marked stomach upset. Her other medications are lisinopril for hypertension and a prenatal vitamin. She would like to become pregnant soon.

Today, her blood pressure is 106/68 mm Hg and pulse rate is 75 beats/min. Her weight is 181 lb (82 kg) (BMI = 28 kg/m²).

How should her antihyperglycemic and antihypertensive medication regimens be modified?

A. Continue lisinopril, dulaglutide, and empagliflozin

B. Continue lisinopril and dulaglutide; stop empagliflozin

C. Discontinue lisinopril, dulaglutide, and empagliflozin; provide intense lifestyle counseling

D. Discontinue lisinopril, dulaglutide, and empagliflozin; start insulin

E. Discontinue lisinopril, dulaglutide, and empagliflozin; start metformin

Answer: D) Discontinue lisinopril, dulaglutide, and empagliflozin; start insulin

ACE inhibitors such as lisinopril should be discontinued before pregnancy because of their teratogenic potential. As GLP-1 receptor agonists and SGLT-2 inhibitors have an unclear safety profile in pregnancy, discontinuation of these agents is recommended. If all current antihyperglycemic medications were stopped, the patient's subsequent hemoglobin A_{1c} level would likely be near 8.0% (64 mmol/mol), a value far above the prepregnancy target. Furthermore, a hemoglobin A_{1c} value as elevated as this patient's on 2 antihyperglycemic agents suggests that the chance of euglycemia without pharmacotherapy is very low. Metformin monotherapy is unlikely to control her hyperglycemia, and her poor tolerance of metformin in the past discourages repeat use. Initiation of insulin therapy now (Answer D) would best prepare her for optimal glycemic control both before and during pregnancy.

Case 3

A 35-year-old woman with a family history of T2DM and a personal history of obesity (BMI = 33 kg/m^2) presents for evaluation after a 100-g oral glucose tolerance test last week resulted in the diagnosis of GDM. Documented glucose values:

> Fasting = 90 mg/dL (5.0 mmol/L)
> 1 hour = 190 mg/dL (10.5 mmol/L)
> 2 hour = 165 mg/dL (9.2 mmol/L)
> 3 hours = 130 mg/dL (7.2 mmol/L)

The patient meets with a registered dietician the day after diagnosis and learns how to perform self-monitoring of blood glucose. Her glucose meter download reveals that fasting glucose measurements have been performed 3 times (range: 80-92 mg/dL [4.4-5.1 mmol/L]), and 1-hour postprandial measurements have been performed 3 times (range: 130-140 mg/dL [7.2-7.8 mmol/L]). She shares her frustration with blood glucose monitoring, as it is painful and inconvenient to perform frequently.

Which of the following is the best next step for this patient's glycemic management?

A. Continue self-monitoring of blood glucose (fasting and 1 hour after each meal); ask patient to return in 1 week

B. Transition to CGM; conduct a diet review and schedule follow-up in 1 week

C. Transition to CGM; start insulin injections

D. Reduce frequency of self-monitoring of blood glucose to fasting and 1 hour after the largest meal of the day

E. Transition to CGM; start insulin pump

Answer: B) Transition to CGM; conduct a diet review and schedule follow-up in 1 week

A recent United Kingdom-based randomized controlled trial comparing intermittently scanned CGM with self-monitoring of blood glucose in 100 women with GDM found that CGM use (Answer B) was linked to lower odds of macrosomia (odds ratio of 5.62 comparing self-monitoring of blood glucose with intermittently scanned CGM),

as well as improved fasting and postprandial hyperglycemia.[13] A similar observation was noted in a prospective cohort study of 340 women in China; intermittently scanned CGM use was associated with improved glycemic control and lower variability.[12] Moreover, this cohort study connected CGM use with a lower risk of neonatal hypoglycemia and LGA, as well as a lower maternal risk of preeclampsia, cesarean delivery, and preterm delivery.[12]

Case 3 (continued)

The patient begins using rtCGM and returns in 1 week (*Figure 7, following page*); she has not had symptoms of hypoglycemia.

Which of the following is the best recommendation?

A. Immediately treat all glucose values that are <63 mg/dL (<3.5 mmol/L)

B. Stop CGM use when her current sensor expires

C. Continue CGM use; review data and provide tips to reduce these types of events

D. Eat protein before bedtime to prevent hypoglycemia

E. Replace sensor after every episode of hypoglycemia

Answer: C) Continue CGM use; review data and provide tips to reduce these types of events

The asymptomatic sharp, "V"-shaped deflection that occurred during sleep most likely represents a pressure-induced sensor attenuation and not authentic hypoglycemia. CGMs are preferentially placed on the upper extremity to optimize accuracy, and pressure-induced sensor attenuations commonly occur when the CGM user turns during sleep onto the arm where the CGM is located. Thus, this patient should continue CGM use and her provider should give her tips to reduce these types of events (Answer C).

Figure 7. The Patient's CGM Tracing on a Day With a Nocturnal Hypoglycemia Alert

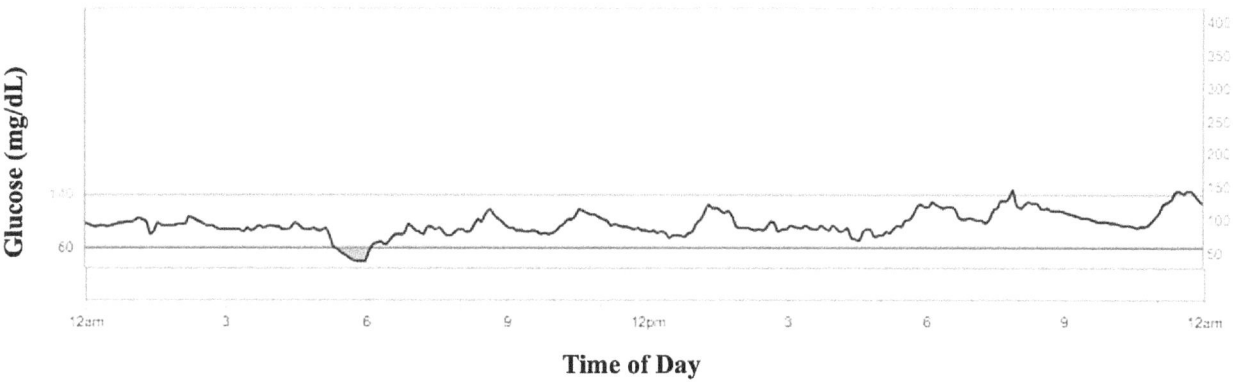

[Color—Print (Color Gallery page CG27) or web & ePub editions]

Key Learning Points

- Pregnancies complicated by diabetes confer an increased risk of adverse maternal outcomes (eg, severe hypoglycemia, preeclampsia) and neonatal complications (eg, perinatal mortality, hypoglycemia requiring NICU admission).

- Gestational changes in insulin resistance confer an increased risk of hypoglycemia and hyperglycemia.

- Preconception counseling is crucial to ensure that individuals of childbearing potential understand glycemic and health goals before pregnancy, and to optimize pregestational control of diabetes and other health issues with medications safe in pregnancy.

- CGM use in pregnancy improves glycemic control and maternal and neonatal outcomes while lowering self-care burden in a cost-saving fashion.

- Commercially available HCL systems may need to be considered for off-label use in select pregnant individuals and by experienced providers after careful discussion of risks, benefits, and alternatives, as well as strategies to optimize pump use and algorithms.

- Individuals with GDM should undergo oral glucose tolerance testing between 4 and 12 weeks postpartum due to a 10-fold greater risk of developing T2DM.

References

1. Benhalima K, Beunen K, Siegelaar SE, et al. Management of type 1 diabetes in pregnancy: update on lifestyle, pharmacological treatment, and novel technologies for achieving glycaemic targets. *Lancet Diabetes Endocrinol.* 2023;11(7):490-508. PMID: 37290466

2. Murphy HR, Feig DS, Sanchez JJ, de Portu S, Sale A; CONCEPTT Collaborative Group. Modelling potential cost savings from use of real-time continuous glucose monitoring in pregnant women with type 1 diabetes. *Diabet Med.* 2019;36(12):1652-1658. PMID: 31162713

3. Majidi S, Ebekozien O, Noor N, et al; T1D Exchange Quality Improvement Collaborative Study Group. Inequities in health outcomes in children and adults with type 1 diabetes: data from the T1D Exchange Quality Improvement Collaborative. *Clin Diabetes.* 2021;39(3):278-283. PMID: 34421203

4. ElSayed NA, Aleppo G, Aroda VR, et al; American Diabetes Association. 15. Management of diabetes in pregnancy: standards of care in diabetes-2023. *Diabetes Care.* 2023;46(Suppl 1):S254-S266. PMID: 36507645

5. García-Patterson A, Gich I, Amini SB, Catalano PM, de Leiva A, Corcoy R. Insulin requirements throughout pregnancy in women with type 1 diabetes mellitus: three changes of direction. *Diabetologia.* 2010;53(3):446-451. PMID: 20013109

6. O'Malley G, Ozaslan B, Levy CJ, et al. Longitudinal observation of insulin use and glucose sensor metrics in pregnant women with type 1 diabetes using continuous glucose monitors and insulin pumps: the LOIS-P Study. *Diabetes Technol Ther.* 2021;23(12):807-817. PMID: 34270347

7. Murphy HR, Elleri D, Allen JM, et al. Pathophysiology of postprandial hyperglycaemia in women with type 1 diabetes during pregnancy. *Diabetologia.* 2012;55:282-293. PMID: 22080230

8. Kaur RJ, Smith BH, Ozaslan B, et al. Hypoglycemia in prospective multicenter study of pregnancies with pre-Existing type 1 diabetes on sensor-augmented pump therapy: the LOIS-P Study. *Diabetes Technol Ther.* 2022;24(8):544-555. PMID: 35349353

9. Feig DS, Donovan LE, Corcoy R, et al; CONCEPTT Collaborative Group. Continuous glucose monitoring in pregnant women with type 1 diabetes (CONCEPTT): a multicentre international randomised controlled trial. *Lancet.* 2017;390(10110):2347-2359. PMID: 28923465

10. Polsky S, Garcetti R, Pyle L, Joshee P, Demmitt JK, Snell-Bergeon JK. Continuous glucose monitor use with and without remote monitoring in pregnant women with type 1 diabetes: a pilot study. *PLoS One.* 2020;15(4):e0230476. PMID: 32298269

11. Battelino T, Danne T, Bergenstal RM, et al. Clinical targets for continuous glucose monitoring data interpretation: recommendations from the International Consensus on Time in Range. *Diabetes Care.* 2019;42(8):1593-1603. PMID: 31177185

12. Yu F, Lv L, Liang Z, et al. Continuous glucose monitoring effects on maternal glycemic control and pregnancy outcomes in patients with gestational diabetes mellitus: a prospective cohort study. *J Clin Endocrinol Metab.* 2014;99(12):4674-4682. PMID: 25057872

13. Majewska A, Stanirowski PJ, Tatur J, et al. Flash glucose monitoring in gestational diabetes mellitus (FLAMINGO): a randomised controlled trial. *Acta Diabetol.* 2023;60(9):1171-1177. PMID: 37160787

14. Lee TTM, Collett C, Bergford S, et al; AiDAPT Collaborative Group. Automated insulin delivery in women with pregnancy complicated by type 1 diabetes. *N Engl J Med.* 2023;389(17):1566-1578. PMID: 37796241

15. Levy CJ, Kudva YC, Ozaslan B, et al. At-home use of a pregnancy-specific zone-MPC closed-loop system for pregnancies complicated by type 1 diabetes: a single-arm, observational multicenter study. *Diabetes Care.* 2023;46(7):1425-1431. PMID: 37196353

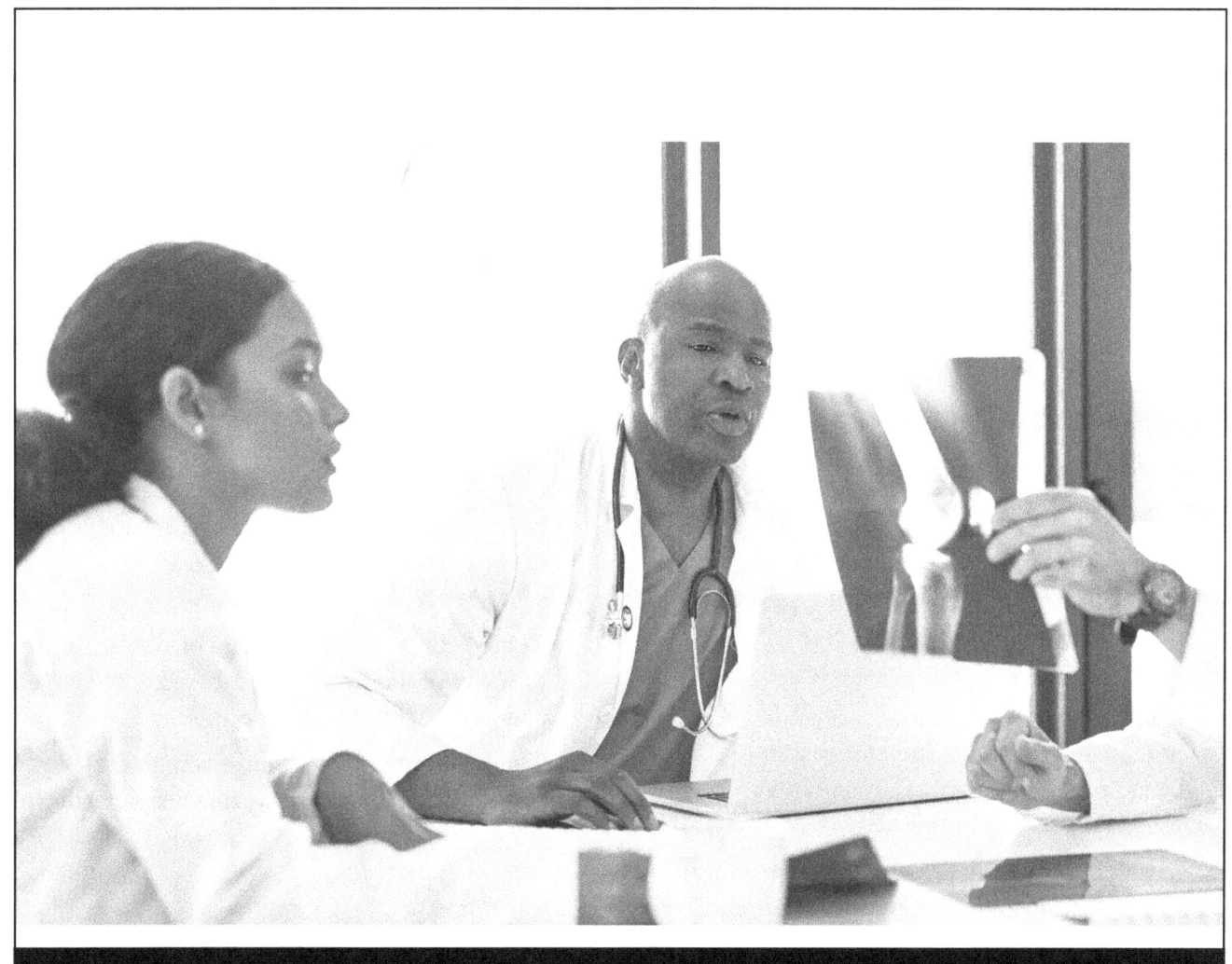

GENERAL
ENDOCRINOLOGY

Recognition and Management of Pseudoendocrine Disorders

Michael T. McDermott, MD. Division of Endocrinology, Metabolism, and Diabetes, University of Colorado Denver School of Medicine, Aurora, CO; Email: michael.mcdermott@cuanschutz.edu

Educational Objectives

After reviewing this chapter, learners should be able to:

- Review the nonspecific symptoms and testing protocols that have been proposed for the diagnosis of the most common pseudoendocrine disorders.

- Discuss the non–evidence-based and potentially harmful treatments that have been proposed for the most common pseudoendocrine disorders.

- Develop a practical, personalized approach to the evaluation and management of patients with pseudoendocrine disorders.

Significance of the Clinical Problem

Pseudoendocrine disorders are often diagnosed by nonendocrinologists, including people without a medical or health care degree, who promote non–evidence-based diagnosis and treatment suggestions from multiple nonvalidated, non-evidence-based sources. People diagnosed with pseudoendocrine disorders frequently present to endocrinologists requesting further evaluation or treatment of these pseudodisorders with diagnostic or treatment modalities that have no evidence for efficacy or safety and may even be harmful.[1-4]

Practice Gaps

- Providers and trainees have little education or training on recognition and interpretation of the proposed, nonvalidated tests for pseudoendocrine disorders.

- There is little or no education or training on how to avoid non–evidence-based, ineffective, and potentially harmful treatments.

- There is scant, if any, training on how to successfully care for vulnerable people with the respect and compassion necessary for positive outcomes.

Discussion

Over the past 30 years, we have seen a disturbing proliferation of print, broadcast, and internet claims and advertisements concerning fabricated diseases that have no actual scientific or credible clinical evidence for their existence and for which unproven and potentially harmful remedies are openly shilled for profit. We have seen practitioners proclaim themselves to be experts in hormonal therapy without any formal training and confidently promote hormone treatments without adequate endocrine evaluations. We have heard practitioners make astonishing promises regarding the benefits of herbal, supplemental, and other unproven therapies that they themselves sell in their offices and/or online. We have witnessed people being given harmful and even dangerous products that contain animal whole-organ (most commonly thyroid and/or adrenal) extracts or hormonal injections that produce highly elevated levels of sex hormones, especially testosterone) without any concern for short-term safety or long-term outcomes. And we have heard about the surprisingly high costs incurred by people who have visited these practitioners and had no beneficial or even frankly concerning results, despite being promised symptom improvement, safety, and full insurance coverage.[1-4]

What is our responsibility as concerned practitioners and citizens in the face of these rogue practitioners and practices? We clearly have a primary obligation to protect our patients and communities from these unscrupulous, charlatan practitioners and the unproven, costly, and sometimes dangerous treatments they promote. We can do this through one-on-one, in-person education with our patients. We should inform patients that misinformation is commonly present on the internet and direct them to view credible professional websites such as those of the Hormone Foundation (Endocrine Society), American Thyroid Association, and Mayo Clinic.

More broadly, however, we should seek opportunities to bring these issues to the attention of the general public. For example, I was interviewed on a local television station about testosterone therapy. During this brief interview, I informed the listeners that low testosterone levels are often a manifestation of more serious underlying medical conditions or of medications, that treatment of these conditions should be the primary focus of therapy, and that low testosterone levels caused by these conditions are often restored to normal, without a need for lifelong testosterone replacement therapy, if the underlying medical conditions are appropriately managed.

We can encourage our local and national professional organizations (state medical societies, American Medical Association [AMA], American College of Physicians [ACP], Endocrine Society, American Association of Clinical Endocrinologists [AACE], and American Thyroid Association [ATA]) to publish fact sheets, official statements, and guidelines regarding these types of practices. And we can write editorials and commentaries

in our local newspapers. One particularly well-written piece by Dr. Lisa Pryor was published in the *New York Times* (January 5, 2018) and was entitled "How to Counter the Circus of Pseudoscience."[5]

Another option is to report rogue practitioners and practices to the local state medical board. A small group of Colorado physicians reported a local physician who was treating patients who complained of fatigue with a combination of high-dosage prednisone and desiccated thyroid extract without testing for either adrenal insufficiency or hypothyroidism prior to initiating this aggressive therapy. I was asked to testify in court regarding this case. The outcome was removal of his medical license; he subsequently retired.

As physicians, we have much more influence over these issues than anyone else in our communities. The public listens to physicians; what we say makes a difference.

Definition of Pseudoendocrine Disorder

The term *pseudoendocrine disorder* does not have one clear and distinct definition.[1] The term could be used in reference to people who believe they have an endocrine or metabolic disorder because of information they received from a health care provider, personal trainer, family member, or friend and, despite previously appropriate normal testing, they request further unwarranted testing of their endocrine system or their hormones. It may apply to patients who have read about endocrine disorders (real and unproven) in books or on the internet and may have even ordered hormone or metabolic testing online. It also refers to those who have been given "endocrine" diagnoses by providers based on symptoms alone without validated hormone testing. It also refers to patients with endocrine or metabolic conditions that were diagnosed correctly (or not) by other providers and who are treated for these conditions with excessive hormone doses or with unproven, inappropriate, and even dangerous medications. Alternatively, an endocrine diagnosis may have erroneously been made as a result of lab assay error due to supplements and other conditions that adversely affect the accuracy of various tests.[1]

Case 1

A 47-year-old woman has been experiencing fatigue for about 15 years but describes "total exhaustion" that has been progressive over the past year. She does not sleep well but does not snore. Her appetite is poor. She only eats full meals occasionally but snacks frequently throughout the day. Mild weight gain (5 lb [2.3 kg]) has occurred in the past year. She cannot exercise due to fatigue. She requests to be treated for adrenal fatigue for which she has tested positive.

Her medical history includes mononucleosis at age 18 years. She takes occasional prescription pain medication.

On physical examination, her blood pressure is 128/70 mm Hg and pulse rate is 80 beats/min. Her height is 68 in (172.7 cm), and weight is 157 lb (71.2 kg) (BMI = 23.9 kg/m²). Orthostatic vital signs are normal. Examination findings are normal.

Full-day salivary cortisol profile, which she brings with her, is interpreted as documenting "adrenal fatigue."

Nonvalidated testing protocols and non–evidence-based treatment for adrenal fatigue have been promoted by which of the following persons with significant public influence?

A. Anthony Fauci

B. Donald Trump

C. Dr. Oz

D. Tom Cruise

Answer: C) Dr. Oz

Dr. Oz invited Dr. Robert Vigersky, MD, then President of the Endocrine Society, to appear on his TV show and debate the evidence for (Dr. Oz) and against (Dr. Vigersky) the validity of adrenal fatigue as an authentic evidence-based medical condition. To my knowledge, Dr. Fauci, Donald Trump, and Tom Cruise have not spoken publicly about adrenal fatigue.

Case 1 (continued)

Which of the following is the most potentially harmful treatment currently proposed for adrenal fatigue?

A. Licorice root, which may cause hypertension

B. Adrenal extracts, which may cause central adrenal insufficiency

C. Creatine supplements, which may cause kidney damage

D. Adrenal support supplements containing amino acids and vitamins

Answer: B) Adrenal extracts, which may cause central adrenal insufficiency

One of the proposed treatments for the pseudoendocrine disorder "adrenal fatigue" is "adrenal support" with supplements that contain extracts from animal adrenal glands (Answer B). These supplements contain actual steroid hormones, in unknown amounts, that can suppress the hypothalamic-pituitary-adrenal axis. This suppression causes secondary adrenal insufficiency, which can be life-threatening. Excess licorice root (Answer A) can cause hypertension, but this is not the most potentially harmful of the choices. Creatine supplements (Answer C) seldom cause kidney damage.

What Is Adrenal Fatigue?

Proposed by James L. Wilson in his 2001 book, "Adrenal Fatigue: The 21st Century Stress Syndrome," adrenal fatigue is suggested to develop when the adrenal glands become unable to produce adequate amounts of adrenal hormones to deal with the daily stresses of life.[1] It is said to occur in people who have chronic high stress (mental, emotional, or physical) in their work and/or family life. It is characterized by nonspecific symptoms such as fatigue, sleep disturbances, difficulty coping, body aches, digestive problems, and dependency on caffeine. Numerous practitioners and websites falsely promote this pseudoendocrine condition. Adrenal fatigue was featured on Dr. Oz on October 22, 2015.

How is Adrenal Fatigue Diagnosed?

Affected people are encouraged to self-diagnose adrenal fatigue based on symptoms using scoring systems that are available on websites. Providers or patients themselves can also order a salivary cortisol profile in which multiple salivary cortisol samples are collected throughout the day and submitted to a lab for analysis (for a price). If the salivary cortisol concentrations fall below a normative line, the diagnosis of adrenal fatigue is said to be confirmed.[1,6]

Is Adrenal Fatigue a Real Condition?

Adrenal fatigue has never been scientifically proven to exist.[1,6-8] Symptom scoring systems or salivary cortisol profiles have never been tested scientifically or validated as tools to evaluate function of the hypothalamic-pituitary-adrenal axis. As clinician-scientists, we must be open to novel ideas and proposals. But rigorous verification by well-designed and well-conducted scientific investigations must still be the standard by which we evaluate and clinically apply new and innovative ideas. It is not sufficient, where patients' health and well-being are concerned, to simply propose a hypothesis and apply it without diligent scientific investigation.[1,6-8]

How Is Adrenal Fatigue Treated?

Proposed treatments start with a healthy well-balanced diet, regular exercise, good sleep habits, stress reduction, and cessation of smoking and alcohol use.[9] Most of us would never object to any of these measures; this is the same advice we give to almost all patients. But adrenal fatigue websites and promoters also suggest that patients use reflexology, take licorice root, or use a variety of supplements that are claimed to improve adrenal function. However, there are also recommendations for and links to purchase "real" or "raw" adrenal extracts that contain bovine adrenal glandular extracts.[10] The obvious potential for these products to cause secondary adrenal insufficiency is clearly a major concern.

What Measures Have Been Taken to Educate the Public About the Adrenal Fatigue Myth?

The Endocrine Society (Hormone Foundation) has taken the lead in opposing promotion of adrenal fatigue.[7] The website and printed literature provide clear warnings, such as "No scientific proof exists to support adrenal fatigue as a true medical condition"; "Doctors are concerned that if you are told you have this condition, the real cause of your symptoms may not be found and treated correctly"; "Doctors urge you not to waste precious time accepting an unproven diagnosis such as 'adrenal fatigue' if you feel tired, weak, or depressed. If you have these symptoms, you may have adrenal insufficiency, depression, obstructive sleep apnea, or other health problems. Getting a real diagnosis is very important to help you feel better and overcome your health problem"; and "If you take adrenal hormone supplements when you don't need them, your adrenal glands may stop working and become unable to make the hormones you need when you are under physical stress. When these supplements are stopped, a person's adrenal glands can remain 'asleep' for months. People with this problem may be in danger of developing a life-threatening condition called adrenal crisis."

The Mayo Clinic website also has the following strong statements[8]: "The term often shows up in popular health books and on alternative medicine websites, but it isn't an accepted medical diagnosis"; and "It's frustrating to have persistent symptoms your doctor can't readily explain. But accepting a medically unrecognized diagnosis from an unqualified practitioner could be worse. Unproven remedies for so-called adrenal fatigue may leave you feeling sicker, while the real cause—such as depression or fibromyalgia—continues to take its toll."

Case 2

A 38-year-old woman is self-referred for hormone evaluation because of chronic progressive fatigue. Fatigue began at age 28 years, one year after the birth of her second child. She also notes hair loss, weight gain, and "brain fog." She is adamant that this is not due to depression.

There is no notable medical history. Her only medication is vitamins.

On physical examination, her blood pressure is 129/74 mm Hg and pulse rate is 74 beats/min. Her height is 67 in (170.2 cm), and weight is 158 lb (71.7 kg) (BMI = 24.8 kg/m^2). Examination findings, including thyroid gland and skin are normal.

She ordered tests online and is asking, "Do I have 'Wilson syndrome' or 'reverse T$_3$ syndrome' and will you treat me?"

Laboratory test results:

TSH = 2.1 mIU/L (0.45-4.5 mIU/L)
Free T$_4$ = 1.0 ng/dL (0.78-1.81 ng/dL)
   (SI: 12.87 pmol/L [10.04-23.30 pmol/L])
Free T$_3$ = 2.4 pg/mL (2.3-4.2 pg/mL)
   (SI: 3.69 pmol/L [3.53-6.45 pmol/L])
Reverse T$_3$ = 23 ng/dL (10-24 ng/dL)
   (SI: 0.35 nmol/L [0.15-0.37 nmol/L])
TPO antibodies, negative
Thyroglobulin antibodies, negative

Which of the following is the nonvalidated proposed pathophysiology of Wilson syndrome?

A. Decreased T$_4$ to T$_3$ conversion due to genetics and/or life experiences

B. Increased T$_3$ to T$_2$ conversion due to genetics and/or life experiences

C. Tissue thyroid hormone resistance due to genetics and/or life experiences

D. Increased albumin affinity for T$_4$ and T$_3$ due to genetics and/or life experiences

Answer: A) Decreased T$_4$ to T$_3$ conversion due to genetics and/or life experiences

The proposed pathophysiology of the pseudoendocrine disorder "Wilson syndrome" is an acquired impairment of the prohormone, T$_4$, into the active thyroid hormone, T$_3$, due to stressful life circumstances, possibly superimposed on a genetic or epigenetic background (Answer A). There is no actual evidence for this pathophysiology or for the existence of this syndrome. There have been no proposals or evidence that these individuals have impaired T$_3$ to T$_3$ conversion, thyroid hormone resistance, or high albumin affinity for T$_4$ or T$_3$.

Case 2 (continued)

Which of the following is the nonvalidated proposed pathophysiology of reverse T$_3$ syndrome?

A. Increased reverse T$_3$ increases hepatic metabolism of T$_3$

B. Increased reverse T$_3$ competes with T$_3$ for binding to the thyroid hormone receptor

C. Increased reverse T$_3$ suppresses TSH synthesis and secretion by the pituitary gland

D. Increased reverse T$_3$ increases hepatic metabolism of cortisol

Answer: B) Increased reverse T$_3$ competes with T$_3$ for binding to the thyroid hormone receptor

The proposed pathophysiology of the pseudoendocrine disorder "reverse T$_3$ syndrome" is that impaired T$_4$ to T$_3$ syndrome not only results in low serum T$_3$ levels but also causes high levels of reverse T$_3$, which then completes for T$_3$ binding to the thyroid hormone receptor, thereby further decreasing T$_3$ action. The well-documented fact that T$_3$ has a 100-fold higher affinity for the T$_3$ receptor than does reverse T$_3$ indicates that reverse T$_3$ cannot outcompete T$_3$ for occupancy of the T$_3$ receptor. There have been no proposals or evidence that reverse T$_3$ increases hepatic T$_3$ metabolism, suppresses TSH synthesis or secretion, or increases hepatic metabolism of cortisol.

What Is Wilson Syndrome?
Proposed by E. Denis Wilson in 1990, Wilson syndrome is suggested to be present when people develop chronically impaired conversion of T$_4$ to T$_3$ as a prosurvival adaptation in response to stress.[1] Susceptible people include famine survivors or their descendants (Scotch, Irish, Russian, Native American); holocaust survivors or their descendants; survivors of divorce, death of a loved one, or stress (family or job); chronic dieters;

yeast suffers; and people with hypoglycemia, eating disorders, and sleep disorders. Wilson syndrome is diagnosed by taking axillary temperature with a mercury thermometer every 3 hours starting 3 hours after waking up; the body temperature readings are averaged over several normal days. If the mean body temperature is 1 degree or more below normal, the person "may" have Wilson syndrome. The diagnosis does not involve testing TSH or thyroid hormone levels.[1]

What Is the Proposed Treatment of Wilson Syndrome?

The suggested treatment of Wilson syndrome involves cycling the body temperature up to normal with "proper T_3 thyroid supplements" (dosages up to 100 mcg daily) and then cycling down again. The cycle is repeated until the body temperature remains normal after stopping T_3 supplements; this typically takes 3 to 4 cycles but may involve 11 to 12 cycles in difficult cases.[1]

What Measures Have Been Taken to Educate the Public About the Wilson Syndrome Myth?

Dr. Denis Wilson was sanctioned by the Florida Board of Medicine after a 50-year-old woman died of cardiac complications while on excessive amounts of thyroid hormone prescribed by Wilson. In 1992, the Florida Board of Medicine accused him of "fleecing" patients with a "phony diagnosis." The Board and Wilson agreed to a 6-month suspension of his medical license, after which Wilson agreed to attend 100 hours of continuing medical education, submit to psychological testing, and pay a $10,000 fine before resuming practice. (Reference: State of Florida, Department of Health. February 12, 1992. Final Order Number: DPR9200039ME.)

The American Thyroid Association states emphatically on its website that there is no scientific evidence to support the existence of Wilson syndrome and that the proposed treatment is unsafe and frankly dangerous.[11]

Vignette Follow-Up
This patient listened carefully. She agreed that Wilson syndrome and/or reverse T_3 syndrome

may not be the cause of her symptoms and agreed not to pursue the liothyronine dosage escalation protocol recommended on the Wilson syndrome website. Her symptoms improved but did not completely resolve. She agreed to continue healthy lifestyle measures and stress reduction as the primary management approach to her symptoms.

How Is Reverse T_3 Syndrome Different From Wilson Syndrome?

Reverse T_3 syndrome, which is similar to Wilson syndrome, was proposed in a 2016 book and website "Stop the Thyroid Madness."[12] The proposal was that impaired T_4 to T_3 conversion not only reduces serum T_3 levels but further that T_4 is diverted into excess amounts of reverse T_3 that then competes with T_3 for the T_3 receptor, further reducing peripheral tissue access to T_3 action. Not only is there no scientific evidence to support the existence of this condition, well-documented, published evidence proves that T_3 has 100-fold higher affinity for the thyroid hormone receptor than does reverse T_3 and therefore excess reverse T_3 is not able to impair T_3 binding.[13,14] The book also proposes ways to "flush reverse T_3 out of the body."

Case 3

Via an email through the electronic health record patient portal, a 65-year-old man writes, "Recently I increased my thyroid dose from 200 mcg to 300 mcg daily due to fatigue and dizzy spells. My symptoms improved. Please renew my prescription for 300 mcg. By the way, I have read on the internet that low dose naltrexone can cure Hashimoto thyroiditis. My naturopath agreed. Please call in a prescription for that also." He has had no clinic visits for the past 6 years.

Which of the following is the proposed mechanism for the beneficial effects claimed regarding low-dosage naltrexone?

A. It increases the serum testosterone-to-estradiol ratio

B. It increases the serum and tissue cortisol-to-aldosterone ratio

C. It increases the serum and tissue T_3-to-T_4 ratio

D. It suppresses multiple processes underlying autoimmunity

Answer: D) It suppresses multiple processes underlying autoimmunity

Because products of proopiomelanocortin breakdown, including some endogenous opioids, may have some regulatory effects on the immune system, it was proposed, but never proven, that naltrexone, even in low dosages, can suppress autoimmunity. Low-dosage naltrexone does not affect the testosterone-to-estradiol ratio, cortisol-to-aldosterone ratio, or the T_3-to-T_4 ratio.

Case 3 (continued)

What autoimmune or idiopathic disorders have been shown to have beneficial effects from low-dosage naltrexone?

A. Hashimoto thyroiditis

B. None

C. Multiple sclerosis

D. Lung cancer

Answer: B) None

There is no evidence that low-dosage naltrexone has any beneficial effects on autoimmune, neoplastic, or neurodegenerative disorders, including Hashimoto thyroiditis (Answer A), multiple sclerosis (Answer C), or lung cancer (Answer D).

What Is the Rationale Behind Low-Dosage Naltrexone Therapy?

The notion that endogenous opioids and opioid antagonists may have a role in healing and tissue repair led to the use of low-dosage naltrexone as a possible treatment for numerous disorders. Dr. Bernard Bihari, former Instructor in Neurology, Harvard Medical School (1959-1960); Assistant Professor in Psychiatry, Mount Sinai School of Medicine (1968-1980); and Attending Physician, Beth Israel Medical Center, NY (2002-2010), was acclaimed on the internet as the "genius who discovered that a very low dose of naltrexone, a drug that had been approved at a higher dose by the FDA for another purpose entirely, could help people with some of the most difficult-to-treat diseases." Dr. Bihari is featured in a 2002 online video describing his work related to low-dosage naltrexone; an online tribute credits him with improving the lives and relieving symptoms in "tens of thousands (some say hundreds of thousands) of people with multiple sclerosis, rheumatoid arthritis, lupus, HIV/AIDS, autoimmune thyroid disease and even cancer." In her book *Honest Medicine*, Julia Schopick, who does not have a medical degree or known degree in science, proposes low-dosage naltrexone as an "effective, time-tested, inexpensive treatment for life-threatening diseases" to include "multiple sclerosis, epilepsy, liver disease, lupus, rheumatoid arthritis and other disorders."

What Evidence Supports the Efficacy of Low-Dosage Naltrexone?

A 2007 study published in the *American Journal of Gastroenterology* reported improvements in the Crohn's Disease Activity Index during 12 weeks of low-dosage naltrexone treatment and for 4 weeks after stopping the medication in patients with active Crohn disease. Other studies followed with mixed results. However, a 2018 Cochrane Database Systematic Review concluded there is "insufficient evidence to allow any firm conclusions regarding the efficacy and safety of low-dosage naltrexone for patients with active Crohn's disease." There is no valid evidence to support the use of low-dosage naltrexone to treat autoimmune endocrine disorders.[15]

Describe a Reasonable, Compassionate, Patient-Centric Approach to People Who Present With Symptoms Erroneously Attributed to a Pseudoendocrine Diagnosis

All providers will develop their own personalized approach that works best for their patients, but I find it best to always remember 3 crucial points: (1) The patient is not to blame for their diagnosis; like all others, they deserve our full attention and compassion; (2) The patient's quality of life is poor, and they are frustrated; and (3) It is an honor that the patient entrusts me with an opportunity to help them achieve better health and quality of life.

I listen attentively, perform a good physical examination, and offer additional testing if appropriate. I explore nonendocrine and psychiatric contributors to their symptoms. I understand and admit that current testing options do have some limitations. I recommend good nutrition, regular exercise, good sleep habits, and stress reduction for all patients. And I always provide honesty, encouragement, and compassion.[1,9]

Other Potential Pseudoendocrine Disorder Discussion Topics

- Is it true that low testosterone in men can be a phony diagnosis?

- What disorders cause a pseudoendocrine pheochromocytoma picture?

- What disorders can cause a pseudo-Cushing syndrome picture?

- How can estrogens cause false-positive testing for Cushing syndrome?

- Is Hashimoto encephalopathy an accurate diagnosis?

- Biotin interferes with some hormone assays. How significant is this in clinical practice?

Key Learning Points

- *Pseudoendocrine disorder* refers to proposed conditions that have never been scientifically proven to exist but, due to widespread misinformation available on the internet and other media, are relatively commonly diagnosed and treated with equally unproven and sometimes dangerous treatments.

- Adrenal fatigue is a nonexistent condition that supposedly results from adrenal exhaustion and atrophy due to chronic stress and that has been promoted as a potential explanation for a variety of symptoms. Testing consists of nonvalidated online surveys and salivary cortisol profiles, while treatment is not evidence-based, at best, and can be dangerous.

- Wilson syndrome and reverse T_3 syndrome are also nonexistent conditions that supposedly result from impaired T_4 to T_3 conversion and competition of excess reverse T_3 with T_3 for the T_3 receptor. Testing involves measurement of axillary temperature and treatment consists of T_3 therapy, often at very high and dangerous dosages.

- Low-dosage naltrexone therapy has been proposed as a treatment for multiple disorders involving autoimmune conditions and other disorders resulting from aberrant immune mechanisms, but there is no valid evidence that treatment has any benefits.

- People seeking our help for these pseudoendocrine disorders should be informed that much information on the internet is not evidence-based and is not correct; they should consult with and trust their physicians' advice on these matters.

- Management of patients with pseudoendocrine disorders must involve careful listening; patient education; healthy lifestyle measures; and honesty, encouragement, and compassion.

References

1. McDermott MT. *Management of Patients with Pseudo-Endocrine Disorders. A Case-Based Pocket Guide.* Springer Nature; 2019.

2. Warraich H. Dr. Google is a liar. *New York Times.* December 16, 2018.

3. Hellmuth J, Rabinovici GD, Miller BL. The rise of pseudomedicine for dementia and brain health. *JAMA.* 2019;321(6):543-544. PMID: 30681701

4. Schwartz LM, Woloshin S. Low "T" as in "template": how to sell disease. *JAMA Intern Med.* 2013;173(15):1460-1462. PMID: 23939516

5. Pryor L. How to counter the circus of pseudoscience. *New York Times.* January 5, 2018.

6. Cadegiani FA, Kater CE. Adrenal fatigue does not exist: a systematic review. *BMC Endocr Disord.* 2016;16(1):48. PMID: 27557747

7. Bancos I, Haines MS, Wexler J, eds. Adrenal fatigue. Endocrine Society. January 25, 2022. Accessed January 18, 2024. https://www.endocrine.org/patient-engagement/endocrine-library/adrenal-fatigue

8. Kearns A. Is there such a thing as adrenal fatigue? Mayo Clinic. April 16, 2022. Accessed January 18, 2024. https://www.mayoclinic.org/diseases-conditions/addisons-disease/expert-answers/adrenal-fatigue/faq-20057906

9. Muller RS. Making a difference in adrenal fatigue. *Endocr Pract.* 2018;24(12):1103-1105. PMID: 30289314

10. Akturk HD, Chindris AM, Hines JM, Singh RJ, Bernet VJ. Over-the-counter "adrenal support" supplements contain thyroid and steroid-based adrenal hormones. *Mayo Clin Proc.* 2018;93(3):284-290. PMID: 29502560

11. American Thyroid Association. American Thyroid Association Statement on "Wilson's Syndrome." American Thyroid Association. May 24, 2005. Accessed January 18, 2024. https://www.thyroid.org/american-thyroid-association-statement-on-wilsons-syndrome/]

12. Stop the Thyroid Madness. Reverse T3 (also called reverse triiodothyronine). Accessed January 21, 2024. https://stopthethyroidmadness.com/reverse-t3/.

13. Schuster LD, Schwartz HL, Oppenheimer JH. Nuclear receptors for 3,5,3'-triiodothyronine in human liver and kidney: characterization, quantitation and similarities to rat receptors. *J Clin Endocrinol Metab.* 1979;48(4):627-632. PMID: 219002

14. Schmidt RL, LoPresti JS, McDermott MT, Zick SM, Straseski JA. Does reverse triiodothyronine testing have clinical utility? An analysis of practice variation based on order data from a national reference laboratory. *Thyroid.* 2018;28(7):842-848. PMID: 29756541

15. Parker CE, Nguyen TM, Segal D, MacDonald JK, Chande N. Low dose naltrexone for induction of remission in Crohn's disease. *Cochrane Database Syst Rev.* 2018;4(4):CD010410. PMID: 29607497

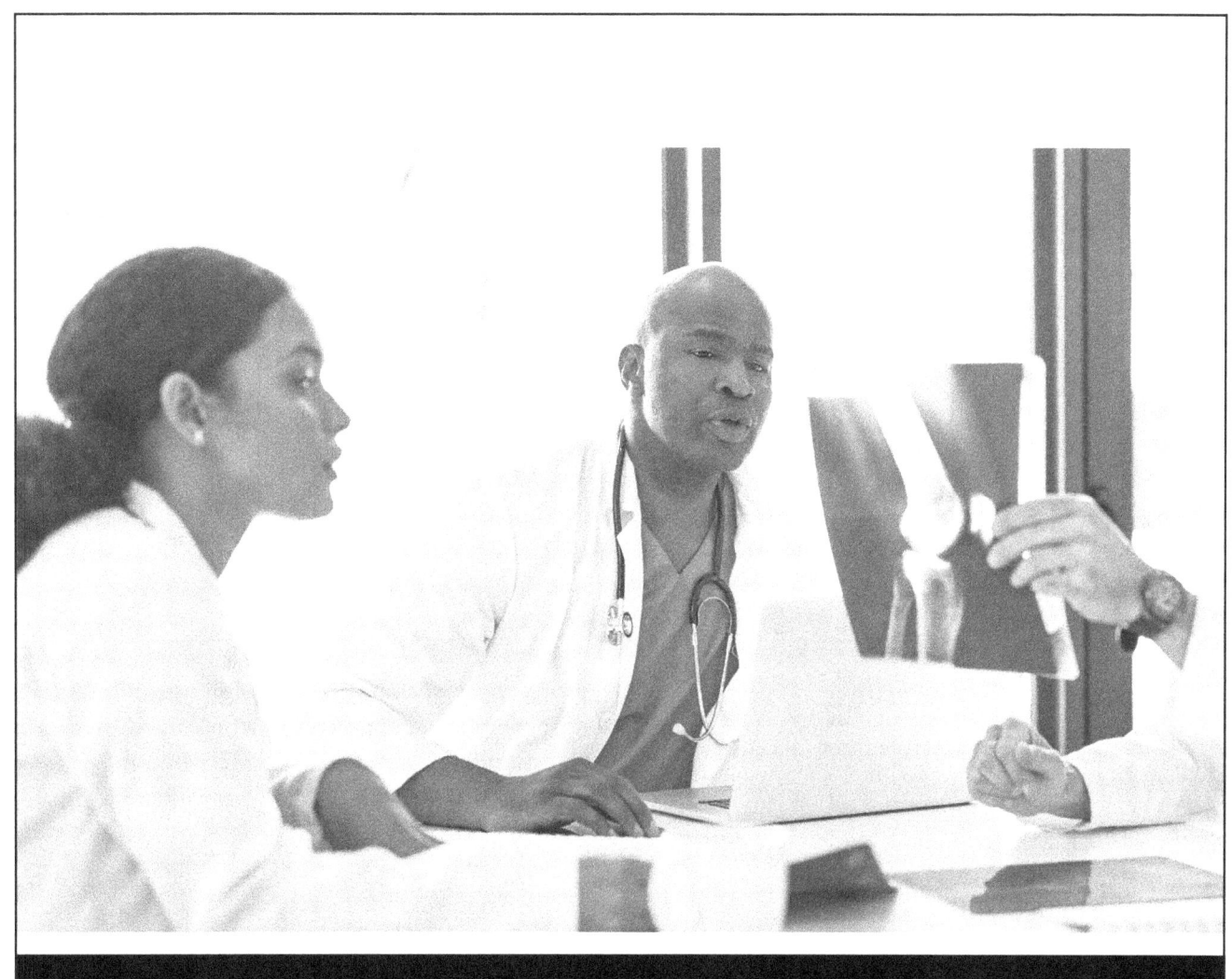

NEUROENDOCRINOLOGY AND PITUITARY

Cancer Risk in Growth Hormone Deficiency and Excess: Growth Hormone–Insulinlike Growth Factor System and Carcinogenesis

Cesar Luiz Boguszewski, MD, PhD. Endocrine Division (SEMPR), Department of Internal Medicine, Federal University of Parana, Curitiba, Brazil; Email: cesar.boguszewski@hc.ufpr.br, clbogus@uol.com.br

Educational Objectives

After reviewing this chapter, learners should be able to:

- Describe the experimental, epidemiological, and clinical evidence that suggests a permissive role of the growth hormone–insulinlike growth factor (GH-IGF) system in carcinogenesis.

- Evaluate cancer risk in persons with acromegaly.

- Identify individuals at higher risk of tumor recurrence, primary cancer, or second neoplasia treated with recombinant human growth hormone (rhGH).

Significance of the Clinical Problem

The components of the GH-IGF system exert contrasting effects in the mechanisms of carcinogenesis. While GH, IGFs, and convertases inhibit apoptosis and promote cell proliferation, differentiation, and angiogenesis, IGF-binding proteins, proteases, and IGF-2 receptors protect against tumor progression by inhibiting mitogenesis and stimulating apoptosis. Curiously, GH stimulates both IGF-2 and IGF binding protein-3 production, simultaneously inducing signaling pathways for cell proliferation that compete with others for cell death. The final effect of these opposed forces is critical for normal and abnormal cell growth.[1]

In genome-wide association studies, GH-induced intracellular signaling pathways have been strongly associated with breast cancer susceptibility, while increased tumoral GH receptor expression has been associated with mortality in prostate, endometrial, ovarian, bladder, gastric, and triple-negative breast cancer.[2] Epidemiological studies in the general population have documented an association between high-normal IGF-1 levels with the development of common malignancies. Furthermore, studies performed in animal models and human populations with genetic defects associated with severe GH deficiency or GH resistance (Laron syndrome) show an absence or very low prevalence of malignancies in these groups.[1,2]

Due to the experimental, epidemiological, and observational data linking the GH-IGF system with tumor development, there have been longstanding concerns about cancer risks in patients with acromegaly and in children and adults treated with recombinant human rhGH. GH-IGF signaling pathways have been tested as potential targets for cancer therapy.

Practice Gaps

- The link between GH-IGF excess and carcinogenesis risk in patients with acromegaly, particularly in relation to colorectal and thyroid cancer, is still a matter of debate, and screening with colonoscopy and thyroid ultrasonography is a controversial issue.

- While use of rhGH in children and adults is safe regarding cancer risk in most circumstances, the decision to recommend treatment for individuals at very high risk is challenging.

- Data from survivors of pediatric or adult cancers who are treated with rhGH during adulthood are scarce, and the risk of replacement therapy in these patients remains unclear.

Discussion

Cancer Screening in Persons With Acromegaly

In the pioneering study by Mustacchi and Shimkin in 1957, 13 cancers were detected in 223 patients with acromegaly followed up over 14 years, with not a single case of colorectal or thyroid cancer. These observations led the authors to conclude against a strong influence of GH on cancer initiation in humans.[3] Since then, studies examining the malignancy risk in persons with acromegaly have continuously led to conflicting findings, particularly in relation to colorectal and thyroid cancer, making cancer screening in these patients highly controversial.[4,5]

Experimental data have suggested that high endocrine or autocrine GH levels contribute to neoplastic colon growth by the inactivation of tumor-suppressor genes, suppression of apoptosis, and stimulation of epithelial-to-mesenchymal transition.[1,2] Many other factors, unrelated to GH-IGF status, may contribute to cancer risk in persons with acromegaly, including variable cancer prevalence in control populations in different countries, genetic and/or epigenetic events that predispose to the development of new neoplasms in persons with pituitary tumors, surveillance bias, and presence of comorbidities, such as insulin resistance and diabetes.[4,5] In addition, improvement in acromegaly management has increased life expectancy in patients who attain normal GH and IGF-1 levels, and longer lifespans are associated with more deaths due to age-related (and not GH-related) cancers.[6]

In the last published document from the Acromegaly Consensus Conference held in 2022, there was no consensus on whether colonoscopy should be performed in all patients at the time acromegaly is diagnosed, regardless of age.[7] Colorectal cancer is the third most commonly diagnosed malignancy in the general population and is the fourth leading cause of cancer-related deaths worldwide. However, its incidence, mortality, and trends show significant variations both regionally and across countries, with numbers rising in many low- and middle-income countries and decreasing or remaining stable in most developed countries, where rates remain among the highest in the world. Genetic, ethnic, environmental, and especially dietary factors are important determinants of colorectal cancer, which most often begins as a precancerous polyp that undergoes malignant transformation in approximately 10 to 15 years.[4,7] Thus, all these factors known to influence the development of colorectal cancer in the general population should be considered when epidemiologic studies are performed in specific populations, such as in individuals with acromegaly. In our hands, the indication for screening colonoscopy in asymptomatic patients with acromegaly follows the same rules as for the general Brazilian population. If the first exam is normal, colonoscopy is repeated every 10 years. It is repeated at shorter intervals (between 3 and 5 years) in cases of abnormal colonoscopy findings, when IGF-1 remains persistently elevated, or in the presence of risk factors or family history of colorectal cancer.[4]

For all other malignancies, including thyroid cancer, the Acromegaly Consensus Conference 2022 concluded that screening must follow the same guidelines as those for the general population.[7] Recently, we performed a prospective, cross-sectional study to evaluate the prevalence of differentiated thyroid cancer in acromegaly. Seventy-one consecutive patients with acromegaly and 57 patients with other non–GH-producing pituitary adenomas (35 prolactinomas, 7 corticotropinomas, and 15 nonfunctioning pituitary adenomas) underwent thyroid ultrasonography by the same examiner and ultrasound-guided FNA biopsy when indicated. To our surprise, differentiated thyroid cancer was not detected in any of the patients with acromegaly, whereas 2 patients with non–GH-producing pituitary adenomas were diagnosed with differentiated thyroid cancer (confirmed histologically after surgery).[8] Our results do not support routine screening for thyroid cancer in persons with acromegaly and reinforce the recommendations made by the last Consensus Conference.

Safety of GH Therapy in Children and Adults

The wide availability of rhGH has expanded its clinical prescriptions beyond replacement therapy in children with GH deficiency to those in which pharmacological dosages are used in children with short stature and growth restriction of other etiologies, with approved indications varying among countries.[2] Of particular concern is the use of rhGH in patients harboring conditions associated with inherited risk of malignancies and neoplasms.[1,2] Replacement therapy with rhGH is indicated in adults with hypopituitarism and severe GH deficiency, which in many cases is caused by tumors in the hypothalamic-pituitary region.[1,2]

With advances in oncological treatment, there has been a substantial increase in the number of cancer survivors who develop GH deficiency related to the malignancy or as an adverse consequence of surgeries, radiation, and immuno- and/or chemotherapies.[2]

A consensus workshop was held by the Growth Hormone Research Society in 2021 to address the safety of rhGH therapy in survivors of cancer and intracranial tumors and in patients with cancer predisposition syndromes.[2] The main key statements from the consensus document are as follows: (1) current evidence does not support an association between rhGH replacement therapy and primary tumor or cancer recurrence in survivors with GH deficiency; (2) specific effects of rhGH replacement on the risk of secondary neoplasia are minor in comparison to host and tumor treatment-related factors; (3) current evidence does not support an association between rhGH treatment and increased mortality from cancer among childhood cancer survivors with GH deficiency; (4) after careful individual risk-benefit analysis, rhGH replacement might be considered in adult cancer survivors with GH deficiency (either with childhood- or adult-onset cancer) whose cancer is in remission; (5) a decision to prescribe rhGH in patients with GH deficiency who have breast, colon, prostate, or liver cancer in remission should be made on a case-by-case basis after detailed counseling about risks and benefits and in close consultation with the treating oncologist; (6) rhGH dosing and monitoring in cancer survivors follow the general recommendations as for other groups, but closer vigilance is required to avoid overtreatment; (7) timing of rhGH initiation following completion of cancer treatment of an intracranial tumor depends on many factors and should be individualized as a joint decision among treating physicians, patient, and caregivers. This period may be as early as 3 months in children with radiologically proven stable craniopharyngiomas who have significant growth failure and metabolic disturbance and up to at least 5 years in adults with a history of solid tumor such as breast cancer; (8) in children with cancer predisposition syndromes, rhGH is usually contraindicated but it may be cautiously considered in particular patients with proven GH deficiency.[2]

Recent data obtained from 2 noninterventional studies from Novo Nordisk (NordiNet International Outcome Study [IOS]) and the American Norditropin Studies: Web-Enabled Research [ANSWER]) with 37,702 patients did not document increased mortality related to rhGH treatment in patients categorized in low-, intermediate-, or high-risk groups.[9] In this study, adverse events reported after age 20 years were excluded from the analysis. Neoplasms were documented in 0.03%, 0.2%, and 1.75% of the low-, intermediate-, and high-risk groups, respectively.[9]

In contrast, data from the Safety and Appropriateness of Growth Hormone Treatments in Europe (SAGhE study) have alerted clinicians to the increased mortality associated with rhGH therapy in certain groups of patients with an inherent risk related to the underlying diagnosis.[10] From this observational study involving 24,232 patients treated with rhGH during childhood with up to 25 years of follow-up, cause-specific mortality from diseases of the circulatory and hematological systems was increased in all risk groups. In contrast, all-cause mortality was strongly related to underlying diagnosis, with the treatment being safe in children with isolated GH deficiency, idiopathic short stature, born small-for-gestational-age, or mild skeletal dysplasia. In contrast, increased mortality was observed in patients treated with rhGH who were classified as being at high risk, including individuals with multiple pituitary hormone deficiencies, severe cerebral and extracerebral malformation, severe chronic pediatric diseases, genetic diseases (neurofibromatosis type 1, Turner syndrome, Noonan syndrome, and Prader-Willi syndrome), malignancies, Langerhans cell histiocytosis, chronic kidney failure, after bone marrow or solid transplant, and syndromes with known increased risk for malignancies (Bloom syndrome, Fanconi syndrome, and Down syndrome and chromosomal breakage), reinforcing that the indication for rhGH

must be considered judiciously and rhGH may be contraindicated in groups at very high risk.[10]

In adults with GH deficiency, rhGH is generally considered a safe replacement therapy in relation to cancer risk, even in patients older than 60 years, as indicated by recent data collected from 2 observational, noninterventional, multicenter registry studies of Novo Nordisk.[11] However, previous observations from the KIMS Database showed that adverse events related to glucose metabolism, cardiovascular diseases, and neoplasms are more frequent in patients older than 65 years.[12] It has been claimed that these conflicting results were not related to rhGH therapy itself, but rather due to differences in methodologies (including more or less intense surveillance in older patients) and in the characteristics of the studied populations.[2,11]

rhGH is contraindicated in any patient with GH deficiency with active malignancy. In those cancer survivors who are in remission, the therapeutic decision should follow a careful risk-benefit analysis. In addition, rhGH therapy should be discontinued if any clinically significant tumor progression or relapse is observed.[13]

Clinical Case Vignettes
Case 1

A 32-year-old man is diagnosed with acromegaly due to a pituitary macroadenoma measuring 1.8 cm in largest diameter, with no cavernous sinus invasion or suprasellar extension. Time elapsed between the start of his symptoms (acral and dental arch changes, increased weight, carpal tunnel syndrome, low back pain, excessive sweating) and the diagnosis was approximately 3 years. He has had sporadic tenesmus and hematochezia. He smokes cigarettes (15 pack-years) and has a family history of a second cousin with gigantism.

On physical examination, he has no goiter, acanthosis nigricans, or skin tags.

Laboratory test results:

GH = 48 ng/mL (<5 ng/mL) (SI: 48 µg/L [<5 µg/L])
IGF-1 = 1.4 ng/mL (117-329 ng/mL) (SI: 178 nmol/L
  [15.3-43.1 nmol/L])

Which of the following is the best next step in this patient's evaluation?

A. Thyroid ultrasonography

B. PSA and prostate ultrasonography

C. Colonoscopy

D. Low-dose chest CT

Answer: C) Colonoscopy

According to the World Health Organization, the purpose of screening is to identify individuals in an apparently healthy population who are at higher risk of a health problem or condition, so that early treatment or intervention can be offered, thereby reducing the incidence and/or mortality of the health problem or condition within the population.[14] Accordingly, screening tests, examinations, or procedures are used to find diseases in individuals who have no symptoms, and in the case of malignancy, to increase the chance of finding cancers early, when they are small, have not spread, and are easier to treat. This concept is different from diagnostic testing that focuses on determining the cause of a person's symptoms. The patient in this vignette is not asymptomatic, as he has sporadic tenesmus and hematochezia. Thus, colonoscopy (Answer C) in this context should not be seen as a screening test, but rather a diagnostic procedure. In asymptomatic patients of his age, the indication for colonoscopy is controversial, with some advocating to perform the procedure at diagnosis in all patients with acromegaly and others following the same guidelines recommended for the general population that take age into account.[5]

Due to his age, there is no recommendation to screen for prostate and lung cancer (Answers B and D).

Thyroid ultrasonography (Answer A) is not routinely recommended in patients with acromegaly if physical examination does not detect a palpable goiter or other cervical abnormality.[7]

Case 1 (continued)

The patient undergoes transsphenoidal surgery, with pathology confirming a GH-secretory pituitary adenoma. After 4 months, the GH nadir on oral glucose tolerance testing is 1.61 ng/mL (1.61 µg/L) and the IGF-1 concentration is 449 ng/mL (115-307 ng/mL) (SI: 58.8 nmol/L [15.1-40.2 nmol/L]). Somatostatin receptor ligand therapy is initiated. At the time of colonoscopy, 3 colon hyperplastic polyps are removed.

Which of the following is the best advice?

A. Repeat colonoscopy in 1 year

B. Repeat colonoscopy in 3 to 5 years

C. Repeat colonoscopy in 10 years

D. No need to repeat colonoscopy if he remains asymptomatic

Answer: B) Repeat colonoscopy in 3 to 5 years

When a polyp is detected in the first examination, a second colonoscopy should be done in an interval of 3 to 5 years, depending on the number, size, and histology of the resected lesion. The interval for a second examination in patients with a normal initial colonoscopy and persistently elevated GH and IGF-1 levels is not well defined, but most experts suggest 5 years as a reasonable approach. In patients with a normal initial colonoscopy and controlled disease thereafter, the recommended follow-up is the same as it is for the general population.[4,7]

Case 2

A 43-year-old man with obesity (BMI = 44.5 kg/m²) is diagnosed with a macroprolactinoma measuring 3.7 cm in largest diameter, with right cavernous sinus invasion (Knosp 3) and filling the suprasellar cistern with compression and upwards displacement of the optic chiasma. Visual field testing is normal.

Laboratory test results:

Serum prolactin = 10.4 ng/mL (4-19 ng/mL)
(SI: 0.45 nmol/L [0.17-0.82 nmol/L])
Total testosterone = 88 ng/dL (249-836 nmol/L)
(SI: 3.1 nmol/L [8.6-29.0 nmol/L])
IGF-1 = 57.9 ng/mL (101-267 ng/mL)
(SI: 7.6 nmol/L [13.2-35.0 nmol/L])
Free T$_4$, normal
Morning cortisol, normal

He is treated with cabergoline with gradual dosage titration up to 3 mg weekly, and after 6 months, pituitary MRI demonstrates 40% tumor volume reduction and his prolactin and total testosterone concentrations are 286 ng/mL and 328 ng/dL (12.4 nmol/L and 11.4 nmol/L, respectively). He has fatigue, low mood, and impaired memory. He lacks energy to perform daily activities and asks whether he should start treatment with rhGH. Peak GH on insulin tolerance testing is 0.3 ng/mL (0.3 μg/L) and IGF-1 is 49 ng/mL (6.4 nmol/L).

Which of the following statements is most accurate?

A. The diagnosis of GH deficiency is confirmed and rhGH replacement should be initiated at a dosage not based on his body weight with subsequent up-titration

B. rhGH is contraindicated due to the large tumor remnant still present

C. rhGH should not be started before a complete screening for malignancies since the patient is at high risk for cancer

D. Higher dosages of cabergoline will be needed for tumor control if rhGH therapy is initiated

Answer: A) The diagnosis of GH deficiency is confirmed and rhGH replacement should be initiated at a dosage not based on his body weight with subsequent up-titration

GH deficiency in adults is mainly caused by hypothalamic-pituitary lesions and associated treatment with surgery and/or radiotherapy, with pituitary adenomas and craniopharyngiomas accounting for more than half the prevalence of adult GH deficiency. A low IGF-1 value is enough for laboratory diagnosis in patients with well-established genetic/congenital defects affecting GH production, irreversible hypothalamic-pituitary lesions diagnosed in childhood, and in those with panhypopituitarism.[15] This patient in this vignette has low IGF-1 but with only one additional pituitary deficit. Therefore, a provocative GH test is needed to confirm the diagnosis of GH deficiency (peak GH below 3-5 ng/mL [3-5 μg/L]). rhGH replacement in adults is generally initiated at a low dosage, not based on body weight, and then titrated up based on clinical response, adverse events, and serum IGF-1 concentrations (Answer A).[15] Targeting a serum IGF-1 value in the normal range while optimizing growth is recommended,[2] although some clinicians advocate maintaining IGF-1 levels in the lower part of the reference range during treatment in patients at intermediate or high risk for malignancy. rhGH does not interfere with dopamine agonist treatment of prolactinomas, and the presence of a pituitary tumor remnant is not a contraindication to initiating rhGH replacement therapy, with imaging monitoring performed as recommended for patients not receiving rhGH. Likewise, cancer screening should follow the same recommendations as for the general population, with no need for more rigorous surveillance in patients with pituitary adenomas on rhGH treatment.[2]

Key Learning Points

- The GH-IGF system does not cause cancer, but it may have a permissive endocrine/paracrine role in the development and progression of certain types of benign and malignant tumors.

- The risk of colorectal cancer in patients with acromegaly is modest and seems to be influenced by selection, surveillance, and diagnostic workup bias. Cancer-specific mortality rates in acromegaly are similar to those observed in the general population and increased life expectancy of patients with acromegaly is associated with more deaths of age-related, rather than GH-related, malignancies.

- The safety of rhGH replacement therapy in relation to cancer risk is reassuring in most children and adults with GH deficiency receiving treatment according to approved indications, but the use of rhGH must be extremely judicious in patients with an underlying condition associated with high risk of cancer.

References

1. Boguszewski CL, Boguszewski MCDS. Growth hormone's links to cancer. *Endocr Rev.* 2019;40(2):558-574. PMID: 30500870

2. Boguszewski MCS, Boguszewski CL, Chemaitilly W, et al. Safety of growth hormone replacement in survivors of cancer and intracranial and pituitary tumours: a consensus statement. *Eur J Endocrinol.* 2022;186(6):P35-P52. PMID: 35319491

3. Mustacchi P, Shimkin MB. Occurrence of cancer in acromegaly and in hypopituitarism. *Cancer.* 1957;10(1):100-104. PMID: 13413804

4. Boguszewski CL, Ayuk J. Management of endocrine disease: acromegaly and cancer: an old debate revisited. *Eur J Endocrinol.* 2016;175(4):R147-R156. PMID: 27089890

5. Terzolo M, Puglisi S, Reimondo G, Dimopoulou C, Stalla GK. Thyroid and colorectal cancer screening in acromegaly patients: should it be different from that in the general population? *Eur J Endocrinol.* 2020;183(4):D1-D13. PMID: 32698136

6. Bolfi F, Neves AF, Boguszewski CL, Nunes-Nogueira VS. Mortality in acromegaly decreased in the last decade: a systematic review and meta-analysis. *Eur J Endocrinol.* 2018;179(1):59-71. PMID: 29764907

7. Giustina A, Biermasz N, Casanueva FF, et al; Acromegaly Consensus Group. Consensus on criteria for acromegaly diagnosis and remission. *Pituitary.* 2024;27(1):7-22. PMID: 37923946

8. Spricido IY, Feckinghaus CM, Silva RHM, Mesa Junior CO, Boguszewski CL. Prevalence of thyroid cancer in patients with acromegaly and non-growth hormone secreting pituitary adenomas: a prospective cross-sectional study. *Growth Horm IGF Res.* 2021;56:101378. PMID: 33486451

9. Sävendahl L, Polak M, Backeljauw P, et al. Long-term safety of growth hormone treatment in childhood: two large observational studies: NordiNet IOS and ANSWER. *J Clin Endocrinol Metab.* 2021;106(6):1728-1741. PMID: 33571362

10. Sävendahl L, Cooke R, Tidblad A, et al. Long-term mortality after childhood growth hormone treatment: the SAGhE cohort study. *Lancet Diabetes Endocrinol.* 2020;8(8):683-692. PMID: 32707116

11. Biller BMK, Höybye C, Ferran JM, Kelepouris N, Nedjatian N, Olsen AH, Weber MM, Gordon MB. Long-term effectiveness and safety of GH replacement therapy in adults ≥60 years: data from NordiNet® IOS and ANSWER. *J Endocr Soc.* 2023;7(6):bvad054. PMID: 37197408

12. Feldt-Rasmussen U, Wilton P, Jonsson P; KIMS Study Group; KIMS International Board. Aspects of growth hormone deficiency and replacement in elderly hypopituitary adults. *Growth Horm IGF Res.* 2004;14(Suppl A):S51-S58. PMID: 15135778

13. Boguszewski CL. Safety of long-term use of daily and long-acting growth hormone in growth hormone-deficient adults on cancer risk. *Best Pract Res Clin Endocrinol Metab.* 2023;37(6):101817. PMID: 37643936

14. World Health Organization. Screening programmes: a short guide. Increase effectiveness, maximize benefits and minimize harm. February 6, 2020. Available at https://www.who.int/europe/publications/i/item/9789289054782

15. Yuen KCJ, Johannsson G, Ho KKY, Miller BS, Bergada I, Rogol AD. Diagnosis and testing for growth hormone deficiency across the ages: a global view of the accuracy, caveats, and cut-offs for diagnosis. *Endocr Connect.* 2023;12(7):e220504. PMID: 37052176

Diagnosis of Cushing Disease in the Era of Corticotropin-Releasing Hormone Shortage

Frederic Castinetti, MD, PhD. Department of Endocrinology, Aix Marseille University, Assistance Publique Hopitaux de Marseille, Marseille, France; Email: Frederic.castinetti@ap-hm.fr

Educational Objectives

After reviewing this chapter, learners should be able to:

- Identify situations in which dynamic testing is needed in ACTH-dependent Cushing syndrome (CS).

- Identify the optimal diagnostic strategy, including dynamic testing and intrapetrosal sinus sampling (IPSS), for severe and nonsevere ACTH-dependent CS.

Significance of the Clinical Problem

ACTH-dependent CS accounts for more than 80% of cases of CS. It may be due to a corticotroph pituitary tumor or to ectopic ACTH secretion from a neuroendocrine tumor. While diagnostic management has long been based on a combination of hormonal parameters (especially after dynamic tests) and imaging, the recent worldwide shortage of CRH must lead endocrinologists to think differently (ie, to determine the situations in which dynamic tests are needed and the optimal approach that would help them make the right diagnosis and propose the best therapeutic option). Finally, this combined approach has led to questioning the role of bilateral IPSS, long considered the gold standard of the diagnostic algorithm. An incorrect diagnosis may lead to inappropriate management in terms of follow-up (imaging) or treatment (surgery vs cortisol-lowering medications). This chapter will discuss the merits and pitfalls of currently available dynamic tests, other parameters that could be useful in making a correct diagnosis, and the role of bilateral IPSS in this setting. Indeed, the lack of CRH availability also raises questions about the accuracy of bilateral IPSS without stimulation or with desmopressin.

Practice Gaps

- The best diagnostic method to distinguish Cushing disease (CD) from ectopic ACTH secretion (EAS) has not been defined. It has long been based on CRH-stimulation testing, but the worldwide shortage of CRH requires endocrinologists to redefine their diagnostic procedures.

- The exact role of the 2 remaining tests, desmopressin-stimulation and high-dose dexamethasone-suppression tests, is uncertain, mainly because the literature reports controversial results on diagnostic accuracy. In addition, many physicians, thinking in a semiautomated fashion, believe that the diagnosis should always include dynamic testing and forget to consider the whole story, as clues can facilitate the diagnosis even without these dynamic tests.

- While IPSS could be considered the gold standard, most series report its benefits after CRH stimulation, which also raises the question of its role now that CRH is scarce.
- IPSS requires an expert neuroradiology team, and it is necessary to define how the diagnostic procedure should be performed when IPSS is not available or the situations in which this procedure is not useful.

Discussion

The steps to diagnose CS are based on an established diagnosis of hypercortisolism, which will not be discussed in this chapter. Rather, the focus here is on the next steps: the differential diagnosis between CD (ie, ACTH-dependent CS due to a corticotroph pituitary tumor) and EAS (ie, ACTH-dependent CS due to a neuroendocrine tumor). While several expert centers emphasize the need for dynamic testing, recent guidelines for the diagnosis of CD acknowledge the following: (1) no test has 100% accuracy for the differential diagnosis between CD and EAS; (2) the whole story, including epidemiology, comorbidities, and hormone concentrations, should be considered; and (3) IPSS should be considered the gold standard for this approach, especially when pituitary MRI shows a mass smaller than 6 mm.[1] The role of IPSS has been challenged by a recent study showing that a combination of CRH-stimulation testing, desmopressin-stimulation testing, pituitary MRI, and thin-slice whole-body CT could avoid the use of IPSS in 47% of cases of ACTH-dependent CS.[2]

However, this approach is no longer feasible due to the CRH shortage. In addition to imaging, which remains mandatory in the diagnostic process (thin-slice whole-body CT and pituitary MRI), only 2 dynamic tests can still be used: the desmopressin-stimulation test and the high-dose dexamethasone-suppression test (in its longer 48-hour version or its short overnight version). Each of these tests has advantages and disadvantages. The interpretation of the high-dose dexamethasone-suppression test is based on the expression of glucocorticoid receptors (with a sustained ability to decrease ACTH secretion) in corticotroph tumors, while interpretation of the desmopressin-stimulation test is based on expression of vasopressin receptors (V2 and V1b, with an ability to stimulate ACTH secretion). These receptors should not be expressed in ACTH-secreting neuroendocrine tumors. Unfortunately, well-differentiated neuroendocrine tumors may express these receptors, leading to false-positive results when trying to confirm the diagnosis of CD.[1]

These tests should typically be performed as a second-line approach when the etiology of ACTH-dependent CS is uncertain. Whether these tests are necessary thus depends on the possibility of distinguishing CD from EAS at baseline with classic biochemical and hormonal parameters. Only a few studies have tried to analyze these differences and have shown that some parameters, mainly related to the severity of the presentation, could help in the diagnostic process.[3] While CD usually presents as an indolent disease with a delay of several years before proper diagnosis, EAS can present with severe life-threatening hypercortisolism, difficult-to-control hypertension and diabetes, and profound hypokalemia (potassium <2.8 mEq/L [>2.8 mmol/L]).[4] Consistent with this, the 24-hour urinary free cortisol excretion is greater than 5 times the upper normal limit in all cases of EAS. Add to this the fact that 80% of CD cases are reported in females, while the sex ratio is closer to 50/50 in EAS, and this means that male patients with a severe presentation of ACTH-dependent CS and a 24-hour urinary free cortisol excretion greater than 5 times the upper normal limit usually have EAS.[5] Instead of dynamic testing, thin-slice whole-body CT should be performed promptly to search for the source of ACTH secretion, and cortisol-lowering medications should be started immediately. However, because EAS accounts for only 20% of cases of ACTH-dependent CS and severe presentations of EAS occur in less than 50% of affected patients in modern series, this situation would be seen in only 10% of all patients with ACTH-dependent CS.

In most cases, the presentation is indolent with mild comorbidities such as controlled hypertension and diabetes and moderate or absent hypokalemia. This scenario, accounting for 90% of ACTH-dependent CS cases, requires that indolent EAS be distinguished from "classic" CD. Indolent EAS can be observed with a variety of neuroendocrine tumors such as bronchial carcinoid, thymic, or intestinal neuroendocrine tumors or pheochromocytoma; interestingly, EAS can also be occult with negative imaging in 15% to 20% of cases.[5] This common situation requires an appropriate diagnostic algorithm, including dynamic testing. Few large studies have evaluated the benefit of each of these tests.[6] The main difficulties are the different thresholds and the hormone being evaluated (ACTH and/or cortisol), which probably explains the wide range of diagnostic accuracy in the literature. Barbot et al compared the diagnostic accuracy of high-dose dexamethasone-suppression testing and desmopressin-stimulation testing in a large series of 170 patients, including 21 with EAS. With a sensitivity of 83% and a specificity of 62%, the desmopressin-stimulation test appeared to be less accurate than the high-dose dexamethasone-suppression test (sensitivity of 88%, specificity of 90%, with a cortisol decrease threshold above 52.7% to confirm the diagnosis of CD).[7] In a recent series of 323 patients with ACTH-dependent CS, including 78 with EAS, the high-dose dexamethasone-suppression test had a diagnostic accuracy of 77% (sensitivity = 75%; specificity = 85%), with a cortisol-suppression criterion of more than 69% in favor of CD. Desmopressin-stimulation testing was not performed in this series.[8] Finally, Frete et al documented a sensitivity of 73% and specificity of 98% using a combined approach of dynamic tests and imaging with a double criterion of 33% increase in ACTH and 18% increase in cortisol.[2] The threshold used in these series obviously defines the choice of better sensitivity or specificity in the diagnosis of CD, but it is true that even the series in favor

of a given test cannot consider it to be the gold standard. A combined score designed by machine learning could account for the epidemiology, severity of comorbidities, hormone secretion, imaging, and dynamic tests to move forward in this difficult diagnostic situation. This was done in a series of 264 patients with CD and 47 patients with EAS, analyzing age, sex, BMI, disease duration, morning cortisol, serum ACTH, 24-hour urinary free cortisol, serum potassium, high-dose dexamethasone-suppression testing, low-dose dexamethasone-suppression testing, and MRI. Interestingly, the best model used serum potassium, MRI, and serum ACTH (no dynamic test) and showed 95% sensitivity and 71.4% specificity in the validation dataset. However, this model did not include desmopressin-stimulation testing and CT. This strategy clearly requires further validation before it can be used regularly.[9]

Imaging remains one of the cornerstones of the diagnostic process in ACTH-dependent CS. Frete et al have shown the advantages of systematic imaging with thin-slice whole-body CT and pituitary MRI.[2] However, each of these modalities has limitations. Pituitary MRI is equivocal or negative in up to 40% of patients with CD and it may be falsely positive in 10% of patients. Some promising results have been shown with the use of ^{11}C-methionine PET-MRI, and this remains limited to a small number of centers worldwide. Thin-slice whole-body CT detects about 50% of tumors; DOTATATE PET-CT, based on somatostatin receptor type 2 expression by the neuroendocrine tumor, identifies 57% to 70% of neuroendocrine tumors with ectopic ACTH secretion, with an increasing rate of efficacy with duration of follow-up.[10,11] The systematic use of DOTATE PET-CT in patients with both negative CT and MRI could be an option, although this imaging modality could be expensive in some countries and, probably cannot reach the diagnostic accuracy of IPSS.

Finally, while some authors argue that IPSS should no longer be considered the gold standard in the absence of CRH, the results of the largest series published on the use of IPSS questioned the benefit of the additional step of stimulation, particularly with desmopressin. More than 15 years ago, we and others reported the efficacy of desmopressin as a stimulating agent to enhance the efficacy of IPSS in a manner comparable to that of CRH. In the original studies, based on a total of 80 patients, desmopressin proved useful in correcting the diagnosis in 12 patients, where the diagnosis of CD was confirmed by a central-to-peripheral ratio greater than 3 after stimulation.[6] Recently, Chen et al questioned the benefit of desmopressin stimulation compared with the unstimulated accuracy of IPSS. In a large series of 226 patients with CD and 24 patients with EAS, the sensitivity of IPSS was 94.7% without stimulation (central-to-peripheral ratio better than 1.4 favoring CD), while it increased to 97.8% after stimulation (ratio >2.8). The specificity was 100% whether stimulated or not, and desmopressin was useful in 6 patients with a questionable finding on pituitary imaging with a mass smaller than 6 mm.[12] Of note, some authors recommend measuring prolactin in parallel with ACTH as a marker of optimal catheter position, but this approach remains controversial. Overall, these rates are much higher than rates of any other test used in the diagnostic process of ACTH-dependent CS, either alone or in combination, and suggest that even in the absence of CRH, IPSS should still be considered the gold standard for patients in whom the diagnosis remains uncertain despite taking into account epidemiology, comorbidities, diagnostic delay, hormone secretion, imaging, and dynamic testing when available.

Conclusions

The etiologic diagnosis of ACTH-dependent hypercortisolism can be challenging. However, clinical clues can easily guide the diagnosis. This is especially true in severe forms of hypercortisolism, where EAS is the most common etiology and should prompt whole-body imaging rather than dynamic testing. Because EAS can also cause mild cortisol hypersecretion mimicking CD, selection of the proper diagnostic approach is important.

Some have recently proposed relying solely on dynamic testing (CRH and desmopressin) and imaging (chest CT and pituitary MRI), but the worldwide shortage of CRH should cause clinicians to rethink diagnostic strategy. While high-dose dexamethasone-suppression and desmopressin-stimulation testing have been suggested, data in the literature are scarce and sometimes contradictory. This means that bilateral IPSS, either with baseline ACTH measurements or after desmopressin stimulation, should still be considered the gold standard in patients with ACTH-dependent CS of uncertain etiology. Imaging is obviously still necessary, but mild forms of ACTH-dependent CS are usually due to small lesions (or nonvisible tumors despite the latest imaging modalities), and this may lead to false-negative imaging results. A correct etiologic diagnosis remains of utmost importance, as it guides the optimal therapeutic strategy.

Clinical Case Vignettes

Case 1

A 60-year-old man presents to the emergency department because of severe abdominal pain. He has lost 13.2 lb (6 kg) in the last 2 months (current BMI = 23 kg/m^2). He has no relevant personal or family medical history and takes no medications.

His clinical examination reveals hypertension (170/100 mm Hg) and easy bruising, which he reports has been present for 2 months.

Laboratory test results (sample drawn in the emergency department):

> Blood glucose = 40 mg/dL (70-99 mg/dL) (SI: 2.2 mmol/L [3.9-5.5 mmol/L]) (with ketosis)
> Potassium = 2.7 mEq/L (3.5-5.0 mEq/L) (SI: 2.7 mmol/L [3.5-5.0 mmol/L])

Abdominal CT shows bilateral adrenal hyperplasia and a suspicious 15-mm nodule in the right lower lobe of the lung. After appropriate intravenous administration of potassium and insulin, he is transferred to the endocrinology department, where hormones are measured:

Urinary free cortisol = 1721 μg/24 h (<87 μg/24 h) (SI: 4750 nmol/d [<240 nmol/d])

ACTH (2 measurements) = 110 and 130 pg/mL (10-60 pg/mL) (SI: 24.2 and 28.6 pmol/L [2.2-13.2 pmol/L])

Cortisol (2 measurements) = 44.6 and 50.8 μg/dL (5-25 μg/dL) (SI: 1230 and 1401 nmol/L [137.9-689.7 nmol/L])

Which of the following additional dynamic tests should be performed now?

A. 1-mg overnight dexamethasone-suppression test

B. Desmopressin-stimulation test

C. High-dose dexamethasone-suppression test

D. Low-dose dexamethasone-suppression test

E. No additional testing required now

Answer: E) No additional testing required now

Given the clinical presentation and the values of urinary free cortisol and blood ACTH and cortisol, there is no need to confirm the diagnosis of CS with an additional test (thus, Answer E is correct and Answers A, B, C, and D are incorrect). The patient has presented with severe hypercortisolism that requires urgent management and no time should be wasted on additional hormone measurements. In these life-threatening situations, imaging should be performed to look for the etiology of ACTH-dependent hypercortisolism.

Case 1 (continued)

Which of the following is this patient's most likely diagnosis?

A. ACTH-dependent hypercortisolism due to stress

B. ACTH-secretion due to bilateral adrenal hyperplasia

C. CD

D. EAS

E. Glucocorticoids

Answer: D) EAS

Severe hypercortisolism is usually due to EAS, most frequently caused by small cell lung carcinoma. Hypercortisolism due to EAS can also be observed in patients with thymic or genitourinary tract neuroendocrine tumors, or less frequently, medullary thyroid carcinoma. The signs usually appear rapidly through a catabolic presentation (weight loss, proximal myopathy in 70% cases), in contrast to the classic presentation of CS and its progressive onset. Hypokalemia with a potassium value less than 2.8 mEq/L (<2.8 mmol/L) is reported in more than 70% of affected patients and is associated with hypertension (89%) and diabetes (65%). Urinary free cortisol is reported to be greater than 5 times the upper normal limit in 70% cases.[4] Only a few studies have compared the profile at diagnosis of patients with CD with that of patients with EAS. For instance, Attri et al compared 23 patients with EAS with 76 patients with CD. Patients with EAS less frequently presented with weight gain (52% vs 87%) and more frequently presented with hypokalemia (82% vs 21%; mean potassium value = 2.8 vs 3.9 mEq/L [2.8 vs 3.9 mmol/L]) and suboptimally controlled diabetes (hemoglobin A_{1c} = 7.7% vs 6.8% [61 vs 51 mmol/mol]). The rate of diabetes was close to 50% in both groups. Finally, the mean ACTH value was greater than 90 pg/mL (>19.8 pmol/L) in 83% vs 34% in patients with EAS vs CD, respectively.[3] In this vignette, the patient's CT showed a suspicious lung nodule, and the most likely diagnosis is thus EAS due to a small cell lung carcinoma (Answer D).

Case 2

A 47-year-old woman is having difficulty losing weight. She has gained 11 lb (5 kg) in the last 5 years despite intensive diet and physical activity. She has been treated with a combination of 2 antihypertensive drugs (ACE inhibitor and calcium channel antagonist) for 2 years. She has no other relevant medical history. She presents with irregular menses (last 12 months) and thinks she has increased facial hair. She has purple striae on her abdomen, easy bruising, and leg muscle weakness. Her primary care physician reassured her that she is probably entering menopause.

Laboratory test results:

> Blood potassium = 3.8 mEq/L (SI: 3.8 mmol/L)
> ACTH (8 AM) = 15 pg/mL (SI: 3.3 pmol/L)
> ACTH (12 AM) = 17 pg/mL (SI: 3.7 pmol/L)
> Cortisol (8 AM) = 16.3 µg/dL (SI: 450 nmol/L)
> Cortisol (12 AM) = 10.1 µg/dL (SI: 280 nmol/L)

An overnight 1-mg dexamethasone-suppression test results in a cortisol value of 5.4 µg/dL (150 nmol/L) (confirmed with 2nd measurement = 5.0 µg/dL [138 nmol/L]). Two 24-hour urinary free cortisol measurements have a mean value 2.3 times the upper normal limit.

Which of the following assumptions is correct?

A. The diagnosis of CD is certain

B. The diagnosis of CS is not yet certain

C. The patient has ACTH-independent hypercortisolism

D. The patient has either CD or indolent EAS

Answer: D) The patient has either CD or indolent EAS

The combination of 2 screening tests (1-mg overnight dexamethasone-suppression test and urinary free cortisol measurement [repeated]) confirms the diagnosis of CS. The ACTH concentration suggests the patient has ACTH-dependent CS. While her most likely diagnosis given her age and clinical presentation should be CD, indolent EAS cannot be ruled out at this stage (thus, Answer D is correct and Answers A, B, and C are incorrect).

Case 2 (continued)

Whole-body CT shows moderate bilateral adrenal hyperplasia and no anomalies. Pituitary MRI findings are normal. Desmopressin-stimulation testing shows a 10% increase in both ACTH and cortisol. A high-dose dexamethasone-suppression test is not performed.

Which of the following assumptions is correct?

A. CT findings rule out EAS

B. Desmopressin-stimulation test result rules out CD

C. Diagnosis of CD is possible

D. Diagnosis of EAS due to an indolent neuroendocrine tumor is certain

E. Pituitary MRI findings rule out CD

Answer: C) Diagnosis of CD is possible

The imaging in this case does not exclude any diagnosis. Pituitary MRI findings are considered normal in up to 40% of patients with CD, and CT identifies only 50% of neuroendocrine tumors that cause EAS (thus, Answers A and E are incorrect). Desmopressin-stimulation testing is positive when ACTH and cortisol increase, but the threshold for defining positivity varies across studies, from 20% to 50%. Moreover, desmopressin-stimulation testing can be positive in up to 20% of patients with EAS and can be negative in up to 20% of patients with CD (thus, Answer B is incorrect). At that stage, there is still uncertainty between CD and indolent ectopic ACTH secretion (thus, Answer C is correct and Answer D is incorrect).

Case 2 (continued)

Which of the following is the best next step in this patient's management?

A. Bilateral IPSS with desmopressin stimulation

B. Bilateral IPSS without desmopressin stimulation

C. Cortisol-lowering drugs

D. DOTATATE PET-CT

E. Explorative transsphenoidal surgery

Answer: A) Bilateral IPSS with desmopressin stimulation

The lack of ACTH response to desmopressin renders stimulation useless during IPSS. The etiology remains unknown in this patient because the imaging is normal (thus, Answers C and E are incorrect). Although DOTATATE PET-CT (Answer D) could be an option, the possibility of identifying a neuroendocrine tumor is less than 60%, which makes it less likely than IPSS to identify the etiology, even without stimulation (thus, Answer A is correct).

Case 3

A 60-year-old woman presented with hypertension and diabetes mellitus 3 years ago and now requires 3 antihypertensive medications and 2 antidiabetes medications. She has a history of mild hypokalemia and was not tested for CS until recently when she became concerned about easy bruising and purple striae. She is moderately overweight (BMI = 27 kg/m²).

Laboratory test results:

> Blood potassium = 3.5 mEq/L (3.5-5.0 mEq/L) (SI: 3.5 mmol/L [3.5-5.0 mmol/L])
> Cortisol following 1-mg overnight dexamethasone-suppression test = 2.9 μg/dL (SI: 80 nmol/L)
> Mean of 3 measurements urinary free cortisol = 83 μg/24 h (40-80 μg/24 h) (SI: 230 nmol/24 h [110-220 nmol/24 h])
> Mean of 3 late-night salivary cortisol measurements = 0.09 μg/dL (<0.08 μg/dL) (SI: 2.5 nmol/L [<2.4 nmol/L])
> ACTH (2 measurements) = 45 and 60 pg/mL (15-45 pg/mL) (SI: 9.9 and 13.2 pmol/L [3.3-9.9 pmol/L])

MRI of the pituitary gland shows a suspicious 3-mm enhancement in the right wing of the pituitary gland. Findings on thoracoabdominal CT are normal.

Desmopressin-stimulation testing documents a 60% increase in ACTH and 53% increase in cortisol. A high-dose dexamethasone-suppression test results in 58% cortisol suppression.

Which of the following is this patient's most likely diagnosis?

A. CD

B. EAS due to an indolent neuroendocrine tumor

C. Nonneoplastic hypercortisolism

Answer: A) CD

The first diagnostic steps in this case led to 3 positive results (1-mg overnight dexamethasone-suppression test, 24-hour urinary free cortisol measurement, and late-night salivary cortisol measurement). ACTH is not decreased, which favors ACTH-dependent CD. Given this patient's sex and clinical presentation, the most likely diagnosis is CD (Answer A). However, the MRI findings are equivocal, and the results of the second-line tests (desmopressin-stimulation test and high-dose dexamethasone-suppression test) are discordant. The result of desmopressin-stimulation testing favors CD, while the result of high-dose dexamethasone-suppression test favors EAS (Answer B). There is no evidence for a nonneoplastic hypercortisolism (Answer C).

Case 3 (continued)

IPSS is performed with desmopressin stimulation. Baseline values are first obtained without desmopressin stimulation. Desmopressin is then injected, and measurements are taken 5 and 15 minutes after injection. Results of IPSS:

Location of sampling	Time		
	Baseline	5 minutes	15 minutes
Right petrosal ACTH	65 pg/mL (SI: 14.3 pmol/L)	280 pg/mL (SI: 61.6 pmol/L)	265 pg/mL (SI: 58.3 pmol/L)
Left petrosal ACTH	60 pg/mL (SI: 13.2 pmol/L)	170 pg/mL (SI: 37.4 pmol/L)	150 pg/mL (SI: 33.0 pmol/L)
Peripheral ACTH	55 pg/mL (SI: 12.1 pmol/L)	80 pg/mL (SI: 17.6 pmol/L)	80 pg/mL (SI: 17.6 pmol/L)

Which of the following assumptions is correct?

A. Desmopressin stimulation did not provide any additional information compared with information available for baseline

B. IPSS findings are consistent with EAS

C. The increase in ACTH (ratio) greater than 3 after desmopressin is consistent with CD

D. The probability that the pituitary tumor is in the right wing of the pituitary is 100%

Answer: C) The increase in ACTH (ratio) greater than 3 between petrosal and peripheral after desmopressin is consistent with CD

In the largest series published on IPSS, Chen et al found that a ratio of 1.4 (petrosal ACTH-to-peripheral ACTH) at baseline and a ratio of 2.8 after desmopressin stimulation favored CD. While this patient's baseline ratio is not in favor of CD, Chen et al showed that desmopressin stimulation was able to correct the diagnosis in 10% of cases (thus, Answer A is incorrect). The ratio obtained in this case after stimulation favors CD (thus, Answer C is correct and Answer B is incorrect). However, even if the ratio were higher in the right wing, it would not confirm the location of the pituitary tumor (thus, Answer D is incorrect).

Key Learning Points

- Dynamic testing is not necessary in patients with severe life-threatening hypercortisolism. The urgency is to control cortisol hypersecretion to improve comorbidities. The priority is imaging to find the tumor.

- While a proportion of patients with EAS develop severe hypercortisolism, small tumors with mild hypercortisolism can cause symptoms similar to those of Cushing disease. In this setting, dynamic testing is necessary.

- Because of the lack of CRH, the diagnostic approach for patients with ACTH-dependent CS should include epidemiology, clinical presentation, imaging, and dynamic testing (ie, desmopressin-stimulation testing and high-dose dexamethasone-suppression testing). Both tests have merits and pitfalls and neither is 100% accurate (approximately 20% false-positive results and 20% false-negative results).

- In patients with a doubtful etiologic diagnosis, IPSS by an experienced operator remains the gold standard. The lack of CRH availability should prompt the use of desmopressin as a secretagogue, although 20% of patients have a tumor that does not respond to desmopressin. Interestingly, recent large-scale data support the accuracy of IPSS even without stimulation.

References

1. Fleseriu M, Auchus R, Bancos I, et al. Consensus on diagnosis and management of Cushing's disease: a guideline update. *Lancet Diabetes Endocrinol.* 2021;9(12):847-875. PMID: 34687601

2. Frete C, Corcuff JB, Kuhn E, et al. Non-invasive diagnostic strategy in ACTH-dependent Cushing's syndrome. *J Clin Endocrinol Metab.* 2020;105(10):dgaa409. PMID: 32594169

3. Attri B, Goyal A, Kalaivani M, et al. Clinical profile and treatment outcomes of patients with ectopic ACTH syndrome compared to Cushing disease: a single-center experience. *Endocrine.* 2023;80(2):408-418. PMID: 36609908

4. Davi MV, Cosaro E, Piacentini S, et al. Prognostic factors in ectopic Cushing's syndrome due to neuroendocrine tumors: a multicenter study. *Eur J Endocrinol.* 2017;176(4):453-461. PMID: 28183788

5. Young J, Haissaguerre M, Viera-Pinto O, Chabre O, Baudin E, Tabarin A. Management of endocrine disease: Cushing's syndrome due to ectopic ACTH secretion: an expert operational opinion. *Eur J Endocrinol.* 2020;182(4):R29-R58. PMID: 31999619

6. Castinetti F, Lacroix A. Is desmopressin useful in the evaluation of Cushing syndrome? *J Clin Endocrinol Metab.* 2022;107(11):e4295-e4301. PMID: 36103267

7. Barbot M, Trementino L, Zilio M, et al. Second-line tests in the differential diagnosis of ACTH-dependent Cushing's syndrome. *Pituitary.* 2016;19(5):488-495. PMID: 27236452

8. Elenius H, McGlotten R, Nieman LK. Ovine CRH stimulation and 8 mg dexamethasone suppression tests in 323 patients with ACTH-dependent Cushing's syndrome. *J Clin Endocrinol Metab.* 2023;109(1):e182-e189. PMID: 37531629

9. Lyu X, Zhang D, Pan H, Zhu H, Chen S, Lu L. Machine learning models for differential diagnosis of Cushing's disease and ectopic ACTH secretion syndrome. *Endocrine.* 2023;80(3):639-646. PMID: 36933156

10. Senanayake R, Gillett D, MacFarlane J, et al. New types of localization methods for adrenocorticotropic hormone-dependent Cushing's syndrome. *Best Pract Res Clin Endocrinol Metab.* 2021;35(1):101513. PMID: 34045044

11. Hayes AR, Grossman AB. Distinguishing Cushing's disease from the ectopic ACTH syndrome: needles in a haystack or hiding in plain sight? *J Neuroendocrinol.* 2022;34(8):e13137. PMID: 35980277

12. Chen S, Chen K, Wang S, et al. The optimal cut-off of BIPSS in differential diagnosis of ACTH-dependent Cushing's syndrome: is stimulation necessary? *J Clin Endocrinol Metab.* 2020;105(4):dgz194. PMID: 31758170

Challenges in the Diagnosis and Management of Non-neoplastic Hypercortisolism

James W. Findling, MD. Medical College of Wisconsin, Milwaukee, WI; Email: jfindling@mcw.edu

Educational Objectives

- Recognize findings in the history, physical examination, and routine laboratory test results that may raise suspicion for non-neoplastic hypercortisolism and describe clinical disorders that have been reported to cause sustained or intermittent activation of the hypothalamic-pituitary-adrenal (HPA) axis.

- Contrast tests of HPA-axis function in patients with neoplastic hypercortisolism from those in patients with non-neoplastic hypercortisolism.

- Differentiate the ACTH/cortisol responses to desmopressin in patients with neoplastic hypercortisolism from those in patients with non-neoplastic hypercortisolism.

If you have never missed the diagnosis of Cushing syndrome or been humbled by trying to determine its cause, you should refer all your patients with suspected hypercortisolism to someone who has.

Significance of the Clinical Problem

The diagnosis and differential diagnosis of neoplastic hypercortisolism (Cushing syndrome) is one of the most challenging problems in clinical medicine. Many of the clinical features of Cushing syndrome, including obesity, hypertension, diabetes, and low bone density, are very commonly seen in general clinical practice. The development of more sensitive and specific laboratory tests to assess HPA function and new diagnostic thresholds has resulted in the recognition of milder degrees of hypercortisolism. The increasing recognition of the negative cardiometabolic effects of milder degrees of cortisol excess without the overt clinical findings of Cushing syndrome has led to more screening for endogenous hypercortisolism in patients with adrenal nodular disease, osteoporosis, and metabolic syndrome. It has been well known for many years that intermittent or sustained activation of the HPA axis caused by inflammatory (chronic kidney disease), chemical (alcohol), physical (chronic intense exercise/starvation), and psychological (major depression) stimuli may cause clinical and biochemical findings that are indistinguishable from those of neoplastic hypercortisolism. With increased diagnostic screening for hypercortisolism, non-neoplastic hypercortisolism (initially called pseudo-Cushing syndrome) has emerged as an even more important consideration.[1,2]

Practice Gaps

- Current guidelines for the diagnostic evaluation of suspected hypercortisolism include 24-hour urinary free cortisol (UFC) measurement, late-night salivary cortisol measurement, and the overnight 1-mg dexamethasone-suppression test (DST). All these tests have imperfections: UFC—very bad sensitivity; late-night salivary cortisol—great sensitivity for ACTH-dependent Cushing syndrome but poor sensitivity for adrenal-dependent Cushing syndrome; and DST—great sensitivity but suboptimal specificity. Moreover, patients with non-neoplastic hypercortisolism may have late-night salivary cortisol, DST, and UFC results that are indistinguishable from those of neoplastic hypercortisolism. The diagnostic evaluation may also be compromised by surreptitious use of glucocorticoids, use of medications that affect diagnostic testing (oral contraceptives or drugs that alter dexamethasone clearance), proximal stress in the evening, improper test execution, and problematic hormone assays.

- Incidental nonfunctioning adrenal and pituitary imaging abnormalities (often the segue to testing) are seductive traps, even for experienced clinicians. Although the desmopressin-stimulation test has emerged now as the most widely used test to distinguish non-neoplastic hypercortisolism from true pathologic Cushing syndrome, it needs more extensive investigation with better standardization of reference intervals using reliable, harmonized ACTH and cortisol assays in diverse populations.

Discussion

Non-neoplastic hypercortisolism (the term *pseudo-Cushing syndrome* is confusing) was initially reported many years ago. These are patients who have biochemical evidence of ACTH-dependent hypercortisolism, due either to sustained or intermittent activation of the HPA axis, who often have clinical and physical features of hypercortisolemia. *Table 1* summarizes the causes of endogenous hypercortisolism. It is important to understand that there are often subtle and sometimes not-so-subtle clues that may help clinicians realize that the dysregulated cortisol hypersecretion may have a nonpathologic cause. *Table 2* (*following page*) provides some clues to help distinguish neoplastic from non-neoplastic

hypercortisolism. The clinical case vignettes in this chapter emphasize how a good history and examination, simple routine laboratory studies, and more specific diagnostic tests are needed to distinguish neoplastic hypercortisolism (true Cushing syndrome for the traditionalists) from non-neoplastic hypercortisolism (pseudo-Cushing syndrome for the medical historians).

Table 1. Causes of Endogenous Hypercortisolism

Neoplastic hypercortisolism	Non-neoplastic hypercortisolism

ACTH-secreting neoplasm
• Pituitary (Cushing disease)
• Ectopic
Adrenal nodular disease
• Adenoma/carcinoma
• Bilateral nodular disease
  ○ Primary pigmented micronodular
  ○ Macronodular
	Cushing phenotype
	• Alcohol-induced
	• Chronic kidney disease stages 4-5
	• Neuropsychiatric disorders
	• Suboptimally controlled diabetes mellitus
	• Pregnancy
	• Glucocorticoid resistance
	NonCushing phenotype
	• Starvation equivalent disorders
	• Relative energy deficiency in sports
	• Eating disorders (anorexia/bulimia)

Reprinted from Findling JW & Raff H. *Journal of the Endocrine Society*, 2023; 7(8): bvad087. © The Authors. Published by Oxford University Press on behalf of the Endocrine Society.[2]

Causes of Non-neoplastic Hypercortisolism With a Cushing Syndrome Phenotype

Alcohol-Induced Hypercortisolism

Alcohol-induced hypercortisolism is an underappreciated, reversible cause of Cushing syndrome. Alcohol intake acutely increases cortisol secretion, and persons with an alcohol use disorder have increased indices of cortisol secretion compared to control. The mechanism of the hypercortisolism is predominately centrally mediated due to increases in hypothalamic corticotropin-releasing hormone and pituitary ACTH. Altered peripheral hepatic cortisol metabolism may also contribute to the dysregulated cortisol secretion, and most patients with alcohol-induced hypercortisolism have evidence of liver function abnormalities (AST > ALT). In addition, patients with alcohol-induced liver disease have an increase in hepatic cortisol production due to induction of 11β-hydroxysteroid dehydrogenase type 1 gene expression, thereby converting more cortisone to cortisol in the liver.

Persons with alcohol-induced hypercortisolism have clinical and biochemical features indistinguishable from those of persons with neoplastic hypercortisolism, and hypercortisolism remits quickly after abstention from alcohol. Despite the increase in alcohol consumption in the United States, there had been only 1 report of alcohol-induced hypercortisolism in the past 20 years. In 2023, our group reported 8 patients with alcohol-induced hypercortisolism and summarized the previous literature.[3] Patients with alcohol-induced hypercortisolism had elevations of liver function enzymes, with AST uniformly greater than ALT—a common problem in patients with more advanced alcohol-induced liver disease. Not surprisingly, patients often underreport their alcohol consumption, which can result in a missed diagnosis. If patients report daily alcohol consumption and/or have AST > ALT, then further investigation is warranted. Blood phosphatidylethanol levels are helpful to quantify the amount of alcohol consumed.[4] Blood phosphatidylethanol measures a group of phospholipids formed in the presence of ethanol and is a biomarker of alcohol intake. Phosphatidylethanol has a 4- to 10-day half-life with a 2- to 4-week window of detection that is prolonged in patients with excessive alcohol intake. The patient described in Case 1 denied any alcohol use until confronted with the phosphatidylethanol level and the history of alcohol intoxication while driving was discovered. To provide further evidence of non-neoplastic hypercortisolism, a desmopressin-stimulation test showed no increase in ACTH/cortisol in the patient described in Case 1. In contrast to most patients with Cushing disease,

Table 2. Clinical and Laboratory Differences in Neoplastic vs Non-neoplastic Hypercortisolism

Clinical and laboratory parameters	Neoplastic hypercortisolism	Non-neoplastic hypercortisolism
History		
Alcohol ≥2/d	---	+++
Hypertension	+++	+++
Type 2 diabetes	++	+/–
Low bone density with fractures	+++	---
Physical examination		
Cushingoid facies	+++	+
Dorsocervical fat	++	+
Cutaneous wasting	+++	+
Myopathy	+++	+
Laboratory test results		
Chronic kidney disease stages 1-3	+	+
Chronic kidney disease stages 4-5	+	+++
Liver ALT > AST	+++	+
Liver AST > ALT	---	+++
Late-night salivary cortisol >5 times upper normal limit	+++	+
Morning cortisol after DST >5 µg/dL (>138 nmol/L)	++	++
UFC >4 times upper normal limit	+++	+
Positive desmopressin stimulation	+++	---

Reprinted from Findling JW & Raff H. *Journal of the Endocrine Society*, 2023; 7(8): bvad087. © The Authors. Published by Oxford University Press on behalf of the Endocrine Society.[2]

patients with alcohol-induced hypercortisolism have consistently been shown to have an absent ACTH response to desmopressin.[3,5] Interestingly, the old dexamethasone–corticotropin-releasing hormone test was not helpful in distinguishing alcohol-induced hypercortisolism from neoplastic hypercortisolism.[3]

Chronic Kidney Disease

Some features of Cushing syndrome are frequently encountered in patients with end-stage kidney failure, including hypertension, diabetes, and low bone density. Mild biochemical hypercortisolism is almost ubiquitous in chronic kidney disease.[6] The glucocorticoid-mediated features of kidney failure are centrally, ACTH-driven so these patients have normal or elevated ACTH levels. There is decreased sensitivity to glucocorticoid negative feedback and reduction in the activity of 11β-hydroxysteroid dehydrogenase type 1 in the kidney. Patients with stage 5 chronic kidney disease almost always have abnormal DST results.[7] In addition, many patients with stage 5 chronic kidney disease exhibit increases in late-night salivary cortisol and some also have very abnormal diurnal rhythms. Late-night salivary cortisol has been shown by some to be inversely correlated with the degree of chronic kidney disease, and persons with even stage 3 and 4 may have altered circadian rhythms.[6,8] A normal urinary cortisol value in patients with stage 3 to 4 chronic kidney disease is difficult to interpret. There are currently no published data on the desmopressin-stimulation test in chronic kidney disease. In our experience, these patients exhibit no increase in ACTH/cortisol after desmopressin (*see Case 2*).

Neuropsychiatric Disorders

Many neuropsychiatric disorders, including major depression, anxiety/panic disorders, obsessive/compulsive disorders, schizophrenia, and autism spectrum disorder, have been reported to be associated with markers of increased HPA-axis activity.[9] Of course, true Cushing syndrome is frequently associated with significant neuropsychiatric challenges and neurocognitive dysfunction. The consensus is that the desmopressin-stimulation test is the best diagnostic tool to distinguish non-neoplastic hypercortisolism due to psychiatric disorders from neoplastic hypercortisolism.[10]

Suboptimally Controlled Type 2 Diabetes

There are varied opinions about whether patients with suboptimally controlled diabetes may have chronic HPA-axis activation.[11] Of course, the magnitude of the suboptimal glycemic control and the presence of inflammatory complications such as chronic kidney disease may be significant factors. Most reports have demonstrated only mild increases in cortisol dysregulation. Currently, there is a large multicenter study identifying the prevalence of abnormal DST results in patients with suboptimally controlled type 2 diabetes and the possible impact of glucocorticoid receptor antagonism for glycemic control in those with adrenal dependent hypercortisolism. Again, the desmopressin-stimulation test is a good resource to confirm the presence or absence of true Cushing syndrome.

Glucocorticoid Resistance

Pathogenic variants in the *NR3C1* gene that encodes the glucocorticoid receptor protein may cause glucocorticoid resistance and an unexplained increase in cortisol production.[12] Not surprisingly, these patients lack features of glucocorticoid excess; however, due to increases in ACTH and the maintenance of androgen and mineralocorticoid sensitivity, they may have hyperandrogenism resulting in hirsutism and oligomenorrhea mimicking polycystic ovary disease. Excessive adrenal mineralocorticoid secretion may cause hypertension with hypokalemia. Although this is a rare familial disorder with both autosomal dominant and recessive forms being described, a French study showed a prevalence of heterozygous *NR3C1* variants of nearly 5% among patients with adrenal hyperplasia, UFC elevation, and abnormal DST results.[13] For those clinicians who want to cling to the term pseudo-Cushing syndrome, I would suggest that they hang their hats here. I am embarrassed to say that I have never diagnosed this disorder—which almost certainly means that I have missed it.

Pregnancy

The final trimester of pregnancy is a hypercortisolemic state that is driven by increases in ACTH. There are many possible contributing factors: secretion of both corticotropin-releasing hormone and ACTH from the placenta, progesterone-driven glucocorticoid antagonism, and a decrease in glucocorticoid negative feedback. It seems likely that this increase in bioactive cortisol has some metabolic benefit in pregnancy. The increases in cortisol secretory tests are usually mild during pregnancy and can usually easily be distinguished from pathologic Cushing syndrome on clinical grounds.

Causes of Non-neoplastic Hypercortisolism Without a Cushing Phenotype

Starvation equivalent disorders, where energy expenditure exceeds energy intake, results in activation of the HPA axis, which is demonstrated by increases in UFC and late-night salivary cortisol and abnormal results on DST. In patients with eating disorders, several mechanisms for the HPA-axis activation have been suggested. Increased hypothalamic Corticotropin-releasing hormone secretion insensitive to glucocorticoid negative feedback is an important cause.[14] Depression and anxiety are also comorbid events associated with eating disorders that may contribute to the pathophysiology of the HPA axis. Even with weight recovery and amelioration of the pathophysiological findings in anorexia nervosa, some patients still have dysregulated cortisol secretion. One radical hypothesis is that the increased HPA axis activity has a neurologic basis and is not just due to the energy-deficient state.

Another example of a starvation equivalent disorder is illustrated in Case 3 and is referred to as relative energy deficiency in sport. In one study, mild hypercortisolism was documented in more than 20% of elite athletes and was sometimes associated with other markers of energy deficiency.[15] Of course, these patients should rarely be confused with patients who have true Cushing syndrome. Although the physical examination in Case 3 should have eliminated any concern about pathologic Cushing syndrome, the low testosterone and possible abnormality on pituitary imaging led clinicians down a rabbit hole of testing HPA-axis function. Severe caloric restriction in men (as in women) results in a very significant decrease in the hypothalamic-pituitary-gonadal axis function and activation of the HPA axis. Patients with starvation equivalent disorders have an absent ACTH response to desmopressin.

Distinguishing Neoplastic From Non-neoplastic Hypercortisolism: Clinical and Biochemical Studies

History, Examination, and Routine Laboratory Tests

Most importantly, a good history of the evolution of the patient's signs and symptoms is always needed. Patients who drink alcohol daily should be carefully evaluated. Patients with severe neuropsychiatric disorders or longstanding or very poorly controlled diabetes should have either very significant clinical features of the Cushing syndrome or unequivocal elevations of HPA-axis function before the diagnosis of neoplastic hypercortisolism can be confirmed. Significant elevations of late-night salivary cortisol (>5 times the upper normal limit) or UFC (>4 times the upper normal limit) usually support diagnosis of neoplastic hypercortisolism (*Table 2*). DST is not very helpful here. Of course, be prepared for patients (who are well-informed from social media) who raise concern about intermittent or cyclical Cushing syndrome.

Imaging

Neither pituitary nor adrenal imaging should be used alone to confirm the presence of neoplastic hypercortisolism. Ephemeral small pituitary imaging abnormalities are so common in practice (especially when the interpreting radiologist sees that the reason for the MRI is "Cushing syndrome") that these findings must be taken in context. Two of the patients with non-neoplastic hypercortisolism presented in this chapter had subtle, vague pituitary imaging abnormalities that led to angst for the patients and their clinicians. It has also been shown that inferior petrosal sinus sampling cannot differentiate patients with Cushing disease, control patients, and those with non-neoplastic hypercortisolism. Since some patients with Cushing disease have adrenal nodules, it should not be shocking that some with non-neoplastic hypercortisolism also harbor adrenal nodules. An adrenal nodule was found in 25% of the patients reported with alcohol-induced hypercortisolism.

Desmopressin-Stimulation Test

The lack of availability of corticotropin-releasing hormone has led to increased interest in the use of the desmopressin-stimulation test to help diagnose

Box. Morning Desmopressin-Stimulation Test Protocol

Protocol

- Study should begin before 9:00 AM
- Indwelling intravenous catheter inserted; then wait 10 minutes before first blood draw
- Measurements at each study timepoint
  - *Plasma ACTH and serum cortisol
  - *Blood pressure and pulse rate
- After baseline blood draw, infuse desmopressin acetate 10 mcg (2.5 mL) intravenously over 60 seconds followed by a 2-mL saline flush
- Draw blood samples for plasma ACTH and cortisol at −15 min, 0 min (baseline), + 10 min, +20 min, +30 min, +45 min, +60 min

Note: Adverse effects of desmopressin may include flushing, increased respiratory rate, and hypotension (rare). If hypotension occurs, immediately notify physician. Hypotension may cause a false-positive result. Patients should restrict fluid intake to 40 oz (1.2 L) for the next 24 hours.

Interpretation: positive response

- Increase in plasma ACTH above baseline >30 pg/mL (>6.6 pmol/L)[a] or peak ACTH >70 pg/mL (>15.4 pmol/L)
- Increase in serum cortisol[b] >6 μg/dL (>166 nmol/L) or peak >18 μg/dL (>497 nmol/L)

[a] Percentage increase over baseline is used by some (ranging from 35%-150%); a positive delta ACTH has been reported to be anywhere between 27-37 pg/mL (5.9-8.1 pmol/L)

[b] Percentage increase over baseline is used by some (ranging from 20%-40%); cortisol cutoffs depend on the assay method used

---

Cushing syndrome (*Box*).[1,2] Desmopressin is a vasopressin analogue that is relatively specific to the V2 receptor that mediates antidiuresis and hemostasis. It has relatively weak affinity for the V3 receptor that stimulates pituitary ACTH. ACTH-secreting pituitary tumors (and some ectopic ACTH-secreting tumors) may have aberrant expression of V3 and V2 receptors. Most patients with pituitary ACTH-secreting tumors exhibit a prompt and vigorous ACTH and cortisol response to desmopressin. In contrast, normal individuals and patients with non-neoplastic hypercortisolism have an absent response. Now used routinely during inferior petrosal sinus sampling, desmopressin has been shown to be as good as corticotropin-releasing hormone.

The desmopressin-stimulation test is easy to execute, but there are some caveats. The test should always be done in the morning and start before 9:00 AM. The ACTH response in patients with neoplastic hypercortisolism occurs very quickly and postdesmopressin ACTH should be secured no later than 10 minutes. Fluid restriction (we recommend 40 oz or 1.2 L) should be recommended for 24 hours after the study. Some patients notice a decrease in urine output and, unfortunately, increase their fluid intake, possibly leading to hyponatremia.

Interpretation of the desmopressin-stimulation test is a work in progress. Please be advised that there will be some patients with neoplastic hypercortisolism who may not have a response, and this test cannot be used to reliably distinguish Cushing disease from ectopic ACTH. Moreover, a few patients with non-neoplastic hypercortisolism (<10% in one series) exhibit a positive ACTH response. There is NO substitution for good clinical judgement in this setting.

In my experience (which is largely confirmed by ROC curves from the current literature), the absolute change in ACTH from baseline is the criterion that achieves the best sensitivity and specificity. Published results suggest that an ACTH increase of anywhere from 27 to 37 pg/mL (5.9-8.1 pmol/L) (we currently use 30 pg/mL [6.6 pmol/L]) or a peak ACTH concentration greater than 70 pg/mL [>15.4 pmol/L]) are the best criteria. The cortisol increase is usually greater than 6 μg/dL (>165.5 nmol/L) in patients with Cushing disease. Many reports have advocated percentage changes in ACTH/cortisol, but I am skeptical: for example, a small increase in ACTH (eg, 20 to 32 pg/mL [4.4-7.0 pmol/L] reflecting >50% increase) may be interpreted as a positive response.

Regardless, the results of desmopressin-stimulation testing must be interpreted cautiously in the context of a thorough clinical evaluation with consideration of the patient's history, examination, comorbid conditions, medications, routine laboratory test results, modern biochemical studies of HPA-axis function, and the pretest probability of true Cushing syndrome.

Clinical Case Vignettes

Case 1

A 33-year-old man is referred for evaluation of persistent hypercortisolism after removal of a benign 3.4-cm left adrenal adenoma. After an automobile accident 2 years earlier, a left adrenal nodule was identified. He was referred to another endocrinologist, and laboratory studies had shown elevations of late-night salivary cortisol and an abnormal result from overnight 1-mg DST. UFC was normal and, the plasma ACTH concentration was 12 pg/mL (2.7 pmol/L). One year after adrenalectomy (no postoperative adrenal insufficiency was seen), he wants another opinion. He has had rapid weight gain (11 lb [5 kg] since his adrenal surgery), muscle weakness and paresthesias, easy bruising, and facial rounding and plethora. He has hypertension that is well controlled with lisinopril and prediabetes (hemoglobin A_{1c} = 5.7% [39 mmol/mol]). He does not drink alcohol or smoke cigarettes. There is no known family history of an endocrine disorder.

On physical examination, he appears slightly cushingoid. His blood pressure is 128/84 mm Hg, and pulse rate is 105 beats/min. BMI is 26 kg/m^2. Spider telangiectasias are noted on his chest. He has a resting tremor but no focal neurologic findings.

Proximal muscle weakness and decreased ankle jerk with diminished proprioception are noted.

Laboratory test results:

> Electrolytes, normal
> Liver function enzymes (AST, ALT), elevated
> Late-night salivary cortisol = 0.94 μg/dL
> (<0.12 μg/dL) (SI: 25.8 nmol/L [<3.2 nmol/L])
> Cortisol after 1-mg DST = 19.1 μg/dL (<1.8 μg/dL)
> (SI: 513 nmol/L [<50 nmol/L])
> Plasma ACTH = 101 pg/mL (10-50 pg/mL)
> (SI: 22.4 pmol/L [2.2-11.0 pmol/L])

Findings on pituitary MRI and chest and abdominal CT are normal.

Which of the following studies should be recommended?

A. PET/CT DOTATATE scan

B. Repeated liver function tests

C. Inferior petrosal sinus ACTH sampling

D. High-dose DST

E. Desmopressin-stimulation test

Answer: B) Repeated liver function tests and E) Desmopressin-stimulation test

Case 1 (continued)

Repeated liver enzyme measurements (similar values to previous tests):

> AST = 191 U/L (<35 U/L) (SI: 3.91 μkat/L
> [<0.58 μkat/L])
> ALT = 56 U/L (<30 U/L) (SI: 0.94 μkat/L
> [<0.50 μkat/L])

Insurance refuses PET/CT DOTATATE imaging. Inferior petrosal sinus sampling is scheduled. High-dose DST is not done.

Desmopressin-stimulation test results:

> Basal ACTH = 63 pg/mL (SI: 13.9 pmol/L)
> Cortisol = 19.5 μg/dL (SI: 538 nmol/L)

Both values decrease after 10 mcg of desmopressin acetate.

Which of the following investigations should be recommended now?

A. Retrieve emergency department records after his automobile accident 2 years ago

B. Perform inferior petrosal sinus sampling as scheduled

C. Measure blood concentration of phosphatidylethanol

D. Perform liver biopsy

E. Refer the patient to another endocrinologist

Answer: A) Retrieve emergency department records after his automobile accident 2 years ago and C) Measure blood concentration of phosphatidylethanol

The patient's blood phosphatidylethanol concentration was 788 ng/mL (>200 ng/mL consistent with heavy alcohol consumption). Inferior petrosal sinus sampling was canceled. Emergency department records from his automobile accident showed that he had blood alcohol concentration of 0.276 g/dL. After an intervention with the patient, he acknowledged consuming 8 to 12 drinks daily for at least 10 years.

Case 2

A 54-year-old woman has been referred by her nephrologist to help with the differential diagnosis of ACTH-dependent Cushing syndrome. She has stage 5 chronic kidney disease and has been receiving hemodialysis 3 times weekly for 5 years. She has had an unexpected 11-lb (5-kg) weight gain in the last 2 years with worsening hypertension. She now requires 4 antihypertensive medications (clonidine, furosemide, hydralazine, metoprolol). She has prediabetes with a modest increase in her hemoglobin A_{1c} over the past year from 5.8% to 6.2% (40 to 44 mmol/mol). She has obstructive sleep apnea treated with continuous positive airway pressure for the past 3 years. She has a history of low bone density, but she has not sustained any fractures. She states she does not drink alcohol.

Because her nephrologist thought she looked a little cushingoid, you had recommended the following studies prior to today's appointment:

> Late-night salivary cortisol = 0.26 μg/dL
> (<0.12 μg/dL) (SI: 7.3 nmol/L [<3.2 nmol/L])
> Cortisol after 1-mg DST = 5.1 μg/dL (<1.8 μg/dL)
> (SI: 138 nmol/L [<50 nmol/L])
> Plasma ACTH = 77 pg/mL (10-50 pg/mL)
> (SI: 17 pmol/L [2.2-11.0 pmol/L])

Routine laboratory test results on a nondialysis day:

> Potassium = 5.1 mEq/L (3.5-5.0 mEq/L)
> (SI: 5.1 mmol/L [3.5-5.0 mmol/L])
> Creatinine = 8.9 mg/dL (0.6-1.1 mg/dL)
> (SI: 787 μmol/L [53.0-97.2 μmol/L])
> Liver enzymes, normal

Pituitary MRI documents a subtle 2-mm hypoenhancement in the left pituitary.

On physical examination, her blood pressure is 156/96 mm Hg and pulse rate is 84 beats/min. Her BMI is 28.9 kg/m². She has slight facial rounding and increased supraclavicular and dorsocervical fat accumulation. There is cutaneous wasting with skin fold thickness in the dorsum of the hand of less than 2 mm. The rest of her examination findings are normal.

Which of the following is the best next step in this patient's management?

A. Inferior petrosal sinus sampling

B. Referral to a pituitary neurosurgeon

C. High-dose DST

D. Desmopressin-stimulation test

E. CT of chest/abdomen

Answer: D) Desmopressin-stimulation test

Desmopressin-stimulation testing documented a basal ACTH concentration of 48 pg/mL (10.6 pmol/L) and a cortisol concentration of 21 μg/dL (567 nmol/L), which decreased after 10 mcg of intravenous desmopressin.

Case 3

A 39-year-old man is referred because of hypercortisolemia. One year ago, he had a very low testosterone measurement with low-normal gonadotropins and normal prolactin. A 3-mm hypoenhancing lesion was seen in the left pituitary gland. Testosterone was initiated. After a curbside phone conversation, you suggest to the referring physician that hypercortisolism should be excluded and you recommend the following lab work:

> Plasma ACTH = 62 pg/mL (10-50 pg/mL)
> (SI: 13.8 pmol/L [2.2-11.0 pmol/L])
> Late-night salivary cortisol = 0.46 µg/dL
> (<0.12 µg/dL) (SI: 12.7 nmol/L [<3.2 nmol/L])
> Cortisol after 1-mg DST = 6.6 µg/dL (<1.8 µg/dL)
> (SI: 178 nmol/L [<50 nmol/L])

He relates a history of intense daily exercise. He runs 90 to 100 miles weekly, bikes 4 miles daily, and lifts weights 45 to 60 minutes daily. He is on a very strict diet to maintain his body weight less than 170 lb (<77 kg). He has no history of diabetes or hypertension. He has never had a fracture.

On physical examination, his blood pressure is 115/70 mm Hg and pulse rate is 53 beats/min. BMI is 21.3 kg/m². He is lean, very well-muscled, and well-virilized and has little subcutaneous tissue. His veins are prominent. There are no physical features of hypercortisolism. He has no gynecomastia and normal genitalia. Onychomycosis is noted on his toenails.

You suggest he markedly decrease his exercise program and then re-investigate HPA-axis function, but he declines.

Which of the following investigations is the best next step?

A. Inferior petrosal sinus sampling for ACTH

B. Desmopressin-stimulation test

C. High-dose DST

D. Dexamethasone–corticotropin-releasing hormone test

E. CT of the abdomen/chest

Answer: B) Desmopressin-stimulation test

Desmopressin-stimulation testing showed a basal ACTH concentration of 55 pg/mL (12.1 pmol/L) and cortisol concentration of 18.5 µg/dL (510 nmol/L), and both decreased after 10 mcg of intravenous desmopressin.

Key Learning Points

- The clinical and biochemical findings of non-neoplastic hypercortisolism may overlap those of neoplastic hypercortisolism. After a thorough history and physical exam, your clinical judgement and experience should help guide your interpretation of all lab and imaging studies.

- Due to the increased screening for possible HPA-axis hyperfunction in patients with incidental adrenal or pituitary imaging abnormalities, osteoporosis, and metabolic syndrome, non-neoplastic hypercortisolism has emerged as a more important consideration.

- Alcohol use disorder is underappreciated due to the underreporting of alcohol consumption by some patients. If a patient consistently has elevated liver function enzymes with AST greater than ALT, further investigation should be considered. The measurement of blood phosphatidylethanol may help identify a patient with excessive alcohol consumption.

- The lack of an acute ACTH and cortisol response to desmopressin may help to confirm non-neoplastic hypercortisolism.

- There are many causes of non-neoplastic hypercortisolism. Alcohol-induced hypercortisolism and stage 5 chronic kidney disease are 2 of the more common causes. Surely many more causes are yet to be characterized.

- It seems possible that pharmacotherapies to either lower cortisol or block its biologic action may have a role in some non-neoplastic hypercortisolemic conditions.

References

1. Findling JW, Raff H. Differentiation of pathologic/neoplastic hypercortisolism (Cushing syndrome) from physiologic/non-neoplastic hypercortisolism (formerly known as pseudo-Cushing syndrome). *Eur J Endocrinol.* 2017;176(5):R205-R216. PMID: 28179447

2. Findling JW, Raff H. Recognition of nonneoplastic hypercortisolism in the evaluation of patients with Cushing syndrome. *J Endo Soc.* 2023;7(8):bvad087. PMID: 37440963

3. Surani A, Carroll TB, Javorsky BR, Raff H, Findling JW. Alcohol-induced Cushing syndrome: report of eight cases and review of the literature. *Front Endocrinol.* 2023;14:1199091. PMID: 37409223

4. Isaksoon A, Walther L, Hansson T, Andersson A, Alling C. Phosphatidylethanol in blood (B-PEth): a marker of alcohol use and abuse. *Drug Test Anal.* 2011;3(4):195-200. PMID: 21438164

5. Coiro V, Volpi R, Capretti L, Caffarri G, Chiodera P. Desmopressin and hexarelin tests in alcohol-induced pseudo-cushing's syndrome. *J Intern Med.* 2000;247(6):667-673. PMID: 10886488

6. Raff H, Trivedi H. Circadian rhythm of salivary cortisol, plasma cortisol, and plasma ACTH in end-stage renal disease. *Endocr Connect.* 2013;2(1):23-31. PMID: 23781315

7. Wallace EZ, Rosman P, Toshav N, Sacerdote A, Balthazar A. Pituitary-adrenocortical function chronic renal failure: studies of episodic secretion of cortisol and dexamethasone suppressibility *J Clin Endocrinol Metab.* 1980;50(1):46-51. PMID: 7350187

8. Cardoso EM, Arregger AL, Budd D, Zucchini AE, Contreras LN. Dynamics of salivary cortisol in chronic kidney disease patients at stages 1 through 4. *Clin Endocrinol (Oxf).* 2016;85(2):313-319. PMID: 26800302

9. Jacobson L. Hypothalamic-pituitary-adrenocortical axis: neuropsychiatric aspects. *Compr Physiol.* 2014;4(2):715-738. PMID: 24715565

10. Malerbi DA, Fragoso MC, Vieira Filho AH, Brenlha EM, Mendoca BB. Cortisol and adrenocorticotropin response to desmopressin in women with Cushing's disease compared with depressive illness. *J Clin Endocrinol Metab.* 1996;81(6):2233-2237. PMID: 8964857

11. Raff H, Magill SB. Is the hypothalamic-pituitary-adrenal axis disrupted in type 2 diabetes mellitus? *Endocrine.* 2016;54(2):273-275. PMID: 27696230

12. Charmandari E, Kino T, Ichijo T, Chrousos GP. Generalized glucocorticoid resistance: clinical aspects, molecular mechanisms, and implications of a rare genetic disorder. *J Clin Endocrinol Metab.* 2008;93(5):1563-1572. PMID: 18319312

13. Vitellius G, Trabado S, Hoeffel C, et al; Investigators of the MUTA-GR Study. Significant prevalence of *NR3C1* mutations in incidentally discovered bilateral adrenal hyperplasia: results of the French MUTA-GR Study. *Eur J Endocrinol.* 2018;178(4):411-423. PMID: 29444898

14. Schorr M, Miller KK. The endocrine manifestations of anorexia nervosa: mechanisms and management. *Nat Rev Endocrinol.* 2017;13(3):174-186. PMID: 27811940

15. Stenqvist TB, Torstveit MK, Faver J, Melin AK. Impact of a 4-week intensified endurance training intervention on markers of relative energy deficiency in sport (RED-S) and performance among well-trained male cyclists. *Front Endocrinol (Lausanne).* 2020;11:512365. PMID: 33101190

Radiation Therapy in the Management of Cushing Disease and Acromegaly

Moisés Mercado, MD. Endocrine Research Unit, Hospital de Especialidades, Centro Médico Nacional Siglo XXI, Instituto Mexicano del Seguro Social, National Autonomous University of México, México City, Mexico; Email: mmercadoa@yahoo.com, moises.mercado@endocrinologia.org.mx

Educational Objectives

After reviewing this chapter, the learner should be able to:

- Explain the value of radiation therapy (RT) as a treatment alternative in patients with Cushing disease and acromegaly.

- Describe the basic technical aspects of modern RT modalities.

- List the indications of the different RT modalities for patients with Cushing disease and acromegaly.

- Guide appropriate clinical and biochemical follow-up of patients with acromegaly and Cushing disease who have received RT.

- Minimize the risks of RT adverse effects by choosing the right modality for each patient.

Significance of the Clinical Problem

The exact role of RT in the treatment of patients with pituitary tumors is contraoversial. With the emergence of ever more sophisticated pharmacological treatments, RT is being used less frequently in developed countries because of the long time required to achieve an objective response and the risk of adverse effects. However, in developing countries where the resources to cover the expense of these costly, frequently lifelong pharmacological treatments is limited, RT is undoubtedly a cost-effective alternative. Modern RT has evolved considerably over the past 30 years.[1] Improvements in patient immobilization methods have resulted in a significant reduction in major adverse effects such as damage to the optic apparatus and brain necrosis.[1] Even nonstereotactic, conformal RT now has a very reasonable safety profile.[1] Radiation delivery systems have also improved. Thus, modern RT can be classified as follows:

1. *Conformal fractionated RT*

2. *Stereotactic RT*

   a. *Fractionated stereotactic radiotherapy (FSRT)*

   b. *Stereotactic radiosurgery (SRS)*

      i. *Linear accelerator CyberKnife (LINAC)*

      ii. *Gamma Knife (^{60}Co gamma-emitting sources)*

Factors that must be considered when deciding which RT modality should be used in each patient include tumor volume, distance to the optic chiasm, cavernous sinus invasion, and the presence of comorbidities.[1] SRS is ideal for biochemically active, relatively small lesions, located at least 3 mm away from the optic chiasm.[1,2] Larger lesions, particularly when close to the optic apparatus are better treated with FSRT.[1,2]

Although old conventional RT has been associated with an increased mortality rate, particularly from cerebrovascular causes, this does not seem to be the case when using modern FSRT or SRS.[1,2]

RT is seldom used as a primary treatment in patients with acromegaly. Although various acromegaly treatment consensus guidelines consider RT as a third-line therapy, depending on the circumstances of each patient, it can reasonably be used as a second choice if transsphenoidal surgery has failed to achieve clinical and biochemical goals.[3] Both FSRT and SRS can achieve strict biochemical control criteria (random GH <1 ng/mL, nadir postglucose GH <0.4 ng/mL, and normal age-adjusted IGF-1) in a substantial number of patients: 20% after 1 year, 40% after 3 years, 60% after 5 years, and 80% after 10 years.[4,5] Patients are usually treated pharmacologically with somatostatin receptor ligands (SRLs), dopamine agonists, or the GH-receptor antagonist pegvisomant, each one alone or in different combinations, while awaiting the therapeutical effect of RT.[1,2] The most common, and to a certain extent unavoidable, adverse effect is the induction of hypopituitarism.[6] Some evidence suggests that SRS results in a lower rate of hypopituitarism that FSRT.[5,6] Ten years after RT, virtually all patients have at least 1 pituitary hormone deficiency and more than 65% have at least 2 deficiencies.[5,6] Other more serious adverse effects, such as damage to the optic apparatus and cognitive impairment due to brain necrosis, are currently seen in less than 1% of patients.[1-6] The cumulative risk for the development of secondary intracranial neoplasms is 2% at 12 years in patients treated with conventional RT.[7] In the case of SRS or FSRT, the incidence of secondary tumors is even lower.[7] The most common secondary tumor types are sarcomas, meningiomas, and gliomas.[7]

Both FSRT and SRS are effective in patients with Cushing disease and are usually administered as a second-line therapy if transsphenoidal surgery has failed to achieve biochemical remission.[8] Remission rates are as high as 60% to 70% after 1 to 2 years of follow-up, but in contrast to what happens to patients with acromegaly, recurrence is not infrequent (up to 20%).[8] SRS, and to a lesser extent FSRT, is frequently used to manage patients with persistent Cushing disease who develop Nelson syndrome after bilateral adrenalectomy, both preventively and therapeutically.[8]

Practice Gaps

- Modern RT is highly effective in patients with pituitary tumors, particularly in functioning neoplasms such as GH- and ACTH-secreting adenomas. Unfortunately, the long time required to document an objective response and the likelihood of severe adverse effects have made practicing endocrinologists somehow reluctant to choose radiation as a therapeutic option.

- Many practicing endocrinologists are not aware of the improvements made to patient immobilization techniques and radiation delivery systems that have made RT an effective and reasonably safe therapeutic strategy.

- In-training endocrinologists should realize that RT is part of the multimodal treatment for acromegaly and Cushing disease.

Discussion
Technical Aspects

Modern, conventional, conformal external beam RT delivers photons generated by a linear accelerator.[1,8] Patients are immobilized using a customized plastic mask that limits movement to 2 to 5 mm.[1,8] Three-dimensional localization of the tumor is achieved using CT or MRI, which provides accurate visualization of the lesion and allows homogeneous distribution of the radiation dose within the target.[1,8] Radiation beams are conformed to the shape of the tumor (hence the term *conformal*) by means of a multileaf collimator.[1,8] Radiation doses range from 40 to 55 Gy and are delivered in daily 1.5 to 2 Gy fractions over 5 to 6 weeks.

Stereotactic RT can be administered either as a single large dose in 1 session (SRS) or as several fractions delivered daily over several weeks (FSRT).[1,8] SRS uses either gamma-emitting [60]Co (Gamma Knife) or a linear accelerator (LINAC, CyberKnife) as radiation sources. In the case of Gamma Knife SRS, a hemispherical array of 192 sources of ^{60}Co converge on a central point of the radiation target (isocenter), which is reached through a collimator metal helmet attached to the patient's head.[1,8] CyberKnife SRS uses a LINAC mounted on a mobile robotic arm and an image-guided robotic system.[1,8] Stereotactic RT uses more precise immobilization techniques than conventional RT that limits movement to 1 to 2 mm.[1,8] SRS delivers single radiation doses of 15 to 25 Gy in one session, whereas FSRT delivers daily 1.5 to 2 Gy fractions over 5 to 6 weeks for a total dose of 45 to 55 Gy.[1,8] SRS should not be used in patients harboring tumors located closer than 3 mm from the chiasm to avoid damage to the optic apparatus.[1,8]

Cushing Disease

Conventional RT

According to a recent meta-analysis of 29 studies comprising 721 patients with Cushing disease, 405 of whom had previously undergone transsphenoidal surgery, conventional external beam RT resulted in an overall remission rate of 66% (95% CI, 58-75) and a recurrence rate of 26% (95% CI, 58-75).[9] Although children have a somewhat higher remission rate than adults (82% [95% CI, 68-99] vs 70% [95% CI, 60-83]), they also show a higher recurrence rate (55% [95% CI, 28-100] vs 31% [95% CI: 13-77]).[9] Biochemical remission is more likely in patients who had previously undergone surgical treatment and in those who received radiation doses higher than 45 Gy, but no other statistically significant predictors of remission have been found.[9] The analyzed studies were relatively small (<50 patients) and highly heterogenous regarding methodological design and biochemical remission criteria.[9] Urinary free cortisol is the most commonly used biochemical parameter to assess

remission, and it usually decreases by 50% of the pretreatment value 6 to 12 months after radiation.[9] The median time to reach a normal urinary free cortisol is 2 years.[9] Hypopituitarism is the most frequent adverse effect and 40% of patients require at least 2 hormone replacements at 10 years.[9] The most common pituitary hormone deficiency is GH, followed by LH and FSH.[9] With current radiation techniques, the incidence of optic neuropathy is 0% to 4%, whereas brain necrosis occurs in less than 2%.[9]

Stereotactic RT

A pooled analysis of 10 studies published between 2007 and 2021, comprising 777 patients with Cushing disease treated with SRS (9 studies with Gamma Knife and 1 study with CyberKnife) and followed for a mean of 5.05 ± 1.9 years reveals that this treatment alternative is reasonably effective and safe.[8] The mean radiation dose was 26.9 ± 3.8 Gy, and all the studies used as remission criterion the normalization of the urinary free cortisol, with a few of them using the overnight low-dose dexamethasone-suppression test as well.[8] The mean initial biochemical remission rate was 60% ± 17.8% (range, 42%-81%), whereas the long-term remission rate was 53.2% ± 13.4% (range, 27.9%-71.4%).[8] The mean time to remission was 1.5 ± 0.8 years (range, 0.8-3.5 years), and the recurrence rate was 15.5% ± 11.3% (range, 10%-36%).[8]

Perhaps the fact that most corticotrope tumors causing Cushing disease are microadenomas located safely far from the optic chiasm has made radiation oncologists prefer SRS over FSRT.[9-13] Therefore, information regarding the efficacy and safety of FSRT is scarce. In the relatively few patients who have been treated with this RT modality, radiation doses vary between 40 and 50 Gy divided in daily fraction delivered over 4 to 6 weeks.[9-13] More than 70% of these patients achieve biochemical remission within 1.5 to 3 years of treatment, and there are no data regarding recurrence rates.[9-13]

A few patients with Cushing disease have been managed with RT without first having had pituitary surgery.[9-13] Remission and recurrence rates, as well as the time to remission, are very similar to figures reported in patients radiated after transsphenoidal surgery.[9-13] Factors that would favor choosing RT as a first-line treatment for Cushing disease include tumor predominantly located within the cavernous sinus that is inaccessible by surgery, cardiopulmonary comorbidities conferring a high anesthetic risk, and patient`s preference.[9-13]

Nelson Syndrome

Approximately one-third of patients with Cushing disease who undergo bilateral adrenalectomy for hypercortisolism control develop Nelson syndrome, currently also known as corticotroph tumor progression syndrome.[12,14] This condition results from the expansion of a residual ACTH-secreting adenoma due to the loss of negative feedback inhibition previously exerted by the high serum cortisol levels.[12,14] The very high circulating ACTH levels (usually 200-800 pg/mL [44-176 pmol/L]) result in skin hyperpigmentation, whereas the expanding pituitary mass can sometimes lead to vision abnormalities due to compromise of the optic apparatus. Although still a matter for debate, corticotroph tumor progression syndrome appears to be more frequent in younger patients with Cushing disease (<35 years old).[12,14]

Gamma Knife SRS is currently the most common radiation method used to treat corticotroph tumor progression syndrome, although a few patients have been treated with FSRT with equal success rates.[12,14] Local tumor control is achieved in 92% to 100% of patients, and 64% to 92% show evidence of tumor shrinkage.[12,14] Although SRS results in a significant reduction in circulating ACTH in virtually all patients, only 10% to 30% achieve normal levels.[12-14] The use of prophylactic RT before bilateral adrenalectomy to prevent the development of corticotroph tumor progression syndrome is still controversial and should be indicated on an individual basis.[12,14]

Acromegaly

Conventional RT

A pooled analysis of 13 studies published between 2000 and 2019, comprising 1104 patients with acromegaly treated with conventional external beam RT, revealed that a median of 17%, 31%, and 53% achieved a normal age-adjusted IGF-1 concentration at 1 to 3, 5, and 10 years, respectively.[15] Radiation doses varied between 50 and 60 Gy, and in more than 85% of the cases, RT was administered as adjuvant therapy after failed transsphenoidal surgery.[15] The proportion of patients achieving a basal GH concentration less than 2.5 ng/mL (<2.5 µg/L) was 50% to 60% at 5 years and 70% to 80% at 10 years. A basal GH value less than 1 ng/mL (<1 µg/L) is achieved by 40% to 50% of patients at 5 years and by 60% to 70% of patients at 10 years, whereas a normal IGF-1 concentration is reached in 20% to 40% of patients at 2 to 5 years and by 60% to 80% after more than 10 years following radiation.[15] Thus, the proportion of patients achieving biochemical goals increases over time. Patients need to be treated pharmacologically with SRLs, dopamine agonists, or pegvisomant while awaiting therapeutic response.[1,2] It was once thought that previous use of SRL renders patients radiation-resistant, and although this has never been proven objectively, it is customary to hold these medications 2 months before RT.[1,2] The most consistent adverse effect in patients with acromegaly receiving RT is hypopituitarism.[1,2,6,15] After 10 years of RT, 40% to 50% of patients develop hypogonadotropic hypogonadism, 50% have central hypocortisolism, 65% to 70% have central hypothyroidism, and 60% have at least 2 pituitary hormone deficiencies.[1,2,6,15]

The heterogeneous response rate to RT results from several factors, including the variability of radiation protocols, the different biochemical remission criteria used in each study, and the length of follow-up. Published studies use different GH and IGF-1 assays, from polyclonal radioimmunoassays to monoclonal ultrasensitive immunoassays. A GH value less than 2.5 ng/mL (<2.5 µg/L) by polyclonal radioimmunoassay probably equates to less than 1 ng/mL (<1 μg/L) when using a new-generation ultrasensitive immunoassay.

Stereotactic RT

Singh et al recently reported the results of a meta-analysis that evaluated the outcome of patients with acromegaly treated with SRS between 2001and 2020.[4] The meta-analysis included 20 studies that comprised 1533 patients, 85% of whom had previously undergone transsphenoidal surgery. More than 80% were treated with Gamma Knife SRS at doses that varied between 15 and 45 Gy.[4] IGF-1 normalization was achieved by 20% to 70% at 5 years and by 45% to 86% at 10 years.[4] A greater than 20% reduction in tumor size was documented in 65% to 100% of patients, and 85% to 100% achieve tumor stability.[4] New pituitary hormone deficiencies were identified in 35% to 70% of patients, whereas the incidence of new vision deficits, mostly attributed to cranial nerve II neuropathy, was 2.7% (95% CI, 1.3-4.2).[4] Neither cases of cognitive impairment due to brain necrosis nor cerebrovascular events have been recorded.[4]

Compared with the number of studies evaluating the efficacy and safety of SRS, there have been relatively few assessing FSRT in patients with acromegaly.[4,5] A meta-analysis of 4 of these studies published between 2009 and 2016 comprising 132 patients who were followed for a median of 4.5 years (range, 1.9-12.6) reveals that this RT modality is somewhat less effective than SRS.[5] Median radiation doses among these 4 studies ranged from 50 to 54 Gy, administered in 25 to 30 fractions over 4 to 5 weeks.[5] Biochemical remission rates, usually defined as the achievement of a normal age-adjusted IGF-1 concentration, varied between 17% and 38%, whereas a greater than 20% reduction in tumor size was seen in 54% of patients.[5] No major adverse effects related to optic apparatus injury, brain necrosis, or cerebrovascular accidents were recorded.[5] New-onset hypopituitarism was identified in 8% to 38% of patients.[5]

Clinical Case Vignettes
Case 1

A 61-year-old man was diagnosed with acromegaly 20 years ago.

Initial laboratory test results at the time of diagnosis:

> Basal GH = 11.3 ng/mL (SI: 11.3 μg/L)
> Postglucose GH = 6.1 ng/mL (SI: 6.1 μg/L)
> IGF-1 = 3.5 times the upper normal limit
> Prolactin = 15 ng/mL (3-20 ng/mL) (SI: 0.65 nmol/L [0.13-0.87 nmol/L])
> Morning cortisol = 17 μg/dL (15-25 μg/dL) (SI: 469.0 nmol/L [413.8-689.7 nmol/L])
> LH = 2.9 mIU/mL (2.0-10.0 mIU/mL) (SI: 2.9 IU/L [2.0-10.0 IU/L])
> FSH = 4.2 mIU/mL (2.0-10.0 mIU/mL) (SI: 4.2 IU/L [2.0-10.0 IU/L])
> Total testosterone = 233 ng/dL (300-950 ng/dL) (SI: 8.09 nmol/L [10.41-32.97 nmol/L])
> TSH = 1.2 mIU/L (0.3-3.0 mIU/L)
> Free T_4 = 1.0 ng/dL (0.6-1.5 ng/dL) (SI: 12.9 pmol/L [7.7-19.3 pmol/L])

MRI of the sellar region showed a left, 1.1-cm (largest diameter) isointense lesion that did not invade the cavernous sinus. He declined transsphenoidal surgery and was started on octreotide LAR, 20 mg monthly. After 12 years of adequate tumoral and hormonal control on this SRL dosage (IGF-1, 0.9 to 1.2 times the upper normal limit), his GH and IGF-1 began to rise again; therefore, the dosage was increased to 30 mg monthly. Cabergoline, 3 mg weekly, was later added. His IGF-1 concentration, however, kept increasing and reached a value 2 times the upper normal limit.

Follow-up MRI now shows persistence of an 8-mm isointense lesion. Headaches and arthralgias have recently recurred (*Figure 1, following page*). He declines transsphenoidal surgery again, and he does not have access to either pasireotide or pegvisomant.

Figure 1. Gadolinium-Enhanced, Coronal Section, T1 MRI Showing a Left 8-mm Hyperintense Lesion

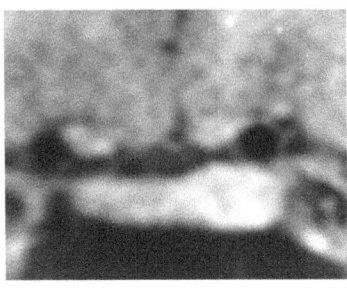

[Color—Print (Color Gallery page CG28) or web & ePub editions]

Which of the following is the best course of action in this case?

A. Perform conformal RT, total dose 15 Gy over 3 weeks

B. Perform Gamma Knife SRS, single 22 Gy dose

C. Perform conformal RT, 80 Gy over 4 weeks

D. Maintain octreotide LAR and switch from cabergoline to bromocriptine, 10 mg nightly

E. Maintain cabergoline and increase octreotide LAR dose to 60 mg monthly

Answer: B) Perform Gamma Knife SRS, single 22 Gy dose

Case 1 (continued)

Which of the following is the best follow-up for this patient?

A. Stop all medications, evaluate GH-IGF-1 axis yearly

B. Measure GH and IGF-1 every 3 months; increase injection interval progressively (and eventually discontinue) if GH and IGF-1 are within therapeutic target

C. Perform pituitary MRI every 3 months for the first year, then yearly

D. Perform neuropsychological testing every 6 months for the next 2 years

E. Maintain cabergoline indefinitely

Answer: B) Measure GH and IGF-1 every 3 months; increase injection interval progressively (and eventually discontinue) if GH and IGF-1 are within therapeutic target

This patient escaped the therapeutic effect of a first-generation SRL after many years of adequate biochemical and tumoral control. He is still reluctant to undergo transsphenoidal surgery and he has no other pharmacological treatment alternatives. Given the small size of the lesion, which is located far from the optic chiasm, SRS is the most appropriate RT modality in this case. The SRL needs to be discontinued at least 2 weeks before RT and then restarted and maintained until the radiation takes effect. The injection interval of the SRL should be increased progressively and eventually discontinued as the GH and IGF-1 levels decrease.

Case 2

A 43-year-old woman has a 10-year history of acromegaly due to an intrasellar, 1.2-cm, GH-producing pituitary tumor. She originally underwent successful transsphenoidal surgery and had been in clinical and biochemical remission until 2 years before consultation, when she presented again with headaches, arthralgias, coarsening of her facial features, and worsening hypertension.

Laboratory test results:

> Basal GH = 7.0 ng/mL (SI: 7.0 µg/L)
> Glucose-suppressed GH = 3.2 ng/mL (SI: 3.2 µg/L)
> IGF-1 = 2.8 times the upper normal limit
> Morning cortisol = 18 µg/dL (15-25 µg/dL) (SI: nmol/L [413.8-689.7 nmol/L])
> Prolactin = 32 ng/mL (3-20 ng/mL) (SI: 1.39 nmol/L [0.13-0.87 nmol/L])
> TSH = 0.1 mIU/L (0.3-3.0 mIU/L)
> Free T$_4$ = 0.45 ng/dL (0.6-1.5 ng/dL) (SI: 5.8 pmol/L [7.7-19.3 pmol/L])
> FSH = 38.0 mIU/mL (2.0-10.0 mIU/mL) (SI: 38.0 IU/L [2.0-10.0 IU/L])
> Estradiol = <10 pg/mL (50-300 pg/mL) (SI: <36.7 pmol/L [183.6-1101.3 pmol/L])

Pituitary MRI showed a 2-cm lesion extending cephalically towards the optic chiasm but without contacting it (distance between chiasma and tumor = 2 mm) (*Figure 2, following page*). Lanreotide autogel was started at a dosage of 120 mg monthly. Six months later, her basal GH concentration was 6.2 ng/mL (6.2 µg/L) and her IGF-1 concentration was 2.1 times the upper normal limit. Cabergoline was added and titrated up to 2.5 mg weekly, but biochemical control was not achieved.

She lives in a country where neither pegvisomant nor pasireotide are available. MRI shows persistence of an 8-mm isointense lesion. She declines transsphenoidal surgery again.

Figure 2. Gadolinium-Enhanced Pituitary MRI, T1 Coronal Section

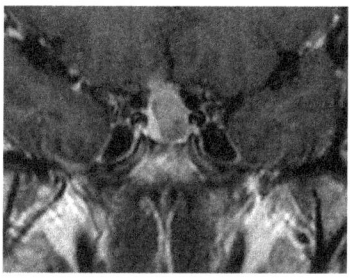

MRI showing a 2-cm, hypointense lesion extending cephalically towards the optic chiasm (distance between chiasma and tumor 2 mm).

Which of the following is the best treatment for this patient?

A. Proceed with surgical reintervention

B. Stop lanreotide and increase the cabergoline dosage to 6 mg weekly

C. Hold pharmacological treatment for 2 weeks and then proceed with FSRT, total fractionated dose 50 Gy

D. Proceed with FSRT, total fractionated dose 87 Gy, while on cabergoline and octreotide

E. Stop cabergoline and lanreotide and start octreotide LAR, 30 mg every 3 weeks

Answer: C) Hold pharmacological treatment for 2 weeks and then proceed with FSRT, total fractionated dose 50 Gy

Case 2 (continued)

Which hormonal replacements does this patient need?

A. Levothyroxine, 75 mcg daily; transcutaneous estradiol; and oral medroxyprogesterone

B. Prednisone, 5 mg daily

C. Desmopressin, 0.1 mg twice daily

D. Hydrocortisone, 10 mg twice daily

E. Liothyronine, 25 mcg daily

Answer: A) Levothyroxine, 75 mcg daily; transcutaneous estradiol; and oral medroxyprogesterone

Two years after achieving postoperative biochemical control, this patient has a clinically significant hormonal and tumoral recurrence. Surgical reintervention is unlikely to solve the problem. Switching her to octreotide and/or adding a dopamine agonist probably will not work. Given the size and location of the pituitary tumor and its proximity to the optic chiasm, the most appropriate RT modality would be either conformal external RT or FSRT. The patient has evidence of central hypothyroidism and has a postmenopausal LH and FSH profile. Levothyroxine should be started, and menopausal estrogen replacement may ameliorate symptoms of acromegaly and even reduce IGF-1 levels due to the induction of a relative GH-resistant state.

Case 3

An 18-year-old man presents with obesity and worsening hypertension.

Laboratory test results:

> Urinary free cortisol = 1075 µg/24 h (SI: 2967 nmol/d)
> Serum cortisol after 1 mg dexamethasone = 14.8 µg/dL (SI: 408.3 nmol/L)
> ACTH = 71.7 pg/mL (10-40 pg/mL) (SI: 15.8 pmol/L [2.2-8.8 pmol/L])
> Serum cortisol after 8 mg dexamethasone = 17 µg/dL (SI: 469.0 nmol/L) (60.4% suppression)

MRI shows a right-sided, 8-mm, hypointense pituitary lesion. He undergoes transsphenoidal surgery and becomes hypotensive 24 hours after the procedure (8 AM cortisol = 1.4 µg/dL [38.6 nmol/L]). The pathology report describes diffuse ACTH immunostaining and a Ki-67 index of 6%. He is discharged on prednisone, 5 mg daily. He loses 17.6 lb (8 kg), and the purple striae improve remarkably. He is able to discontinue prednisone 10 months later. Four years later, his Cushing disease recurs clinically and biochemically, with a urinary free cortisol concentration of 1157 μg/24 h (3193 nmol/d). Follow-up MRI shows a questionable left-sided, 4-mm, hypointense pituitary lesion. He undergoes transsphenoidal surgery again, but this time no adenoma is identified. Ketoconazole is started but is discontinued because of elevated liver enzymes. His blood pressure remains uncontrolled despite 5 antihypertensive medications. He undergoes bilateral adrenalectomy and is started on hydrocortisone and fludrocortisone. He becomes progressively hyperpigmented, and his plasma ACTH concentration increases to 650 pg/mL (143 pmol/L). MRI reveals a 1.8-cm lesion, extending cephalically but without contacting the optic chiasm (distance from chiasma 4 mm) (*Figure 3*).

Figure 3. Gadolinium-Enhanced Pituitary MRI, T1 Coronal Section

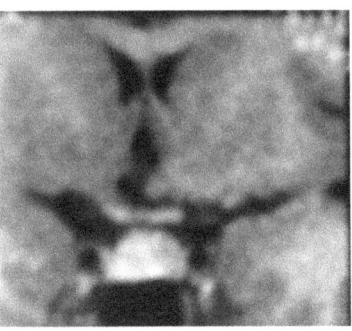

MRI showing a 1.8-cm lesion extending cephalically but without contacting the optic chiasm (distance between chiasma and tumor 4 mm).

[Color—Print (Color Gallery page CG28) or web & ePub editions]

Which of the following statements is true regarding RT for this patient?

A. Gamma Knife SRS is contraindicated because of the distance between the tumor and the optic apparatus

B. His condition cannot be treated with RT because of the risk of brain necrosis

C. He could be treated with either SRS or FSRT

D. Any RT modality in this scenario puts him at risk for malignant tumor transformation

E. RT would be ineffective unless the patient undergoes surgical debulking of the pituitary lesion

Answer: C) He could be treated with either SRS or FSRT

Case 3 (continued)

Which of the following is the best option for monitoring this patient?

A. Serial ACTH measurement

B. Urinary free cortisol measurement every 6 months

C. Morning serum cortisol measurements

D. Yearly low-dose dexamethasone-suppression test

E. Brain CT every 6 months

Answer: A) Serial ACTH measurement

This patient developed Nelson syndrome after bilateral adrenalectomy. Although his original ACTH-secreting tumor grew considerably after adrenalectomy, the lesion remained far enough from the optic chiasm to allow SRS. He does not have any particular risk factors for developing post-RT brain necrosis or RT-induced malignant transformation. Although, at least in theory, the smaller the radiation target, the more effective RT should be, there is no evidence that reducing tumor mass by surgical debulking is necessary to obtain a positive therapeutic response. Patients such as this one should be followed by periodical ACTH measurement, because ACTH concentrations tend to correlate with tumor size. Measuring serum or urinary cortisol is pointless because the patient already underwent bilateral adrenalectomy. The imaging method of choice to monitor the ACTH-secreting tumor is MRI.

Case 4

A 36-year-old woman presents with symptoms and signs of Cushing syndrome, which is confirmed by elevated urinary free cortisol excretion and a lack of serum cortisol suppression with low-dose dexamethasone. Her ACTH concentration is in the high-normal range, but pituitary MRI only shows a questionable 4-mm lesion. Bilateral inferior petrosal sinus sampling confirms the diagnosis of Cushing disease. She undergoes transsphenoidal surgery, whereby a small right-sided microadenoma is macroscopically identified by the neurosurgeon. The pathology report describes a basophilic pituitary adenoma with Crooke changes that immunostain diffusely for ACTH and T-Pit. Although she does not develop postoperative hypocortisolism, she is much improved clinically and her urinary free cortisol decreases to 332 µg/24 h (916 nmol/d). Ketoconazole is started at a dosage of 200 mg twice daily, but it is discontinued 6 months later because of hepatotoxicity. Biochemical reevaluation 1 year later reveals a urinary free cortisol value of 657 µg/24 h (1813 nmol/d). Cabergoline, 2 mg weekly, is initiated but she continues to have symptomatic hypercortisolism. Repeat MRI reveals the presence of a 6-mm subinfundibular hypointensity (*Figure 4*). She declines surgical reintervention and is also reluctant to undergo bilateral adrenalectomy.

Figure 4. Gadolinium-Enhanced Pituitary MRI, T1 Coronal Section

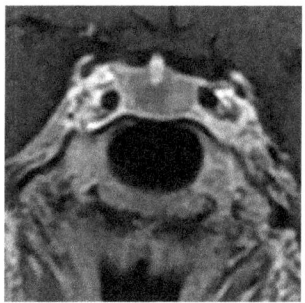

MRI showing a 6-mm subinfundibular hypointense lesion.

Which of the following would be the most appropriate therapeutic strategy?

A. Insist on pituitary surgical reintervention

B. Schedule conformal pituitary RT 50 Gy fractionated over 2 weeks

C. Convince her to undergo bilateral adrenalectomy after prophylactic RT

D. Schedule SRS to the sella with a single 20 Gy dose

E. Convince her to undergo bilateral adrenalectomy without prophylactic RT

Answer: D) Schedule SRS to the sella with a single 20 Gy dose

Which of the following statements is true?

A. All patients with Cushing disease who have persistent, clinically significant postoperative hypercortisolism should be managed with RT

B. Silent corticotroph adenomas, particularly those with Crooke changes, have a high recurrence rate; therefore, some authors recommend prophylactic RT

C. The previous use of ketoconazole limits the efficacy of RT

D. The previous use of dopamine agonists potentiates the efficacy of RT

E. Patients with Cushing disease almost invariably develop central hypogonadism 3 to 6 months after receiving RT

Answer: B) Silent corticotroph adenomas, particularly those with Crooke changes, have a high recurrence rate; therefore, some authors recommend prophylactic RT

Patients with Cushing disease whose tumors have Crooke cell changes are at high risk of recurrence/persistence, to the extent that some authors recommend prophylactic RT, although this is not a generally accepted practice. Late reintervention is not likely to solve the problem and this patient has declined any kind of surgical treatment. RT is an effective and relatively safe alternative for such patients. Although FSRT and conventional RT are viable options, SRS has proven to be more effective and perhaps safer, as it has a better chance of preserving pituitary function. The previous use of dopamine agonists or ketoconazole does not compromise the efficacy of RT.

Key Learning Points

- RT is an effective and reasonably safe alternative for the management of pituitary tumors.

- Factors to be considered when choosing RT strategy:

  - Tumor size, location, and extension

  - Distance to the optic chiasm

  - SRS should be reserved for relatively small lesions, particularly when they invade the cavernous sinus

  - SRS should not be used when the tumor is closer than 3 mm to the optic chiasm

  - RT dose to the optic chiasm should not exceed 8 Gy with any RT modality

  - FSRT or conventional RT using modern immobilization techniques is indicated for patients with large tumors, particularly when invasive, irregularly shaped, and located less than 3 mm from the optic chiasm

  - With current RT methods, the most common adverse effect is new-onset hypopituitarism. Other adverse events such as damage to the optic apparatus, brain necrosis, induction of cerebrovascular accidents, and secondary intracranial neoplasms are rare.

References

1. Minniti G, Scaringi C, Enrici RM. Radiation techniques for acromegaly. *Radiat Oncol.* 2011;6:167.. PMID: 22136376
2. Li X, Li Y, Cao Y, Li P, Liang B, Sun J, Feng E. Safety and efficacy of fractionated stereotactic radiotherapy and stereotactic radiosurgery for treatment of pituitary adenomas: A systematic review and meta-analysis. *J Neurol Sci.* 2017;372:110-116. PMID: 28017195
3. Giustina A, Barkhoudarian G, Beckers A, et al. Multidisciplinary management of acromegaly: a consensus. *Rev Endocr Metab Disord.* 2020;21(4):667-678. PMID: 32914330
4. Singh R, Didwania P, Lehrer EJ, Sheehan D, Sheehan K, Trifiletti DM, Sheehan JP. Stereotactic radiosurgery for acromegaly: an international systematic review and meta-analysis of clinical outcomes. *J Neurooncol.* 2020;148(3):401-418. PMID: 32506372
5. Zheng Q, Huang Y, Lin W, Cai L, Wen J, Chen G. Comparing stereotactic radiosurgery and fractionated stereotactic radiotherapy in treating patients with growth hormone-secreting adenomas: a systematic review and meta-analysis. *Endocr Pract.* 2020 [Online ahead of print] PMID: 32576046
6. Xu Z, Lee Vance M, Schlesinger D, Sheehan JP. Hypopituitarism after stereotactic radiosurgery for pituitary adenomas. *Neurosurgery.* 2013;72(4):630-7; 636-637. PMID: 23277375
7. Yamanaka R, Abe E, Sato T, Hayano A, Takashima Y. Secondary Intracranial Tumors Following Radiotherapy for Pituitary Adenomas: A Systematic Review. *Cancers (Basel).* 2017;9(8):103. PMID: 28786923
8. Ironside N, Chen CJ, Lee CC, Trifiletti DM, Vance ML, Sheehan JP. Outcomes of pituitary radiation for Cushing's disease. *Endocrinol Metab Clin North Am.* 2018;47(2):349-365. PMID: 29754636
9. Abu Dabrh AM, Singh Ospina NM, Al Nofal A, et al. Predictors of biochemical remission and recurrence after surgical and radiation treatments of Cushing disease: a systematic review and meta-analysis. *Endocr Pract.* 2016;22(4):466-475. PMID: 26789343
10. Minniti G, Brada M. Radiotherapy and radiosurgery for Cushing's disease. *Arq Bras Endocrinol Metabol.* 2007;51(8):1373-1380. PMID: 18209876
11. Mehta GU, Ding D, Patibandla MR, et al. Stereotactic radiosurgery for Cushing disease: results of an international, multicenter study. *J Clin Endocrinol Metab.* 2017;102(11):4284-4291. PMID: 28938462
12. Gheorghiu ML. Updates in the outcomes of radiation therapy for Cushing's disease. *Best Pract Res Clin Endocrinol Metab.* 2021;35(2):101514. PMID: 33814300
13. Abdali A, Kalinin PL, Trunin YY, et al. CyberKnife for the management of Cushing's disease: our institutional experience and review of literature. *Br J Neurosurg.* 2021;35(5):578-583. PMID: 33955316
14. Reincke M, Albani A, Assie G, et al. Corticotroph tumor progression after bilateral adrenalectomy (Nelson's syndrome): systematic review and expert consensus recommendations. *Eur J Endocrinol.* 2021;184(3):P1-P16. PMID: 33444221
15. Gonzales-Virla B, Vargas-Ortega G, Martínez-Vázquez KB, et al. Efficacy and safety of fractionated conformal radiation therapy in acromegaly: a long-term follow-up study. *Endocrine.* 2019;65(2):386-392. PMID: 31098940

Approach to the Patient With Hypoglycemia

Alia Munir, MBBCh, PhD. Department of Endocrinology, Royal Hallamshire Hospital, Sheffield Teaching Hospitals NHS Foundation Trust, Sheffield, South Yorkshire, United Kingdom; Email: alia.munir@nhs.net

Educational Objectives

After reviewing this chapter, learners should be able to:

- Describe the problems and complexities of diagnosing and investigating non–diabetes-related hypoglycemia.

- Identify the symptoms of hypoglycemia, what constitutes Whipple triad, and the approach to evaluation of non–diabetes-related hypoglycemia.

- Ideal care and follow-up should be offered in a specialist expert center and discussions should occur within a specialist multidisciplinary team.

Significance of the Clinical Problem

Hypoglycemia can be complex and potentially life-threatening. It requires systematic workup. Non–diabetes-related hypoglycemia is relatively uncommon; a large retrospective review of hospital admissions estimated a frequency of 36 per 10,000 admissions.[1] Reportedly, patients older than 65 years are more likely to have an episode of hypoglycemia.

Broadly, we can divide hypoglycemia into insulin-mediated and insulin-independent forms. Having fulfilled Whipple triad, characterized by hypoglycemia and neuroglycopenic symptoms relieved with the ingestion of carbohydrate, investigations can be undertaken. If an insulin-independent cause is suspected, a battery of tests should be performed to exclude adrenal insufficiency, pituitary hormone deficiencies, liver/kidney failure, critical illness, sepsis, anorexia, identify post bariatric surgeries, mesenchymal tumors with elevated IGF-2 levels, and autoimmune causes (Hirata syndrome with assessment of insulin antibodies or insulin-receptor antibodies). Review of drugs and alcohol intake should also be performed, as it is well known that insulin, glinides, sulfonylureas, and other drugs such as antimalarial agents, quinolones, lithium, angiotensin inhibitors, and nonselective β-adrenergic blockers can be the cause. Ideally, these etiologies should be excluded before evaluating for an endogenous cause.[1,2]

When we refer to *insulin-mediated hypoglycemia*, we are referring to the neuroendocrine tumor insulinoma or islet-cell hyperplasia (nesidioblastosis, a histopathological term), which is sometimes also called noninsulinoma pancreatogenous hypoglycemia syndrome. Insulinoma is a rare functional pancreatic neuroendocrine tumor[3,4] with an incidence of 0.4 per 100,000 patient years. Extrapancreatic insulinoma is even more rare. The clinical effects can be problematic and life threatening. Systematic investigation using evidence-based biochemical testing[5,6] determining the endogenous nature of insulin secretion in predetermined conditions is recommended. Following biochemical confirmation, the tumor should be localized with multimodal imaging, including endoscopic ultrasonography (EUS), and sampling techniques. Newer nuclear imaging techniques offer great promise but have limited availability.[3,4] The condition often requires urgent management to ensure patient safety. Long-term cure with surgery is the optimal outcome. Insulinoma has a 5-year survival of 94% to 100% for the so-called indolent group. However, when metastatic disease is present (10%-15% of cases), 5-year survival is 24% to 67%. In this setting, glycemic and tumor control is paramount with appropriate evidence-based therapy.

Patients should be managed by a specialist expert multidisciplinary clinical team and, when possible, in a center of excellence or with the input of one. Continuous glucose monitoring (CGM) may be useful in patients with insulinoma in the perioperative phase and for those on medical therapies, but it has limitations.[7]

Notably, 5% to 10% of insulinomas are associated with multiple endocrine neoplasia type 1. This diagnosis should be considered in patients with insulinoma who are younger than 35 years.[8,9]

Adult nesidioblastosis is rare and presents clinically and biochemically like insulinoma. Pathogenic variants in 2 known genes cause the diffuse form of nesidioblastosis in adults. There can be symptom overlap, which makes diagnosis difficult. More recently, nesidioblastosis has been associated with bariatric surgery, suggesting a reactive process that alters β-cell regulation in the pancreas. Management includes dietetic measures, diazoxide, and even pancreatectomy, but experience is limited and dependent on case reports and small series.

Practice Gaps

- Correctly defining and classifying hypoglycemia is difficult.

- Lack of experience managing these rare conditions.

- Limited knowledge and access to specific localization and imaging techniques for insulinoma.

- Paucity of evidence for benefit of CGM in patients with hypoglycemia who do not have diabetes.

Discussion

Strategies for Approaching Patients With Non–Diabetes-Related Hypoglycemia

A full history should be taken with pertinent, targeted questions that detail the history of the presenting concern with respect to timing of the hypoglycemic episode, its relationship to meals and exercise, medication history, alcohol use, psychiatric history, history of endocrinopathies (either personal history or an affected family member). The patient's general health should be assessed (whether the patient is well or ill). The possibility of organ failure (eg, liver or kidney) and potential hormone deficiencies should be assessed. A complete examination, specifically looking for organomegaly or potential tumors, can help rule out a paraneoplastic cause. A clinical algorithm for the workup of hypoglycemia is shown in the *Figure* (*following page*).

Hypoglycemia is a clinical syndrome most often defined by a plasma glucose concentration below 70 mg/dL (<3.9 mmol/L), but in most healthy people symptoms are frequently not felt until glucose reaches 55 mg/dL (3.1 mmol/L).[1] The European Neuroendocrine Tumor Society (ENETS) guidelines from 2023 state a blood glucose value less than 45 mg/dL (<2.5 mmol/L) is required for insulinoma diagnosis.[4,5] The glucose cutoff defining hypoglycemia is higher in patients with diabetes mellitus (<70 mg/dL [<4 mmol/L]). However, there is no formal laboratory agreement for a plasma glucose concentration that defines hypoglycemia, but guideline recommendations exist. Clinically, it is a level at which signs or symptoms occur, including impairment of brain function. Therefore, documentation of Whipple triad assists in identification of those patients who should undergo further evaluation. Whipple triad consists of signs or symptoms of hypoglycemia, a low plasma glucose concentration, and resolution of symptoms after ingestion of carbohydrate. Symptoms of hypoglycemia include neuroglycopenic symptoms (brain being deprived of glucose), neurogenic or autonomic, that occur

Figure. Clinical Algorithm for Hypoglycemia Workup

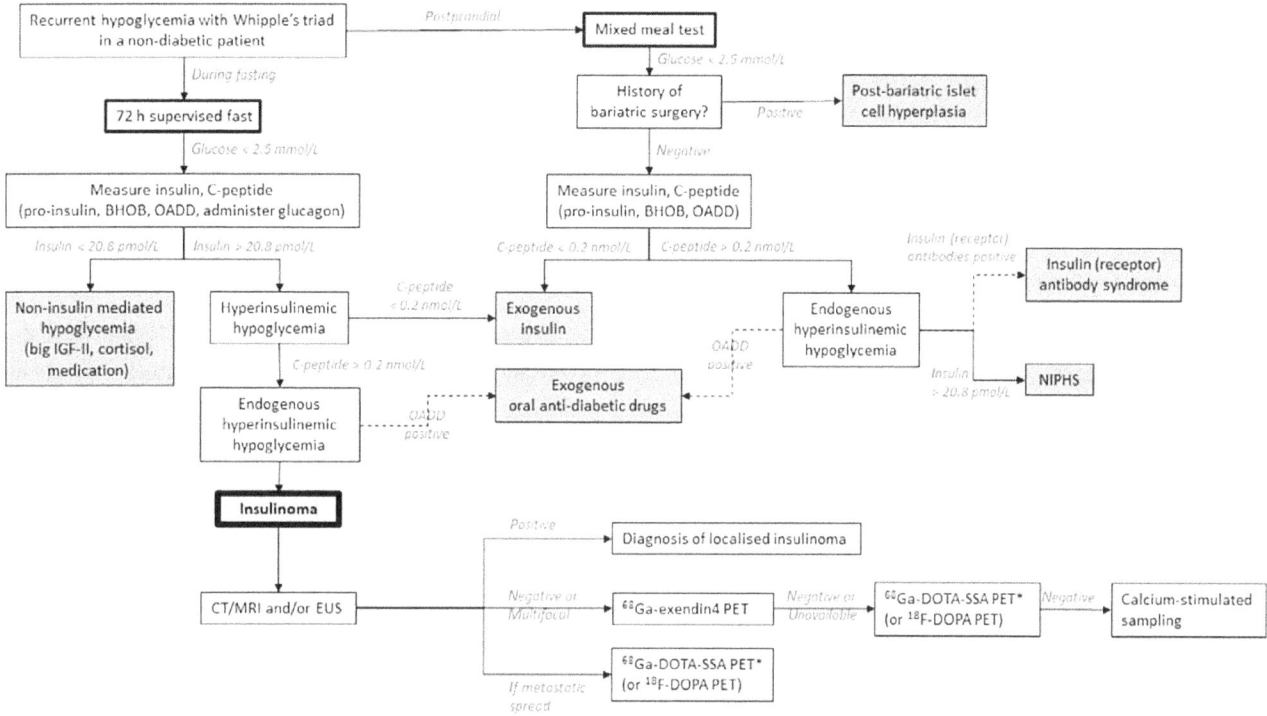

Reprinted from Hofland J et al. J Neuroendocrinol, 2023; 35(8): e13318. © The Authors. Published by John Wiley & Sons Ltd on behalf of the British Society for Neuroendocrinology.[4]

[Color—Print (Color Gallery page CG29) or web & ePub editions]

because of the perception of physiological changes. Behavior changes, confusion, fatigue, seizure, coma, permanent neurological damage, and death can occur. Pallor, palpitations, tremor, anxiety/arousal, and arterial hypertension are adrenergic, with sweating, hunger, and paresthesia occur as part of the cholinergic response. After fulfilling the Whipple triad, rapid confirmation of the diagnosis is important to institute treatment in a timely manner. After a detailed history and examination, one should have established whether the patient with hypoglycemia is well or ill and whether the hypoglycemia is likely to be reactive or related to fasting. In some cases, this may be difficult to ascertain.

Non–Insulinoma-Related Hypoglycemia

Noninsulinoma pancreatogenous hypoglycemia syndrome is rare and typically occurs in the postprandial state. This is considered when the 72-hour fast and imaging are negative and there is endogenous insulin production in a patient who has not had bariatric surgery.

Postbariatric hypoglycemia has the potential complication of postprandial hyperinsulinemic hypoglycemia, most commonly after Roux-en-Y gastric bypass but also after sleeve gastrectomy. The effects of the surgery are believed to mediate hypoglycemia in several ways, including inappropriate hypersecretion of insulin due to the early and higher peak of glucose after eating, cytokine signaling (interleukin 1β), and an increased incretin response.

Non–Islet-Cell Tumor (Paraneoplastic Syndrome)

Paraneoplastic syndrome can be caused by a variety of benign and malignant non–islet-cell tumors, including mesenchymal, epithelial, neuroendocrine, or hematopoietic tumors. These tumors can secrete IGF-2 or the so-called big IGF as the posttranslational precursor. The homology to insulin causes hypoglycemia.

Insulin Autoimmune Hypoglycemia

Insulin autoimmune hypoglycemia can occur in the presence of antibodies against insulin or the insulin receptor, and it is an exceedingly rare cause of hyperinsulinemia hypoglycemia. Mostly reported in Japan and Korea, it is also known as Hirata syndrome.[10] Insulin autoimmune hypoglycemia may be triggered by exposure to drugs or viruses or it can occur spontaneously. Drugs with sulfhydryl groups such as antithyroid medication are postulated to precipitate this condition. Autoantibodies to the insulin receptor usually cause insulin resistance but can rarely cause fasting hypoglycemia.[1]

Other Causes

Sepsis, organ failure, and poor nutrition can all cause hypoglycemia. Severe liver disease impairs gluconeogenesis, and kidney failure reduces insulin clearance and degradation, so there is a relative insulin excess. Alcohol inhibits hepatic gluconeogenesis and glycogenolysis. Some nondiabetes medications have low to moderate evidence that they cause hypoglycemia (eg, indomethacin and quinine).

Basic Biochemical Evaluation

- Complete blood count, urea and creatinine measurement, liver function tests, thyroid function tests, early-morning cortisol, waking salivary cortisol, or short cosyntropin-stimulation test (if indicated), IGF-1, IGF-2 (if weight loss or malignancy is present), IgG insulin/receptor antibodies.

- Measurement of fasting blood glucose, insulin, C-peptide, and proinsulin; sulfonylurea and metiglinide screen; and β-hydroxybutyrate at time of hypoglycemia or during a 72-hour fast.

- Blood should be drawn in a tube with an inhibitor of glycolysis, and there should be no delay before sample processing.

- Data supporting use of CGM at this stage of diagnosis are insufficient but it may be useful.

- Once hormone deficiency and autoimmunity are excluded, a provocative test is recommended to confirm hypoglycemia.

- If there are postprandial symptoms, a mixed-meal test for reactive or postprandial hypoglycemia can be undertaken. This is a nonliquid meal, with blood samples taken every 30 minutes until the patient is symptomatic or for 5 hours. Five percent of patients with insulinoma have postprandial hypoglycemia.

- If fasting (or erratic) symptoms occur, proceed to the gold standard 72-hour fast conducted in a dedicated endocrine ward and adhering to a meticulous protocol. Data show that significant hypoglycemia occurs in 95% of affected patients by 48 hours, but 72 hours firmly excludes endogenous secretion.

- Appropriate biochemical tests to assess hypoglycemia can be performed in an emergency setting.

- Localization imaging (CT, MRI, EUS) is negative in 5% to 10% of patients with insulinoma. Selective arterial calcium stimulation and hepatic venous sampling is less commonly used as it is invasive and may not identify the exact location of the insulinoma. Nuclear imaging (gallium 68 PET/CT) is positive in 25% to 31% of patients with insulinomas, and ^{18}F-DOPA PET-CT or gallium 68 exendin 4 PET-CT, if available, is sensitive in greater than 90% of affected patients but both are not widely used.

- If other techniques fail, intraoperative ultrasonography and palpation may be useful.

- Fifty percent of affected patients note a weight increase.

Management

Dietary Management

Strategies to manage hypoglycemia include eating regular, small meals, with 1 to 2 snacks, and including complex carbohydrates. A late-night or bedtime snack can help.[11] Cornstarch is also sometimes used. Involvement of a specialist dietician is essential, and their guidance should be tailored to the underlying etiology. Management requires expert multidisciplinary team discussion. When a patient is acutely hypoglycemic, they should be treated with 15 to 20 g of rapid-acting carbohydrate, blood glucose should be checked at 10 to 15 minutes. More rapid-acting carbohydrates can be consumed if the glucose concentration is still less than 72 mg/dL (<4 mmol/L). A low-medium glycemic index snack should be eaten when blood glucose is greater than 72 mg/dL (>4 mmol/L). CGM may help patients recognize hypoglycemia early, and it can also be used to set an alarm to warn of falling blood glucose, particularly at night when a bedtime snack may also be recommended. CGM may be especially useful in cases of hypoglycemia unawareness, but further data are needed in this cohort.

In patients who have undergone bariatric surgery, guidance may require adjustment in dietary strategies, such as avoiding consuming liquids when eating and avoiding liquid carbohydrates and rapidly absorbed sugars. Recommendations depend on symptom severity. Dietary strategies include multiple small meals, high-fiber foods, and complex-carbohydrate and protein-rich foods. Lying down after meals may also help. Acarbose, diazoxide, octreotide, pasireotide, and calcium channel blockers have been used off label. Feeding gastrotomy or surgical revision has been performed in patients with refractory hypoglycemia, including

reduction of the gastric restriction and reversal. Pancreatectomy is not generally recommended.[12,13]

Medical Management

Diazoxide, a nondiuretic benzothiadiazide, at dosages of 50 to 600 mg daily (divided into 8 hourly doses), controls insulin secretion by blocking ATP-dependent potassium channels of the β-cells in the pancreas and is usually successful in patients with insulinoma. Dosage escalation may be limited by adverse effects, which occur in up to 80% of treated patients (mainly hirsutism in females, fluid retention, and edema). First-generation somatostatin analogues have a high affinity for somatostatin receptors 2 and 5 and can reduce insulin levels and have antiproliferative effect. However, glucagon levels can be reduced and paradoxical hypoglycemia can occur in patients with insulinomas lacking somatostatin receptor 2 expression, and a dosing trial of short-acting octreotide can be given with glucose monitoring to assess for this before administering a long-acting analogue. If needed, a second-generation agent, off-label pasireotide, can be trialed.[14] In the absence of intravenous glucose, glucagon is available intramuscularly, subcutaneously, and intranasally. Verapamil, phenytoin, and glucocorticoids have also been used.

RZ358, a human monoclonal antibody, binds uniquely to the insulin receptor and is currently being studied in patients with congenital hyperinsulinism. It has reportedly been successful in refractory hypoglycemia in patients with malignant insulinoma.[15]

Everolimus is a mammalian target of rapamycin (mTOR inhibitor) with antitumor activity. It impairs the skeletal muscle and adipose glucose uptake and impairs insulin-related suppression of gluconeogenesis and β-cell insulin secretion. Everolimus is approved for the use in patients with progressive pancreatic neuroendocrine tumors and it decreases insulin secretion. In a small series, a 6.5-month period of abated symptoms was documented with everolimus treatment.

Sunitinib, an oral multitargeted receptor tyrosine kinase inhibitor, is also approved to treat progressive pancreatic neuroendocrine tumors. Sunitinib does not influence insulin and, in fact, reduces blood glucose levels in patients with kidney cancer.

Surgical treatment should be performed by a skilled pancreatic surgeon. EUS, laparoscopy, robot-assisted enucleations are tools. Parenchyma-sparing resections such as enucleation are proposed as the first-line approach when feasible. Avoidance of the Whipple procedure and use of central pancreatectomy is a valuable option for tumors in the neck of the pancreas. Nodal sampling may be needed.[4,5]

EUS-guided ablation with alcohol and radiofrequency ablation is safe and effective for lesions smaller than 2 cm and is possibly an option in those who are not good surgical candidates. However, long-term survival data are needed before this can be recommended.[5] Stereotactic radiotherapy is also promising.

Peptide receptor radionuclide therapy for metastatic disease has been shown to control hypoglycemic syndromes partially or completely in the context of metastatic insulinoma in a retrospective trial.[16]

Streptozotocin is known to be diabetogenic and can be used in high-grade or clinically aggressive insulinomas. For neuroendocrine carcinomas, cisplatin or carboplatin with etoposide is most commonly used. Tolerance to temozolomide with capecitabine has also been shown.

Recently, radioembolization and chemoembolization have been successful in a series of patients.[4]

CGM as a Tool

CGM provides real-time glycemic trends in the interstitial fluid. The potential limitation is accuracy at lower glucose levels. Studies have shown low blood glucose concentrations occur in healthy individuals. Further evidence is needed in people without diabetes.[1]

Clinical Case Vignettes

Case 1

A 42-year-old man with a 6-month history of sweats and lightheadedness is referred for evaluation. Symptoms are relieved with the ingestion of food. He works as a heavy goods vehicle mechanic. His colleague at work has diabetes and thought the patient was having a hypoglycemic episode; the colleague checked the patient's capillary blood glucose concentration, which was low at 40 mg/dL (2.2 mmol/L). He has been snacking and eating regularly to control his symptoms and has gained 11 lb (5 kg).

Which of the following is the best next step in this patient's evaluation?

A. Mixed-meal test

B. 72-hour observed fast

C. MRI of the pancreas

D. CT of the pancreas

E. Sulfonylurea screen

Answer: B) 72-hour fast

This patient's history is consistent with hypoglycemia and proceeding to a fast (Answer B) is the correct approach. In real-world practice in our institution, he would be admitted to the hospital and undergo full testing, starting with a mixed meal (Answer A) followed by a 72-hour fast. Preadmission testing would include blood draw at 9 AM to measure salivary cortisol, hemoglobin A$_{1c}$, and insulin antibodies/receptor antibodies and assess kidney and liver function and complete blood cell count (this testing would be arranged in advance). Imaging (Answers C and D) should be arranged after biochemical confirmation. A sulfonylurea screen (Answer E) would be conducted at the time of the 72-hour fast.

This patient underwent a mixed-meal test (no hypoglycemia and no symptoms) and a 72-hour fast (he developed hypoglycemia and symptoms of sweating and lightheadedness). The results of plasma glucose, insulin, and C-peptide measurement are shown (*Tables 1* and *2 following page*):

Table 1. Patient's Mixed-Meal Test Results

Time (min)	Glc mg/dl/mmol/L	Insulin pmol/L
0	81/ 4.5	30
30	117/ 6.4	348
60	85/ 4.8	317
120	70/ 3.8	225
150	63/ 3.5	150
180	60/ 3.3	83
210	55/ 3.1	49
240	60/ 3.3	50
270	65/ 3.6	67
300	63/ 3.5	31

[Color—Print (Color Gallery page CG29) or web & ePub editions]

Table 2. Patient's 72-Hour Fast Test Results

Time	Glc (mg/dl/mmol/L) Criteria 2.2 mol/L	Insulin Nr 17.8-173 Criteria > 36 pmol/L	C-peptide pmol/L Nr 298-2350 Criteria >200pmol/L
10:00	65/3.6	50.2	391
15:15	45/2.5	49.8	417
18:00	62/3.4	43.3	414
21:00	40/2.3	38.2	401
02:00	38/2.1	36.1	322

Beta hydroxy butyrate 1.4 mmol/L
Sulphonylurea screen neg
IgG Insulin antibodies neg

[Color—Print (Color Gallery page CG29) or web & ePub editions]

Which of the following can be inferred from the biochemical investigations?

A. There is postprandial hypoglycemia

B. There is ketosis

C. There is exogenous administration of insulin although the sulfonylurea screen is negative

D. There is endogenous insulin secretion

E. He has adrenal insufficiency

Answer: D) There is endogenous insulin secretion

There is endogenous insulin secretion (Answer D), as demonstrated by the data from the mixed-meal series that shows an appropriate response of glucose and insulin concentrations when eating but no absolute drop in glucose levels: glucose levels flatten, the insulin level decreases, and there is no hypoglycemia (thus, Answer A is incorrect). The production of endogenous insulin does not cause ketosis and the β-hydroxybutyrate level is low (thus, Answer B is incorrect). The presence of C-peptide means the insulin production is endogenous, which excludes exogenous administration of insulin (Answer C). Adrenal insufficiency (Answer E) is a red herring.

Case 1 (continued)

The patient has CT of the chest, abdomen, and pelvis. This is reviewed by the multidisciplinary team and is reported as negative. *Table 3* shows the predicted changes in parameters for the underlying causes of hypoglycemia.

Which of the following is the best next step in this patient's management?

A. Magnetic resonance cholangiopancreatography

B. EUS

C. Selective intra-arterial injection of calcium with hepatic venous insulin gradients

D. Initiation of a somatostatin analogue

E. Receptor scintigraphy with radiolabeled GLP-1 receptor analogue or ^{68}Ga PET-CT if available

Table 3. Diagnosis of Functioning Pancreatic NETs

Time of Symptoms	Glucose (mmol/L)	C-peptide (nmol/L)	Insulin (pmol/L)	Pro-Insulin (pmol/L)	BHOB (mmol/L)	ΔGlucose after glucagon	Additional parameters	Diagnosis
No symptoms	<2.5	<0.2	<20.8	<5	>2.7	<-1.4	No	Normal
Mainly fasting hypoglycaemia	<2.5	>0.2	>20.8	>5	<2.7	>-1.4	No	Insulinoma
Postprandial hypoglycaemia	<2.5	>0.2	>20.8	>5	<2.7	>-1.4	Bariatric surgery	Post bariatric hypoglycaemia
More often postprandial hypoglycaemia	<2.5	>0.2	>20.8	>5	<2.7	>-1.4	No	NIPHS
Mainly fasting	<2.5	>0.2	>20.8	>5	<2.7	>-1.4	Insulin secretagogues	Exogenous administration with oral compounds
Fasting	<2.5	<0.2	>>20.8	>5	<2.7	>-1.4	NA	Exogenous administration of insulin
Mainly postprandial	<2.5	>>0.2	>>20.8	>>5	>2.7	>-1.4	Anti-insulin antibodies	Anti insulin antibody syndrome
Fasting	<2.5	<0.2	<20.8	<5	<2.7	>-1.4	IGF-2	Non-insulin mediated hypoglycaemia

Reprinted from Hofland J et al. J Neuroendocrinol, 2023; 35(8): e13318. © The Authors. *The Journal of Neuroendocrinology* is published by John Wiley & Sons Ltd on behalf of the British Society for Neuroendocrinology.[4]

Answer: B) EUS

EUS (Answer B) can localize, as well as allow FNA biopsy to confirm the grading of the functional pancreatic neuroendocrine tumor. Receptor scintigraphy with radiolabeled GLP-1 receptor analogue or ^{68}Ga PET-CT (Answer E) is a viable option, but its availability is so limited that it is currently not feasible. Somatostatin analogue therapy (Answer D) is a therapeutic option, but test dosing is recommended first. Oral medical treatment with diazoxide, if tolerated, is a good starting option. Magnetic resonance cholangiopancreatography (Answer A) is incorrect because this technique is used to assess the bile ducts.

EUS locates a single 1-cm lesion in the neck of the pancreas. FNA biopsy histology confirms a well-differentiated neuroendocrine tumor that stains positive for synaptophysin and chromogranin with an ENETS grade of 1 with a Ki67 index less than 1%. Diazoxide is prescribed at a dosage of 100 mg twice daily, and this is well tolerated. Nuclear imaging, in the form of a tektrotyd scan, is performed to detect neuroendocrine tumors (consists of a radioactive tracer attached to octreotide and called ^{99m}Tc-ethylenediammonium diacetate-tricine-hydrazinonictotinamide-Tyr0-octreotide (tektrotyd) single-photon emission CT, and the findings concur with those of EUS with no identified metastatic disease.

Which of the following should be offered to this patient who is well and has a performance status of zero with no comorbidities?

A. The Whipple procedure

B. Peptide receptor radionuclide therapy

C. Everolimus

D. Somatostatin analogue therapy

E. Parenchymal-sparing curative pancreatic surgery with enucleation

Answer: E) Parenchymal-sparing curative pancreatic surgery with enucleation

Although the tumor location in the neck of the pancreas is challenging, the preferred strategy would be parenchymal-sparing curative pancreatic surgery (Answer E). This should be performed by an experienced pancreatic surgeon. Discussion in the expert multidisciplinary team should address planned management of preoperative hypoglycemia, as well as postoperative future glycemia.

Peptide receptor radionuclide therapy (Answer B) and everolimus (Answer C) are indicated in progressive disease, and somatostatin analogue therapy (Answer D) would only be offered after test dosing if diazoxide failed or the patient was intolerant to it. The Whipple procedure (Answer A) is excessive for a 1-cm lesion.

Case 2

A 52-year-old man presents with hypoglycemia, and insulinoma is biochemically proven followed by histopathological confirmation. The patient undergoes pylorus-sparing pancreaticoduodenectomy. Histology shows an ENETS grade 2 neuroendocrine tumor with a Ki67 index of 18%. The patient is well for next 3 years. He then presents to his local clinic for a follow-up appointment, and he has liver metastases and worsening hypoglycemia. Somatostatin analogue therapy is initiated. Unfortunately, radiological progression ensues, and the local team treats him with chemotherapy (capecitabine and streptozotocin). Chemotherapy is interrupted when the patient has a myocardial infarction. After recovering, everolimus is initiated. However, medication is discontinued because he develops limbic encephalitis and is hospitalized. He has worsening hypoglycemia and diazoxide is started with incremental dose adjustments. Hypoglycemia becomes intractable, and intravenous dextrose infusion is initiated by the local team through a peripherally inserted central catheter line. Transarterial chemoembolization is administered for the liver metastases, but this is halted because a liver abscess develops.

The patient is referred to a specialty center for a second opinion after diazoxide is discontinued because of a rash. Intravenous ambulatory dextrose is continued but is cumbersome.

During review by the multidisciplinary team, the patient is noted to have anorexia, weight loss, and a performance status of 2. Tektrotyd scan shows a Krenning score of 4 for avidity in liver metastases.

Which of the following is the best treatment option?

A. Peptide receptor radionuclide therapy

B. Everolimus re-trial

C. Alternative second-generation somatostatin analogue therapy

D. Debulking surgery if possible

E. Chemotherapy re-trial

Answer: A) Peptide receptor radionuclide therapy

Everolimus (Answer B) and chemotherapy (Answer E) were unsuccessful previously, and the patient experienced disease progression while on these agents (albeit, in part due to comorbidities). An alternative second-generation somatostatin analogue (Answer C) currently has limited data and would need to be used off-label if there were no other alternatives. Debulking surgery (Answer D) may be too high risk.

Peptide receptor radionuclide therapy (Answer A) is the best option because the patient has a functional grade 2 pancreatic metastatic neuroendocrine tumor that has progressed. The ENETS guidelines and recent publications support its use in this context. Kidney and liver function monitoring, as well as being able to follow radiation protection advice, is required. The tektrotyd scan showed high avidity, which means he would be a suitable candidate for this therapy. This treatment usually consists of 4 cycles every 8 weeks.

The patient responded rapidly after the first cycle, with improvement in appetite, weight gain, and better control of hypoglycemia. He initially had some nausea, but this was well managed, and he was able to discontinue intravenous dextrose completely. Each cycle included a dose of ^{177}Lu oxodotreotide at 7.4 GBq. Evidence of a radiological response was documented after his third cycle. After completing 4 cycles, his quality of life improved, he returned to a performance status of 0, and he was able to return to work. Peptide receptor radionuclide therapy has evidence for progression-free survival and improvement in quality of life. It is well tolerated with less than a 2% risk of developing myelodysplasia.

Case 3

A 23-year-old woman is admitted to the hospital after a witnessed seizure. Paramedics on the scene document her blood glucose concentration to be 34 mg/dL (1.9 mmol/L). She requires intramuscular glucagon and intravenous dextrose resuscitation. She has a history of gastric surgery, but the details of the surgery are unclear. She is accompanied by her mother.

Her glucose concentration was stable during morning rounds, but later in the afternoon she collapses. Blood draw for urgent biochemistry is done, along with a bedside glucose measurement (34 mg/dL [1.9 mmol/L]). Her laboratory venous blood glucose concentration is 19.8 mg/dL (1.1 mmol/L).

Additional laboratory test results (measured at the same time as blood glucose):

> Insulin = 21.6 µIU/mL (2.6-24.9 µIU/mL)
>   (SI: 50 pmol/L [17.8-173.0 pmol/L])
> C-peptide = 150 pmol/L (370-1470 pmol/L)
> β-Hydroxybutyrate = <0.1 mmol/L (indicating
>   no ketosis)
> Cortisol (8 AM) = 18.1 µg/dL (SI: 499 nmol/L)
> IgG insulin antibodies, normal

Which of the following is the most likely etiology of this patient's hypoglycemia?

A. Endogenous insulin secretion from an insulinoma

B. Surreptitious insulin injection

C. Hirata syndrome

D. Addison disease

E. Dumping syndrome

Answer: B) Surreptitious insulin injection

The low C-peptide value is crucial in this case, as it indicates the patient's hypoglycemia is not from an endogenous source. Given the insulin value is inappropriately high, this is a case of surreptitious insulin administration (Answer B). The history refers to a form of gastric surgery, but it is not clear what type of surgery was performed. If dumping syndrome were the culprit, symptoms would be expected to occur after ingestion of food. Expected laboratory findings would be hypoglycemia and elevated and detectable C-peptide and insulin levels. If she had an insulinoma, C-peptide would be inappropriately elevated.

Addison disease (Answer D) is excluded by the normal morning cortisol, and Hirata syndrome (Answer C) is excluded by normal insulin antibodies.

The patient was given the results and the cause of her hypoglycemia was discussed. She subsequently left the hospital grounds before a psychiatry consultation could take place. She was readmitted to her local hospital with another hypoglycemic episode, and we advised her medical team to send a blood sample for an insulin assay.

This determined the type of exogenous insulin being administered.

Unfortunately, despite best efforts to manage the underlying psychiatric illness, the patient has had another hospital admission with a diazoxide overdose. It is thought she obtained all of the medications in question online.

Key Learning Points

- Hypoglycemia in individuals without diabetes requires careful workup.

- The 72-hour fast is the gold standard test for insulinoma-related hypoglycemia.

- Rare causes of hypoglycemia should be discussed in a specialist multidisciplinary team meeting.

- Newer imaging techniques exist for evaluation of hypoglycemia, and new treatments are available to address hypoglycemia.

References

1. Nirantharakumar K, Marshall T, Hodson J, et al. Hypoglycemia in non-diabetic in-patients: clinical or criminal? *PLoS One.* 2012;7(7):e40384. PMID: 22768352

2. Palani G, Stortz E, Moheet A. Clinical presentation and diagnostic approach to hypoglycemia in adults without diabetes mellitus. *Endoc Pract.* 2023;29(4):286-294. PMID: 36464132

3. Falconi M, Eriksson B, Kaltsas G, et al; Vienna Consensus Conference participants. ENETS consensus guidelines update for the management of patients with functional pancreatic neuroendocrine tumors and non-functional pancreatic neuroendocrine tumors. *Neuroendocrinology.* 2016;103(2):153-171. PMID: 26742109

4. Hofland J, Falconi M, Christ E, et al. European Neuroendocrine Tumor Society 2023 guidance paper for functioning pancreatic neuroendocrine tumour syndromes. *J Neuroendocrinol.* 2023;35(8):e13318. PMID: 37578384

5. Mathew P, Thoppil D. Hypoglycemia. [Updated 2022 Dec 26]. In: StatPearls [Internet]. Treasure Island, FL: StatPearls Publishing; 2024. https://www.ncbi.nlm.nih.gov/books/NBK534841/

6. Cryer PE, Axelrod L, Grossman AB, et al; Endocrine Society. Evaluation and management of adult hypoglycemic disorders: an Endocrine Society clinical practice guideline. *J Clin Endocrinol Metab.* 2009;94(3):709-728. PMID: 19088155

7. Munir A, Choudhary P, Harrison B, Heller S, Newell-Price J. Continuous glucose monitoring in patients with insulinoma. *Clin Endocrinol (Oxf).* 2008;68(6):912-918. PMID: 18088393

8. Hofland J, Refardt JC, Feelders RA, Christ E, de Herder WW. Approach to the patient: insulinoma. *J Clin Endocrinol Metab.* 2024;109(4):1109-1118. PMID: 37925662

9. Klein Haneveld MJ, van Treijen MJC, Pieterman CRC, et al. Initiating pancreatic neuroendocrine tumor (pNET) screening in young MEN1 patients: results from the DutchMEN study group. *J Clin Endocrinol Metab.* 2021;106(12):3515-3525. PMID: 34333645

10. Church D, Cardoso L, Kay RG, et al. Assessment and management of anti-insulin autoantibodies in varying presentations of insulin autoimmune syndrome. *J Clin Endocrinol Metab.* 2018;103(10):3845-3855. PMID: 30085133

11. Hofland J, Refardt JC, Feelders RA, Christ E, de Herder WW. Approach to the patient: insulinoma. *J Clin Endocrinol Metab.* 2024;109(4):1109-1118. PMID: 37925662

12. Foster-Schubert KE. Hypoglycemia complicating bariatric surgery: incidence and mechanisms. *Curr Opin Endocrinol Diabetes Obes.* 2011;18(2):129-133. PMID: 21297468

13. Kefurt R, Langer FB, Schindler K, Shakeri-Leidenmühler S, Ludvik B, Prager G. Hypoglycemia after Roux-En-Y gastric bypass: detection rates of continuous glucose monitoring (CGM) versus mixed meal test. *Surg Obes Relat Dis.* 2015;11(3):564-569. PMID: 25737101

14. Oziel-Taieb S, Maniry-Quellier J, Chanez B, Poizat F, Ewald J, Niccoli P. Pasireotide for refractory hypoglycemia in malignant insulinoma: case report and review of the literature. *Front Endocrinol (Lausanne).* 2022;13:860614. PMID: 35518928

15. Osataphan S, Vamvini M, Rosen ED, et al. Anti-insulin receptor antibody for malignant insulinoma and refractory hypoglycemia. *N Engl J Med.* 2023;389(8):767-769. PMID: 37611129

16. Zandee WT, Brabander T, Blažević A, et al. Symptomatic and radiological response to 177Lu-DOTATATE for the treatment of functioning pancreatic neuroendocrine tumors. *J Clin Endocrinol Metab.* 2019;104(4):1336-1344. PMID: 30566620

Diagnostic Challenges and Individualized Management of Acromegaly

Elena V. Varlamov, MD. Departments of Medicine (Endocrinology, Diabetes, and Clinical Nutrition) and Neurological Surgery, and Pituitary Center, Oregon Health & Science University, Portland, OR; Email: varlamoe@ohsu.edu

Maria Fleseriu, MD. Departments of Medicine (Endocrinology, Diabetes, and Clinical Nutrition) and Neurological Surgery, and Pituitary Center, Oregon Health & Science University, Portland, OR; Email: fleseriu@ohsu.edu

Educational Objectives

After reviewing this chapter, learners should be able to:

- Explain the role and limitations of IGF-1 and GH measurements (random and during oral glucose tolerance testing [OGTT]) in the diagnosis of acromegaly and describe criteria for remission.

- Select medical therapy for acromegaly based on tumor characteristics, IGF-1 and GH concentrations, comorbidities, and patient goals.

- Guide screening and monitoring for complications of acromegaly.

Significance of the Clinical Problem

Acromegaly results from chronic exposure to GH and IGF-1 excess, usually due to a pituitary adenoma, and it is probably underdiagnosed. Despite increased awareness and improvements in diagnostic tools, the overall delay in diagnosis remains significant, approximately 5 to 6 years.[1] Patients with a mild and/or atypical presentation may be missed, resulting in longer exposure to deleterious effects of GH and tumor burden. Untreated or uncontrolled acromegaly has been linked to multisystem complications. Mortality is approximately 2-fold higher than that of the general population, mostly due to cardiovascular disease and malignancies, but mortality can be reduced by treating comorbidities and achieving biochemical control.[2-4] Treatment goals for acromegaly include achieving biochemical control, tumor removal/volume reduction, symptom relief, reversal/improvement of comorbidities, and quality of life improvement.[1] Patient preference should be included in the discussion when choosing treatment options.

First-line treatment is usually transsphenoidal surgery with complete resection or debulking of the GH-producing adenoma by an experienced neurosurgeon.[5] Many somatotroph tumors are large and invasive by the time they are discovered, and therefore they may not be amenable to complete excision and subsequent remission. Younger age and higher preoperative GH concentrations are also associated with lack of surgical remission.[1] Overall surgical remission rates are 75% to 90% for microadenomas and 40% to 60% for macroadenomas.[1] Adjuvant treatment is thus needed in many patients not cured by surgery. Medical therapy is aimed at normalization of IGF-1 (and GH) concentrations, as well as tumor shrinkage or prevention of tumor growth, if needed. Radiotherapy is considered when medical therapy fails or for aggressive adenomas or persistently growing residual masses.[1,5,6]

The idea of personalized management is receiving renewed attention in all rare diseases, but especially in acromegaly. An individualized approach considers tumor type, tumor size, IGF-1 and GH concentrations, symptoms, comorbid conditions, and patient preferences.[7,8] Although biochemical control typically results in significant symptom improvement, the classic "goal" target (normal age- and sex-adjusted IGF-1 concentration and random GH concentration <1 ng/mL [<1.0 μg/L]) can still be associated with persistent signs or symptoms (arthralgias, sweating, fatigue, soft-tissue swelling). Individualized therapy adjustment or combination therapy should be considered in patients with ongoing symptoms. Furthermore, long-term follow-up, including screening for recurrence and regular reassessment of both biochemical control and tumor size, is important.

Practice Gaps

- GH and IGF-1 assays are heterogeneous with varying reference ranges depending on age, sex, and technology used. Discrepancies exist among laboratories, complicating diagnosis and monitoring.

- GH measurements during OGTT have limitations in the diagnosis of mild acromegaly.

- Information that can guide treatment choice or determine prognosis (eg, sparsely vs densely granulated GH-secreting adenomas, presence of somatostatin receptor type 2 or 5) is still missing in many histopathology reports.

- Somatostatin receptor ligand (SRL) monotherapy (eg, octreotide, lanreotide) is effective in less than 50% of patients in unselected populations; thus, patients often require a switch to a different agent, either a multiligand SRL, GH receptor antagonist, or combination therapy. Adjustment of the treatment regimen is sometimes delayed.

- Patients are not systematically screened for acromegaly complications.

Discussion
Difficulties in the Diagnosis of Acromegaly

Challenging diagnostic cases include patients who lack typical clinical features of acromegaly, those whose biochemical test results are inconclusive, or those who do not have a clear pituitary adenoma on MRI. Acromegaly may be suspected based on clinical symptoms and signs (eg, acral enlargement, jaw expansion, excessive sweating, etc) or based on associated health conditions (sleep apnea, glucose intolerance or diabetes mellitus, osteoarthritis, carpal tunnel syndrome, etc) that are sometimes the only obvious manifestations of this disease. Patients presenting with hyperprolactinemia and a pituitary adenoma may have subclinical GH excess due to cosecretion of GH by the adenoma (eg, mixed somatotroph-lactotroph adenoma).

Measurement of IGF-1 is the first step in evaluating symptomatic patients, as well as evaluating a pituitary mass, even in the absence of symptoms.[1,5] Unequivocally and repeatedly elevated IGF-1 values greater than 1.3 times the upper normal limit combined with classic symptoms and signs confirm the diagnosis of acromegaly.[9] Patients who fall outside of these criteria may benefit from additional testing, including OGTT. However, each test has limitations related to established cutoffs, assay performance, and physiologic factors affecting the results.

There is variability of IGF-1 measurements between laboratories and within individuals. A reliable IGF-1 assay should be calibrated to the current international standard (02/254) and have age-adjusted reference ranges established based on a large population sample.[9] "Falsely" elevated IGF-1 concentrations have been attributed to inadequately determined reference ranges.[1,9] Importantly, a variety of physiologic and

Table 1. Factors That Affect IGF-1 and GH Levels

Factors that ↑ IGF-1	Factors that ↓ IGF-1	Factors that ↑ GH	Factors that ↓ GH
• Parenteral testosterone • Pregnancy • Late-stage adolescence • Inadequate limits of normality • Assay interference	• Oral estrogen, selective estrogen receptor modulators • Severe obesity • Prolonged fasting and malnutrition • Liver disease • Kidney disease • Uncontrolled diabetes • Acute illness	• Oral estrogen, midcycle • Poorly controlled diabetes • Kidney failure • Prolonged fasting and malnutrition • Liver disease • Acute critical illness	• Age (postmenopausal) • High BMI

pathologic factors can affect IGF-1 results (*Table 1*).[10,11] Measurement of IGF-1 by tandem mass spectrometry does not appear to be superior to measurement with an immunoassay.[9]

GH assays also exhibit variability in measurements, but more so when the GH concentration is higher. Detection of very low GH levels using modern, ultrasensitive assays has allowed improvement in the sensitivity of the standard OGTT in evaluating acromegaly, and the traditional GH cutoff of 1.0 ng/mL (<1.0 µg/L) has been replaced by 0.4 ng/mL (<0.4 µg/L).[6] However, some patients with mild GH excess may suppress to less than 0.4 ng/mL (<0.4 µg/L) (*Figure 1, following page*).[12] On the contrary, a "positive" OGTT result (GH ≥0.4 ng/mL [≥0.4 µg/L]) has been reported in healthy slim individuals and in women taking oral estrogen. Interestingly, a few patients with acromegaly exhibit a paradoxical GH increase in response to glucose.[1]

When the initial evaluation produces borderline or discrepant results (IGF-1 vs GH) that do not align with clinical picture, re-testing should be undertaken. If clinical suspicion for acromegaly is high despite adequate suppression of GH during OGTT, pituitary MRI should be performed. A "normal" MRI does not exclude the diagnosis of acromegaly. Missed microadenomas, empty sella, and pituitary hypertrophy due to GHRH-secreting tumors or ectopic GH-secreting tumors have also been reported in acromegaly. In cases when the diagnosis still cannot be established, monitoring for biochemical and clinical progression is warranted.[1]

Surgical Remission Criteria

Biochemical remission after surgery is usually defined as a normal IGF-1 value and a random GH value less than 1.0 ng/mL (<1.0 µg/L). This assessment is typically done 12 weeks postoperatively given the gradual decline of IGF-1. Early postoperative drop in GH to less than 0.4 ng/mL (<0.4 µg/L) (day 1-5 after surgery) can predict long-term remission.[9] Discrepant results, most commonly a GH value less than 1 ng/mL (<1.0 µg/L) and an elevated IGF-1 value, may occur postoperatively. This is thought to be related to mild, persistent disease resulting from dysregulation of GH production and tissue responsiveness.[9] OGTT may be helpful in further evaluation of prognosis. However, IGF-1 measurement using assays with robust normative data[13] seems to correlate better with comorbidities than nadir GH concentrations.[5]

Treatment of Persistent Disease After Pituitary Surgery

Persistent disease after surgery is usually treated with medical therapy. Reoperation is less common in patients with acromegaly than in patients with Cushing disease. Radiation therapy can be beneficial in selected patients with resistance to medical therapy, in patients with large residual adenomas after surgery, or in patients with aggressive tumors. Tumor control is more frequently achieved with radiation, and half of patients also achieve long-term biochemical GH control, albeit with hypopituitarism.

Somatostatin Receptor Ligands

SRLs are the preferred initial medical treatment for most patients with acromegaly (*Table 2*).[1,5,9] SRLs include octreotide long-acting release (LAR), lanreotide (depot or prolonged release formulation for subcutaneous injection), oral octreotide capsules, and pasireotide LAR.

Octreotide LAR and lanreotide seem to be equally effective formulations, although studies with generic lanreotide are lacking. However, only 30% to 60% of patients achieve biochemical control with these agents and dosage escalation is often necessary to normalize IGF-1 concentrations. Tumor volume reduction (>20%)

Figure 1. Diagnosis and Management of Acromegaly

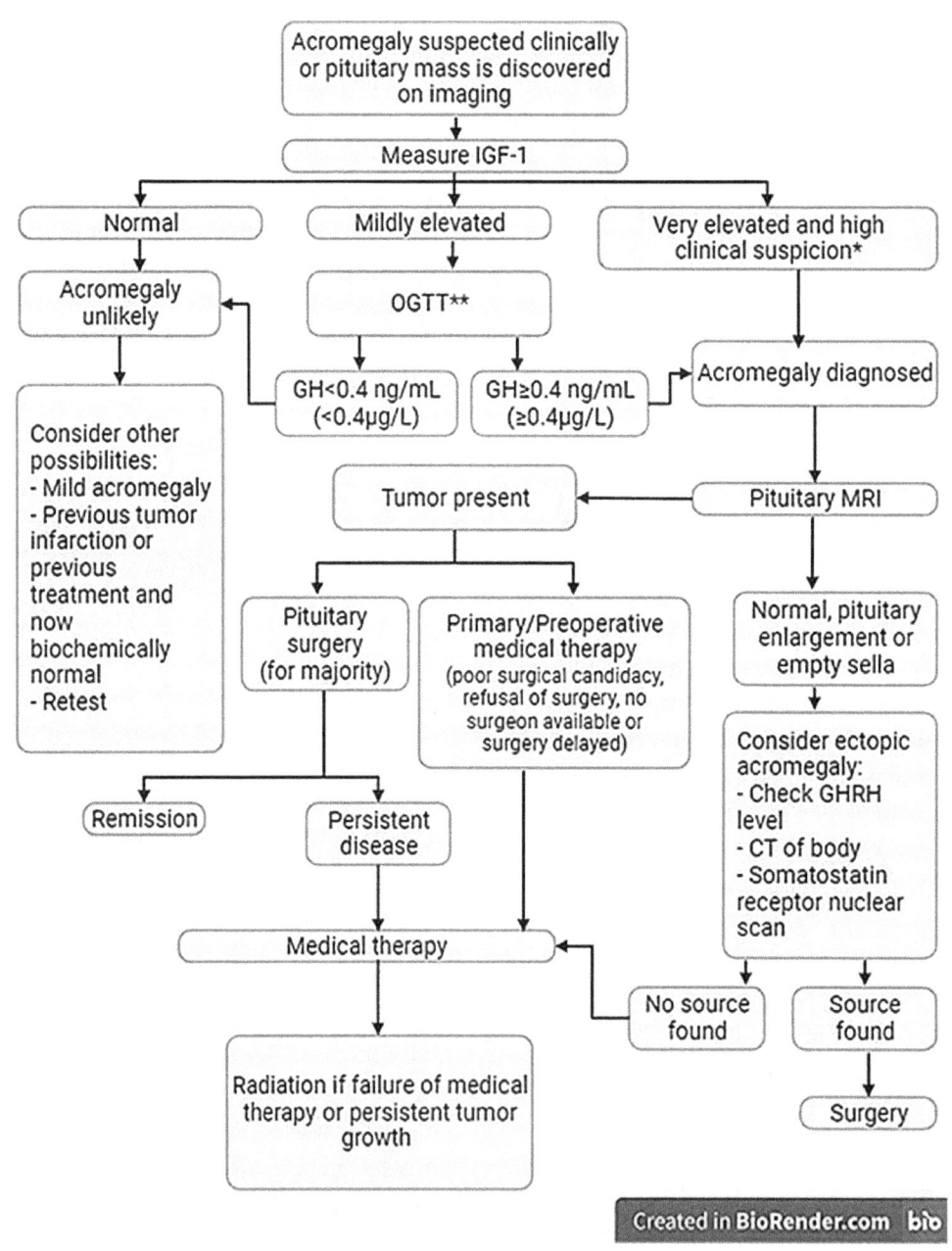

*Consensus[9] recommends IGF-1 >1.3 upper normal limit. **OGTT can show "suppressed" levels (GH <0.4 ng/mL [<0.4 µg/L]) in mild acromegaly and "unsuppressed" levels in patients on oral estrogen and occasionally in slim healthy adults.[9] Adapted from Fleseriu M et al. *Lancet Diabetes Endocrinol*, 2022; 10(11): 804-26. © Elsevier Ltd.[1]

[Color—Print (Color Gallery page CG30) or web & ePub editions]

has been noted in up to 50% of patients.[1] In clinical trials, oral octreotide capsules, the most recently approved SRL, maintained IGF-1 normalization in approximately 60% to 79% of patients naïve to oral octreotide capsules when switched from octreotide or lanreotide.[3,4] Long-term IGF-1 control was similar with injectable SRLs for patients who previously responded to both therapies.[3,4] Treatment convenience and patient satisfaction as demonstrated by acromegaly treatment

Table 2. Summary of Medical Therapies Available for Acromegaly

Class	Agent	Notes	Possible adverse effects
Somatostatin receptor ligands Affinity to somatostatin receptor 2 is the greatest, less so to 5 and 3, less so to 1 and least to 4	Octreotide LAR, 10, 20, 30, or 40 mg every 4 weeks, intramuscularly	• Administered by a health care professional, as it requires reconstitution • Measure IGF-1 1 week before next injection • Monitor IGF-1 3 months after 1st injection/dose adjustment	Gastrointestinal distress cholelithiasis, liver function enzyme elevation, hyperglycemia or hypoglycemia, bradycardia Intolerance to1 drug does not indicate high likelihood of cross-intolerance to other
	Lanreotide Autogel, lanreotide injection: 60, 90, or120 mg every 4 to 8 weeks, deep subcutaneously	• May be self-administered (prefilled syringes) • Measure IGF-1 1 week before next injection • Monitor IGF-1 3 months after 1st injection/dose adjustment	
	Octreotide, 50 to 100 mcg 3 times daily, subcutaneously	• Rarely used alone • Sometimes used for treatment of acromegaly-related headaches	
	Octreotide capsule, 20 mg twice daily, up to 80 mg daily, orally	• Approved for patients controlled on injectable octreotide LAR or lanreotide • Must be taken on empty stomach or 2 hours after meal • Monitor IGF-1 2 to 4 weeks after initiation/dose adjustment	...
Multiligand somatostatin receptor ligand Higher affinity to somatostatin receptor type 5	Pasireotide, 40 or 60 mg every 4 weeks, intramuscularly	• Biochemical control in 20% of cases resistant to first-generation somatostatin receptor ligand • Measure IGF-1 1 week before next injection • Monitor IGF-1 3 months after 1st injection/dose adjustment	Hyperglycemia/diabetes mellitus (~60%), QT prolongation, liver function enzyme elevation
D2 receptor agonist	Cabergoline, 1 to 5 mg weekly, orally	• For mild IGF-1 elevation or in combination therapy • Monitor IGF-1 1 to 3 months after initiation/dose adjustment	Nausea, dizziness, worsening mood disorders and impulse control disorders
GH receptor antagonist	Pegvisomant, 10 to 40 mg daily, subcutaneously Regimens of 2 to 3 times per week can be used (off label)	• Effective in >60% in real-life scenarios • Can improve glycemic control • No antitumor effect • Monitor IGF-1 1 to 3 months after initiation/dose adjustment • GH levels remain elevated and should not be monitored	Liver function enzyme elevation QT prolongation

questionnaire satisfaction (ACRO-TSQ) improved in most patients.[3,4] Thus, oral octreotide capsules are a reasonable option for patients with injection burden, patients with breakthrough symptoms that develop before scheduled injection, and patients whose disease is controlled on injectable SRLs, based on patient preference.[3,4] Resistance to octreotide and lanreotide has been observed in patients with sparsely granulated somatotroph adenomas, somatostatin receptor type 2-negative adenomas, T2-MRI hyperintense adenomas, large and invasive tumors, *AIP* gene pathogenic variants, high Ki67 proliferation index, and age at diagnosis younger than 40 years (*Figure 2*).[1,7]

Pasireotide LAR is a multiligand SRL with higher efficacy than octreotide or lanreotide for biochemical control and tumor shrinkage in approximately 50% of patients. Up to 25% of patients with resistance to octreotide and lanreotide respond to pasireotide. Pasireotide induces hyperglycemia/diabetes in approximately 60% of patients, which is reversible upon discontinuation. If continuation of therapy is strongly preferred, the patient requires close monitoring and the possible addition of metformin, a GLP-1 receptor agonist, or a DPP-4 inhibitor. Older age, abnormal glucose tolerance, and a history of hypertension or dyslipidemia have been identified as predictors of hyperglycemia in patients treated with pasireotide in clinical trials.[14]

Pegvisomant, a GH receptor blocker, induced IGF-1 control in greater than 90% of patients in clinical trials with dosages of up to 40 mg daily. Control rates were lower in real-life observation studies (53%-75%), likely due to lower dosages (14.0-18.2 mg daily on average) and slower titration rates outside of clinical trials.[15] Tumor volume increase was reported in 3% to 7% of patients. Obesity, female sex, and very high baseline IGF-1 may predict poorer response and higher dosages needed to achieve control. Pegvisomant is approved as a first-line treatment in the United States, but it is usually used as a second-line agent. It can be used as first-line therapy in patients with risk factors for resistance to SRL. Notably, pegvisomant can improve fasting and postprandial glycemia, making it more appropriate for patients with diabetes. Additionally, its long half-life (60-138 hours) allows reduced injection frequency (2-3 times weekly), thus lessening the injection burden.

Figure 2. Suggested Algorithm for Medical Management of Acromegaly

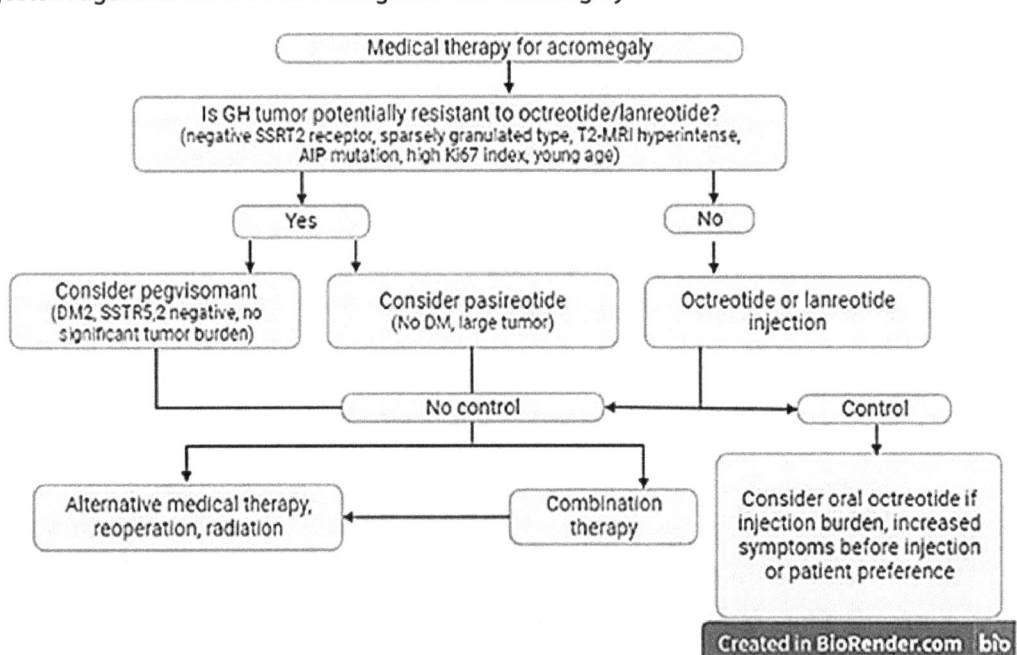

Reprinted from Ting Lim DS & Fleseriu M. *Endocr Pract*, 2022; 28(3): 321-332. © AACE. Published by Elsevier Inc.[7]

[Color—Print (Color Gallery page CG31) or web & ePub editions]

In some studies, dopamine agonists achieve biochemical control in 30% to 40% of patients with mild acromegaly, but with decreased effectiveness over time in some patients and variable degree of tumor shrinkage.[6] Because of limited effectiveness, cabergoline should be used mainly in patients with mild disease or in combination with other agents.

Combination medical therapy is used when (1) monotherapy fails to attain control, (2) when it is necessary to minimize adverse effects by using lower dosages of 2 medications, or (3) when tumor control is needed with an SRL but the SRL alone would not achieve biochemical control. A combination of octreotide or lanreotide and pegvisomant provides 60% to 90% IGF-1 normalization, with lower dosages/fewer pegvisomant injections (once or twice weekly), lower cost, and better tolerability.[1,6,7] With the pasireotide LAR-pegvisomant combination, the pegvisomant dosage can be reduced by up to 66% compared with the octretide/lanreotide-pegvisomant combination. However, it causes double the number of diabetes cases. Close monitoring of liver function enzymes is required. The combination of an SRL and cabergoline is relatively well-tolerated and suitable for patients with very mild IGF-1 elevations. The combination of pegvisomant and cabergoline is considered in case of intolerance to SRLs or unaffordability of SRL-pegvisomant combination. Future studies should determine long-term efficacy and safety of various combination therapies.[5,7]

Primary medical therapy (medication for acromegaly with the hope to avoid surgery) is sometimes considered for patients with smaller tumors without optic chiasm involvement, those who are not surgical candidates or decline surgery, and those with empty sella after "burnt-out" adenoma. Practices differ among countries and centers. SRLs are usually preferred because they can reduce tumor volume and control GH secretion. Pegvisomant for smaller adenomas is also an option, as risk of tumor enlargement is overall low. Use of medical therapy before surgery to improve postoperative biochemical outcomes is controversial and therefore not routinely done.

It has, however, been advocated for patients with uncontrolled hypertension, heart failure, and severe respiratory complications (eg, pharyngeal edema, severe sleep apnea) to possibly reduce perioperative morbidity.

Emerging medical therapies for acromegaly with promising results in phase 3 clinical trials include a nonpeptide selective somatostatin receptor type 2 agonist (paltusotine), taken once daily, and long-acting subcutaneous depot octreotide (CAM2029) once monthly. Temozolomide is rarely used in combination with other medical therapies off-label in aggressive GH-secreting tumors.

In most countries, radiation (conventional and stereotactic) is reserved for patients for whom surgery and medical therapy fail, and it is used as a second-line treatment postoperatively for aggressive somatotroph adenomas. Practices differ among centers and countries depending on availability and cost of therapies. Radiation is slow to act, typically achieving biochemical control in 40% to 60% of patients at 5 years, and it requires bridge medical therapy in the interim. Hypopituitarism develops in 25% to 50% of treated patients at 5 years.[6] Rates of radiation-induced cerebrovascular disease, cranial nerve dysfunction, and secondary tumors appear to be lower when stereotactic techniques are used.[6]

Reoperation is an option for patients whose disease is not controlled on medical therapy after initial surgery and who have a distinguishable tumor that can be resected or for patients with tumor regrowth. Second operations are associated with much lower biochemical control rates than first-line surgery for macroadenomas (~25% of patients) and tumors invading the cavernous sinus. State-of-the-art nuclear medicine diagnostics (eg, ^{11}C-methionine PET-CT), which are not available in all countries, may help visualize residual somatotroph adenomas that are not detected on MRI.[1]

Screening for Complications

A patient with a new diagnosis of acromegaly requires a comprehensive assessment for complications (*Table 3, following page*). Any identified complications should be addressed with appropriate treatment or referral to a specialist. Remission of biochemical disease typically leads to improvement or even complete resolution of complications such as sleep apnea, cardiomyopathy, and insulin resistance; however, musculoskeletal changes and vertebral fractures may persist and even worsen despite remission. Therefore, periodic reassessment of each complication is necessary.[1-3,5]

Clinical Case Vignettes

Case 1

A 23-year-old woman is referred for possible acromegaly with concerns about tall stature, fatigue, irregular menses, facial hair, muscle and joint aches, and night sweats.

Laboratory test results:

> IGF-1 = 445 ng/mL (73-329 ng/mL) (SI: 58.3 nmol/L [9.6-43.1 nmol/L])
> Repeat IGF-1 = 381 ng/mL (SI: 49.9 nmol/L)

On physical examination, her blood pressure is 130/84 mm Hg, and pulse rate is 83 beats/min. Her height is 70 in (177.8 cm), and weight is 184 lb (83.9 kg) (BMI = 26.4 kg/m^2). Her mother's height is 70 in (177.8 cm), and her father's height is 71 in (180.3 cm). There is no hand enlargement, frontal bossing, protruding jaw, or gaps between the teeth. She has oily skin, sweaty palms, and some skin tags.

Additional laboratory test results:

> TSH, normal
> Free T$_4$, normal
> Prolactin, normal

Table 3. Systemic Complications of Acromegaly and Screening Recommendations

Complication	Screening recommendations
Cardiovascular Hypertension, ventricular hypertrophy, valve disease, systolic/diastolic dysfunction, arrhythmias	• Blood pressure, echocardiography, electrocardiography • Referral to cardiology as needed
Respiratory Obstructive and central sleep apnea, rarely respiratory insufficiency	• Questionnaire screens for sleep apnea (eg. Epworth Sleepiness Scale and STOPBang), sleep study if positive screen • Referral to pulmonologist and pulmonary function testing as needed
Neoplastic Colorectal polyps/cancer, thyroid nodules/cancer, breast and kidney cancer	• Colonoscopy (no clear consensus if it is necessary in all patients regardless of age; consider on individual basis in younger patients), thyroid neck exam • Breast and other cancer screening per general population
Musculoskeletal Osteoarthritis, vertebral fractures, and jaw expansion/malocclusion	• Spine x-rays; DXA with trabecular bone score • Biochemical evaluation of bone heath as needed
Metabolic Impaired glucose tolerance, diabetes mellitus, dyslipidemia	• Hemoglobin A$_{1c}$ or OGTT, lipid profile
Neurologic Carpal tunnel syndrome, headache	• Clinical assessment, referral to neurologist, hand surgeon as needed
Quality of life Struggle with body image, physical pain, cognitive dysfunction, treatment burden	• AcroQoL or other assessment instrument for quality of life and treatment satisfaction
Tumor- and treatment-related Hypopituitarism	• Pituitary hormonal workup as needed

Late-night salivary cortisol, 2 normal measurements
Hemoglobin A$_{1c}$ = 5.5% (4.0%-5.6%) (37 mmol/mol [20-38 mmol/mol])

OGTT documents the following GH values: 6.42 ng/mL (6.42 µg/L), 2.03 ng/mL (2.03 µg/L), 1.26 ng/mL (1.26 µg/L), 0.91 ng/mL (0.91 µg/L), and 0.40 ng/mL (0.40 µg/L).

She takes no medications or supplements. Pituitary MRI shows a small area of delayed fill-in on the dynamic sequence along the right inferior portion of the gland, as well as a 2 × 4 × 3-mm nonenhancing lesion posterior to the infundibulum favored to represent Rathke cleft cyst (*Figure 3*).

Which of the following is the best interpretation of these findings?

A. Acromegaly is excluded because GH is suppressed <1 ng/mL (<1 µg/L) on OGTT

B. Acromegaly is unlikely given absence of classic morphological changes

C. Acromegaly is unlikely given no clear adenoma on MRI

D. Patient has ectopic acromegaly given no clear adenoma on MRI

E. Acromegaly is possible despite borderline-normal OGTT

Answer: E) Acromegaly is possible despite borderline-normal OGTT

While OGTT is often used as a confirmatory test for acromegaly, no specific glucose-suppressed value can definitively exclude acromegaly. This patient's GH value was at the cutoff of 0.4 ng/mL (0.4 µg/L). Morphologic changes, while very common, are not always present, particularly in mild acromegaly. Pituitary MRI can also appear normal in patients with acromegaly. No clear adenoma on MRI does not automatically confirm ectopic acromegaly; more tests (GHRH, body imaging) are needed to diagnose ectopic acromegaly. Thus, acromegaly is possible despite borderline-normal OGTT (Answer E).

This patient underwent pituitary surgery, and multiple "white lesions" were removed (per operative report). Final pathology showed foci of pituitary adenoma staining positive for prolactin and GH, most consistent with a mixed somatotroph and lactotroph adenoma supporting the diagnosis of acromegaly. Six weeks after surgery, her IGF-1 value was 232 ng/mL (30.4 nmol/L) and GH value was less than 0.05 ng/mL (<0.05 µg/L). She remains in remission 18 months after surgery.

Figure 3. Patient's Pituitary MRI, Contrast Enhanced

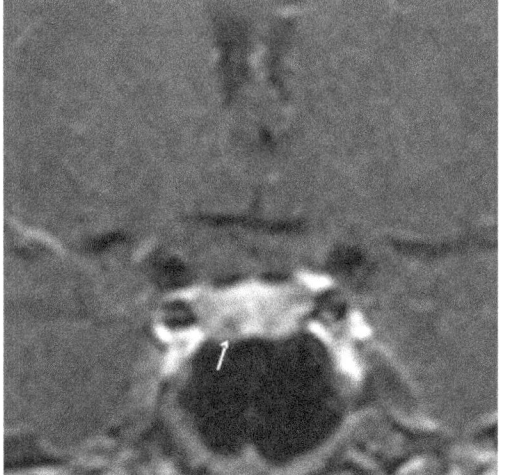

Coronal view

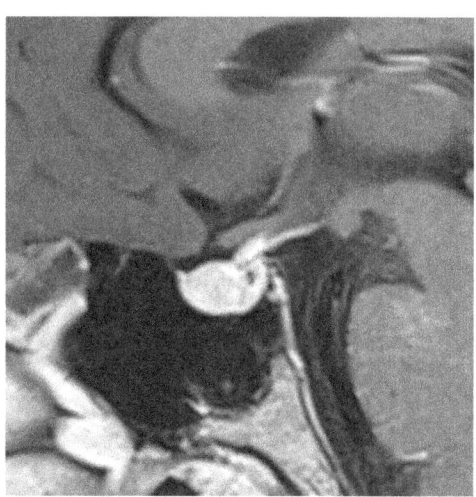

Sagittal view

[Color—Print (Color Gallery page CG31) or web & ePub editions]

Case 2

A 39-year-old woman presents with newly diagnosed acromegaly. She reports increased shoe size and rings no longer fitting. She has prognathism with underbite, headaches, sweating, enlarged tongue, carpal tunnel symptoms, amenorrhea, and hirsutism.

Laboratory test results:

IGF-1 = 1018 ng/mL (59-279 ng/mL)
(SI: 133.4 nmol/L [7.7-36.5 nmol/L])
GH = 22 ng/mL (0.01-3.61 ng/mL) (SI: 22 μg/L
[0.01-3.61 μg/L])
Cortisol (8 AM) = 15.4 μg/dL (5.3-22.5 μg/dL)
(SI: 424.8 nmol/L [146.1-620.5 nmol/L])
ACTH = 17.9 pg/mL (7.2-63.0 pg/mL)
(SI: 3.9 pmol/L [1.6-13.9 pmol/L])
Prolactin = 6.6 ng/mL (2.8-26.0 ng/mL)
(SI: 0.29 nmol/L [0.12-1.13 nmol/L])
TSH = 1.9 mIU/L (0.47-4.68 mIU/L)
Free T$_4$ = 1.37 ng/dL (0.78-2.19 ng/dL)
(SI: 17.6 pmol/L [10.0-28.2 pmol/L])

MRI shows a 2.5-cm macroadenoma with mass effect on the optic chiasm and possible cavernous sinus invasion. Visual fields are normal. She has mild hypertension and mild left ventricular hypertrophy with normal ejection fraction on echocardiography. She has no chest pain, shortness of breath, leg edema, or exercise intolerance. Family history is notable for colon cancer in her father.

Which of the following is the best management recommendation?

A. Perform pituitary surgery as soon as possible

B. Hold off on surgery and initiate octreotide LAR or lanreotide to shrink the tumor; consider surgery if tumor is not responding

C. Hold off on surgery due to left ventricular hypertrophy and initiate pegvisomant to normalize IGF-1; perform surgery when left ventricular hypertrophy resolves

D. Do not recommend surgery because of the low likelihood of cure and start combination therapy with an SRL and pegvisomant

E. Do not recommend surgery because of the low likelihood of cure and recommend radiation

Answer: A) Perform pituitary surgery as soon as possible

First-line treatment of acromegaly is pituitary surgery (Answer A) for most patients, whether the goal is gross total resection or partial debulking of the tumor. Surgery can relieve mass effect and reduce tumor burden. After surgery, adjunctive medical therapy and/or radiation are used for persistent disease. While SRLs can induce tumor shrinkage, it takes months to years and they are not appropriate for a patient with mass effect on the optic chiasm when surgery is available and not contraindicated. Pegvisomant can effectively lower IGF-1, and improvement in cardiomyopathy is expected with biochemical control; however, postponing surgery is not appropriate due to mild left ventricular hypertrophy and otherwise normal cardiac function (unless acute cardiac complications develop). While the likelihood of surgical remission is indeed low for this patient, is it not the reason to recommend against surgery in a patient with optic chiasm compression; additionally, combination therapy is rarely started simultaneously. Radiation is usually a third-line treatment option if the patient is not responding to medical therapy or if the tumor is aggressive, but radiation is not the best choice in those with mass effect on the optic chiasm.

Case 2 (continued)

The patient undergoes pituitary surgery at another institution, and her IGF-1 concentration decreases to 632 ng/mL (82.8 nmol/L) 3 months postoperatively. MRI shows enhancing tissue (14 × 6 × 8 mm) in the right tuberculum sellae (*Figure 4, following page*).

If the pathology report with details on granularity is not available, which of the following is the best recommendation to manage this patient's persistent disease?

A. Octreotide or lanreotide injection

B. Oral octreotide capsules

C. Pasireotide plus pegvisomant

D. Cabergoline

E. Pegvisomant

Answer: A) Octreotide or lanreotide injection

SRLs such as octreotide and lanreotide are usually the first-line treatment unless resistance is highly probable (sparsely granulated somatotroph adenomas, somatostatin receptor type 2-negative adenomas, T2-MRI hyperintense adenomas, large and invasive tumors, *AIP* gene pathogenic variants, high Ki67 proliferation index, and younger age). If a pathology report is not available, a trial of octreotide or lanreotide injections (Answer A) is reasonable.

Pasireotide and pegvisomant (Answer E) are both second-line options, but combination therapy (Answer C) is rarely initiated initially.

Oral octreotide capsules (Answer B) are approved for patients whose disease is controlled on octreotide or lanreotide injections. The capsules can also be considered if injections are burdensome.

Cabergoline (Answer D) is suggested for mild IGF-1 elevation (<1.5 times upper normal limit).

Case 2 (continued)

This patient's IGF-1 remains elevated after 6 months of octreotide treatment, 40 mg every 4 weeks. Pegvisomant, 30 mg 3 times weekly, is added to her regimen of octreotide injections. IGF-1 normalizes. One year after surgery, MRI shows unchanged residual tumor. The patient expresses frustration with multiple injections, but she does not want her disease to become uncontrolled.

How can her regimen be adjusted?

A. Stop pegvisomant, continue octreotide injections

B. Stop both injections, initiate oral octreotide capsules

C. Change octreotide LAR injection to oral octreotide capsules, continue pegvisomant

D. Stop both injections, initiate oral octreotide capsules-cabergoline combination

E. Recommend no changes

Answer: C) Change octreotide LAR injection to oral octreotide capsules, continue pegvisomant

Given this patient's desire to reduce her injection burden, recommending no treatment changes (Answer E) would not be appropriate. Since her disease was not previously controlled on octreotide LAR injection alone (Answer A), it is unlikely to be controlled on only oral octreotide capsules (Answer B), but the capsules are likely to maintain control in combination with pegvisomant (Answer C). The combination of oral octreotide and cabergoline (Answer D) has

Figure 4. Patient's Pituitary MRI, Contrast Enhanced

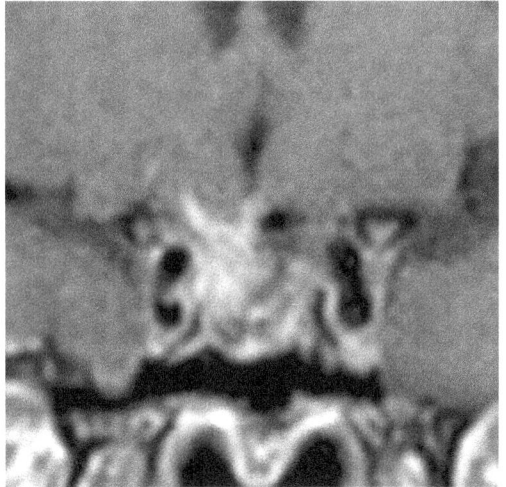

Coronal view

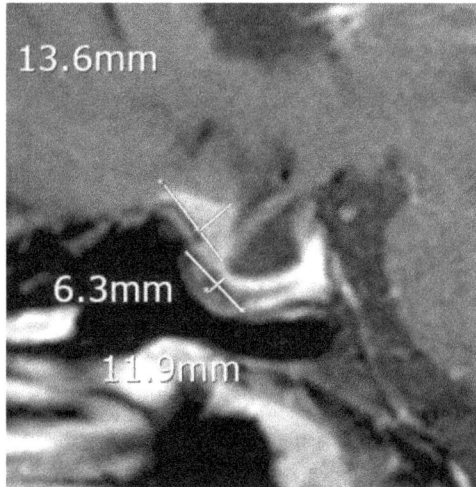

Sagittal view

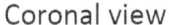

[Color—Print (Color Gallery page CG32) or web & ePub editions]

been studied in just a few patients; however, is also unlikely to main control in highly active biochemical disease. Notably, all combination treatments are used off-label.

Case 2 (continued)

After reviewing her comorbidities, it is noted that she did not have all the recommended screening at diagnosis.

Which of the following tests should be recommended now?

A. Sleep apnea questionnaire, colonoscopy, vertebral x-rays

B. Thyroid ultrasonography, colonoscopy, vertebral x-rays

C. Mammography, colonoscopy, vertebral x-rays

D. Thyroid ultrasonography, vertebral x-rays, hip and knee x-rays

E. No additional testing now

Answer: A) Sleep apnea questionnaire, colonoscopy, vertebral x-rays

Sleep apnea is a very common complication of acromegaly, and every patient should be screened with a questionnaire and referred for a sleep study if there is suspected sleep apnea. Patients with acromegaly are at higher risk of colon cancer; however, mortality rates due to colon cancer are similar to those in the general population. Some experts suggest screening colonoscopy at diagnosis, while others recommend following national guidelines. Since this patient has an additional risk factor for colon cancer—first-degree relative with colon cancer—screening colonoscopy is appropriate despite the patient's younger age (39 years). Thus, this patient should be screened with a sleep apnea questionnaire, colonoscopy, and vertebral x-rays (Answer A).

Thyroid ultrasonography is recommended if thyroid nodule/enlargement is palpated. Mammography is recommended based on standard national/regional guidelines. Joint x-rays are not part of screening recommendations for acromegaly.

Case 3

A 54-year-old woman with seronegative rheumatoid arthritis is found to have a 3.7 × 2.8 × 2.6-cm pituitary macroadenoma with optic chiasm compression during workup for chronic vision changes. (*Figure 5, left, following page*). She has chronic migraines, fatigue, bone aches and muscle cramps and endorses increased ring and shoe size. Her IGF-1 concentration is 412 ng/mL (65-216 ng/mL) (SI: 54.0 nmol/L [8.5-28.3 nmol/L]). The rest of her pituitary function is normal. She undergoes pituitary surgery. Pathologic findings indicate a sparsely granulated somatotroph adenoma. MRI shows postoperative changes with residual tumor (7 × 13 × 15 mm) along the posterior right cavernous sinus. Vision normalizes postoperatively. Her IGF-1 concentration decreases to 240 ng/mL (31.4 nmol/L) 3 months after surgery and to 193 ng/mL (25.3 ng/mL) 6 months after surgery. Two years after surgery, MRI shows residual tumor (*Figure 5, right, following page*). Thyroid and adrenal function remains normal. The patient is not taking glucocorticoids for rheumatoid arthritis. Her hemoglobin A_{1c} value is 5.1% (32 mmol/mol).

Which of the following is the best next step?

A. Continued observation

B. Perform another surgery

C. Administer radiotherapy

D. Initiate an SRL

E. Initiate pegvisomant

Answer: A) Continued observation

This patient remains in remission despite residual tumor. Should IGF-1 or nadir GH on OGTT become elevated, various treatment options may be considered. Surgery (Answer B) with medial wall resection may be considered; however, there is some tumor in the lateral cavernous sinus, which decreases the odds of achieving remission with surgery and comes with risk of cranial nerve dysfunction and diplopia postoperatively.

Figure 5. Patient's Pituitary MRI

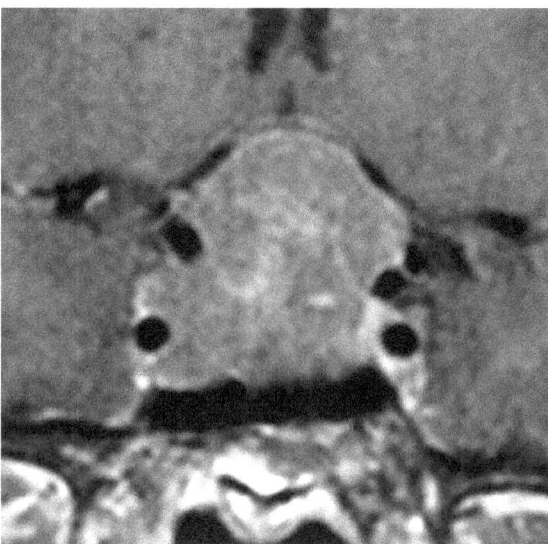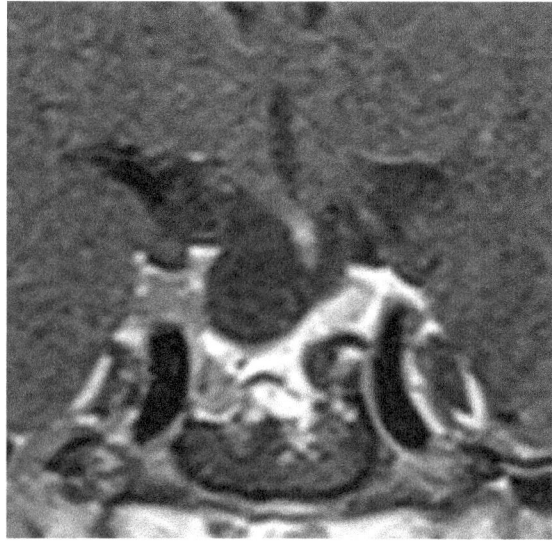

Left, preoperative contrast-enhanced coronal view. Right, postoperative contrast-enhanced coronal view.

SRL therapy (Answer D) is a good option for tumors not completely amenable to surgery, as it allows for control of both IGF-1 and the tumor. In this patient, pasireotide might be discussed first because the tumor is sparsely granulated and patient does not have significant metabolic risk factors.

Pegvisomant (Answer E) is effective for IGF-1 control, but it does not control tumor growth; it would be a good option if used in combination with an SRL.

Radiation (Answer C) would be indicated if there is any tumor growth. This patient has normal pituitary function, and radiation now would increase risk of hypopituitarism.

Key Learning Points

- An elevated IGF-1 value (at least 1.3 times upper limit of normal) in conjunction with classic symptoms and signs usually confirms the diagnosis of acromegaly. A GH value ≥0.4 ng/mL (≥0.4 µg/L) on OGTT using modern GH assays also usually confirms the diagnosis; however, patients with mild acromegaly may have a lower GH concentration (<0.4 ng/mL [(<0.4 µg/L]) on OGTT.

- IGF-1 and GH levels are influenced by different physiologic and pathologic factors and medications. Careful clinical evaluation, repeat testing, and pituitary MRI are necessary for patients in whom suspicion of acromegaly is reasonably high.

- Pituitary surgery is first-line treatment for most patients in the United States. Primary medical therapy is used if surgery is contraindicated, not feasible, or declined by the patient, as well as in patients with "empty sella" and smaller but unresectable adenomas. Preoperative medical therapy may be considered in patients with severe cardiovascular or respiratory complications, but it has not been consistently shown to improve outcomes.

- SRLs (eg, lanreotide and octreotide [injectable and oral]), are commonly implemented as the initial treatment for persistent biochemical/radiologic disease postoperatively. Pegvisomant can be also used as first-line therapy in some patients. If a tumor has characteristics associated with resistance to octreotide and lanreotide, pasireotide LAR could also be first-line medical therapy.

Combination therapy with an SRL and pegvisomant is needed in many patients. Cabergoline is an option in patients with mild acromegaly.

- Radiation therapy is third-line treatment for most patients, particularly those who have large, invasive, or enlarging residual tumors after surgery. Radiation therapy is frequently associated with hypopituitarism, and patients require medical therapy while awaiting effects.

- Screening for comorbidities should be done both at diagnosis and periodically thereafter.

- Quality of life and symptom improvement are important determinants of successful treatment outcomes; clinicians should evaluate symptoms in all patients even after biochemical control is achieved.

Disclosures

MF has received research support to institution from Amryt, Crinetics, Ionis, and Recordati and occasional scientific consulting fees from Amryt, Camurus, Crinetics, Ipsen, and Recordati.

EV received research support to institution from Recordati and Lumiio (Pfizer).

References

1. Fleseriu M, Langlois F, Lim DST, Varlamov EV, Melmed S. Acromegaly: pathogenesis, diagnosis, and management. *Lancet Diabetes Endocrinol.* 2022;10(11):804-826. PMID: 36209758

2. Gadelha MR, Kasuki L, Lim DST, Fleseriu M. Systemic complications of acromegaly and the impact of the current treatment landscape: an update. *Endocr Rev.* 2019;40(1):268-332. PMID: 30184064

3. Giustina A, Barkan A, Beckers A, et al. A consensus on the diagnosis and treatment of acromegaly comorbidities: an update. *J Clin Endocrinol Metab.* 2020;105(4):dgz096. PMID: 31606735

4. Fleseriu M, Biller BMK, Freda PU, Gadelha MR, Giustina A, Katznelson L, et al. A Pituitary Society update to acromegaly management guidelines. *Pituitary.* 2021;24(1):1-13. PMID: 33079318

5. Katznelson L, Laws ER Jr, Melmed S, et al; Endocrine Society. Acromegaly: an Endocrine Society clinical practice guideline. *J Clin Endocrinol Metab.* 2014;99(11):3933-3951. PMID: 25356808

6. Giustina A, Barkhoudarian G, Beckers A, et al. Multidisciplinary management of acromegaly: a consensus. *Rev Endocr Metab Disord.* 2020;21(4):667-678. PMID: 32914330

7. Lim DST, Fleseriu M. Personalized medical treatment of patients with acromegaly: a review. *Endocr Pract.* 2022;28(3):321-332. PMID: 3503649

8. Fleseriu M, Barkan A, Del Pilar Schneider M, et al. Prevalence of comorbidities and concomitant medication use in acromegaly: analysis of real-world data from the United States. *Pituitary.* 2022;5(2):296-307. PMID: 34973139

9. Giustina A, Biermasz N, Casanueva FF, et al; Acromegaly Consensus Group. Consensus on criteria for acromegaly diagnosis and remission. *Pituitary.* 2023 [Online ahead of print] PMID: 37923946

10. Akirov A, Masri-Iraqi H, Dotan I, Shimon I. The biochemical diagnosis of acromegaly. *J Clin Med.* 2021;10(5):1147. PMID: 33803429

11. Schilbach K, Strasburger CJ, Bidlingmaier M. Biochemical investigations in diagnosis and follow up of acromegaly. *Pituitary.* 2017;20(1):33-45. PMID: 28168377

12. Ribeiro-Oliveira A, Jr., Faje AT, Barkan AL. Limited utility of oral glucose tolerance test in biochemically active acromegaly. *Eur J Endocrinol.* 2011;164(1):17-22. PMID: 20926592

13. Bidlingmaier M, Friedrich N, Emeny RT, et al. Reference intervals for insulin-like growth factor-1 (igf-i) from birth to senescence: results from a multicenter study using a new automated chemiluminescence IGF-I immunoassay conforming to recent international recommendations. *J Clin Endocrinol Metab.* 2014;99(5):1712-1721. PMID: 24606072

14. Gadelha MR, Gu F, Bronstein MD, et al. Risk factors and management of pasireotide-associated hyperglycemia in acromegaly. *Endocr Connect.* 2020;9(12):1178-1190. PMID: 33434154

15. Fleseriu M, Fuhrer-Sakel D, van der Lely AJ, et al. More than a decade of real-world experience of pegvisomant for acromegaly: ACROSTUDY. *Eur J Endocrinol.* 2021;185(4):525-538. PMID: 34342594

What to Do? Add Salt, Water, Both, or Neither

Joseph G. Verbalis, MD. Division of Endocrinology and Metabolism, Georgetown University Medical Center, Washington, DC; E-mail: verbalis@georgetown.edu

Educational Objectives

After reviewing this chapter, learners should be able to:

- Explain the rationale for our recent proposal to change the name of *central diabetes insipidus* to *vasopressin deficiency* (AVP-D) and *nephrogenic diabetes insipidus* to *vasopressin resistance* (AVP-R).

- Describe new developments in the differential diagnosis of polyuric disorders, particularly the use of plasma copeptin levels to differentiate among AVP-D, AVP-R, and primary polydipsia.

- Summarize new developments in the diagnosis and treatment of hyponatremic disorders, particularly the syndrome of inappropriate antidiuresis (SIAD).

Significance of the Clinical Problem

Disorders of body fluids are among the most commonly encountered problems in clinical medicine. This is, in large part, because many different disease states can disrupt the finely balanced mechanisms that control the intake and output of water and solute. Because body water is the primary determinant of the osmolality of the extracellular fluid, disorders of water metabolism can be broadly divided into hyperosmolar disorders, in which there is a deficiency of body water relative to body solute, and hypoosmolar disorders, in which there is an excess of body water relative to body solute. Because sodium is the main constituent of plasma osmolality, these disorders are typically characterized by hypernatremia and hyponatremia, respectively.

Practice Gaps

- General unfamiliarity with these disorders by virtue of their relative rarity. Reviewing basic concepts of diagnosis and treatment of AVP-D and AVP-R can enhance an endocrinologist's ability to manage these patients when they present.

- Difficulty with performing water-deprivation tests and the lack of uniform criteria for both executing these tests and interpreting their results. This can be overcome by using newer AVP-stimulation tests with serum copeptin measurements as determinants of adequate or inadequate AVP responses.

- Lack of knowledge about which therapies are suitable for individual patients, including understanding predictors of failure of commonly used therapies such as fluid restriction and isotonic saline administration. Therefore, reviewing basic concepts of diagnosis and treatment of hyponatremia can enhance an endocrinologist's ability to manage these patients when they present.

- There is a general sense that most hyponatremic patients are not affected by modest decreases in serum sodium levels and therefore do not require treatment beyond fluid restriction. There is also concern about the potential production of osmotic demyelination syndrome with overly rapid correction of hyponatremia, which often leads to failure to use more effective methods to correct hyponatremia.

Discussion

Clinical treatment errors have resulted when clinical care providers confuse diabetes insipidus with diabetes mellitus, and there have been several reported fatalities due to withholding inpatient desmopressin therapy. In 2022, an international panel of experts recommended changing the name of diabetes insipidus to AVP-D, previously called central diabetes insipidus, and AVP-R, previously called nephrogenic diabetes insipidus.

Figure 1. Algorithm for Differential Diagnosis of Polyuria–Polydipsia Syndrome

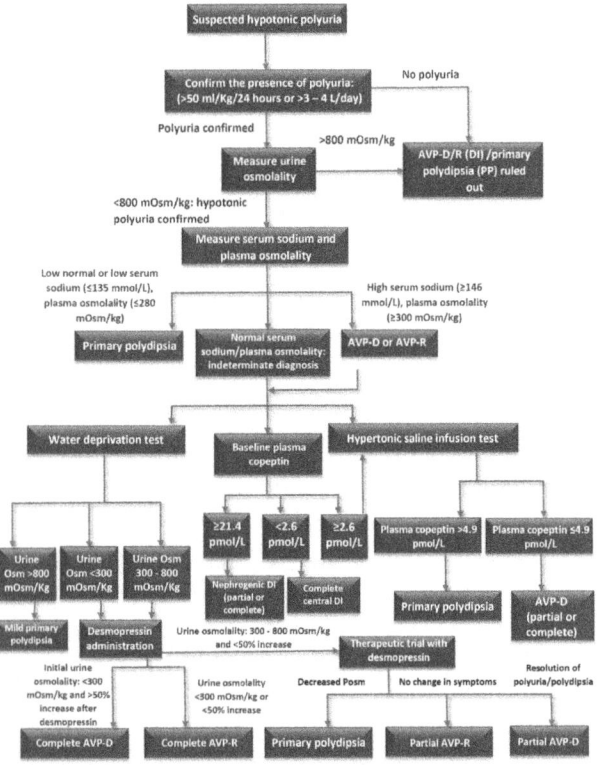

In the first step, polyuria should be confirmed; otherwise polyuria–polydipsia syndrome is excluded and genitourinary (GU) evaluation is needed. In case of polyuria and a urinary osmolality less than 800 mOsm/kg, serum sodium and plasma osmolality are measured. If these concentrations are in the normal range, further differentiation is done using either a classic water-deprivation test or a copeptin-based algorithm (if copeptin measurement is available). Adapted from Gubbi S et al. in Endotext (eds. Feingold KR et al.). © 2000-2024, MDText.com, Inc.

[Color—Print (Color Gallery page CG32) or web & ePub editions]

This recommendation has been endorsed by 8 international endocrine societies and was recently incorporated into the SNOMED International Clinical Terms disease classification system: http://www.snomed.org/.

Appropriate therapy for polyuric disorders is critically dependent on correctly diagnosing AVP-D, AVP-R, or primary polydipsia. The current diagnostic strategy is summarized in *Figure 1*, which will be reviewed during discussion of the clinical vignettes.

Appropriate therapy for hyponatremic disorders is similarly dependent on correctly diagnosing SIAD, hypovolemic hyponatremia, or hypervolemic hyponatremia. The current diagnostic strategy is summarized in *Figure 2* (*following page*), which will be reviewed during discussion of the clinical vignettes.

Clinical Case Vignettes

Case 1

A 77-year-old man is referred by a community endocrinologist for evaluation of possible AVP-D. The patient reports the onset of polyuria and polydipsia 4 years ago after a viral infection that was presumed to be COVID-19 but was never confirmed. The polyuria and polydipsia persisted afterward but have slowly decreased in intensity over time. The patient has kept logs of urine output over the last several months, with values between 2000 and 2875 mL/24 h (weight = 80.1 kg; maximum urine output = 36 mL/kg per 24 h). He notes nocturia once or twice each night and daytime urinary frequency. However, he does not report large volumes of urine with each void. He estimates his fluid intake to be approximately 2.0 L per day. His thirst is described as moderate, and it is usually easily assuaged with small sips of water. He has a long history of bipolar disorder treated with lithium for more than 30 years. When he reported polyuria and polydipsia, his psychiatrist stopped the lithium approximately 1 year ago, without much effect on his polyuria. He also has a history of bladder outlet obstruction, bladder cancer, and benign prostatic hypertrophy currently being treated with tamsulosin, 0.4 mg twice daily. His other medications include quetiapine, 300 mg daily, and atorvastatin, 20 mg daily. Additional testing after an 8-hour overnight fluid deprivation shows the following:

Sodium = 144 mEq/L (SI: 144 mmol/L)
Serum urea nitrogen (BUN) = 24 mg/dL (SI: 8.6 mmol/L)
Creatinine = 1.35 mg/dL (SI: 119.3 μmol/L)
Estimated glomerular filtration rate = 54 mL/min per 1.73 m^2
Plasma osmolality = 301 mOsm/kg (SI: 301 mmol/kg)
Urinary osmolality = 390 mOsm/kg (SI: 390 mmol/kg)
Hemoglobin A$_{1c}$ = 5.9% (41 mmol/mol)
Free T$_4$ = 1.4 ng/dL (SI: 18.0 pmol/L)
TSH = 1.42 mIU/L
Uric acid = 6.3 mg/dL (SI: 374.8 μmol/L)
Lithium chloride = <0.1 mmol/L

Laboratory results are thought to be most consistent with AVP-D.

Which of the following is the best first step to distinguish AVP-R from AVP-D?

A. Overnight fluid-deprivation test

B. Desmopressin challenge

C. Plasma AVP measurement

D. Serum copeptin measurement

Answer: D) Serum copeptin measurement (Answer C is not the best option, but not wrong)

Evaluation consisted of a single morning serum copeptin measurement, which was elevated to 22.8 pmol/L and confirmed the diagnosis of AVP-R. An elevated plasma AVP level has long been a diagnostic feature of AVP-R. But because of variability in immunochemical assays for AVP, formal criteria for making this diagnosis have not been described. The development of the BHRAHMS copeptin assay has enabled formal criteria to be developed, and a cutoff of 21.4 pmol/L in a baseline plasma sample has 100% specificity and sensitivity for this diagnosis, without need for further testing.[1] This case was confusing to the referring endocrinologist because the patient had discontinued lithium

Figure 2. Algorithm for Evaluation and Treatment of Patients With Hypoosmolality

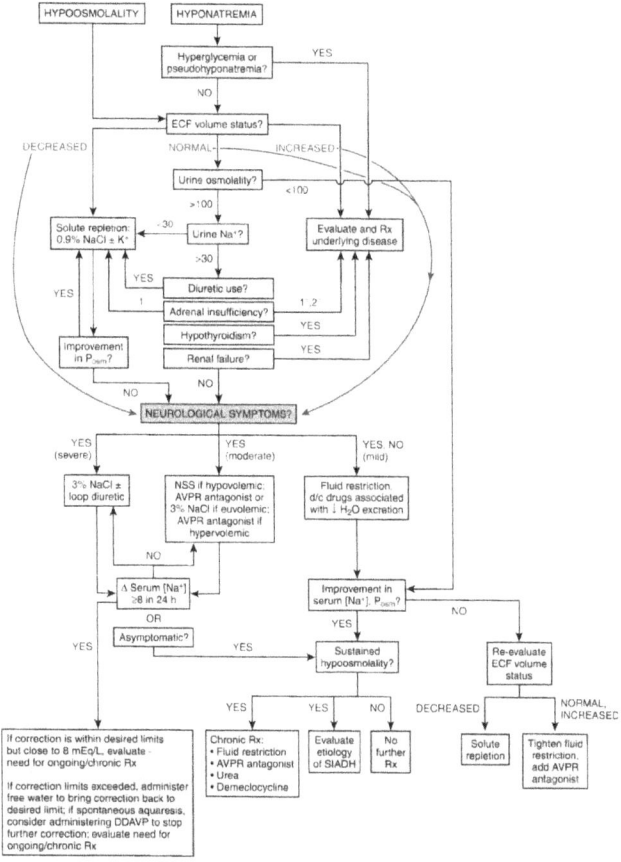

The dark red arrow in the center emphasizes that the presence of CNS dysfunction resulting from hyponatremia should always be assessed immediately, so that appropriate therapy can be started as soon as possible in significantly symptomatic patients, even while the outlined diagnostic evaluation is proceeding. Values for osmolality are in mOsm/kg H$_2$O, and those referring to serum [Na$^+$] are in mmol/L. Abbreviations: Δ, change (in concentration); 1°, primary; 2°, secondary; AVPR, arginine vasopressin receptor; d/c, discontinue; DDAVP, desmopressin; ECF, extracellular fluid volume; Posm, plasma osmolality; Rx, treatment; SIADH, syndrome of inappropriate antidiuretic hormone secretion. Reprinted from Verbalis JG. Hyponatremia and hypoosmolar disorders. In National Kidney Foundation's Primer on Kidney Diseases, 8th edition, edited by Gilbert SJ & Weiner DE. Elsevier Saunders, Philadelphia: 62-70, 2023.

[Color—Print (Color Gallery page CG33) or web & ePub editions]

therapy more than a year ago, and the intercurrent COVID-19 infection raised concern for CNS effects and AVP-D. Polyuria due to impaired urinary concentrating ability occurs in up to 20% of patients treated with long-term lithium therapy; an additional 30% have a subclinical impairment in concentrating ability.[2] These effects are mediated by lithium entry into the principal cells in the collecting tubule via the epithelial sodium channel (ENaC), where lithium inhibits signaling pathways that involve glycogen synthase kinase type 3β (GSK3β), resulting in dysfunction of the aquaporin-2 water channels. Most cases of lithium-induced AVP-R resolve after discontinuation of lithium therapy, but AVP-R often becomes irreversible after many years of use.[3] Although the mechanism is incompletely understood, it is thought to be the result of a chronic tubulointerstitial nephropathy. One potential confounder in this case is the patient's underlying chronic kidney disease, which has been shown to elevate serum copeptin levels.[4] However, this effect is most marked with an estimated glomerular filtration rate less than 50 mL/min per 1.73 m^2, which should not have affected this case.

Case 2

A 54-year-old woman saw an ophthalmologist because of symptoms of haziness in her left eye for the last 6 weeks. Evaluation included a brain MRI that identified a 1.5-cm sellar and suprasellar cystic mass. Following neurosurgical consultation, she underwent endoscopic resection last year. Postoperative course was uneventful without development of AVP-D, and the patient was discharged on postoperative day 3 on hydrocortisone replacement. Pathologic findings were consistent with a Rathke cleft cyst. On postoperative day 5, she developed tremors, restlessness, insomnia, and nausea. Her family reported decreased oral intake of food and fluids. She came to the emergency department on postoperative day 7 and was found to have serum sodium concentration of 111 mEq/L (111 mmol/L). She had no headache, vision changes, focal weakness, numbness or paresthesias, or systemic symptoms. Vital signs were normal.

Laboratory test results in the emergency department:

> Sodium = 111 mEq/L (SI: 111 mmol/L)
> Potassium = 4.1 mEq/L (SI: 4.1 mmol/L)
> BUN = 6 mg/dL (SI: 2.1 mmol/L)
> Creatinine = 0.49 mg/dL (SI: 43.3 μmol/L)
> Glucose = 131 mg/dL (SI: 7.3 mmol/L)
> Plasma osmolality = 231 mOsm/kg (SI: 231 mmol/kg)

> Urine osmolality = 735 mOsm/kg (SI: 735 mmol/kg)
> Urinary sodium (spot urine) = 81 mmol/L
> Total T$_3$ = 118.7 ng/mL (SI: 1.8 nmol/L)

Which of the following is the most likely cause of this patient's hyponatremia?

A. Hyponatremic hyponatremia due to nausea and poor oral intake

B. Secondary adrenal insufficiency due to failure to take hydrocortisone replacement

C. Isolated second phase of a triphasic response

D. Cerebral salt wasting

E. SIAD from postoperative subarachnoid hemorrhage

Answer: C) Isolated second phase of a triphasic response

Transient hyponatremia without preceding or subsequent AVP-D has been reported after transsphenoidal surgery for pituitary microadenomas, and it generally occurs 5 to 10 days postoperatively. The incidence may be as high as 30% when these patients are carefully followed up, although most cases are mild and self-limited.[5] This is due to inappropriate AVP secretion via the same mechanism as in the triphasic response, namely uncontrolled AVP release from the degenerating nerve terminals of damaged AVP neurons in the posterior pituitary.[6] However, in these cases, only the second phase occurs (isolated second phase) because the initial neural lobe or pituitary stalk damage is not sufficient to impair AVP secretion enough to produce clinical manifestations of AVP-D, which requires greater than 80% loss of AVP neuronal cell bodies.

Hypovolemic hyponatremia due to solute deficiency is eliminated by the elevated urinary spot sodium, which is generally less than 30 mmol/L in volume-depleted patients who have not taken diuretics in the last 24 hours.[7] Secondary adrenal insufficiency commonly causes hyponatremia,[8] but rarely causes hyponatremia this severe or such elevated urine osmolality; replacement with stress-dose hydrocortisone is always indicated until serum cortisol levels are reported. Cerebral salt wasting has never been documented after transsphenoidal surgery, and is not supported in this case considering the absence of any signs of volume depletion (hypotension, tachycardia, elevated BUN-to-creatinine ratio).[9] Subarachnoid hemorrhage causes hyponatremia in 50% of cases, and although rare after uncomplicated transsphenoidal surgery, it is usually caused by SIAD[10] and should be evaluated with brain imaging.

Treatment is dependent on neurological symptomatology. In cases of mild asymptomatic hyponatremia, fluid restriction while waiting for depletion of AVP stores in the damaged posterior pituitary terminals is sufficient and generally occurs within 2 to 14 days.[5] However, with more severe symptomatic hyponatremia, treatment should be initiated promptly with therapies effective at rapidly increasing the serum sodium (eg, 3% NaCl, vasopressin receptor antagonists).[7]

Case 3

A 38-year-old woman is admitted to the hospital for progressively altered mental status, disorientation, and confabulatory speech with a serum sodium concentration of 121 mEq/L (121 mmol/L). She has a history of chronic alcoholism, pancreatitis with pseudocyst, eating disorder (bulimia), and hypothyroidism.

Vital signs are stable, and she appears euvolemic on clinical examination. Her weight is 90.2 lb (40.9 kg) (BMI = 14.5 kg/m²). She is not taking antidepressants or diuretics.

Laboratory test results from the emergency department:

Sodium = 121 mEq/L (SI: 121 mmol/L)
Potassium = 2.3 mEq/L (SI: 2.3 mmol/L)
BUN = 7 mg/dL (SI: 2.5 mmol/L)
Creatinine = 0.59 mg/dL (SI: 52.2 μmol/L)
Plasma osmolality, not measured
Urine osmolality, not measured
Urinary sodium, not measured
TSH = 17.1 mIU/L
Bilirubin = 1.6 mg/dL (SI: 27.4 μmol/L)
ALT = 83 U/L (SI: 1.39 μkat/L)

Brain CT documents no acute intracranial abnormality. There is mild global parenchymal volume loss.

Which of the following therapies is the best recommendation at this time?

A. Begin fluid restriction to 800 mL per day

B. Begin isotonic (0.9%) NaCl at 1 L over 1 hour, then 100 mL/h

C. Begin hypertonic (3%) NaCl at 40 mL/h

D. Start NaCl tablets, 1 g 3 times daily with meals

E. Start urea, 15 g orally twice daily

F. Administer tolvaptan, 15 mg orally

Answer: B) Begin isotonic (0.9%) NaCl at 1 L over 1 hour, then 100 mL/h

Urine studies are generally not available for patients presenting to the emergency department with hyponatremia, so initial therapy should be based on clinical characteristics. Despite absence of clinical signs of volume depletion, a patient with chronic alcoholism and an eating disorder should be assumed to be volume depleted until proven otherwise. Hypokalemia in the absence of diuretic therapy is most consistent with solute depletion and is not a common finding in SIAD. Whenever hypovolemic hyponatremia is a possibility, initial treatment with isotonic NaCl (1.0-2.0 L) is appropriate. Improvement in the serum sodium supports the diagnosis, whereas failure to increase the serum sodium indicates a more likely diagnosis of SIAD and the need for fluid restriction or more effective therapies for SIAD (eg, 3% NaCl, vasopressin receptor antagonists, urea).[7]

This patient should be assumed to have chronic hyponatremia based on her history. Treatment of hypovolemic hyponatremia with isotonic saline infusion frequently leads to an overly rapid correction of serum sodium. This is because a large part of the hyponatremia is due to water retention caused by baroreceptor-mediated endogenous AVP secretion. As the extracellular fluid volume is normalized, the stimuli to AVP secretion decreases to the point where a free water diuresis ("aquaresis") occurs.

The resulting free water excretion corrects the serum sodium much more quickly than predicted by the infusion of isotonic NaCl. In such cases, limits to the rate of correction should be observed. For patients not at increased risk for osmotic demyelination syndrome, a correction of 10 to 12 mEq/L (10-12 mmol/L) in the first 24 hours and 18 mEq/L (18 mmol/L) in the first 18 hours is thought to be safe. However, if there are risk factors for osmotic demyelination syndrome (serum sodium <105 mEq/L [<105 mmol/L], hypokalemia, alcoholism, malnutrition, severe liver disease), then the correction should be limited to no more than 8 mEq/L (8 mmol/L) in any 24-hour period.[7] Since this patient has several of the defined osmotic demyelination syndrome risk factors, the initial correction should be stopped after an increase in serum sodium of 8 mEq/L (8 mmol/L). This is accomplished by discontinuing isotonic saline and infusing D5W at a rate to match the urine output. If the urine output is very high, desmopressin should be administered (2 mcg intravenously or subcutaneously every 8 hours) until it is safe to allow the aquaresis to continue.[7] Although recent retrospective reviews have shown the prevalence of osmotic demyelination syndrome to be less than 0.5%,[11] a general consensus of experts is that correction limits should still be observed in patients with serum sodium concentration less than 120 mEq/L (<120 mmol/L) or in patients with osmotic demyelination syndrome risk factors.[12]

Case 4

An 81-year-old man with a history of coronary artery disease status post coronary artery bypass grafting, prediabetes, hypertension, and hyperlipidemia presents for evaluation of chronic hyponatremia. Serum sodium has been documented to be as low as 125 to 128 mEq/L (125-128 mmol/L) since 2015. The patient reported unsteady gait and multiple falls. Past falls have resulted in wrist and multiple rib fractures.

Vital signs are stable and the patient is euvolemic on clinical examination. His weight is 187.6 lb (85.1 kg) (BMI = 28.4 kg/m²). He does not take antidepressants or diuretics. The patient and his wife estimate a fluid intake of 2 L per day, and he does not restrict salt intake.

Laboratory test results:

Sodium = 127 mEq/L (SI: 127 mmol/L)
Potassium = 4.6 mEq/L (SI: 4.6 mmol/L)
BUN =16 mg/dL (SI: 5.7 mmol/L)
Creatinine = 0.92 mg/dL (SI: 81.3 μmol/L)
Plasma osmolality = 270 mOsm/kg (SI: 270 mmol/kg)
Urine osmolality = 397 mOsm/kg (SI: 397 mmol/kg)
Urinary sodium (spot urine) = 73 mmol/L
TSH = 0.58 mIU/L
Fasting plasma glucose = 98 mg/dL (SI: 5.4 mmol/L)
Serum cortisol (8 AM) = 10.4 μg/dL
    (SI: 286.9 nmol/L)

Which of the following tests is the best recommendation?

A. Plasma copeptin measurement

B. Plasma AVP measurement

C. DXA to assess bone mineral density

D. Chest CT

E. 24-Hour urine for sodium excretion

Answer: C) DXA to assess bone mineral density

Chronic hyponatremia is particularly more common in elderly individuals, with reported incidences from 7% to 53% in ambulatory and institutionalized geriatric patients. Epidemiological studies have confirmed a marked age-related increase in the prevalence of hyponatremia.[13] This has been ascribed to multiple factors that impair water homeostasis in elderly persons, including comorbidities such as cardiac, liver, and kidney diseases; drugs such as diuretics and antidepressants; abnormal suppression of thirst by plasma volume expansion; and enhanced osmotically stimulated AVP secretion with an inability to suppress AVP secretion during fluid intake or administration.[13] Thus, the elderly population is at increased risk for disturbances of water homeostasis due to both intrinsic disease and iatrogenic causes.

Although chronic hyponatremia has been described as "asymptomatic" and is largely untreated, the long-term adverse effects of hyponatremia have not been carefully evaluated in controlled studies. Accumulating evidence strongly suggests that chronic hyponatremia is not a benign condition. Recent clinical data have suggested that even mild hyponatremia is associated with increased mortality and has significant unrecognized effects on cognition and gait stability, which is likely related to an observed increased incidence of falls in hyponatremic patients relative to normonatremic patients. Thus, patients with levels of hyponatremia previously considered to be "asymptomatic" have significant cognitive deficits and gait disturbances, both of which can contribute to an increased incidence of falls and subsequent fracture risk, as well as overall increased mortality, in this vulnerable and frail population.

Although the increased susceptibility of hyponatremic patients to falls in itself represents a significant risk factor for fractures because of the age-associated decrease in bone mineral density in elderly patients, this risk would be amplified if hyponatremia aggravates the bone loss in patients with postmenopausal and senile osteoporosis. Studies in experimental animals indicate that hyponatremia causes marked bone loss in a well-established animal model of human SIAD.[14] These results were extended to humans via epidemiological analysis of the NHANES III database, suggesting that osteoporosis occurred at a significantly increased odds ratio in hyponatremic persons older than 50 years compared with incidence in participants with a normal serum sodium concentration. Of note, the mean serum sodium concentration in hyponatremic participants in NHANES III was only 133 ± 0.2 mmol/L, suggesting that even mild hyponatremia is associated with decreased bone mineral density by DXA.[14]

Numerous independent reports have since verified that hyponatremia is associated with increased fracture rates. These include retrospective studies of the incidence of hyponatremia in patients presenting with fractures in Belgium and New York; retrospective analysis of the incidence of fractures in women with early kidney disease in Ireland; and an increased incidence of fractures in elderly individuals with mild hyponatremia in the Netherlands and Argentina.[15] Epidemiological analysis of 2.9 million patients in our health system demonstrated markedly increased odds ratios of both osteoporosis and fragility fractures in patients with hyponatremia, with risks proportional to the duration and severity of hyponatremia.[16] Thus, it is now recognized that hyponatremia represents a significant and independent risk factor for osteoporosis, fractures, and mortality worldwide, particularly in the elderly population.

This patient has already had multiple fragility fractures and reports numerous falls. DXA would provide important information regarding bone mineral density and potential treatment options with antiresorptive therapies, since hyponatremia primarily induces a resorptive osteoporosis.[15]

Key Learning Points

- Understanding of the basic physiology of water homeostasis and the critical role that AVP plays in maintaining normal water balance in turn enables an understanding of the pathogenesis of all disorders of water homeostasis, including AVP-D and AVP-R, and disorders of SIAD and nonosmotic vasopressin secretion.

- Plasma copeptin offers a more reliable measure of AVP secretion that will replace measurement of plasma AVP as a determinant of AVP-D and AVP-R.

- Transient hyponatremia after transsphenoidal surgery is due to an isolated second phase of the triphasic response to pituitary stalk section.

- Well-defined risk factors for osmotic demyelination syndrome have been characterized. In the absence of risk factors, corrections of 10 to 12 mEq/L (10-12 mmol/L) per 24 hours appear to be overwhelmingly safe. However, in patients with any risk factors for osmotic demyelination syndrome, correction limits of 8 mEq/L or less (≤8 mmol/L) per 24 hours should still be observed.

- The greatest risk of overly rapid correction occurs following aquaresis in hypovolemic hyponatremic patients treated with volume repletion (either with normal saline solution or 3% NaCl).

- In most patients, achieving a serum sodium concentration of 130 to 134 mEq/L (130-134 mmol/L) is sufficient to prevent most adverse effects of hyponatremia, including risk of osteoporosis, falls, and fragility fractures. However, in older patients with increased risk of falls and fractures, normalization of serum sodium is preferable.

- All patients with chronic hyponatremia (>1 year duration) should have evaluation of bone quality by DXA and antiresorptive therapy if the hyponatremia cannot be corrected.

References

1. Christ-Crain M, Bichet DG, Fenske WK, Goldman MB, Rittig S, Verbalis JG, Verkman AS. Diabetes insipidus. *Nat Rev Dis Primers*. 2019;5(1):54. PMID: 31395885

2. Grunfeld J-P, Rossier BC. Lithium nephrotoxicity revisited. *Nat Rev Nephrol*. 2009;5(5):270-276. PMID: 19384328

3. Thompson CJ, France AJ, Baylis PH. Persistent nephrogenic diabetes insipidus following lithium therapy. *Scott Med J*. 1997;42(1):16-17. PMID: 9226773

4. Roussel R, Fezeu L, Marre M, et al. Comparison between copeptin and vasopressin in a population from the community and in people with chronic kidney disease. *J Clin Endocrinol Metab*. 2014;99(12):4656-4663. PMID: 25202818

5. Olson BR, Rubino D, Gumowski J, Oldfield EH. Isolated hyponatremia after transsphenoidal pituitary surgery. *J Clin Endocrinol Metab*. 1995;80(1):85-91. PMID: 7829644

6. Ultmann MC, Hoffman GE, Nelson PB, Robinson AG. Transient hyponatremia after damage to the neurohypophyseal tracts. *Neuroendocrinology*. 1992;56(6):803-811. PMID: 1369588

7. Verbalis JG, Goldsmith SR, Greenberg A, et al. Diagnosis, evaluation, and treatment of hyponatremia: expert panel recommendations. *Am J Med*. 2013;126(10 Suppl 1):S1-S42. PMID: 24074529

8. Garrahy A, Thompson CJ. Hyponatremia and glucocorticoid deficiency. *Front Horm Res*. 2019;52:80-92. PMID: 32097946

9. Verbalis JG. The curious story of cerebral salt wasting: fact or fiction? *Clin J Am Soc Nephrol*. 2020;15(11):1666-1668. PMID: 32611661

10. Hannon MJ, Behan LA, O'Brien MMC, et al. Hyponatremia following mild/moderate subarachnoid hemorrhage is due to SIAD and glucocorticoid deficiency and not cerebral salt wasting. *J Clin Endocrinol Metab*. 2014;99(1):291-298. PMID: 24248182

11. George JC, Zafar W, Bucaloiu ID, Chang AR. Risk factors and outcomes of rapid correction of severe hyponatremia. *Clin J Am Soc Nephrol*. 2018;13(7):984-992. PMID: 29871886

12. Sterns RH, Rondon-Berrios H, Adrogue HJ, et al; PRONATREOUS Investigators. Treatment guidelines for hyponatremia: stay the course. *Clin J Am Soc Nephrol*. 2023;19(1):129-135. PMID: 37379081

13. Cowen LE, Hodak SP, Verbalis JG. Age-associated abnormalities of water homeostasis. *Endocrinol Metab Clin North Am*. 2023;52(2):277-293. PMID: 36948780

14. Verbalis JG, Barsony J, Sugimura Y, et al. Hyponatremia-induced osteoporosis. *J Bone Miner Res*. 2010;25(3):554-563. PMID: 19751154

15. Barsony J, Kleess L, Verbalis JG. Hyponatremia is linked to bone loss, osteoporosis, fragility and bone fractures. *Front Horm Res*. 2019;52:49-60. PMID: 32097915

16. Usala RL, Fernandez SJ, Mete M, et al. Hyponatremia is associated with increased osteoporosis and bone fractures in a large US health system population. *J Clin Endocrinol Metab*. 2015;100(8):3021-3031. PMID: 26083821

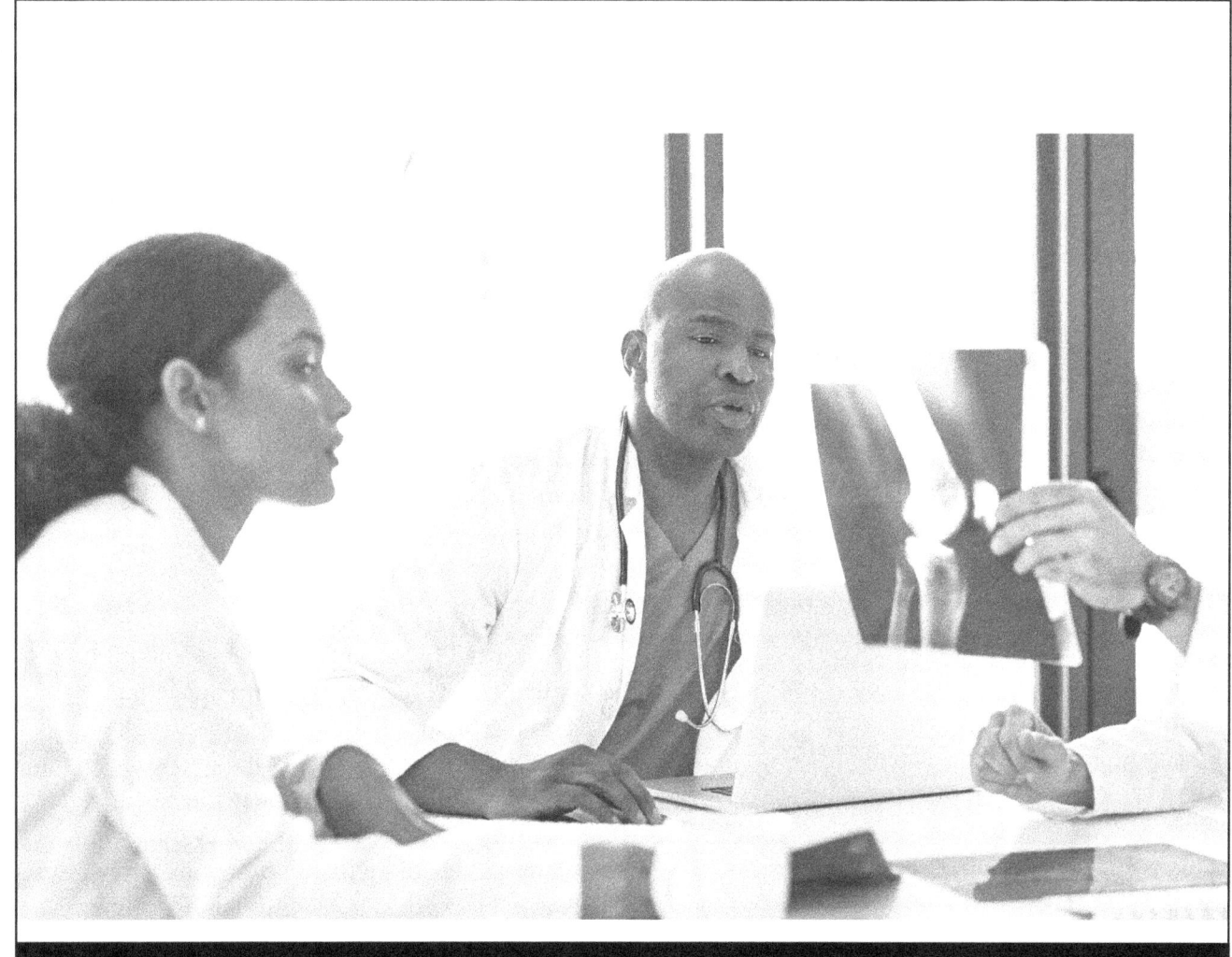

PEDIATRIC
ENDOCRINOLOGY

Approach to Triglyceride Management in Youth

Ambika P. Ashraf, MD. Division of Pediatric Endocrinology and Diabetes, University of Alabama at Birmingham, Birmingham, AL; Email: aashraf@uabmc.edu

Educational Objectives

After reviewing this chapter, learners should be able to:

- Illustrate the pathophysiology of hypertriglyceridemia (HTG).

- Discuss the differential diagnosis of HTG in youth, emphasizing lipid phenotype analysis.

- Explain the pivotal role of diet, lifestyle modifications, and medications in comprehensive management of HTG.

Significance of the Clinical Problem

HTG is typically diagnosed when the fasting plasma concentration of triglycerides (TG) exceeds a specified threshold (eg, >150 mg/dL [>1.7 mmol/L]). There are several classifications for HTG. In this chapter, the classification of HTG follows the 2012 Endocrine Society Guidelines based on concentration of fasting plasma TG: mild HTG (150-199 mg/dL [1.7-2.3 mmol/L]), moderate HTG (200-999 mg/dL [2.3-11.2 mmol/L]), severe HTG (1000-1999 mg/dL [11.2-22.4 mmol/L]), and very severe HTG (≥2000 mg/dL [≥22.4 mmol/L]).[1]

Ideally, TG are measured after a 10- to 12-hour fast. However, from a practical standpoint, a nonfasting sample is becoming an emerging trend. Despite the increase in TG postprandially, other lipid measurements, such as total cholesterol, low-density lipoprotein cholesterol (LDL-C), and high-density lipoprotein cholesterol (HDL-C), exhibit minimal changes in response to an average meal intake in most individuals.[2] TG concentrations on average increase by only 17.7 to 35.4 mg/dL (0.2-0.4 mmol/L) 2 to 6 hours after eating a typical meal. However, in patients with HTG, TG concentrations can increase by up to 4 times following a meal, indicating their inability to clear postprandial lipids.[2] If a nonfasting TG measurement is elevated, fasting TG can be measured.

Plasma TG concentration represents all circulating TG-rich lipoproteins, including chylomicron (originating in the intestine), very low-density lipoprotein (VLDL), and some amount of remnant lipoproteins, namely intermediate-density lipoprotein.[3] In general, chylomicrons and intermediate-density lipoproteins are swiftly removed from the plasma through hydrolysis of TG by lipoprotein lipase (LPL). Thus, in most individuals in the fasting state, the plasma TG concentration reflects the concentration of VLDL. HTG is due to increased production of TG-rich lipoproteins, impaired clearance of TG-rich lipoproteins, or a combination of both factors.

Practice Gaps

- While elevated plasma TG concentration (HTG) is frequently encountered in clinical practice, specific management recommendations are limited. Mild to moderate HTG is a recognized risk factor for premature cardiovascular disease.

- In cases where mild to moderate HTG is observed (ie, in insulin-resistant conditions such as type 2 diabetes), the lipid phenotype is that of combined dyslipidemia characterized by elevated TG, low HDL-C, variable LDL-C, and persistently elevated non–HDL-C.

However, non–HDL-C is not recommended as a therapeutic target by the American Heart Association, American Diabetes Association, or International Society for Pediatric and Adolescent Diabetes.

- The heightened risk of acute pancreatitis associated with severe HTG is acknowledged; however, clear and defined dietary and pharmacotherapeutic approaches for management of severe HTG are currently lacking.

Discussion

Pathophysiology of HTG

Understanding the pathophysiology of HTG, particularly TG metabolism, is crucial for developing effective treatment approaches. Dietary fat is solubilized in the proximal small intestine by the bile acid micelles, which are hydrolyzed into fatty acids and monoacylglycerol. Once absorbed into enterocytes, these are reassembled into triacyl glycerols and ultimately form chylomicrons, which carry apolipoprotein B_{48}, These chylomicrons are then directed to various tissues to serve as an energy source. TG undergo lipid hydrolysis by the LPL enzyme. The remaining chylomicron remnants are taken up by the liver. Synthesis of VLDL by hepatocytes involves deriving TG content from various sources such as chylomicron remnants, free fatty acids, and de novo fatty acids synthesized from carbohydrates. Increased dietary fat and carbohydrate intake, as well as insulin resistance, lead to excessive production of TG-rich VLDL. Subsequently, hepatic lipase further releases free fatty acids from VLDL to produce intermediate-density lipoproteins. Cholesteryl ester transfer protein mediates lipid exchange between HDL and apolipoprotein B–containing lipoproteins, contributing to small, dense atherogenic LDL and reduced HDL in persons with HTG.

Etiology

Etiologies of HTG include genetic and acquired causes (*Table 1, following page*). Some specific primary HTG conditions such as familial HTG, familial combined hyperlipidemia, hypoalphalipoproteinemia, and familial dysbetalipoproteinemia require a secondary factor for the expression of HTG.

Evaluation and Management of HTG

Mild to Moderate HTG

Etiologies of HTG include polygenic HTG and primary HTG. Mild to moderate HTG often results from the cumulative effect of common and rare gene variants[3] triggered or exacerbated by secondary factors. Taking a comprehensive family history regarding dyslipidemia and cardiovascular disease is crucial for evaluating genetic factors and predicting future cardiovascular risk. Non–HDL-C (calculated as total cholesterol minus HDL)[4-6] can be used as a guide for management, particularly in the nonfasting states and in patients with TG concentrations of 400 mg/dL or greater (≥4.5 mmol/L) (as LDL-C cannot be accurately calculated using the Friedewald equation). Alternatively, the blood concentration of atherogenic lipoprotein particles can be assessed by measuring apolipoprotein B. Routine genetic testing is not justified in cases of mild to moderate HTG.

Three aspects of management include lifestyle changes, management of secondary factors, and pharmacotherapy. Lifestyle changes include weight reduction in patients with obesity or overweight. Most patients experience 10% to 70% reduction in TG levels with weight loss. Dietary recommendations are listed in *Table 2* (*following pages*).[7] TG response to dietary changes varies and up to 70% reduction can be observed depending on baseline concentration. Physical activity and exercise recommendations include 60 minutes of moderate to vigorous physical activity daily,[5,8] and these efforts can reduce TG by up to 30%. Secondary causes such as obesity, metabolic syndrome, type 2 diabetes, hypothyroidism, autoimmune conditions, concomitant use of medications must be ruled out and treated if identified.

Table 1. Etiology and Lipid Phenotype of HTG

Disorder	Etiology	Defect	Lipid phenotype	Triggers
Genetic forms of HTG				
Familial chylomicronemia syndrome	Autosomal recessive, monogenic: pathogenic variants in *LPL, APOC2, APOA5, LMF1, GPIHBP1*	Hyperchylomicronemia	TG >1000 mg/dL (>11.2 mmol/L)	Dietary fat
Familial combined hyperlipidemia	Autosomal dominant with variable penetrance	Apolipoprotein B$_{100}$ overproduction	Combined hyperlipidemia TG <500 mg/dL (<5.6 mmol/L)	Can progress to severe HTG in the presence of secondary factors
Familial HTG	Autosomal dominant	Enlarged VLDL	TG <500 mg/dL (<5.6 mmol/L) Normal LDL-C and HDL-C	Can progress to severe HTG in the presence of secondary factors
Dysbetalipoproteinemia	Complex, autosomal recessive	APOE pathogenic variants (E2/E2 genotype)	Equal elevation of TG and cholesterol (remnant particle)	In conjunction with familial combined hyperlipidemia or secondary causes
Familial hypoalphalipoproteinemia	Tangier disease, autosomal dominant LCAT deficiency, autosomal recessive		Elevated TG and low HDL-C TG <500 mg/dL (<5.6 mmol/L)	
Acquired: secondary factors triggering HTG manifestation*				
Multifactorial chylomicronemia syndrome	Multifactorial	Secondary factors*	TG >1000 mg/dL (>11.2 mmol/L)	
Acquired HTG	Polygenic	Secondary factors*	Combined hyperlipidemia TG <500 mg/dL (<5.6 mmol/L)	Can progress to severe HTG in the presence of secondary factors

Abbreviations: HTG, hypertriglyceridemia; LCAT, familial lecithin cholesterol acyltransferase; LDL-C, low-density lipoprotein cholesterol; TG, triglycerides; VLDL, very low-density lipoprotein.

*Secondary factors: obesity or overweight; sedentary habits; highly processed, nutrient-dense food with high-glycemic index or high-fat content; metabolic syndrome; type 2 diabetes; hypothyroidism; metabolic dysfunction-associated steatotic liver disease; kidney disease; alcohol use; chronic inflammatory conditions such systemic lupus erythematosus; concomitant use of medications; and lipodystrophies.

Severe HTG

Etiology of severe HTG includes familial chylomicronemia syndrome and multifactorial chylomicronemia syndrome. The primary management objective is to prevent pancreatitis. In cases of very severe HTG, dietary fat restriction becomes crucial due to accumulation of chylomicrons. Thus, taking in nothing by mouth is very effective in lowering TG. In insulin-resistant or -deficient scenarios, intravenous insulin infusion can significantly decrease the TG concentration (up to 40%).[9,10] Fasting combined with intravenous insulin can lead to an impressive 80% reduction in TG levels within 24 hours.[11] Hospitalization is recommended for patients with abdominal pain and pancreatitis in the presence of very severe HTG. Once the risk for pancreatitis has been addressed, the foundation for management primarily relies on lifestyle interventions. Dietary recommendations for severe HTG include strict fat-reduced diet (10%-15% of total daily calories as fat).[7] Abstaining from alcohol is essential. A 5% to 10% weight reduction is

Table 2. Management of Hypertriglyceridemia

Rule out and manage secondary causes; optimize glycemic control; stop alcohol use (if any)				
Moderate to vigorous physical activity for 1 hour daily				
Weight-loss goal 5%-10% (if patient has obesity or overweight)				
Macronutrient composition: reduce simple sugar and high-glycemic index food intake; reduce fructose intake reduce total carbohydrate intake replace trans and saturated fats with monounsaturated fats, and increase dietary omega-3 fatty acids				
Fasting TG	<500 mg/dL (<5.6 mmol/L)	500-999 mg/dL (5.6-11.2 mmol/L)	1000-1999 mg/dL (11.2-22.4 mmol/L)	>2000 mg/dL (>22.4 mmol/L)
Total dietary fat	No reduction	20%-25% total dietary calories	10%-15% total dietary calories	Nothing by mouth
Dietary added sugars	<6%	<5%	Eliminate	Nothing by mouth
Pharmacotherapy	Statin for increased LDL-C and/or non-HDL-C	Fibrates/omega-3 fatty acids	Fibrates/omega-3 fatty acids	Not effective

Abbreviations: LDL-C, low-density lipoprotein cholesterol; non–HDL-C, non–high-density lipoprotein cholesterol; TG, triglycerides.

suggested if the patient has obesity or overweight. Secondary factors contribute to exacerbation of HTG. Hence, optimizing glycemic control and managing other secondary causes are important.

Pharmacotherapy

Mild to moderate HTG

- **TG <500 mg/dL (<5.6 mmol/L)** Treatment is aimed at reducing the global cardiovascular disease risk. The first treatment target is LDL-C; if LDL-C is close to goal, then non–HDL-C is the target. Drug choice is a statin.

- **TG >500 mg/dL (>5.6 mmol/L)** Treatment is aimed at reducing fasting TG concentration with a fibrate or omega-3 fatty acids.

Severe HTG

- Medications are not useful in patients with familial chylomicronemia syndrome. Fibrates and omega-3 fatty acids can be used in patients with multifactorial chylomicronemia syndrome. However, when the TG concentration exceeds 1770 mg/dL

(>20 mmol/L), fibrates and omega-3 fatty acids show no therapeutic effect.

Clinical Case Vignettes
Case 1

A 15-year-old girl with class 3 obesity (BMI = 44 kg/m²) presents with severe HTG and new-onset type 2 diabetes.

Laboratory test results:

Hemoglobin A_{1c} = 11.4% (101 mmol/mol)
Glucose = 343 mg/dL (SI: 19.0 mmol/L)
Total cholesterol = 415 mg/dL (SI: 10.75 mmol/L)
TG = 4800 mg/dL (SI: 54.2 mmol/L)
HDL-C = 26 mg/dL (SI: 0.67 mmol/L)

She is hospitalized and is placed on nothing-by-mouth status and an insulin drip.

Repeated laboratory test results (after 24 hours):

Total cholesterol = 318 mg/dL (SI: 8.24 mmol/L)
TG = 1300 mg/dL (SI: 14.69 mmol/L)
HDL-C = 34 mg/dL (SI: 0.88 mmol/L)

Basal insulin and a GLP-1 receptor agonist are initiated.

Which of the following lipoproteins is contributing to the elevated cholesterol concentration in this patient?

A. LDL-C

B. VLDL-C

C. Chylomicron

D. Apolipoprotein B$_{48}$

Answer: B) VLDL-C

This patient has acquired severe HTG (TG ≥1000 mg/dL [≥11.2 mmol/L]). Severe HTG is primarily a consequence of substantial accumulation of chylomicrons stemming from impaired activity of the LPL-related TG-clearing system. HTG in this patient with type 2 diabetes is mainly caused by reduced clearance of TG due to defective LPL function in the insulin-resistant or -deficient state, as insulin serves as a cofactor for LPL. This can be considered to be multifactorial chylomicronemia syndrome. The accumulation of chylomicrons in the pancreatic capillary bed can cause abdominal pain, ischemia, and, if left untreated, may progress to pancreatitis. The risk of developing acute pancreatitis rises progressively, with serum TG concentration exceeding 500 mg/dL (>5.6 mmol/L). The risk of pancreatitis is approximately 5% when serum TG exceed 1000 mg/dL (>11.3 mmol/L), and it escalates to 10% to 20% with TG surpassing 2000 mg/dL (>22.6 mmol/L).[12]

In multifactorial chylomicronemia syndrome, there is overproduction of VLDL in the liver due to genetic predisposition, metabolic syndrome, or lifestyle factors such as diet and lack of exercise. Insulin resistance stimulates apolipoprotein B production (structural lipoprotein of the lipid particles). In response, the liver increases the synthesis and secretion of VLDL by assembling free fatty acids and apolipoprotein B. Moreover, hydrolysis of TG in chylomicrons and VLDL by LPL is compromised due to insulin deficiency or resistance, leading to accumulation of VLDL in the bloodstream. A useful clinical tool to identify the predominant TG-containing lipoprotein particles is to calculate the ratio of TG to cholesterol.

Chylomicron has a TG-to-cholesterol ratio of approximately 10:1, whereas VLDL has a TG-to-cholesterol ratio of 5:1. The TG-to-cholesterol ratio in this patient is 1300/318 mg/dL = 4, indicating a substantial concentration of VLDL-C. When a patient has very severe HTG or pancreatitis, it is important to implement nothing-by-mouth status and intravenous fluids to eliminate oral fat intake. Once the TG concentration reduces slowly, foods with low-fat content can be reintroduced and fat content can be increased as tolerated (*Table 2*).

Case 2

A 15-year-old girl with class 3 obesity (BMI = 42 kg/m^2) presents for follow-up of type 2 diabetes. She has a history of severe HTG that required hospitalization with intravenous fluids and an insulin drip. Her current medications include dulaglutide, 3 mg weekly, and insulin glargine, 50 units daily.

Laboratory test results:

> Hemoglobin A$_{1c}$ = 6.7% (50 mmol/mol)
> Glucose = 93 mg/dL (SI: 5.2 mmol/L)
> Total cholesterol = 281 mg/dL (SI: 7.28 mmol/L)
> TG = 225 mg/dL (SI: 2.54 mmol/L)
> HDL-C = 38 mg/dL (SI: 0.98 mmol/L)
> LDL-C = 198 mg/dL (SI: 5.13 mmol/L)
> Non–HDL-C = 243 mg/dL (SI: 6.29 mmol/L)

Family history is notable for premature cardiovascular disease in multiple first-degree relatives.

Which of the following is the best next step in this patient's management?

A. Statin therapy

B. Fenofibrate

C. Dietary fat at 15% of total daily calories

D. Omega-3 fatty acids

Answer: A) Statin therapy

This patient has mild-to-moderate HTG (TG = 150-999 mg/dL [1.7-11.2 mmol/L]). Her lipid phenotype is that of combined hyperlipidemia (elevated TG, low HDL-C, and variable concentrations of LDL-C). Scenarios of mild-to-moderate HTG mostly represent VLDL elevations secondary to increased VLDL synthesis in the liver. This is in contrast to scenarios of higher TG concentrations (eg, Case 1), where it is usually due to TG-clearance issues secondary to dysfunction of the LPL complex.

In this patient, HTG is predominantly attributed to the cumulative effects of obesity, insulin resistance, sedentary habits, and type 2 diabetes. As previously mentioned, the excessive production of free fatty acids from the diet, free fatty acid release from visceral adipose tissue, and increased apolipoprotein B_{100} from the liver all contribute to heightened VLDL synthesis. Additionally, clearance of TG is somewhat diminished due to the defective LPL function in the insulin-resistant state, as insulin serves as a cofactor for LPL.

Mild-to-moderate HTG can progress to severe HTG in the event of secondary causes promoting HTG.

The primary objective in this patient's management is to prevent cardiovascular disease. Mild-to-moderate HTG is considered an independent risk factor for cardiovascular disease.[2,13] Given her elevated LDL-C and non–HDL-C, a statin (Answer A) is the treatment of choice.

When the TG concentration is less than 500 mg/dL (<5.6 mmol/L), the focus is not to prevent pancreatitis. Therefore, neither fibrates (Answer B) nor omega-3 fatty acids (Answer D) are indicated.

Fat restriction (Answer C) is not indicated in patients with TG concentrations less than 500 mg/dL (<5.6 mmol/L). However, it is crucial to reduce added sugars (*Table 2*). Optimizing management of secondary causes such as diabetes, obesity, and insulin resistance is critical in such patients.

Case 3

A 29-day-old, full-term neonate has a blood sample resembling "creamy tomato soup."

Initial laboratory test results:

> Total cholesterol = 895 mg/dL (SI: 23.18 mmol/L)
> TG = 16,300 mg/dL (SI: 184.19 mmol/L)
> HDL-C = 8 mg/dL (SI: 0.21 mmol/L)

There is no family history of pancreatitis, HTG, or other disorders. Initial management includes dextrose-containing intravenous fluids while not feeding the patient orally. On the fourth hospital day, the baby's serum TG concentration has decreased to 1480 mg/dL (16.72 mmol/L).

Which of the following is the best recommendation for nutrition in this patient?

A. Start fish oil supplementation of feeds

B. Feed regular formula with medium-chain triglyceride supplementation

C. Continue feeding breast milk

D. Reduce total fat intake to <15% of total calories

Answer: D) Reduce total fat intake to <15% of total calories

This infant has early-onset, severe HTG (TG ≥1000 mg/dL [≥11.2 mmol/L]) in the neonatal period, indicating the baby has familial chylomicronemia syndrome. Early-onset, severe HTG typically results from autosomal recessive, monogenic loss-of-function pathogenic variants in the *LPL* gene (95%) or in genes related to its function (eg, *APOC2, APOA5, LMF1, GPIHBP1,* and *GPD1*), which affect regulation of the catabolism of TG-rich lipoproteins.[3]

The management objective is to prevent pancreatitis with a treatment target of reducing the TG concentration to less than 1000 mg/dL (<11.2 mmol/L). Acute management includes placing the patient on nothing-by-mouth status and starting intravenous dextrose to avoid further chylomicron load from dietary sources. Dietary fat restriction (Answer D) is the key in any case of hyperchylomicronemia. The cornerstone of long-term management involves limiting fat intake to less than 10% to 15% of dietary calories while ensuring sufficient calories for growth. Given breast milk's higher fat content (4.2%-4.5% fat per 100 mL), it is not recommended. Similarly, regular formula is also not an option because it also has high fat content.

Medium-chain triglycerides (chain length of C10-12) (Answer B) can be directly absorbed into the portal vein without forming chylomicrons. They do not require LPL for absorption. Medium-chain triglycerides are suitable for oral supplementation of fat calories. Commercially available amino acid formulas can be supplemented with medium-chain triglycerides in this scenario.

When the TG concentration exceeds 1770 mg/dL (>20 mmol/L), fibrates show no therapeutic benefit.

Omega-3 fatty acids are ineffective in managing LPL deficiency. In fact, the use of fish oil supplements in this scenario can increase TG concentrations by contributing to total fat intake. For instance, the administration of a 1-g fish oil capsule would require a reduction in dietary fat content by 1 g to adhere to the recommended daily fat allowance. In older children, a pancreatic lipase inhibitor, such as orlistat, may provide additional benefits in conjunction with a fat-restricted diet.

Key Learning Points

Insulin resistance significantly contributes to the phenotypic expression of HTG, except in familial chylomicronemia syndrome. Therefore, lifestyle and dietary modifications form the cornerstone of HTG management.

- When the TG concentrations are less than 500 mg/dL (<5.6 mmol/L), the associated risk shifts towards atherogenicity. In such cases, it is recommended to lower non–HDL-C or LDL-C through statin use.

- When the TG concentration surpasses 500 mg/dL (>5.6 mmol/L) due to saturated or deficient LPL activity, the risk for acute pancreatitis escalates.

- Current medications exhibit limited efficacy when the TG value exceeds 2000 mg/dL (>22.6 mmol/L).

References

1. Berglund L, Brunzell JD, Goldberg AC, et al., Evaluation and treatment of hypertriglyceridemia: an Endocrine Society clinical practice guideline. *J Clin Endocrinol Metab.* 2012;97(9):2969-2989. PMID: 22962670

2. Nordestgaard BG, Varbo A. Triglycerides and cardiovascular disease. *Lancet.* 2014;384(9943):626-635. PMID: 25131982

3. Hegele RA, Ginsberg HN, Chapman MJ, et al; European Atherosclerosis Society Consensus Panel. The polygenic nature of hypertriglyceridaemia: implications for definition, diagnosis, and management. *Lancet Diabetes Endocrinol.* 2014;2(8):655-666. PMID: 24731657

4. Frontini MG, Srinivasan SR, Xu J, Tang R, Bond MG, Berenson GS. Usefulness of childhood non–high density lipoprotein cholesterol levels versus other lipoprotein measures in predicting adult subclinical atherosclerosis: the Bogalusa Heart Study. *Pediatrics.* 2008;121(5):924-929. PMID: 18450895

5. Expert Panel on Integrated Guideleins for Cardiovascular Health and Risk Reduction in Children and Adolescents; National Heart, Lung, and Blood Institute, Expert panel on integrated guidelines for cardiovascular health and risk reduction in children and adolescents: summary report. *Pediatrics.* 2011;128(Suppl 5):S213-S256. PMID: 22084329

6. Daniels SR, Greer FR; Commitee on Nutrition, Lipid screening and cardiovascular health in childhood. *Pediatrics.* 2008;122(1):198-208. PMID: 18596007

7. Virani SS, Morris PB, Agarwala A, et al. 2021 ACC expert consensus decision pathway on the management of ASCVD risk reduction in patients with persistent hypertriglyceridemia: a report of the American College of Cardiology Solution Set Oversight Committee. *J Am Coll Cardiol.* 2021;78(9):960-993. PMID: 34332805

8. Ashraf AP, Sunil B, Bamba V, et al. Case studies in pediatric lipid disorders and their management. *J Clin Endocrinol Metab.* 2021;106(12):3605-3620. PMID: 34363474

9. Valaiyapathi B, Sunil B, Ashraf AP. Approach to hypertriglyceridemia in the pediatric population. *Pediatr Rev.* 2017;38(9):424-434. PMID: 28864733

10. Valaiyapathi B, Ashraf AP. Hospital management of severe hypertriglyceridemia in children. *Cur Pediatr Rev.* 2017;13(4):225-231. PMID: 29345595

11. Rodríguez Santana,Y, Roman AN, Saez IG et al.,Treatment of severe hypertriglyceridemia with continuous insulin infusion. *Case Rep in Critical Care.* 2011;293917. PMID: 24804116

12. Scherer J, Singh VP, Pitchumoni CS, Yadav D. Issues in hypertriglyceridemic pancreatitis: an update. *J Clin Gastroenterol.* 2014;48(3):195-203. PMID: 24172179

13. Arca M, Veronesi C, D'Erasmo L, et al; Local Health Units Group. Association of hypertriglyceridemia with all-cause mortality and atherosclerotic cardiovascular events in a low-risk Italian population: the TG-REAL retrospective cohort analysis. *J Am Heart Assoc.* 2020; 9(19):e015801. PMID: 32954906

Challenges for Pediatric and Adult Endocrinologists in the Diagnosis and Management of Individuals With a Variant in Sex Development

Martine Cools, MD, PhD. Department of Pediatrics, Division of Pediatric Endocrinology, Ghent University Hospital, and Department of Internal Medicine and Pediatrics, Ghent University, Ghent, Belgium; Email: martine.cools@ugent.be

Educational Objectives

After reviewing this chapter, learners should be able to:

- Skillfully approach parents of a newborn with a potential variant in sex development (VSD) and design a diagnostic plan.

- Explain the ethical concerns related to genital surgery in childhood and legislative initiatives on this matter.

- Develop a medical management plan for adolescents who have complete androgen insensitivity syndrome (CAIS), or a 45,X/46,XY VSD, and who transition to adult care.

- Recall gonadal germ-cell cancer (GCC) risk in children and adults who have a VSD and Y-chromosomal material, estimate this risk in various diagnostic groups, and develop an individualized gonadal management plan.

Significance of the Clinical Problem

Management of VSDs poses important challenges to health care providers for several reasons. First, VSDs are rare, heterogenous congenital conditions, making it difficult for health care providers to gain sufficient experience and expertise. Second, having a VSD affects a person's body development and physical health, but it may also heavily impact their mental well-being, even many years after the initial diagnosis. Third, VSDs have low visibility in our society, and many affected individuals prefer to keep their condition private. Nonetheless, information and openness have been related to positive outcomes. Fourth, the importance of transition to adult endocrine care and long-term follow-up have only recently received more attention. As a result, many adult care providers are not yet familiar with VSDs, and the related comorbidities, long-term outcomes, and health risks in adult life are understudied. Lastly, management of VSDs in childhood, and in particular genital surgery at an early age, have become very controversial and are high on the political agenda both in the United States and Europe.

The birth of a child with a genital variation is often a traumatic experience for parents, especially if it is not possible to register a sex for the baby without further technical investigations and/ or when contacts with medical staff immediately after birth are suboptimal. Qualitative research has shown that the information and support received from the medical team around the time of birth often have a lifelong impact on parents' ability to cope with their child's condition and to openly discuss the condition with their child and increase resilience.

Most VSDs are thought to be of genetic origin. Surprisingly, despite major advances in genome-wide sequencing technologies, the etiology of approximately 50% of 46,XY VSDs remains unexplained.

Genital surgery in infancy or childhood to make the genital appearance more typical male-looking or female-looking has been the cornerstone of management for decades. This approach has been vigorously criticized because it interferes with the individual's right to make a personal and independent choice in the future. However, the alternative option for the patient—to grow up with a sometimes very marked genital difference—has not been studied regarding its potential effect on mental well-being and identity development. In practice, this choice is not straightforward for many affected children and their parents. The debate surrounding genital surgery before an age at which an individual can give personal informed consent has led to a tense relationship between health care providers and some activist movements. Progress in this matter can only be reached through collaborative initiatives, self-criticism, and mutual respect, with improved patient care as a common goal. Traditionally, care for individuals who have a VSD has focused on pediatric and adolescent age groups. With many adolescents being lost to follow-up as they age, the importance of transition to adult care is receiving more attention. Some VSDs are associated with life-threatening comorbidities, such as aortic root dilation in men and women who have a 45,X/46,XY sex chromosomal DSD, or severe hyposplenism in individuals who have monoallelic or biallelic *NR5A1* variants. Other health problems may result from medications that need to be taken lifelong (eg, low BMD in individuals who need hormone replacement therapy, or hypertension and obesity in those who need hydrocortisone treatment).

Most individuals who have a VSD and Y-chromosomal material in their (gonadal) karyotype are at increased risk to develop a GCC (mostly seminoma/dysgerminoma) in early adulthood. This risk must be balanced against the functional capacity of the gonad in terms of hormone production and fertility. Based on this balance in individual patients, a process of shared decision-making can further guide gonadal management, which can vary from prophylactic gonadectomy to careful surveillance of retained gonads. Pediatric and adult endocrinologists must have a sound understanding of GCC risk in the various VSD diagnostic groups to coordinate the gonadal management plan.

Practice Gaps

- Approaching parents of a newborn with atypical-looking genitalia in a sensitive way and determining how and when to refer their baby for diagnostic workup.

- Including the young child's voice in medical decision-making around genital surgery in the absence of evidence supporting the benefits of growing up with a genital difference.

- Learning about specific comorbidities related to 46,XY VSDs that can develop in adulthood.

- Determining whether to screen for these comorbidities and whether to take any preventive measures.

- Evaluating options for girls who have vaginal hypoplasia.

- In the context of increased GCC risk in individuals who have a VSD, determining how to weigh the GCC risk against benefits of leaving gonads in place and how to organize a safe follow-up plan beyond childhood.

Discussion

Having a VSD can be very impactful for children, adolescents, and adults. Some of the challenges are growing up with a genital difference, learning that one's karyotype or internal genital structures are not congruent with an aspect of the external genitals or one's gender identity, and dealing with infertility. To fully support their children on this journey, it is crucial that parents effectively cope with their child's condition and do not experience the neonatal period as traumatic. Health care providers can contribute positively by emphasizing that the baby is in good health and by providing clear and transparent information. Health care providers should communicate with nonstigmatizing words and a gender-neutral and logic vocabulary to describe the genital structures of the newborn (eg, use the external genitalia score [EGS]). Validated reference values for the EGS are helpful in deciding whether a baby should be referred for specialized diagnostic workup.[1] An example of transparent and sensitive communication with parents can be found at https://starship.org.nz/guidelines/differences-of-sex-development-atawhai-taihemahema/.

Registration of the newborn's sex is not an emergency, and the decision to raise a child with a genital difference as a girl or as a boy requires an individualized approach, tailored to the needs of individual families. Considerations are the precise diagnosis, the presence or absence of specific genital structures (eg, testes, uterus), the expected gender identity, the capacity of the gonads to produce sex steroids, and importantly, parental preferences and beliefs, which may be influenced by culture or religion.

Genital surgery in infancy or childhood to align the genital aspect with the sex registered at birth has traditionally been a component of VSD care, as it is believed to facilitate psychosocial adaptation of the child and to promote coping with the condition. However, activist movements across the world, supported by human rights bodies, have argued that this practice impedes the ability of the affected individual to make an autonomous decision on whether surgery is needed. This is problematic, given that genital surgery is complex, technically difficult, and risks altering genital sensitivity. In addition, the sex registered at birth does not necessarily coincide with future gender

identity. Some affected individuals have stated that because they had genital surgery in childhood, they feel as if their body was "not good enough" and/or had to be altered to be socially acceptable. However, many studies surveying adolescents and adults who have a VSD have shown that most affected individuals prefer having had genital surgery in childhood.[2] Importantly, there are no outcome studies assessing the impact of growing up with a genital difference on self-esteem, body image, and (gender) identity development. Many health care providers who specialize in VSD care underscore the importance of individualized decision-making with families for good outcomes, and point out that from their experience, living with a genital difference can cause severe distress in children. A recent collaboration between our VSD expert center, a human rights specialist, and an intersex activist has identified some crucial aspects that have not been considered in existing legislative initiatives on this topic. These include the potential mental distress that some children experience due to the genital difference, and the fact that receiving high-quality care is of equal importance for a favorable outcome as whether genital surgery was performed in childhood. These aspects of care should be an integral part of any further legislation developed on this matter.[3]

When the phenotype and hormonal results point towards a specific diagnosis, Sanger sequencing is the most appropriate genetic test beyond karyotyping. Most specialized centers in high-income countries offer whole-exome sequencing–based gene panels and high-resolution arrays to determine the diagnosis at the molecular genetic level, which is important to guide management and inform parents on an eventual familial risk. However, even with the most advanced technologies, a molecular diagnosis can only be reached in about 50% of patients with 46,XY VSD. Whole-genome sequencing, which can reveal intronic variants, has not yet been introduced in most clinical diagnostic genetic services, but it can sometimes be performed in a research context. The apolipoprotein D test is an in vitro assay that allows assessment of androgen signaling in genital skin fibroblasts. This test is especially informative in patients who are suspected of having CAIS or partial androgen insensitivity (PAIS) but in whom Sanger sequencing of the androgen receptor gene reveals no pathogenic variants. Most recently, this test, in combination with whole-exome sequencing, has led to the identification of the first androgen receptor cofactor required for accurate androgen signaling. Pathogenic variants in the *DAAM2* gene (dishevelled-associated activator of morphogenesis 2) lead to androgen resistance. This has mechanistically been explained by loss of dihydrotestosterone-induced, actin-dependent androgen receptor polymerization, together with polymerase II, in transcriptional droplets that are required for transcription of androgen receptor target genes.[4] This is a significant breakthrough, as pathogenic variants in the androgen receptor gene can only be found in approximately 20% of individuals with a clinical phenotype of PAIS.

Medical care for individuals who have a VSD has, for a long time, been the almost exclusive domain of pediatric endocrinologists, and many adolescents are lost to follow-up at the age of transition to adult care. Scarce long-term outcome studies and large-scale collaborations, such as the International Registries for Rare Conditions Affecting Sex Development and Maturation (https://sdmregistries.org/), have shown that VSDs can be associated with severe comorbidities, mental health problems, or adverse effects from certain medications.[5,6] Thus, many individuals with a VSD require expert medical care that is continued into adulthood. For example, adults who have congenital adrenal hyperplasia are at increased risk for developing hypertension, obesity, or metabolic syndrome, which has been related to the lifelong exposure to slightly supraphysiological corticosteroid doses. Men and women who have 45,X/46,XY sex chromosomal DSD have cardiac, kidney, and liver problems and hearing loss to the same extent as what is observed in women who have Turner syndrome, and they should be offered the same preventive health measures and surveillance protocols.[7,8] Some

genes involved in gonadal development are also relevant for the development and/or functioning of other organ systems. A typical example is *WT1* (WT1 transcription factor). Intron 9 splice site variants in *WT1* cause Frasier syndrome, which is characterized by 46,XY gonadal dysgenesis, and focal segmental glomerulosclerosis, often requiring kidney transplant in the second or third decade of life. *NR5A1* has been shown to be involved in gonadal, adrenal, and spleen development. Individuals who have a VSD due to monoallelic *NR5A1* pathogenic variants, as well as their asymptomatic family member carriers, are at increased risk of severe hyposplenism and require prophylactic measures to protect them from life-threatening bacterial infections.[9]

Individuals who have a VSD and Y-chromosomal material are at increased risk for developing an invasive gonadal GCC, mostly seminoma/dysgerminoma. These GCCs are preceded for many years by an in situ neoplastic lesion, termed germ-cell neoplasia in situ (GCNIS) in the testis and gonadoblastoma in the dysgenetic gonad. Extrapolation of epidemiological data obtained in the typical male population suggests an expected peak incidence of seminoma between age 15 and 40 years. The overall risk across diagnostic groups has been estimated to be around 30%. Therefore, until 2000, prophylactic gonadectomy was routinely performed at diagnosis in all patients, usually in childhood or adolescence. Subsequent epidemiological research and increased insight in the pathogenesis of these GCCs has allowed for better risk stratification. Conditions associated with gonadal dysgenesis have a risk of GCC up to 60% in some cases, particularly in patients with Frasier syndrome. Conditions resulting from disorders in testosterone biosynthesis or action are characterized by normal embryonic testis development and have a much lower risk, although exact incidence data are still lacking. Severely dysgenetic gonads (eg, in women who have complete gonadal dysgenesis) are nonfunctional in terms of hormone or gamete production. This, in combination with high GCC risk, justifies prophylactic gonadectomy at an early age. Men with partial gonadal dysgenesis are almost invariably sterile, but they often do not need hormone replacement therapy until well into adult life. If brought into a stable scrotal position, their testes can be easily palpated and readily visualized on ultrasonography. A testicular biopsy to detect GCNIS can be performed as an extra safety measure in late adolescence, often combined with testicular semen extraction. In such cases, a careful surveillance program seems appropriate, although no research has investigated the required modalities of such a program. In individuals who have a disorder of testosterone biosynthesis, the approach must be individualized as well. Given the low GCC risk at a young age and yet uncertain gender identity, prophylactic gonadectomy in childhood must be avoided. Gonadectomy may be necessary in early puberty to avoid virilization in affirmed girls when pubertal testosterone effects are expected (eg, in 17β-hydroxysteroid dehydrogenase deficiency or 5α-reductase deficiency). Alternatively, GnRH analogues can be given to temporarily to block puberty, for example, when gender identity is not yet clear.[10]

The best studied condition associated with adult GCC risk is CAIS. Endogenous testosterone production in CAIS is important, as the aromatase enzyme CYP19A1 converts excess testosterone into estradiol, allowing for breast development, female fat distribution, and acquisition of bone density. Whether an optimal peak bone mass can be acquired in women who have CAIS and preserved gonads is unknown, as androgenic effects are by definition lacking and bone remodeling relies on the combined effects of estrogens and androgens. Overall, the trophic effects of estradiol and IGF-1 on bone are thought to be more important than androgenic effects.

No cases of invasive GCC have been reported in children with AIS and given the importance of endogenous testosterone production for pubertal development, prophylactic gonadectomy in childhood is not indicated. Studies in adolescent and adult women who have CAIS suggest the risk of developing GCNIS is 5% to 10%, and the risk of seminoma not higher than 1% to 2%.[11] These

data need to be confirmed in larger series, as such studies are hampered by low case numbers because of the former practice of performing gonadectomy in childhood.

In our center, whether to perform prophylactic gonadectomy in young adult women who have CAIS is the subject of a dedicated shared decision-making process. Given the low chance of developing an invasive GCC and the possibility to benefit from endogenous testosterone production, most young adult women who have CAIS decide to further postpone gonadectomy and to participate in a surveillance program. Such a program consists of annual MRI and a blood screen for tumor markers (α-fetoprotein and β-hCG). Unfortunately, the resolution of MRI images is insufficient to detect GCNIS in abdominal testes, so the purpose of imaging is to visualize an invasive GCC at the earliest possible stage. Classic tumor markers have a very low sensitivity to detect GCC. A diagnostic test based on the detection of specific micro-RNAs secreted by seminomatous embryonic stem cells (MiR-371a-3p, 373- 3p, and 367-3P) can detect invasive GCC with 90% sensitivity and 91% specificity. Unfortunately, the test cannot detect the precursor GCNIS lesion.[12] This test is about to become commercially available.

As outlined in the preceding text, given the known combined androgenic and estrogenic effects on bone, it is important to prospectively screen for osteoporosis in all women who have CAIS—both those with gonads in place and those who rely on hormone replacement therapy. As more women with CAIS now have preserved gonads, it may become possible in the near future to study the natural evolution of bone mineral density, metabolism, and other sexually dimorphic traits in aging women. Women who have CAIS have a short (usually not more than 1 to 2 cm) blind-ending vagina. Vaginal dilation is the first-choice method to address vaginal hypoplasia. When well-counseled and emotionally prepared, almost all women (90%-96%) will be able to achieve anatomic and functional success by primary vaginal dilation.[13]

Clinical Case Vignettes

Case 1

On day 1 of life, a newborn with typical male-looking genitals is determined to have no palpable gonads. This is the first child of Belgian parents.

Does this baby need urgent workup for a possible VSD?

A. Yes

B. No, testes can spontaneously descend in the first 3 months after birth

C. It is best to reassess the baby in 1 week, and then decide about referral

D. No, this baby needs referral to a urologist for orchidopexy; undescended testes occurs in 1% of male newborns, no specific workup is needed

Answer: A) Yes

This baby's EGS is 9/12. The cut-off score for further investigations to exclude a VSD is 10.5. Thus, the baby needs urgent workup for a possible VSD (Answer A).

Case 1 (continued)

Which of the following is highest in the differential diagnosis list for this newborn?

A. Bilateral testicular regression

B. Congenital hypogonadotropic hypogonadism

C. Congenital adrenal hyperplasia in a 46,XX individual

D. 45,X/46,XY

E. Partial gonadal dysgenesis

Answer: C) Congenital adrenal hyperplasia in a 46,XX individual

Apart from the fact that congenital adrenal hyperplasia in a 46,XX individual (Answer C) is the most frequent cause of this phenotype, it is crucial not to forget about this possibility because late diagnosis can lead to a life-threatening shock. Appropriate treatment must be initiated as soon as possible. A prompt diagnosis of congenital adrenal

hyperplasia can also avoid problems with sex assignment.

Case 1 (continued)

The diagnosis of congenital adrenal hyperplasia is confirmed on day 4 of life based on a 46,XX karyotype (quantitative PCR), adrenal and pelvic ultrasonography (enlarged adrenals, normal ovaries, and visible uterus), and hormone values (elevated ACTH, 17-hydroxyprogesterone, and androstenedione).

Should this child be registered as male or female sex?

A. Male sex

B. Female sex

C. Discuss both options with the parents, ask their opinion, weigh pros and cons of each option, and assess whether a decision can be made that is supported by the parents and the medical team

D. Recommend the parents raise the child as gender-neutral, so that they can make a personal decision later without bias

E. I don't know

Answer: C) Discuss both options with the parents, ask their opinion, weigh pros and cons of each option, and assess whether a decision can be made that is supported by the parents and the medical team

Most girls and women with congenital adrenal hyperplasia express a female gender identity, although there is evidence that the strength of that identity may be reduced.[14] Current guidelines recommend female sex registration at birth for 46,XX individuals with congenital adrenal hyperplasia (including in severely virilized individuals). However, research has shown that gender dysphoria and gender change are more frequent (up to 10%) in the most virilized individuals and that the long-term outcomes of genital surgery as they relate to sexual function are suboptimal in women who were most virilized at birth. Also, there is wider acceptance of nonbinary gender identities in some cultures; and there have been reports of satisfactory outcomes of 46,XX individuals with congenital adrenal hyperplasia who were raised as males. Keeping all options fully open for the child to make a personal choice regarding future gender identity requires deferral of irreversible genital surgery such a clitoris glans reduction. Although scientific data are still lacking, it is commonly anticipated that psychosocial adaptation of a child to a marked incongruence between bodily sex characteristics and sex of rearing is not straightforward and may even be problematic and cause mental harm to the child. In view of this, some parents may prefer to raise their fully virilized child as a boy in the first years of life to facilitate coping, until a stable gender identity emerges and a decision on genital surgery can include the voice of the maturing child. Thus, a decision on sex registration should always be the result of a genuine shared decision-making process, weighing all options, and should be tailored to the needs and beliefs of individual families (Answer C).

After a process of shared decision-making, the parents decided to register a female sex for this child and to abstain from genital surgery given the uncertain gender outcome. At age 3 years, the girl became very distressed about her genital appearance, up to the point that both the parents and the medical team feared that further deferral of genital surgery might cause irreversible mental harm. At age 3.5 years, genitoplasty was performed, which consisted in opening the phallic urethra to the perineum, bringing the meatus in a typical female position and hiding the enlarged phallus in the prepubic fat, creating minor labia of the preputial skin, and leaving a part to cover the glans, which was not reduced in size. Vaginoplasty was not performed. Mental well-being of the child has strongly improved following this surgery, but long-term follow-up is not available yet.[3]

Case 2

On day 1 of life, a newborn is observed to have isolated penoscrotal hypospadias. The EGS is 10/12. This is the second child of healthy Belgian parents, and pregnancy and delivery were uneventful. The child is referred for further workup.

Figure 1. Family Pedigree and Laboratory Test Results (Sample Drawn at Age 20 Days)

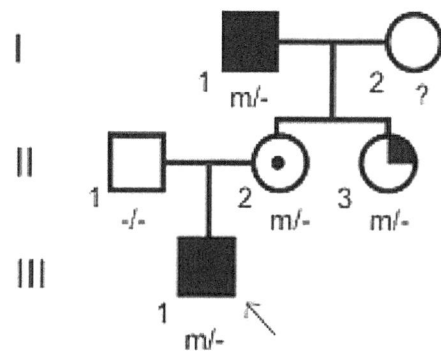

Test	Result	Age-specific reference	SI
Platelet count (10E3/µL)	684	217-497	684 10E9/L
LH (mU/mL)	8.7	1-9	8.7 IU/L
FSH (mU/L)	5.3	1.5-12	5.3 IU/L
Testosterone (ng/dL)	184	NA	6.38 nmol/L
Androstenedione (ng/dL)	89	22-122	3.1 nmol/L
DHT	54	30-120	1.83 nmol/L
AMH (µg/L)	61	62-130	435 pmol/L

Baetens D et al. Orphanet J Rare Dis, 2014; 9: 209. BioMed Central Ltd., part of Springer Nature.[15]

[Color—Print (Color Gallery page CG34) or web & ePub editions]

The baby's karyotype is 46,XY.

Should further genetic testing be performed to exclude a VSD?

A. No, everything is normal, the boy is not suspected to have a VSD

B. Yes, proceed with Sanger sequencing of the *AR* gene

C. Yes, proceed with whole-exome sequencing

D. Yes, proceed with whole-genome sequencing

E. Yes, proceed with Sanger sequencing of the *NR5A1* gene

Answer: E) Yes, proceed with Sanger sequencing of the NR5A1 gene

A recent large study of 193 boys with hypospadias has revealed that genome-wide genetic screening in patients with isolated hypospadias is unlikely to reveal pathogenic variants in VSD-related genes.[16] However, as noted in the pedigree, the child's aunt has primary ovarian insufficiency. Primary ovarian insufficiency has been associated with familial pathogenic *NR5A1* variants, and given the particular family context and marginally low serum antimullerian hormone, sequencing of *NR5A1* (Answer E) is indicated. Given the potential comorbidities associated with *NR5A1* haploinsufficiency (infertility, GCC, possibly imminent primary ovarian insufficiency in the mother) associated with *NR5A1* variants, it is important not to miss this diagnosis.

A heterozygous pathogenic variant in *NR5A1* (predicted to result in loss-of-function) was confirmed: c.630-637 del, leading to a truncated protein p.(Tyr211Profs*12) (NM_004959.5 reference sequence). The same variant was also documented in the child's mother, grandfather, and aunt. The child's mother was referred to a gynecologist for assessment of ovarian reserve. No signs of imminent primary ovarian insufficiency were detected.

Case 2 (continued)

Knowing that this baby has a VSD, which of the following is the best approach to long-term GCC risk management?

A. Bilateral orchidectomy

B. Bilateral testicular biopsy before age 1 year and annual ultrasonography thereafter

C. Bilateral testicular biopsy between age 2 to 5 years and annual ultrasonography thereafter

D. Annual ultrasonography from puberty onwards and bilateral testicular biopsy in late adolescence

E. No monitoring necessary (no increased GCC risk in VSD related to NR5A1 pathogenic variants)

Answer: D) Annual ultrasonography from puberty onwards and bilateral testicular biopsy in late adolescence

Given that there is full testicular differentiation, the baby has adequate testicular function (based on phenotype and lab results), and the testes are in scrotal position, GCC risk is low, especially in childhood. Reliable data on GCC risk in adulthood, specifically for men who have *NR5A1* loss-of-function variants, are lacking, but the risk is thought to be considerably higher than in the typical male population. Epidemiologic data suggest a peak incidence for seminoma between 15 and 40 years. Scrotal gonads can be safely monitored by regular self-palpation and annual ultrasonography. Bilateral testicular biopsies at the end of puberty have a high likelihood of detecting GCNIS if present, and biopsy at this time presents the opportunity to combine this procedure with testicular semen extraction, if desired (Answer D).

Case 2 (continued)

For which other health problems or comorbidities should family members be screened?

A. Assess spleen anatomy and function to exclude functional hyposplenism in all family members, including asymptomatic family member carriers and regardless of whether they have a VSD phenotype

B. Assess spleen anatomy and function to exclude functional hyposplenism in all family members who have a VSD phenotype

C. Perform a low-dose cosyntropin-stimulation test to exclude adrenal insufficiency in all family members regardless of whether they have a VSD phenotype (also in asymptomatic family members who are carriers)

D. Perform a low-dose cosyntropin-stimulation test to exclude adrenal insufficiency in all family members who have a VSD phenotype

E. Perform a low-dose cosyntropin-stimulation test and assess spleen anatomy and function to exclude both functional hyposplenism and adrenal insufficiency in all family members regardless of whether they have a VSD phenotype

Answer: A) Assess spleen anatomy and function to exclude functional hyposplenism in all family members, including asymptomatic family member carriers and regardless of whether they have a VSD phenotype

NR5A1 is required for activation of TLX1, an embryonic enhancer of splenic cell differentiation and proliferation. A recent study has revealed that functional hyposplenism is frequently associated with heterozygous *NR5A1* pathogenic variants, both in individuals who have or do not have a VSD.[9] Individuals with hyposplenism require prophylactic measures to protect them against life-threatening infections with encapsulated bacteria (*Figure 2*). Thus, all family members, including asymptomatic family member carriers and regardless of whether they have a VSD phenotype, should have assessment of spleen anatomy and function to exclude functional hyposplenism (Answer A). Although sporadically described, there are currently no data that suggest a likely co-occurrence of adrenal insufficiency in individuals who have monoallelic pathogenic *NR5A1* variants. Very few patients with biallelic

NR5A1 pathogenic variants have been described, but assessment of both adrenal and splenic function is recommended in those individuals. In the literature, individuals who are homozygous for a pathogenic *NR5A1* variant have asplenism or very severe hyposplenism.

Case 3

A 15-year-old girl with a tentative diagnosis of Mayer-Rokitansky-Küster-Hauser (MRKH) syndrome is referred to discuss vaginoplasty. The diagnosis was made by her mother's gynecologist, who had examined the patient because of primary amenorrhea despite of breast development starting at age 10 years. Upon physical examination, this gynecologist had found that she had a blind-ending vagina of 1 cm depth. In addition, no uterus could be detected on abdominal ultrasonography.

Figure 2. Spleen Function in Individuals With NR5A1 Variants

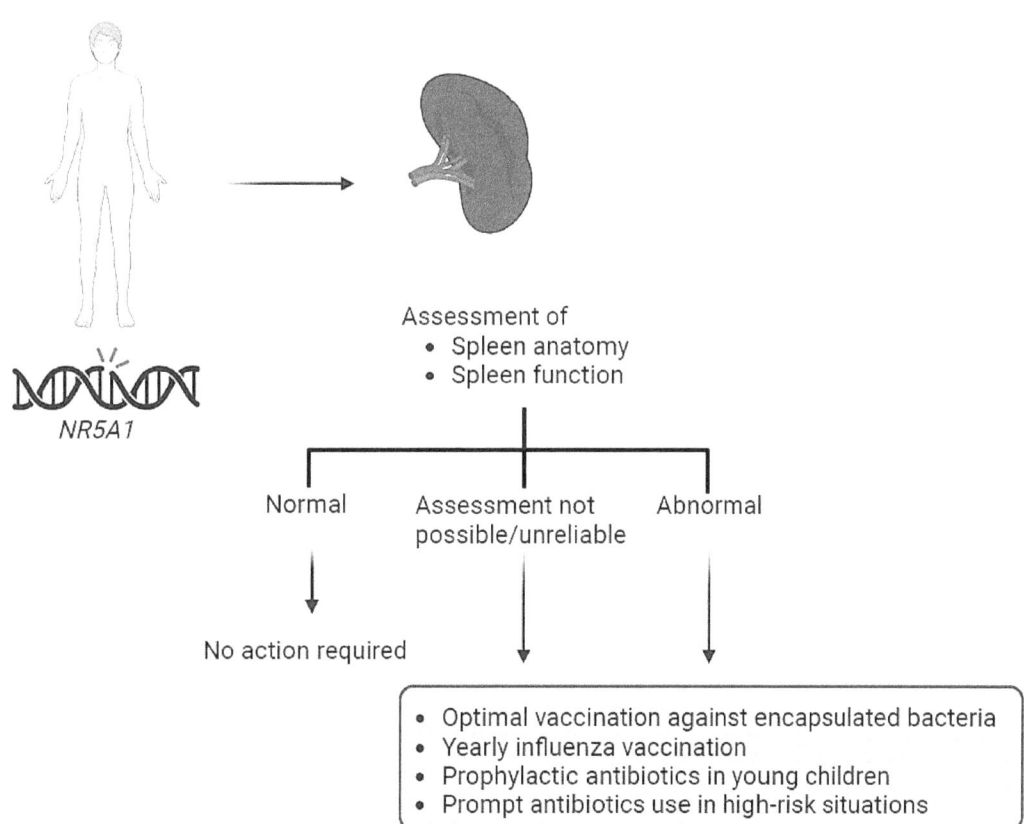

Is there anything else that needs to be done? Is the proposed management of vaginal hypoplasia appropriate?

A. The diagnosis is clear; she needs a vagina to have satisfactory sexual intercourse and vaginoplasty is the best method to create a functional vagina of satisfactory depth; adherence to vaginal self-dilation methods is generally very poor, especially in adolescent girls

B. The diagnosis is clear; however, vaginal dilation therapy is the first-line approach for vaginal hypoplasia, as it has a high success rate provided that motivation is good and sufficient support is provided

C. Pelvic MRI should be done to confirm the diagnosis of MRKH; vaginal dilation rather than vaginoplasty is the first-line approach for vaginal hypoplasia

D. Pelvic MRI should be done to confirm the diagnosis of MRKH; additional investigations are required to distinguish between MRKH type 1 and type 2 (MURCS); the options of vaginoplasty and vaginal dilation therapy should be discussed with the patient as they are equally successful regarding anatomical depth and functional outcome

E. A blood test to assess gonadal function and conventional karyotype analysis are needed before MRKH can be diagnosed; vaginal dilation therapy is the first-line approach for vaginal hypoplasia as it has a high success rate, provided that motivation is good and sufficient psychosocial support is offered; a clear diagnosis must be established first and psychosocial support should be provided to process the diagnosis

Answer: E) A blood test to assess gonadal function and conventional karyotype analysis are needed before MRKH can be diagnosed; vaginal dilation therapy is the first-line approach for vaginal hypoplasia as it has a high success rate, provided that motivation is good and sufficient psychosocial support is offered; a clear diagnosis must be established first and psychosocial support should be provided to process the diagnosis

Although much rarer, CAIS presents in the same way as MRKH. Both conditions can be easily distinguished by karyotype analysis (46,XY and 46,XX) and by gonadotropins, sex steroid concentration, and antimullerian hormone concentration (in CAIS: moderately increased LH, testosterone within the reference range for males, antimullerian hormone about 100-fold the female range; in MRKH: normal gonadotropins, normal ovarian function, antimullerian hormone within the female reference range). Thus, Answer E is correct. Management of vaginal hypoplasia can be considered when the patient is ready, but there is no urgency. It is the patient's personal choice to start or defer this treatment. Vaginal dilation therapy is the first-line approach to manage vaginal hypoplasia, both in MRKH and in CAIS. This treatment has a very high success rate (>90%) in highly motivated women and when supported by a pelvic floor physiotherapist and a psychologist or sexologist. Best results are seen in girls 16 years and older and/or those who would like to engage in vaginal intercourse in the near future.

In this vignette, the patient's karyotype was 46,XY. Hormonal results were consistent with the diagnosis of complete androgen insensitivity syndrome. She chose to defer vaginal dilation therapy. Infertility and gonadal GCC risk were discussed with her.

Case 3 (continued)

Which of the following is the best advice regarding management of gonads in this patient?

A. There is no increased risk for GCC in CAIS, so the topic does not need to be discussed

B. There is a rapid decline in germ-cell count in aging girls who have CAIS; thus, gonadectomy should be performed as soon as possible and testicular tissue should be cryopreserved for later fertility purposes

C. There is an increased risk for GCC in CAIS, but the risk is much lower than in girls who have complete gonadal dysgenesis; gonadectomy should be discussed, as well as the alternative option to keep the testes in place if the patient has annual follow-up visits for surveillance of GCC risk

D. She is end-pubertal; because breast development and bone mass acquisition are complete, GCC risk will start to rise; gonadectomy and estradiol replacement therapy should be recommended

E. She is end-pubertal; because breast development and bone mass acquisition are complete, GCC risk will start to rise; gonadectomy and testosterone replacement therapy should be recommended, as she has been exposed to high testosterone levels throughout puberty

Answer: C) There is an increased risk for GCC in CAIS, but the risk is much lower than in girls who have complete gonadal dysgenesis; gonadectomy should be discussed, as well as the alternative option to keep the testes in place if the patient has annual follow-up visits for surveillance of GCC risk

The risk of invasive GCC in adult women who have CAIS is indeed much lower than in patients with a VSD associated with gonadal dysgenesis, and is probably not higher than 1% to 2%. The preinvasive lesion GCNIS is found more often (in 5%-10%), but it is likely that not all of these lesions will develop into a seminoma because of the lack of a trophic androgenic effect. However, it is important to discuss the limitations of a surveillance program consisting of annual MRI and blood screen for tumor markers (Answer C). Such a surveillance program can be a burden for a teenager, and she should be informed that the resolution of MRI is insufficient to detect GCNIS. Classic tumor markers, such as α-fetoprotein and β-hCG have a very low sensitivity to detect seminomas. Development of a new test, based on the detection of specific microRNAs secreted by embryonic stem cells, is underway but this test will also not detect GCC at a preinvasive GCNIS stage.

Cryopreservation of testicular tissue for fertility purposes is not yet recommended. Most tubules in testes of adult women with CAIS are Sertoli cell only, and remaining germ cells are likely to have undergone (epi)genetic changes equipping them with extra survival and/or proliferation capacity. In addition, all ongoing transplant experiments and all in vitro techniques using immature human testicular tissue have thus far resulted in massive loss of spermatogonial stem cells.

Key Learning Points

- The first contacts with the medical team often have a lifelong impression on parents of a newborn who has a VSD, and these early interactions may determine acceptance of and coping with the condition and the sharing of information with their child.

- Genital surgery before an age at which a child can give personal informed consent is highly controversial, and it should be avoided whenever possible. However, raising a child with a genital difference is not easy and can sometimes cause mental harm. Threats to physical, but also to mental, health are criteria to be discussed in the shared decision-making process when genital surgery is being considered. In any case, the decision should be an individualized one, and blunt legislation that forbids all forms of genital surgery for children upon the age of maturity would cause much harm to these children.

- Most adolescents who have a VSD require follow-up that continues into adulthood. Some VSDs are associated with severe comorbidities. Adult endocrinologists should have a sound knowledge of VSDs and organize follow-up and, when indicated, targeted screening tests to detect comorbidities and take preventive measures if needed.

- Individuals who have a VSD and a Y chromosome in their (gonadal) karyotype are at increased risk of gonadal GCC. The risk can differ among the various diagnostic groups and this should be reflected in the proposed surveillance actions. In AIS, the risk is low, and girls with AIS can benefit from endogenous testosterone production. Most adolescent girls with AIS prefer to keep their gonads. Pros and cons of various treatment options should be discussed, and the patient, family, and medical team should come to an informed decision regarding gonadectomy or starting a surveillance program at the end of puberty.

- Pathogenic variants in the genes encoding androgen receptor cofactors can cause PAIS or CAIS.

- Vaginal dilation therapy is the first-choice treatment for vaginal hypoplasia, but this needs to be supported by a psychologist/sexologist and a pelvic-floor physiotherapist.

References

1. van der Straaten S, Springer A, Zecic A, et al. The External Genitalia Score (EGS): a European multicenter validation study. *J Clin Endocrinol Metab.* 2019;105(3):dgz142. PMID: 31665438

2. Meyer-Bahlburg HFL. The timing of genital surgery in somatic intersexuality: surveys of patients' preferences. *Horm Res Paediatr.* 2022;95(1):12-20. PMID: 35045418

3. Cools M, Verhagen E, Hoebeke P, Van Hoecke E, Cannoot P. Working towards convergence of the clinical management of differences of sex development/intersex conditions and the human rights framework: a case study. *Clin Endocrinol (Oxf).* 2023 [Online ahead of print] PMID: 38059612

4. Knerr J, Werner R, Schwan C, et al. Formin-mediated nuclear actin at androgen receptors promotes transcription. *Nature.* 2023;617(7961):616-622. PMID: 36972684

5. Cools M, Nordenström A, Robeva R, et al; COST Action BM1303 working group 1. Caring for individuals with a difference of sex development (DSD): a consensus statement. *Nat Rev Endocrinol.* 2018;14(7):415-429. PMID: 29769693

6. Falhammar H, Claahsen-van der Grinten H, Reisch N, et al; dsd-LIFE group. Health status in 1040 adults with disorders of sex development (DSD): a European multicenter study. *Endocr Connect.* 2018;7(3):466-478. PMID: 29490934

7. Debo B, Van Loocke M, De Groote K, De Leenheer E, Cools M. Multidisciplinary approach to the child with sex chromosomal mosaicism including a Y-containing cell line. *Int J Environ Res Public Health.* 2021;18(3):917. PMID: 33494433

8. Gravholt CH, Andersen NH, Conway GS, et al. Clinical practice guidelines for the care of girls and women with Turner syndrome: proceedings from the 2016 Cincinnati International Turner Syndrome Meeting. *Eur J Endocrinol.* 2017;177(3):G1-G70. PMID: 28705803

9. Cools M, Grijp C, Neirinck J, et al. Spleen function is reduced in individuals with NR5A1 variants with or without DSD: a cross-sectional study. *Eur J Endocrinol.* 2024;190(1):34-43. PMID: 38128121

10. van der Zwan YG, Biermann K, Wolffenbuttel KP, Cools M, Looijenga LH. Gonadal maldevelopment as risk factor for germ cell cancer: towards a clinical decision model. *Eur Urol.* 2015;67(4):692-701. PMID: 25240975

11. Barros BA, de Oliveira LR, Surur CRC, Barros-Filho AA, Maciel-Guerra AT, Guerra-Junior G. Complete androgen insensitivity syndrome and risk of gonadal malignancy: systematic review. *Ann Pediatr Endocrinol Metab.* 2021;26(1):19-23. PMID: 33819955

12. van Agthoven T, Looijenga LHJ. Accurate primary germ cell cancer diagnosis using serum based microRNA detection (ampTSmiR test). *Oncotarget.* 2017;8(35):58037-58049. PMID: 28938535

13. Committee on Adolescent Health Care. ACOG Committee Opinion No. 728: mullerian agenesis: diagnosis, management, and treatment. *Obstet Gynecol.* 2018;131(1):e35-e42. PMID: 29266078

14. Claahsen-van der Grinten HL, Speiser PW, Ahmed SF, et al. Congenital adrenal hyperplasia-current insights in pathophysiology, diagnostics, and management. *Endocr Rev.* 2022;43(1):91-159. PMID: 33961029

15. Baetens D, Mladenov W, Dell Chiaie B, et al. Extensive clinical, hormonal and genetic screening in a large consecutive series of 46,XY neonates and infants with atypical sexual development. *Orphanet J Rare Dis.* 2014;9:209. PMID: 25497574

16. Tack LJW, Spinoit A-F, Hoebeke P, et al. Endocrine outcome and seminal parameters in young adult men born with hypospadias: a cross-sectional cohort study. *EBioMedicine.* 2022;81:104119. PMID: 35759917

Approach to the Patient With Delayed Puberty

Francesco d'Aniello, MD. Bambino Gesù Children's Hospital, Rome, Italy, and Centre for Endocrinology, William Harvey Research Institute, Queen Mary University of London, London, United Kingdom; Email: francesco.daniello@opbg.net

Sasha R. Howard, MBBS, PhD. Centre for Endocrinology, William Harvey Research Institute, Barts and the London School of Medicine and Dentistry, Queen Mary University of London, London, United Kingdom; Email: s.howard@qmul.ac.uk and sasha.howard@nhs.net

Educational Objectives

After reviewing this chapter, readers should be able to:

- Identify and correctly diagnose causes of delayed puberty (DP).

- Recommend the most appropriate test to differentiate different forms of hypogonadism.

- Manage and treat patients with different etiologies of DP.

Significance of the Clinical Problem

Puberty is defined as a process of physical maturation leading to the attainment of adult height and body proportions, together with the development of the gonads with secondary sexual characteristics and the ability to reproduce.[1] Puberty onset is marked in males by attainment of testicular volume of 4 mL (Tanner genital stage 2) and in females by the initiation of breast development (Tanner breast stage 2). The timing of the physiological onset of puberty varies widely in both genders, but certain age thresholds have been established to define both precocious and delayed pubertal onset. Thus, DP is defined as the onset of puberty at 2 to 2.5 SD later than the mean age for the general population, which corresponds to approximately 14 years of age for males and 13 years of age for females. In addition, DP may also encompass older children with delayed pubertal progression, a diagnosis that is aided by the use of puberty nomograms.

The etiology of DP is complex, but it is usually divided into 3 main categories: Self-limited delayed puberty (SLDP, also known as constitutional delay of growth and puberty), hypergonadotropic hypogonadism, and hypogonadotropic hypogonadism, which can be further divided into functional, acquired, and congenital causes (congenital hypogonadotropic hypogonadism [CHH]).[2,3] Differentiation of these underlying conditions can be challenging, especially with respect to distinguishing SLDP from CHH, the presentations of which share many features.

The management of DP depends on the underlying cause. Treatment of SLDP typically involves either expectant observation or short courses of low-dosage sex steroid supplementation. In cases of permanent hypogonadotropic or hypergonadotropic hypogonadism, a more intricate and comprehensive approach is required to facilitate the development of secondary sexual characteristics and optimize fertility potential. At the same time, functional forms of hypogonadism often benefit from therapies that address the underlying cause.

Practice Gaps

- There is no single clinical or biochemical marker that clearly distinguishes SLDP from CHH.

- Due to their relatively high cost and poor availability in some centers, useful biochemical parameters, such as inhibin B and antimullerian hormone (AMH), are less commonly used for diagnostic purposes.

- Many clinicians lack of knowledge about these conditions and their underlying causes.

- Not many countries have national registries for congenital and syndromic causes of hypogonadotropic and hypergonadotropic hypogonadism, which can facilitate understanding and best practice management of these conditions.

Discussion

Etiology and Epidemiology

Self-Limited Delayed Puberty

The most prevalent cause of DP is SLDP. Delayed pubertal onset is more common in males, and up to 83% of boys with DP have SLDP, while 30% to 55% of girls with DP have SLDP.[3,4] SLDP has been linked to negative health consequences such as short stature, lower bone mineral density, and impaired psychosocial well-being.[5] Most patients with SLDP have a family history of DP (50%-75%).[6] Thus, although SLDP remains a diagnosis of exclusion, a positive family history of DP and the absence of pathological conditions, or signs, and symptoms are suggestive of this diagnosis.

Congenital Hypogonadotropic Hypogonadism

Hypogonadotropic hypogonadism is due to deficiency of GnRH from the hypothalamus, or alternatively due to a pituitary disorder, either of which results in deficiency of gonadotropin hormone production. Hypogonadotropic hypogonadism may be due to a congenital hypothalamic or pituitary disorder—either with gonadotropin deficiency as the only phenotype or with multiple pituitary hormone deficiencies and/or syndromic clinical phenotypes—or it may be due to acquired central dysfunction caused by irradiation, tumors, trauma, or vascular lesions.

CHH has an approximate prevalence of 1 in 4000 to 1 in 15,000.[7,8] A marked male preponderance (~4:1) in CHH has been consistently reported.[9] Despite recent genetic discoveries, the pathophysiological basis of CHH remains unclear in about 40% to 50% of individuals. More than 60 genes have been associated with CHH.[1] Kallmann syndrome, characterized by hypogonadotropic hypogonadism and anosmia, represents the most common form of CHH, constituting 60% of cases. However, there is wide variability in the CHH phenotype, ranging from severe or complete gonadotropin deficiency with lack of pubertal development to partial forms with entry into puberty followed by arrest of pubertal progression. This range of severity is secondary to varying molecular mechanisms and incomplete penetrance. Some patients may even experience reversal of the CHH phenotype after treatment.[10]

Functional Hypogonadotropic Hypogonadism

Chronic disease, malnourishment, excessive exercise, psychological or emotional stress can cause a maturational delay in the hypothalamic-pituitary-gonadal axis resulting in DP with low levels of gonadotropins—a condition called functional hypogonadotropic hypogonadism. A comprehensive medical history should include evidence of ongoing health problems, caloric intake, extent of physical exercise, and presence of chronic diseases (eg, inflammatory bowel disease or celiac disease). Any of these elements could suggest transient or secondary hypogonadotropic hypogonadism.

Hypergonadotropic Hypogonadism

Hypergonadotropic hypogonadism occurs in approximately 7% of male patients and 25% of female patients with DP.[3] It is characterized by primary gonadal insufficiency, which results in increased gonadotropin concentrations due to the absence of negative feedback. Klinefelter syndrome in males and Turner syndrome in females are the most common chromosomal anomalies causing hypergonadotropic hypogonadism. Both syndromes are caused by an abnormal number of X chromosomes or structural abnormalities of the X chromosome with an increased risk of autoimmune, metabolic, and cardiovascular disorders and certain cancers.[11,12]

Klinefelter syndrome (47,XXY) occurs in 1 in 667 live births. While most individuals with this syndrome experience spontaneous puberty at a typical age, DP may be observed in persons with a more complex karyotype, such as 48,XXYY, 48,XXXY, and 49,XXXXY. Most patients with Klinefelter syndrome, even those with normal onset of puberty, tend to become testosterone deficient by the time they reach Tanner stages 4 to 5 as a result of secondary regression. In nonmosaic forms of the condition, testicular volume rarely exceeds 6 mL. However, only 10% of boys between the ages of 10 and 14 years are diagnosed in a timely manner, with many individuals only referred to an endocrinologist in later adulthood.[11]

In women, Turner syndrome occurs with an incidence of about 1 in 2500 liveborn females.[12] In women with a classic 45,X karyotype, the ovaries are typically "streak gonads," made up of minimal amounts of connective tissue with no, or few atresic, follicles. Partial absence of or a structurally abnormal X chromosome, such as an isochromosome or ring chromosome, or mosaicism is also seen in patients with this condition with variable phenotypic features. While most affected women experience no pubertal development and primary amenorrhea, the degree of ovarian dysfunction and the extent of defects vary. Thus, some individuals (particularly those with mosaicism) undergo normal pubertal development (21%-50%) but later experience secondary amenorrhea.

Primary gonadal insufficiency may also be due to monogenic or syndromic causes, testicular regression or torsion in males, autoimmune ovarian disease in females, or childhood cancer in males or females treated with gonadotoxic chemotherapy such as alkylating agents, or radiation.

Diagnosis

One of the main challenges that clinicians face in the diagnosis of DP is distinguishing between SLDP and CHH, which is particularly difficult during adolescence. For many individuals with CHH, the condition is diagnosed during the second or third decade of life. Nevertheless, some clinical features allow detection of this condition earlier in childhood, particularly in males, such as cryptorchidism (undescended testis) or micropenis (stretched penile length <2 SD below mean for age). Additionally, during the infantile period of "mini-puberty" (which occurs approximately during the first 2 to 6 months of life), low or undetectable gonadotropins (LH and FSH) and sex steroid concentrations can indicate the absence of the physiological activation of the gonadal axis and biochemically confirm the diagnosis of CHH.[1] In adolescence, there are additional clinical, biochemical, and radiological features that can help to obtain a clearer picture of etiology. Patients with SLDP often have a degree of delayed skeletal maturation during childhood and thus tend to be shorter than both their peers and patients with CHH in adolescence.[13] Thus, bone age is often delayed to a greater extent in patients with SLDP. Another clinical element that can help to distinguish these 2 conditions is that adrenarche usually occurs later in persons with SLDP than in those with CHH. However, the most relevant clinical features to discriminate CHH from SLDP remain the so-called "red flags," which are listed in *Table 1* (*following page*).

When evaluating DP, laboratory testing should include measurements of gonadotropin concentrations and basal testosterone (for males) and estradiol (for females). LH and FSH concentrations are particularly helpful in determining whether the cause of hypogonadism is primary, in which case their basal concentrations are increased (hypergonadotropic hypogonadism). Basal LH and FSH are not as useful in the differential diagnosis of functional hypogonadotropic hypogonadism, SLDP, and CHH, where gonadotropin concentrations may be similarly low or undetectable. In these cases, stimulation tests such as gonadotropin response to GnRH and testosterone response to hCG can be of some utility, but they lack the sensitivity and specificity to effectively differentiate these conditions.

Table 1. Clinical "Red Flag" Signs of CHH

Sex	Clinical features
Males only	Cryptorchidism (unilateral or bilateral)
	Micropenis (stretched penile length <2 SD below mean for age)
Males and females	Anosmia
	Synkinesis (mirror movements)
	Cleft lip and/or palate
	Dental anomalies
	Skeletal anomalies
	Hearing loss (sensorineural)
	Iris coloboma
	Kidney agenesis

Inhibin B is a promising biochemical parameter to distinguish CHH from SLDP. Recent results suggest a cutoff of less than 61 pg/mL to enable identification of CHH in males, with a sensitivity and specificity of 90% and 83%, respectively.[4] There are insufficient data in females for the utility of inhibin B. Another proposed strategy is to use a combination of different tools to increase diagnostic accuracy; for example, the combination of a testicular volume cutoff of 1.1 mL together with a peak LH cutoff of 4.3 mIU/mL (4.3 IU/L) following GnRH stimulation and basal inhibin B concentrations. Recent research has highlighted the potential for kisspeptin-stimulation testing to diagnose CHH in adolescents and young adults, but this is currently only available in a research setting.

In addition, when hypogonadotropic hypogonadism is suspected, MRI of the pituitary gland and olfactory bulbs could confirm the diagnosis if anatomical abnormalities are found. For females, pelvic ultrasonography scan can help with both diagnosis and treatment by looking at the development of the uterus and ovaries.

Testes ultrasonography is useful for location of undescended testes and accurate sizing.

When hypergonadotropic hypogonadism is suspected, karyotype analysis is crucial because the most common causes to be confirmed (or excluded) are Turner and Klinefelter syndromes. For women, informative insights may be gained through autoantibody screening and AMH measurement. The former helps with the diagnosis when an autoimmune etiology is suspected, while the latter is a valuable parameter to establish the ovarian reserve in patients with primary ovarian insufficiency.

Over the past few decades, significant progress has been made in understanding genetic basis of CHH and Kallmann syndrome, as well as, more recently, monogenic causes of SLDP and primary ovarian insufficiency.[1] However, variable penetrance, oligogenicity, and complexity of gene-environment interactions in all of these conditions add to the complexity of phenotypic prediction by genetic testing alone.

Treatment

Treatment to induce or complete puberty is commonly considered for adolescents who either have significantly delayed or arrested puberty, or who have been diagnosed with a permanent underlying cause for their hypogonadism. Therapeutic regimens depend on the underlying diagnosis and differ between males and females (*Tables 2 and 3, following page*).

In SLDP, monitoring without intervention may be appropriate in situations where pubertal onset is late but may occur spontaneously. However, this decision should be made in conjunction with the patient and their family and should be reconsidered if no, or suboptimal, pubertal development is seen over 6 to 12 months of monitoring.

However, adolescents with SLDP can experience significant anxiety about body image in terms of physical size, short stature, and pubertal immaturity, and can experience decreased self-esteem, withdrawal from sporting activities, and difficulties with psychosocial and peer

Table 2. Medications to Treat DP in Male Patients

Drugs	Induction of puberty	
	SLDP	CHH/primary hypogonadism
Testosterone	*Enanthate, cypionate, and propionate (intramuscular)* • Not recommended before age 13.5 years • Initial dose: 50-100 mg once every 4 weeks for 3 to 6 months (not exceeding 100 mg) Minimal data available on other formulation (transdermal preparations and undecanoate)	*Enanthate, cypionate, and propionate (intramuscular)* • Recommended from age 12.0 years • Initial dose: 50 mg once every 4 weeks; progressive increase with 50 mg every 6 to 12 months; after reaching 150 mg, decrease interval to 2 to 3 weeks • Adult dosage 250 mg once every 2 to 4 weeks *Undecanoate* • Data on patients 17 years and older[14] • Transdermal • Initial dose: 10-20 mg daily; increasing doses over 1 to 3 years
Pulsatile GnRH (subcutaneous pump) **CHH only**	NA	Initial dose: 5-25 ng/kg per pulse every 90-120 min; increase to 25-600 ng/kg per pulse
hCG (subcutaneous or intramuscular) plus recombinant FSH (subcutaneous) **CHH only**	NA	hCG: 500 to 3000 IU/once to twice weekly rhFSH: 75-225 IU 3 times weekly (adjusted based on serum testosterone/FSH concentrations)

Table 3. Medications to Treat DP in Female Patients

Drugs	Induction of puberty	
	SLDP	CHH/primary hypogonadism
Estrogens (17β-estradiol)	*Transdermal patch* • Not recommended before age 13 years • Initial dose: 1/8-1/4 of 25 mcg 24-hour patch; increase by 1/8-1/4 patch after 6 months *Oral* • Initial dose: 0.5 mg (1/2 tablet) alternate days or 5 mcg/kg daily; increase to 0.5 mg (1/2 tablet) or 10 mcg/kg daily after 6-12 months	*Transdermal patch* • Not recommended before age 11 years • Initial dose: as per SLDP • Increase as per SLDP until 1 full patch *Oral* • Initial dose: as per SLDP, increase by 5 mcg/kg every 6-12 months until dose of 1 mg (1 tablet) daily
Estrogens (oral ethinylestradiol)	Initial dose: 2 mcg daily, increase to 4 mcg daily after 6 months	Initial dose: 2 mcg daily, increase by 2 mcg every 6 months until 10 mcg daily
Progestins *Introduced once adult uterine growth achieved*[14]	Not applicable	Norethisterone: 5 mg Utrogestan: 200 mg once daily Medroxyprogesterone acetate: 5 mg once daily
Combination preparations *Introduced once adult uterine growth achieved*	Not applicable	Transdermal or oral (eg, Evorel sequi, Elleste-Duet)

relationships. These issues may prompt clinicians to consider commencing therapy in patients with this diagnosis.

In males with SLDP, the most commonly used regimen is a time-limited course of low-dosage testosterone given as intramuscular depot preparations of a testosterone ester. At a starting dosage of 50 mg given once every 4 weeks for 3 to 6 months, increased height velocity (without advanced bone age) with promotion of sexual maturation can be achieved, often with improvement in psychosocial parameters. Further treatment courses may be given with dose escalation as required. In males, a key clinical confirmation of the diagnosis of SLDP is an increase in testicular volume in response to this therapy, indicating the development of the patient's endogenous pubertal gonadotropin production stimulating testicular growth (which will not occur in response to exogenous testosterone only). In contrast, males with CHH do not respond to exogenous testosterone with testicular growth, and testes remain small and immature. In patients with SLDP, alternatives to intramuscular testosterone are also used, including transdermal or oral preparations of testosterone or aromatase inhibitors, but these have fewer data to support their efficacy.

In females with suspected SLDP, equivalent short courses of sex steroids can be given as transdermal or oral 17β- estradiol. In both males and females, monitoring LH, FSH, estradiol, and testosterone in response to these therapies is important, as is clinical assessment of Tanner staging and growth. In females, pelvic ultrasonography to monitor uterine growth is also important.

In DP due to functional causes, the principal treatment strategy is to improve the underlying condition or environmental driver of DP. However, in certain cases, particularly chronic illnesses where treatment has already been optimized, sex steroid therapy may be required in males and females to support progress through puberty.

In permanent hypogonadism, if the diagnosis is made in a timely fashion, therapy to induce puberty can be commenced before the patient has officially developed DP. In females from age 11 years and in males from 12 years, slowly increasing dosages of sex steroids can mimic the gradual physiological rise in these hormones over 2 to 4 years in healthy adolescents. Timely diagnosis and treatment to induce puberty can be beneficial for sexual, bone, and metabolic health and can help minimize the psychological sequelae of DP. International guidelines are available for pubertal induction regimens with estradiol for females with primary ovarian insufficiency (including Turner syndrome)[12] and congenital or acquired hypogonadotropic hypogonadism.[10] For males with anorchia (eg, due to testicular

regression syndrome), induction of puberty with testosterone uses a similar regimen to that used for classic testosterone induction of puberty in males with CHH,[10] commenced at a low dosage with incremental dose increases to an adult dosage over 2 to 3 years. In patients who present or are diagnosed later with permanent hypogonadism (ie, older than 15 years in females or 17 years in males), a quicker progressing regimen is possible to prevent further delay in the development of sexual maturity.[14] Management priorities are somewhat different in adolescent males with Klinefelter syndrome, as most men with this condition enter puberty but many do not complete it. Thus, testosterone supplementation is introduced at the time when low testosterone concentrations or symptoms of hypogonadism are identified.[11] In all patients with permanent or longstanding hypogonadism, attention must be given to maintenance of good bone health, and psychological support should be provided for the adolescent or young adult and their family who are navigating the issues of fertility optimization and preservation and associated comorbidities.

In males with CHH, an emerging paradigm is the use of gonadotropins to induce puberty in place of testosterone. The hypothesis is that replacement of gonadotropins will allow stimulation of testicular growth and maturation, with endogenous production of testosterone and the potential for spermatogenesis, none of which are possible with exogenous testosterone replacement alone, as well as improved quality of life in this patient group. Use of either GnRH or combined gonadotropin regimens with recombinant FSH and hCG in adolescents with CHH, as opposed to waiting until fertility is desired to offer these medications, is increasing and has been shown to be well-tolerated with effective outcomes for testicular and penile development, serum testosterone concentrations, and sperm production.[15] Long-term studies, with longitudinal data collection via international electronic registries, are required to assess whether gonadotropin treatment in puberty in males with

CHH improves fertility (live birth rate) and long-term health and psychosocial outcomes.

Clinical Case Vignettes

Case 1

A 15-and-6/12-year-old boy is referred for short stature, low BMI, and lack of pubertal development. He was born at term after an uneventful pregnancy. He was delivered by emergency caesarean due to fetal bradycardia without complications. He was small-for-gestational-age with a birth weight of 5.6 lb (2.56 kg) (–2.05 SDS). During childhood, he developed multiple allergies and eczema, was small compared to his peers, and was a picky eater. Inquiry into his family history revealed that both his mother and father are below average height (respectively, –1.42 and –1.8 SDS), and his uncle was treated for delayed pubertal onset. The patient reports a normal sense of smell.

On physical examination, his height is 59.5 in (151.2 cm) (–2.6 SDS), arm span is 59.6 in (151.5 cm), weight is 85.8 lb (38.9 kg) (–2.4 SDS), and BMI is 14.0 kg/m^2 (–1.3 SDS). He has 4-mL testes bilaterally with a pubertal Tanner stage of G2, P2, A2. No dysmorphic features are noted.

Laboratory test results:

Total testosterone = 25.9 ng/dL (247.8-835.7 ng/dL) (SI: 0.9 nmol/L [8.6-29.0 nmol/L])
LH = <1.0 mIU/mL (1.7-8.6 mIU/mL) (SI: <1.0 IU/L [1.7-8.6 IU/L])
FSH = 1.8 mIU/mL (1.5-12.4 IU/L) (SI: 1.8 IU/L [1.5-12.4 IU/L])
IGF-1 = 224.4 ng/mL (129.0-486.3 ng/mL) (SI: 29.4 nmol/L [16.9-63.7 nmol/L])
Prolactin, normal
Thyroid function tests, normal
Full blood count, normal
Liver and kidney function, normal

His bone age is 12.9 years (chronologic age, 15.6 years).

Which of the following is the best next step in this patient's management?

A. Assess GH production by stimulation testing
B. Measure inhibin B and AMH and monitor growth and pubertal development over 6 months
C. Refer to a dietician to achieve a healthy body weight
D. Discharge to family practitioner for follow-up
E. Perform a karyotype analysis to exclude Klinefelter syndrome

Answer: B) Measure inhibin B and AMH and monitor growth and pubertal development over 6 months

This teenage boy presents with clinical findings that are highly suggestive of SLDP. Still, some features overlap with possible partial or functional hypogonadotropic hypogonadism. Being chronically underweight could partially explain DP and low gonadotropin concentrations (functional hypogonadism). However, his almost undetectable serum testosterone and low testicular volume are the main concerns in this clinical picture, and further evaluation is required to distinguish SLDP from CHH.

His baseline inhibin B and AMH were measured (Answer B) (215 pg/mL [215 ng/L] and 43 ng/mL [307.1 pmol/L], respectively), and the values indicated good Sertoli-cell function and made CHH a less likely diagnosis. After 3 months, a GnRH test was performed, which demonstrated a robust pituitary LH response to stimulation (19.9 mIU/mL [19.9 IU/L]), increasing the likelihood of SLDP.

Evaluating GH production (Answer A) in this case may not be necessary. It is highly probable that his short stature is familial. Both parents have below-average adult height. Despite being underweight, he has reasonable IGF-1 concentrations and is not short for his bone age (height for bone age: –0.4 SDS, which gives him a predicted adult height above his target height). For all these reasons, we would not suggest GH testing as a first step in this case.

Similarly, advising him to follow a nutritional plan to gain weight (Answer C) could be an accompanying intervention but not the primary one.

Patients with Klinefelter syndrome (Answer E) usually have spontaneous onset of puberty with normal early progression, followed by a progressive arrest of testicular growth. Affected individuals often have distinctive clinical features, with a tendency to be taller than their peers, with an arm span 2 to 3 cm greater than their height.

Referring him back to his family doctor for follow-up (Answer D) would be unwise without first ruling out possible organic causes and the potential need for hormone replacement therapy.

During follow-up over the next 6 months, his testosterone concentrations remained low with a small but gradual increase in testicular volume. In such cases, and depending on the patient's wishes, a short course of testosterone for 3 to 6 months can enhance the endogenous production of testosterone. Endogenous testosterone concentrations should be rechecked after stopping treatment. In this case, the patient's testosterone concentrations after 6 months of testosterone therapy normalized on a morning sample (322.8 ng/dL [11.2 nmol/L], 1 month after his last injection of intramuscular testosterone), and his gonadotropins rose into the age-appropriate range. His testicular volume reached adult size (20 mL) over the next 18 months, and he attained his midparental target height by age 18 years.

Case 2

A 17-year-old boy presents with suspected GH deficiency due to a suboptimal response to a glucagon-stimulation test. He recently stopped going to the gym because he is unable to work out due to low muscle strength. He is often told he looks younger than his age. The patient's sense of smell is intact. At age 18 months, he was treated for bilateral cryptorchidism with orchidopexy. His father has some memories of being a "late bloomer."

On physical examination, his auxological parameters are within the average range. His height is 67.4 in (171.1 cm) (−0.7 SDS), and weight is 134.3 lb (60.9 kg) (−0.3 SDS). His Tanner staging is G2, P2, A2 with a testicular volume of 3 mL bilaterally.

Laboratory test results:

Total testosterone = 14.4 ng/dL (237.8-835.7 ng/dL) (SI: <0.5 nmol/L [8.6-29.0 nmol/L])
LH = <0.1 mIU/mL (1.7-8.6 mIU/mL) (SI: <1.0 IU/L [1.7-8.6 IU/L])
FSH = <1.0 mIU/mL (1.5-12.4 mIU/mL) (SI: <1.0 IU/L [1.5-12.4 IU/L])
Inhibin B = 56.9 pg/mL (25.0-325.0 pg/mL) (SI: 56.9 ng/L [25.0-325.0 ng/L])
AMH = 25.6 ng/mL (6.4-156.8 ng/mL) (SI: 182.9 pmol/L [46.0-1120.0 pmol/L])
IGF-1 = 352.0 µg/L (129.0-487.5 µg/L) (SI: 46.1 nmol/L [16.9-63.9 nmol/L])
Prolactin, normal
Thyroid function tests, normal
Full blood count, normal
Liver and kidney function, normal

His bone age is delayed at 15.5 years (chronologic age, 17.0 years). Findings on brain MRI are normal. Testicular ultrasonography shows small but structurally normal gonads (right, 2.8 mL; left, 3.4 mL). A GnRH test shows a flat response, with low peak gonadotropin concentrations after stimulation (LH = 2.4 mIU/mL [2.4 IU/L]; FSH = 4.6 mIU/mL [4.6 IU/L]).

Which of the following is this patient's most likely diagnosis?

A. Functional hypogonadotropic hypogonadism
B. GH deficiency
C. Acquired hypogonadotropic hypogonadism
D. SLDP
E. CHH

Answer: E) CHH

This young man has multiple clinical, biochemical, and radiological characteristics typical of CHH (Answer E). He also has a suggestive finding in his medical history: bilateral surgically treated cryptorchidism, one of the clinical "red flags" for CHH. Moreover, he presents with an androgen deficiency-like clinical picture: fatigue with difficulty gaining muscle mass and small testicular volumes with delayed Tanner staging. Furthermore, his testosterone and gonadotropin concentrations are undetectable.

Functional hypogonadotropic hypogonadism (Answer A) is unlikely, as it is usually associated with an inflammatory or chronic illness or, more commonly in women, being underweight or overtraining.

GH deficiency (Answer B) is unlikely. He is not short and his IGF-1 concentration is in the reference range. The explanation for the suboptimal response to glucagon-stimulation testing is that GH testing is less sensitive when circulating testosterone concentrations are low (sensitivity is increased with sex steroid "priming").

Acquired hypogonadotropic hypogonadism (Answer C) is unlikely because there is no history of damage to the pituitary gland (radiation, chemotherapy, or local surgery). In addition, there is a reassuringly normal brain MRI, which can help to exclude this diagnosis.

SLDP (Answer D) is a less probable diagnosis than CHH in this case. Although SLDP is the most common etiology of late pubertal onset in males, by the age of 17 years the risk of CHH increases markedly, as most boys with SLDP have entered puberty by this age. While there is a family history of DP in a parent, this can also be seen in patients with CHH.[13] Usually, patients with SLDP tend to be shorter and weigh less at presentation and tend to respond to GnRH testing (although this is not always the case, particularly in younger unprimed patients). Inhibin B, an important biomarker to distinguish SLDP from CHH, is usually greater than 100 pg/mL (>100 ng/L) in those with SLDP.[4]

Case 2 (continued)

Which of the following is the optimal course of action in this patient's management?

A. Start testosterone treatment

B. Start gonadotropin treatment (hCG alone)

C. Start gonadotropin treatment (hCG + recombinant FSH)

D. Pretreat him with recombinant FSH for 2 months and then start him on combined treatment with recombinant FSH + hCG

Answer: D) Pretreat him with recombinant FSH for 2 months and then start him on combined treatment with recombinant FSH + hCG

When CHH is diagnosed in male adolescents, 2 treatment modalities can be considered. The first is classic therapy with sex steroids (testosterone in males [Answer A]) at increasing dosages to induce puberty. While gradually increasing dosages are important for optimal puberty outcomes, the pace can be accelerated in older adolescents to avoid contributing to a further delay in development.[14] The second treatment modality is induction of puberty with gonadotropins (Answers B and C), which has the advantage of promoting testicular maturation and the potential for facilitating fertility.[10] These are increasingly being used in place of testosterone and are effective and well-tolerated.

In view of this patient's low testicular volume and low inhibin B concentration—both suggestive of testicular immaturity—he is started on recombinant FSH alone for 2 months to increase Sertoli cell numbers (thus "priming" the testes) and then started on combined therapy with recombinant FSH and hCG (Answer D). The guidelines for treatment differ between different centers (see the United Kingdom protocol for an example (https://www.bsped.org.uk/media/1989/protocol-for-induction-of-puberty-with-gonadotropins-in-males-with-gnrh-or-gonadotropin-deficiency_bsped_website-002.pdf).

After one year of therapy, the patient has a testicular volume of 15 mL bilaterally (increase in volume confirmed by ultrasonography: right, 11.7 mL; left, 14.7 mL). He has testosterone and FSH concentrations in the reference range (markers of good response to appropriate treatment). His inhibin B concentration has increased to 218.2 pg/mL (218.2 ng/L) and AMH has decreased to 3.6 ng/mL (25.7 pmol/L), indicating testicular maturation. As a further diagnostic test, treatment is suspended for a short period and endogenous testosterone and gonadotropin concentrations are measured. Testosterone is undetectable with low LH and FSH, so the diagnosis of CHH is confirmed. Therapy is recommended with either gonadotropins or testosterone undecanoate.

Case 3

A 15-and-6/12-year-old girl is referred for primary amenorrhea and short stature. She had some pubertal development with axillary hair and initial breast development, and her primary care provider previously advised that she should give it more time as she is likely to be a "late developer" like her mother (who had menarche at age 14 years). However, the patient and her mother are worried about her childish appearance and that she is not progressing through puberty. She was born at term after a healthy pregnancy; amniocentesis was performed because of increased nuchal thickness on antenatal scans, but this showed a normal karyotype. Apart from a history of recurrent urinary tract infections, she feels well, is very active, and loves sports.

On physical examination, she is short (58.7 in [149.2 cm] [−2.2 SDS]) and at the lower end of her familial target height (62 ± 3.1 in [157.5 ± 8 cm]). Her mother's height is 60.2 in (153 cm) (−1.8 SDS), and her father's height is 68.9 in (175 cm) (−0.5 SDS)]. She is of average weight (112.4 lb [51 kg] [−0.5 SDS]). Her Tanner staging is B3 (with hypoestrogenized areolae), P3, A2-3. There are no obvious dysmorphic features except for low-set ears.

Results from previous laboratory testing:

> Estradiol = 6.5 pg/mL (0-26.7 pg/mL)
>   (SI: 24.0 pmol/L [0-98.0 pmol/L])
> LH = 4.2 mIU/mL (2.0-8.0 mIU/mL) (SI: 4.2 IU/L
>   [2.0-8.0 IU/L])
> FSH = 15.6 mIU/mL (3.0-10.0 mIU/mL)
>   (SI: 15.6 IU/L [3.0-10.0 IU/L])
> Thyroid function tests, normal
> Blood count, normal
> Liver and kidney function, normal

Her bone age is delayed at 12.3 years (chronologic age, 15.5 years). Her height for bone age is −1.3 SDS.

Which of the following is the best next step in this patient's care?

A. Repeat karyotype analysis (peripheral blood)

B. Confirm the primary care provider's diagnosis of SLDP and treat with a short course of estradiol therapy

C. Perform brain MRI

D. Prescribe a combined oral contraceptive pill

E. Perform an autoimmune screen

Answer: A) Repeat karyotype analysis (peripheral blood)

This girl has some features suggestive of Turner syndrome. It is important to emphasize that amniocentesis has a percentage of false-negative results, particularly in individuals who have some form of genetic mosaicism. Some features in her history may seem reassuring at first (a mother with a delayed age at menarche and parents being of below-average height). However, in a girl with short stature and primary amenorrhea who has not entered or is not progressing through puberty, particularly if she has high gonadotropins concentrations with low or undetectable estradiol, it is advisable to perform karyotype analysis (Answer A).

A diagnosis of SLDP (Answer B) is not impossible, but this is a diagnosis of exclusion and requires further evaluation before it can be confirmed.

Brain MRI (Answer C) is not indicated in a patient such as this who likely has primary ovarian insufficiency (with a biochemical picture of low or undetectable estradiol with raised FSH).

Starting a combined oral contraceptive (Answer D) before having a clear diagnosis is not the best next step. It is good practice to perform pelvic ultrasonography to measure uterine dimensions before introducing progesterone.

Performing an autoimmune screen (Answer E) is important in girls with a clinical picture of primary ovarian insufficiency, but it is not the first-line investigation to perform in this case.

Karyotype analysis was repeated, with 100 leukocytes examined, and the karyotype

45,X/46,XX confirmed a diagnosis of mosaic Turner syndrome. Further blood tests confirmed elevated gonadotropins (FSH = 23.0 mIU/mL [23.0 IU/L]) with low inhibin B (<9.8 pg/mL [<9.8 ng/L]) and AMH (3.3 ng/mL [23.6 ng/mL]) concentrations, confirming a low ovarian reserve. Ultrasonography of the abdomen and pelvis demonstrated a malformation of the urinary tract (horseshoe kidneys), which was most likely the cause of the recurrent urinary tract infections. Her care was transferred to a multidisciplinary Turner syndrome clinic (including endocrinology, psychology, cardiology, urology/gynecology specialists) to provide holistic care for the patient and her family.

Case 4

A 16-year-old girl with a recent spontaneous fracture has been referred for suspected idiopathic juvenile osteoporosis. She felt a sharp pain in her wrist while playing tennis. Plain x-ray confirmed a fracture of the distal radius and showed generalized demineralization of the surrounding bone tissue. Recent DXA shows a Z-score of –2.6 SD at the femoral neck and –1.6 SD at the lumbar spine. Her mother explains that the patient has asthma; she is worried that the use of inhaled corticosteroids could have caused the low bone density (she uses 100 mcg, 2 puffs twice daily of beclomethasone dipropionate). Despite developing breasts at age 12 years, the patient has not had her first period. Her mother is concerned that the patient has lost weight over the last few years. The patient is reluctant to talk about this and appears cross with her mother, withdrawing from the conversation. Family history is unremarkable.

On physical examination, her height is 66.3 in (168.4 cm) (+0.9 SDS), weight is 106.3 lb (48.2 kg) (–1.0 SDS) (BMI = 17.0 kg/m² [–1.6 SDS]). A previous weight measurement from her primary care physician's clinic shows she has lost 14.3 lb (6.5 kg) in the previous 4 months. Tanner staging is B3, P2, A2. She has no dysmorphic features.

Laboratory test results:

> Estradiol = 0.7 pg/mL (0-26.7 pg/mL) (SI: 65.0 pmol/L [0-98.0 pmol/L])
> LH = 1.1 mIU/mL (2.0-8.0 mIU/mL) (SI: 1.1 IU/L [2.0-8.0 IU/L])
> FSH = 1.6 mIU/mL (3.0-10.0 mIU/mL) (SI: 1.6 IU/L [3.0-10.0 IU/L])
> Inhibin B = 215 pg/mL (<224 pg/mL) (SI: 215 ng/L [<224 ng/L])
> AMH = 1.5 ng/mL (0.3-6.2 ng/mL) (SI: 10.7 pmol/L [2.1-44.3 pmol/L])
> Prolactin, normal
> Thyroid function tests, normal
> Liver and kidney function, normal
> Complete blood cell count, normal

Her bone age is 14.5 years (chronologic age, 16.3 years). Pelvic ultrasonography shows a peripubertal uterus (fundus-to-cervix ratio >1) with a longitudinal diameter of 40 cm and endometrial thickness of 3 mm.

Which of the following is the best course of action for this patient?

A. Start replacement therapy with gonadotropins to treat CHH

B. Start a bisphosphonate to treat idiopathic juvenile osteoporosis

C. Evaluate her nutritional status, mood, and eating behaviors to assess for functional hypogonadotropic hypogonadism

D. Start estradiol valerate to improve bone density

E. Modify her asthma therapy to address corticosteroid-induced osteoporosis

Answer: C) Evaluate her nutritional status, mood, and eating behaviors to assess for functional hypogonadotropic hypogonadism

In this case, the patient has some suggestive features and history that should lead one to evaluate for functional hypogonadotropic hypogonadism (Answer C). Especially in the absence of features suggestive of organic causes (anosmia, cleft lip/palate, etc), it is important to exclude conditions that could lead to functional inactivation of the hypothalamic-pituitary axis, such as chronic diseases, excessive physical exercise, and reduced caloric intake. This girl has a low BMI and, importantly, has lost a marked amount of weight over recent months. Her mother's concerns about her eating habits and the patient's reluctance to discuss this require a more in-depth review with respect to possible disordered eating habits.

The potential diagnosis of CHH has not been entirely excluded, but therapy to induce puberty with gonadotropins (Answer A) is not an available option in female patients. Furthermore, in a girl with primary amenorrhea, excluding functional causes of hypogonadism related to weight loss/reduced energy availability is essential before suggesting a diagnosis of permanent hypogonadism.

Idiopathic juvenile osteoporosis (Answer B) is unlikely given that it tends to have a more precocious onset and that recent weight loss, associated with hypogonadism, could instead explain the reduced bone health of patients with inadequate estrogen exposure. Thus, bisphosphonates are not indicated because there are more appropriate therapeutic options to treat reduced bone density during adolescence; for example, management of the underlying eating disorder or replacement of estrogen to treat suspected functional hypogonadism. However, in this case, given the strong suspicion of an eating disorder, treatment with estradiol valerate (Answer D) is not the first choice. In fact, according to consensus guidelines, the primary management of amenorrhea secondary to low caloric intake is to improve the patient's weight, which allows the endogenous gonadal axis to recover. In addition, another partially reassuring element is the DXA result. According to the 2019 official position of the International Society for Clinical Densitometry, the recommended scanning site to evaluate during growth remains the posterior-anterior spine (while the femoral neck site is only used in specific cases such as severe scoliosis or positioning difficulties). this patient's spine Z-score is low, but not significantly so (not below −2.0 SD), and it tends to improve with appropriate treatment and the resulting alignment of bone age with chronologic age.

Finally, although inhaled corticosteroids have been associated with reduced bone density in the literature, this patient is taking a low dosage, which is not likely to be sufficient to affect bone density and cause corticosteroid-induced osteoporosis (Answer E).

The patient and family were informed of the possible cause of her condition, and she accepted a referral to the eating disorder service. At subsequent follow-up visits, she was documented to be slowly gaining weight. After a year of appropriate management, her BMI had increased to 19.2 kg/m² (−0.7 SDS) and there was further progression of pubertal development to B3-4, P4, A3. At age 17.4 years, she had menarche and her estradiol and gonadotropins returned to the normal range, confirming the initial hypothesis of functional hypogonadism associated with abrupt weight loss.

Key Learning Points

- DP can be the presentation of a primary gonadal disorder or a temporary or permanent deficiency of central (hypothalamic-pituitary) reproductive hormones.

- Diagnosis of the underlying cause of DP requires careful attention to the patient's medical history; clinical, biochemical, and radiologic features; genetic investigations; and frequently a period of monitoring of pubertal progress with or without intervention.

- Successful treatment of DP depends on understanding the underlying condition, and therapy ranges from monitoring only to managing an underlying disorder in functional hypogonadism to hormone replacement (commonly sex steroids and, more recently, gonadotropins in CHH).

References

1. Howard SR, Dunkel L. Delayed puberty-phenotypic diversity, molecular genetic mechanisms, and recent discoveries. *Endocr Rev.* 2019;40(5):1285-1317. PMID: 31220230

2. Palmert MR, Dunkel L. Clinical practice. Delayed puberty. *N Engl J Med.* 2012;366(5):443-453. PMID: 22296078

3. Sedlmeyer IL, Palmert MR. Delayed puberty: analysis of a large case series from an academic center. *J Clin Endocrinol Metab.* 2002;87(4):1613-1620. PMID: 11932291

4. Varimo T, Miettinen PJ, Kansakoski J, Raivio T, Hero M. Congenital hypogonadotropic hypogonadism, functional hypogonadotropism or constitutional delay of growth and puberty? An analysis of a large patient series from a single tertiary center. *Hum Reprod.* 2017;32(1):147-153. PMID: 27927844

5. Zhu J, Chan Y-M. Adult consequences of self-limited delayed puberty. *Pediatrics.* 2017;139(6):e20163177. PMID: 28562264

6. Sedlmeyer IL, Hirschhorn JN, Palmert MR. Pedigree analysis of constitutional delay of growth and maturation: determination of familial aggregation and inheritance patterns. *J Clin Endocrinol Metab.* 2002;87(12):5581-5586. PMID: 12466356

7. Laitinen E-M, Vaaralahti K, Tommiska J, et al. Incidence, phenotypic features and molecular genetics of Kallmann syndrome in Finland. *Orphanet J Rare Dis.* 2011;6:41. PMID: 21682876

8. Fromantin M, Gineste J, Didier A, Rouvier J. Impuberism and hypogonadism at induction into military service. Statistical study. *Probl Actuels Endocrinol Nutr.* 1973;16:179-199. PMID: 4147392

9. Swee DS, Quinton R. Managing congenital hypogonadotrophic hypogonadism: a contemporary approach directed at optimizing fertility and long-term outcomes in males. *Ther Adv Endocrinol Metab.* 2019;10:2042018819826889. PMID: 30800268

10. Boehm U, Bouloux PM, Dattani MT, et al. Expert consensus document: European Consensus Statement on congenital hypogonadotropic hypogonadism--pathogenesis, diagnosis and treatment. *Nat Rev Endocrinol.* 2015;11(9):547-564. PMID: 26194704

11. Zitzmann M, Aksglaede L, Corona G, et al. European academy of andrology guidelines on Klinefelter syndrome endorsing organization: European Society of Endocrinology. *Andrology.* 2021;9(1):145-167. PMID: 32959490

12. Gravholt CH, Andersen NH, Conway GS, et al; International Turner Syndrome Consensus Group. Clinical practice guidelines for the care of girls and women with Turner syndrome: proceedings from the 2016 Cincinnati International Turner Syndrome Meeting. *Eur J Endocrinol.* 2017;177(3):G1-G70. PMID: 28705803

13. Aung Y, Kokotsis V, Yin KN, et al. Key features of puberty onset and progression can help distinguish self-limited delayed puberty from congenital hypogonadotrophic hypogonadism. *Front Endocrinol (Lausanne).* 2023;14:1226839. PMID: 37701896

14. Howard SR, Quinton R. Outcomes and experiences of adults with congenital hypogonadism can inform improvements in the management of delayed puberty. *J Pediatr Endocrinol Metab.* 2023;37(1):1-7. PMID: 37997801

15. Alexander EC, Faruqi D, Farquhar R, et al. Gonadotropins for pubertal induction in males with hypogonadotropic hypogonadism: systematic review and meta-analysis. *Eur J Endocrinol.* 2024;190(1):S1-S11. PMID: 38128110

Recurrent Fractures in Children

Natalie Hecht Baldauff, DO, MBA. UPMC Children's Hospital of Pittsburgh. Pittsburgh, PA; Email: natalie.baldauff@chp.edu

Educational Objectives

After reviewing this chapter, learners should be able to:

- Illustrate clinical findings and fracture characteristics that should prompt an evaluation for primary and secondary osteoporosis.

- Explain the appropriate stepwise workup for children with clinically significant fractures.

- Identify patients who should be treated with bisphosphonates.

Significance of the Clinical Problem

Fractures are common in children; therefore, it can be clinically challenging to distinguish those who have underlying primary and secondary osteoporosis from those who do not. Differentiating normal childhood fractures from primary and secondary forms of osteoporosis in children is essential to prevent consequences of untreated bone fragility, including long-term deformities and decreased quality of life.

In 2013, the International Society for Clinical Densitometry (ISCD) published revised criteria to define pediatric osteoporosis as (1) bone mineral density (BMD) Z-score ≥ –2 and a clinically significant fracture history (defined as 2 or more long bone fractures before age 10 years or 3 or more long bone fractures before age 19 years); or (2) 1 or more vertebral compression fracture occurring in the absence of high-energy trauma or local disease, irrespective of the BMD Z-score.[1] This definition has been largely successful in preventing overdiagnosis of osteoporosis and inappropriate pharmacologic treatment in otherwise healthy children. However, strict adherence to the ISCD criteria may miss clinically relevant bone fragility in high-risk children, for whom a single fracture can be associated with significant morbidity. There are also pitfalls with using BMD Z-scores, as these can differ by up to 2 SD depending on the reference database used.[2] For these reasons, it is essential to consider underlying chronic disease states, bone-toxic medications, family history, and the clinical and radiographic features of the fracture to ensure an accurate diagnosis of primary or secondary osteoporosis.

Practice Gaps

- Understanding what constitutes a "low-trauma fracture" and fracture characteristics that should prompt a bone health evaluation.

- Understanding limitations of DXA in children.

- Early identification of individuals at high risk for secondary osteoporosis, including children with inflammatory disorders, hematological/oncological disorders, kidney disease, and neuromuscular disorders and those being treated with bone-toxic medications.

Discussion

The overall incidence of a normally active child sustaining a fracture between birth and 16 years is between 10% and 25% (42% to 64% for boys and 27% to 40% for girls).[3-5] The age at peak incidence is 13 for boys and 10 for girls, and fractures of the distal radius and/or ulna are the most common sites for all pediatric age groups.[6] Several factors contribute to the higher prevalence of fractures in otherwise healthy children. First, during rapid childhood growth, the metaphysis of bones is thinner and cortical porosity is higher compared with that in adults, leading to transient cortical weakness. There is also an 8-month delay between peak growth velocity and peak bone mineral accrual, with the peak bone mineral accretion rate occurring at 12.5 ± 0.90 years in girls and 14.1 ± 0.95 years in boys of European ancestry.[7] Peak bone mass occurs between the end of the second decade and early third decade of life, highlighting the importance of the pubertal years for future bone health.

Nonaccidental trauma should be considered in any child who presents with fractures, especially children who are very young (<2 years of age) or are nonambulatory. There is not a single exam or radiographic finding that differentiates nonaccidental trauma from osteogenesis imperfecta (OI) and other primary osteoporotic bone diseases. In very young children, a classic metaphyseal lesion, a fracture through the metaphyseal region of the long bones near the growth plate, is caused by torsion and traction and is suggestive of abuse. Fractures of the ribs, scapula, spinous processes, and sternum are also highly concerning for abuse. Bruising in children younger than 9 months or bruising in unusual locations such as the back, ears, and genitals is highly suspicious of abusive injury. Other red flags for abusive injury include retinal hemorrhages, fractures in various stages of healing, a vague or inconsistent history, and a delay in seeking medical care.

OI, a genetic disorder of connective tissue, is caused by abnormalities in processing or synthesis of type I collagen. Radiographic findings that are suggestive of OI include osteopenia on skeletal survey, long bone diaphysis fractures or deformities, multiple thoracolumbar compression deformities, and multiple Wormian bones. Wormian (or intrasutural) bones are supernumerary bones that form due to extra ossification centers in the cranium, typically in the lambdoidal and coronal sutures. They can be seen in several disorders, including OI and craniosynostosis, although larger

numbers of Wormian bones (>10) are commonly associated with OI. Exam findings concerning for connective tissue disease include short stature, blue-gray sclerae, dentinogenesis imperfecta, and ligamentous laxity. Blue-gray sclerae, present in some subtypes of OI, occur due to thinness and transparency of the defective collagen fibers, which allows for visualization of the pigmented uvea. This finding can be normal in infants and young children who have thinner sclerae, as well as in acquired conditions such as iron deficiency anemia.

Assessing fracture characteristics is a key part of the initial evaluation of a child with recurrent fractures. The degree of trauma required to cause the fracture is a key part of this evaluation. The 2013 ISCD criteria exclude fractures sustained in motor vehicle accidents and those from falls from above 3 m (10 feet), as fractures are expected to occur under these circumstances. Mild to moderate trauma is much more difficult to define, and studies to further explore this are lacking in the pediatric population. For children with chronic diseases that increase the risk of bone fragility, including those treated with long-term glucocorticoids, more conservative criteria have been used. In this population, a fracture occurring at standing height or less at walking speed or less has been used to define a low-trauma fracture.[8]

Bone densitometry is a key part of the evaluation for a child with clinically significant fractures; however, this should always be used as part of a larger comprehensive workup and clinical evaluation. The lumbar spine (L1-L4) and total body less head are the preferred skeletal sites for measuring bone mineral content (BMC) and areal BMD measurements in children. This differs from measurement in adults in whom the preferred sites are the lumbar spine and hip. In 2019, the ISCD pediatric position statement was updated to endorse the use of alternative sites, including the proximal femur, one-third radius, and lateral distal femur. The proximal femur is ideal for children with reduced weight bearing who will need ongoing monitoring in adulthood. Lateral distal femur measurement correlates well with risk of lower-extremity fragility fractures and is the ideal site for children with orthopedic hardware or positioning difficulties (including secondary to severe scoliosis).

DXA should be done in a patient who may benefit from intervention and in those for whom BMD trajectory can be used to inform treatment decisions. DXA is the preferred method for assessing BMC and areal BMD; however, as areal BMD is calculated as the BMC divided by the scanned area, it can lead to artificially low BMD Z-scores in children with short stature and pubertal delay. There are 2 height adjustment approaches to address this discrepancy. The first is using height-for-age Z-score adjusted BMD Z-scores and the second is calculation of lumbar spine bone mineral apparent density (BMAD). BMAD uses a transformation of bone area to estimate the volume of each individual vertebra (L1-L4), which allows for approximation of the effects of bone depth and body size.[9] Additional imaging, including thoracolumbar spine radiographs and a skeletal survey should also be considered depending on the clinical context. Taken together, imaging provides supporting evidence to guide the need for further workup in uncertain and puzzling cases.

In the cases that follow, a multifaceted approach to the evaluation and treatment of children with recurrent fractures will be discussed. The workup of a child with recurrent fractures should aim to identify those with primary and secondary osteoporosis and prevent unnecessary workup in otherwise healthy children. The goal of care is to facilitate timely intervention and prevent major osteoporotic fractures in children with skeletal fragility.

Clinical Case Vignettes

Case 1

A 4-month-old baby girl with a medical history notable for 36-week prematurity and right pelvic kidney presents to the emergency department of a small community hospital because of right leg swelling. X-rays obtained in the emergency department show a right femur fracture and possible healing left femur fracture. Her caregivers are unaware of known trauma. She is transferred to the local children's hospital for further evaluation. According to her parents, there were concerns for a skeletal dysplasia on prenatal ultrasonography. Her long bones were noted to be short (<5th percentile) and her femurs appeared curved. As there was no family history of bone fragility fractures or skeletal dysplasias, her parents declined prenatal genetic testing. She was born via spontaneous vaginal delivery and there were no postnatal complications. She passed her newborn hearing screen. She has been meeting age-appropriate milestones and is bottlefed with milk-based formula.

Physical examination is notable for a length of 54 cm (0.02%, Z-score −3.54), weight of 4.64 kg (0.69%, Z-score −2.46), large anterior and posterior fontanelle without evidence of craniotabes, down-slanting palpebral fissures, and white sclerae. She has no bruising on exam.

Which of the following is the most appropriate next step in this patient's evaluation?

A. Obtain a skeletal survey

B. Assess for disorders of mineral homeostasis (serum and urinary calcium and phosphate, serum creatinine, urinary creatinine, PTH, alkaline phosphatase, 25-hydroxyvitamin D, and 1,25-dihydroxyvitamin D)

C. Obtain DXA

D. Assess for underlying acute or chronic systemic illness (complete blood count, celiac screening, inflammatory markers, and thyroid function tests)

E. Order genetic testing for OI

Answer: A) Obtain a skeletal survey

A skeletal survey (Answer A) is the appropriate next step in this child's evaluation. Because limited imaging was done at the outside facility, additional imaging is needed to assess for clinically unsuspected fractures, as well as possible skeletal abnormalities, particularly given the prenatal history. After assessing for possible nonaccidental trauma, the next step is to assess for disorders of bone mineral metabolism such as rickets (vitamin D dependent, hypophosphatemic, etc) and hypophosphatasia. Testing for underlying acute or chronic systemic illness is also important in the initial evaluation of a patient with multiple fractures, but these conditions would be less likely in this patient who has been an otherwise healthy infant. Baseline bone densitometry is part of the initial diagnostic workup for a child with multiple fractures; however, the reference data for infants younger than 1 year are scarce. Additionally, significant disparity between available databases further complicates use in young children. Reference data for children aged 1 to 5 years were recently published.[10] Genetic testing for OI, as well as other less common skeletal dysplasias, could both be considered in this patient, although neither would be part of this patient's initial assessment.

A skeletal survey showed a nondisplaced oblique fracture of the proximal diaphysis of the right femur and bowing of the left femur without acute or healing fracture. Imaging also showed a subtle cortical irregularity in the right lateral ninth rib and compression deformities at T8, T9, T10, and L1. Wormian bones were present and diffuse osteopenia was noted. Head CT showed a mild right occipital depressed skull fracture and again showed the presence of multiple Wormian bones. Laboratory studies were notable for normal complete blood cell count, comprehensive metabolic panel, magnesium, phosphate, 25-hydroxyvitamin D, and PTH. Subsequent genetic testing showed a heterozygous pathogenic variant in *COL1A2* (c.3106G>T, p.G1036C), consistent with a diagnosis of OI type IV with dentinogenesis imperfecta.

Case 1 (continued)

The patient is now 6 months old, and her parents bring her to an outpatient follow-up appointment to discuss treatment and long-term management. She has not had any additional fractures since her hospitalization. She has mild gross motor delay but is progressing developmentally. Her linear growth rate has been normal, but her height Z-score remains quite low (−3.5). Her weight has been maintained at the 1st percentile. Treatment is initiated with intravenous bisphosphonates (zoledronic acid).

Which of the following would be the most significant therapeutic benefit of bisphosphonate therapy in this patient?

A. Prevention of new fractures

B. Improvement in linear growth

C. Reshaping vertebral compression fractures over time

D. Prevention of scoliosis

E. Improved mobility and attainment of gross motor milestones

Answer: C) Reshaping vertebral compression fractures over time

Bisphosphonates, derivatives of inorganic phosphate, bind to hydroxyapatite crystals with high affinity and act to inhibit calcification and hydroxyapatite resorption, leading to suppressed bone resorption. Second- and third-generation bisphosphonates (alendronate, risedronate, ibandronate, pamidronate, and zoledronic acid) have nitrogen-containing side chains that selectively inhibit farnesyl pyrophosphate synthase within osteoclasts, leading to osteoclast apoptosis.[11] Bisphosphonates are the treatment mainstay in children with OI. It is well established that bisphosphonate therapy increases lumbar spine BMD and leads to reshaping of vertebral compression fractures (Answer C), particularly with early treatment initiation. Given that this patient was found to have multilevel compression deformities, treatment initiation will have a positive therapeutic outcome. A recent meta-analysis showed a lower fracture risk in bisphosphonate-treated individuals,[12] although results from other studies have shown conflicting results on reduction of fracture incidence.[13] Data on improvements in growth, function, and bone pain have not been conclusive.[14] Therapy has not been shown to prevent development of scoliosis in children with OI but may slow progression in children with more severe forms of OI.

Case 2

A 9-year-11-month-old boy with a medical history of obesity presents to the emergency department with back pain for approximately 36 hours. The day before presentation, he tripped and fell onto his knees and felt a "pop" in his back. He presents for further evaluation because of persistent pain with walking. Spine films reveal compression fractures at T6, T7, T8, L2, and L3. He has never had long bone fractures. His review of systems is notable for intermittent abdominal pain but is otherwise negative. He is described as a sedentary child who does not play sports. His dietary recall is normal with adequate dietary sources of calcium and vitamin D. His weight is 115.3 lb (52.3 kg) (98th percentile), height is 55.0 in (139.8 cm) (63rd percentile), and there has been no recent linear growth deceleration or weight loss.

Physical examination findings are notable for mild tenderness over the midthoracic spine but are otherwise normal. Dentition is normal.

A skeletal survey shows compression fractures and diffuse demineralization, particularly of the spine and pelvis. There are no new or healing long bone fractures and no other bony abnormalities. Spine MRI shows biconcave compression deformities at T2, T4, T6, T7, T8, T9, T11, T12, L2, and L3. A neurosurgeon evaluates the patient and recommends conservative (nonsurgical) management.

Initial laboratory test results:

> Calcium = 9.2 mg/dL (2.3 mmol/L)
> Phosphate = 5.5 mg/dL (SI: 1.78 mmol/L)
> Magnesium = 2.1 mg/dL (SI: 0.86 mmol/L)
> Alkaline phosphatase = 282 U/L (SI: 4.71 μkat/L)
> PTH = 21 pg/mL (SI: 2.23 pmol/L)
> 25-Hydroxyvitamin D = 28 ng/mL (SI: 69.9 nmol/L)
> 1,25-Dihydroxyvitamin D = 58 pg/mL (SI: 150.8 pmol/L)

Which of the following is the most important next step in this patient's evaluation and management?

A. Obtain a DXA scan to assess baseline bone densitometry

B. Assess for an underlying acute or chronic systemic illness (complete blood cell count, celiac disease screening, inflammatory markers)

C. Refer to medical genetics for further evaluation of underlying genetic causes of osteoporosis; begin supplemental calcium and vitamin D

D. Assess bone turnover markers (osteocalcin, bone-specific alkaline phosphatase, propeptides of type 1 collagen, telopeptides of type 1 collagen)

Answer: B) Assess for an underlying acute or chronic systemic illness (complete blood cell count, celiac screening, inflammatory markers)

The most appropriate next step in this patient's evaluation is to rule out underlying acute or chronic inflammatory conditions that may be associated with pathologic vertebral fractures (Answer B). Although pediatric vertebral fractures are rare in the absence of high-velocity trauma, they are present in 16% of children at the time of acute lymphoblastic leukemia diagnosis[15] and can also be seen in inflammatory conditions such as ulcerative colitis and Crohn disease. Long-term treatment with systemic corticosteroids is a risk factor for development of vertebral fractures. Baseline bone densitometry is an appropriate part of this patient's workup, but it should not be done before evaluation for underlying systemic illness. Similarly, evaluation of primary osteoporosis may be warranted in this child if the initial evaluation rules out disorders of mineral metabolism, as well as acute and chronic systemic illness. Supplemental calcium and vitamin D are not indicated for this patient who has normal labs and adequate dietary sources of both calcium and vitamin D. Finally, bone turnover markers are not part of a standard workup for children with suspected osteoporosis.

Bone turnover markers correlate with growth velocity, making their use as a measure of bone remodeling more challenging. A recent review by Landang et al[16] provides an excellent summary of their use in pediatrics.

Case 2 (continued)

Additional laboratory studies are notable for a normal complete blood cell count and inflammatory markers and negative celiac screening. DXA (GE Lunar iDXA) shows a lumbar spine BMD of 0.528 g/cm^2 (Z-score, –1.9) and total body less head BMD of 0.580 g/cm^2 (Z-score –1.7). Follow-up imaging shows interval healing of the midthoracic and upper lumbar compression fractures. The patient is attending physical therapy regularly and is pain free. He is evaluated by medical genetics, and subsequent testing shows a pathogenic variant in *PLS3* (c.1377+2T>G), which results in aberrant mRNA processing and is consistent with a diagnosis of X-linked osteoporosis.

The patient presents in the outpatient endocrine clinic to review laboratory results, genetic testing, and diagnostic imaging.

Which of the following is the most appropriate treatment plan for this patient?

A. Continue physiotherapy and low-impact activities

B. Repeat DXA in 1 year and begin bisphosphonate therapy when the BMD Z-score is less than –2.0

C. Begin treatment with zoledronic acid, 0.05 mg/kg intravenously every 6 months

D. Begin treatment with alendronate, 35 mg orally once weekly

E. Optimize nutrition and ensure appropriate intake of calcium and vitamin D

Answer: C) Begin treatment with zoledronic acid, 0.05 mg/kg intravenously every 6 months

The most appropriate therapy for this child who has sustained multiple low-trauma vertebral compression fractures is treatment with intravenous bisphosphonates, either zoledronic acid (Answer C) or pamidronate. Although oral bisphosphonates can be used in pediatrics and have been shown to increase BMD in patients with primary[14] and secondary osteoporosis,[17] only intravenous bisphosphonates have been shown improvement in vertebral height/vertebral body reshaping. Both physiotherapy and adequate intake of calcium and vitamin D may be beneficial for this patient, but neither is appropriate treatment for a child with this medical history. Finally, based on the 2013 ISCD Position Statement, the presence of 1 or more vertebral compression fracture, defined as greater than 20% loss of vertebral height ratio using the Genant semiquantitative method, is diagnostic of osteoporosis regardless of BMD Z-score.

PLS3, located on chromosome Xq23, encodes plastin-3, an actin-bundling protein, and has been recently identified as a gene associated with primary osteoporosis. The specific mechanisms by which *PLS3* pathogenic variants cause osteoporosis have not yet been fully deciphered.[18] Males with primary osteoporosis due to *PLS3* pathogenic variants present with both long bone and vertebral fractures without other extraskeletal manifestations typically seen in OI such as joint hyperlaxity, short stature, blue sclerae, and dentinogenesis imperfecta. Affected females have a variable phenotype ranging from mild osteopenia to childhood onset osteoporosis.

Case 3

An 18-year-old woman with a medical history of epilepsy, spastic quadriplegic cerebral palsy, and gastrostomy tube dependence presents to the endocrinology outpatient clinic after sustaining a left proximal femur fracture from an unknown mechanism of injury. The day before presentation, her nurse heard a "pop" in the left leg when positioning her for a bath, but she did not have any unusual fussiness in the immediate hours after this event. The following day, her mother noticed decreased range of motion of the left lower extremity and irritability during routine care. This femur fracture is the patient's third lifetime fracture. Her first fracture at age 2 years (a spiral tibia and fibula fracture) occurred with minimal trauma. Her second fracture, a Salter Harris I of the left distal tibia, occurred at age 7 years after she fell out of bed. Menarche was at age 12 years, and she has been on intramuscular depot medroxyprogesterone acetate since age 14 years because of painful menstrual periods. Her other medications are pantoprazole, phenobarbital, and levetiracetam. She receives gastrostomy tube feedings with a plant-based formula that provides adequate dietary calcium, phosphate, and vitamin D; however, she has recently struggled with feeding intolerance, and both weight and BMI are less than the 3rd percentile.

Which of the following sets of laboratory findings is most likely in this patient?

Answer	Calcium	PTH	Bone-specific alkaline phosphatase	25-Hydroxy-vitamin D
A.	↔	↔	↑	↓
B.	↔	↔	↑	↔
C.	↑	↓	↔	↔
D.	↓	↑	↑	↓
E.	↓	↑	↔	↔

Answer: D) Calcium, decreased; PTH, increased; bone-specific alkaline phosphatase, increased; 25-hydroxyvitamin D, decreased

This patient's epilepsy is currently managed with phenobarbital and levetiracetam. Levetiracetam has not been shown to have deleterious effects on bone when used as monotherapy, although data in pediatric patients remain sparse.[19] Phenobarbital, along with phenytoin, carbamazepine, and oxcarbazepine, increases the activity of cytochrome P450 enzymes. The cytochrome p450 enzyme, CYP24A1, catalyzes the conversion of both 25-hydroxyvitamin D and 1,25-dihydroxyvitamin D to inactive metabolites. The decrease in 1,25-dihydroxyvitamin D may lead to reduced calcium absorption, secondary hyperparathyroidism, and increased bone resorption. The patient has also had difficulty with feeding tolerance, which may be further impairing absorption of calcium, phosphate, and vitamin D. Therefore, the most likely laboratory profile is hypocalcemia, secondary hyperparathyroidism, elevated alkaline phosphatase due to high bone turnover, and low 25-hydroxyvitamin D levels (Answer D).

Case 3 (continued)

Additional evaluation includes DXA (GE Lunar iDXA). The lumbar spine BMD is 1.176 gm/cm^2 (Z-score, –0.1) and total body less head BMD is 0.840 gm/cm^2 (Z-score, –1.6). She does not have evidence of compression fractures. Supplemental calcium and cholecalciferol are initiated and she is evaluated by gastroenterology to optimize her feeding regimen and address her feeding intolerance. Follow-up laboratory studies show normalized values, and her weight has improved although BMI remains low for age. She continues to struggle with feeding intolerance. She remains on pantoprazole, levetiracetam, and phenobarbital. Due to concerns for bone loss with long-term use, medroxyprogesterone acetate is discontinued following the fracture, and normal monthly menstrual periods resume within 3 months.

The patient and her mother return for follow-up to discuss ongoing management.

Which of the following treatment plans is most appropriate for this patient?

A. Continue supplemental calcium and vitamin D, repeat laboratory tests in 6 months, and repeat DXA in 1 year

B. Initiate bisphosphonate therapy

C. Discuss changing anticonvulsant therapy with the neurology team

D. Repeat DXA in 1 year with plans to begin bisphosphonate therapy if Z-scores have worsened or remain below average

E. Discontinue supplements because laboratory values have normalized, repeat laboratory tests in 6 months, and repeat DXA in 1 year

Answer: B) Initiate bisphosphonate therapy

Although this patient has normal bone densitometry in the total body less head and lumbar spine, she has sustained 3 fractures, 2 of which occurred with minimal trauma. Additionally, she has multiple risk factors that will continue to affect her BMD, including spastic quadriparesis/nonambulatory status, long-term treatment with anticonvulsant drugs and proton-pump inhibitors, and recent feeding intolerance that has affected her overall nutritional status. For this reason, bisphosphonate therapy (Answer B) is the most appropriate treatment for this patient. Children with chronic disease and neuromuscular disorders can sustain osteoporotic fractures with BMD Z-scores greater than –2, which highlights the possible pitfalls with strict adherence to the 2013 ISCD criteria. Additionally, obtaining accurate BMD measurements in children with cerebral palsy can be challenging due to joint contractures, scoliosis, and hip dysplasia. Lateral distal femur DXA measurements correlate well with lower-extremity fracture risk in nonambulatory children and may be a preferred site in this population if reference data are available.[20] Individuals with contractures and other neuromuscular disabilities can be comfortably positioned for this imaging.

Ongoing calcium and vitamin D supplementation is recommended due to continued issues with feeding intolerance and ongoing treatment with phenobarbital. As this patient has been stable from an epilepsy standpoint, adjustment to her anticonvulsant regimen may not be in her best interest and would not negate the need for osteoporosis management.

Key Learning Points

*   The initial assessment of a young child with multiple fractures should aim to exclude nonaccidental trauma and disorders of bone mineral metabolism and facilitate (when appropriate) the diagnosis of the underlying genetic etiology. Radiographic findings of osteopenia on skeletal survey, long-bone diaphysis fractures or deformities, multiple thoracolumbar compression deformities, and multiple Wormian bones are highly concerning for OI.

*   Vertebral compression fractures are diagnostic of osteoporosis, regardless of the BMD Z-score. These fractures can be seen in children with chronic disease, particularly those treated with glucocorticoids, as well as in children with primary osteoporosis. Presence of vertebral compression fractures warrants consideration of treatment with bisphosphonates.

*   Children with neuromuscular disorders may have multiple risk factors for secondary osteoporosis, including limited/no weight bearing and use of bone toxic medications. In this population, multiple fractures can lead to significant morbidity; therefore, strict adherence to the ISCD criteria should not be used. The lateral distal femur can be used for BMD measurement in this population, particularly if other sites cannot be used due to difficulty with positioning or the presence of orthopedic hardware.

References

1. Bishop N, Arundel P, Clark E, et al. Fracture prediction and the definition of osteoporosis in children and adolescents: the ISCD 2013 Pediatric Official Positions. *J Clin Densitom.* 2014;17(2):275-280. PMID: 24631254
2. Kocks J, Ward K, Mughal Z, Moncayo R, Adams J, Högler W. Z-score comparability of bone mineral density reference databases for children. *J Clin Endocrinol Metab.* 2010;95(10):4652-4659. PMID: 20668038
3. Landin LA. Fracture patterns in children. Analysis of 8,682 fractures with special reference to incidence, etiology and secular changes in a Swedish urban population 1950-1979. *Acta Orthop Scand Suppl.* 1983;202:1-109. PMID: 6574687
4. Landin LA. Epidemiology of children's fractures. *J Pediatr Orthop B.* 1997;6(2):79-83. PMID: 9165435

5. Cheng JC, Shen WY. Limb fracture pattern in different pediatric age groups: a study of 3,350 children. *J Orthop Trauma*. 1993;7(1):15-22. PMID: 8433194

6. Larsen AV, Mundbjerg E, Lauritsen JM, Faergemann C. Development of the annual incidence rate of fracture in children 1980-2018: a population-based study of 32,375 fractures. *Acta Orthop*. 2020;91(5):593-597. PMID: 32500789

7. Weaver CM, Gordon CM, Janz KF, et al. The National Osteoporosis Foundation's position statement on peak bone mass development and lifestyle factors: a systematic review and implementation recommendations. *Osteoporos Int*. 2016;27(4):1281-386. PMID: 26856587

8. Ward LM, Ma J, Lang B, et al. Bone morbidity and recovery in children with acute lymphoblastic leukemia: results of a six-year prospective cohort study. *J Bone Miner Res*. 2018;33(8):1435-1443. PMID: 29786884

9. Kindler JM, Lappe JM, Gilsanz V, et al. Lumbar spine bone mineral apparent density in children: results from the bone mineral density in childhood study. *J Clin Endocrinol Metab*. 2019;104(4):1283-1292. PMID: 30265344

10. Kalkwarf HJ, Shepherd JA, Fan B, et al. Reference ranges for bone mineral content and density by dual energy x-ray absorptiometry for young children. *J Clin Endocrinol Metab*. 2022;107(9):e3887-e3900. PMID: 35587453

11. Drake MT, Clarke BL, Khosla S. Bisphosphonates: mechanism of action and role in clinical practice. *Mayo Clin Proc*. 2008;83(9):1032-1045. PMID: 18775204

12. Shi CG, Zhang Y, Yuan W. Efficacy of bisphosphonates on bone mineral density and fracture rate in patients with osteogenesis imperfecta: a systematic review and meta-analysis. *Am J Ther*. 2016;23(3):e894-e904. PMID: 25844482

13. Hald JD, Evangelou E, Langdahl BL, Ralston SH. Bisphosphonates for the prevention of fractures in osteogenesis imperfecta: meta-analysis of placebo-controlled trials. *J Bone Miner Res*. 2015;30(5):929-933. PMID: 25407702

14. Dwan K, Phillipi CA, Steiner RD, Basel D. Bisphosphonate therapy for osteogenesis imperfecta. *Cochrane Database Syst Rev*. 2016;10(10):Cd005088. PMID: 27760454

15. Halton J, Gaboury I, Grant R, et al. Advanced vertebral fracture among newly diagnosed children with acute lymphoblastic leukemia: results of the Canadian Steroid-Associated Osteoporosis in the Pediatric Population (STOPP) research program. *J Bone Miner Res*. 2009;24(7):1326-1334. PMID: 192102218

16. Ladang A, Rauch F, Delvin E, Cavalier E. Bone turnover markers in children: from laboratory challenges to clinical interpretation. *Calcif Tissue Int*. 2023;112(2):218-232. PMID: 35243530

17. Ward L, Tricco AC, Phuong P, Cranney A, Barrowman N, Gaboury I, et al. Bisphosphonate therapy for children and adolescents with secondary osteoporosis. *Cochrane Database Syst Rev*. 2007;2007(4):Cd005324. PMID: 17943849

18. Zhong W, Pathak JL, Liang Y, et al. The intricate mechanism of PLS3 in bone homeostasis and disease. *Front Endocrinol (Lausanne)*. 2023;14:1168306. PMID: 37484945

19. Gözükızıl ST, Aydın Z, Yalçın AD. Relationship between bone density and levetiracetam monotherapy in epilepsy patients. *Clin Neurol Neurosurg*. 2022;218:107270. PMID: 35623138

20. Henderson RC, Berglund LM, May R, et al. The relationship between fractures and DXA measures of BMD in the distal femur of children and adolescents with cerebral palsy or muscular dystrophy. *J Bone Miner Res*. 2010;25(3):520-526. PMID: 19821773

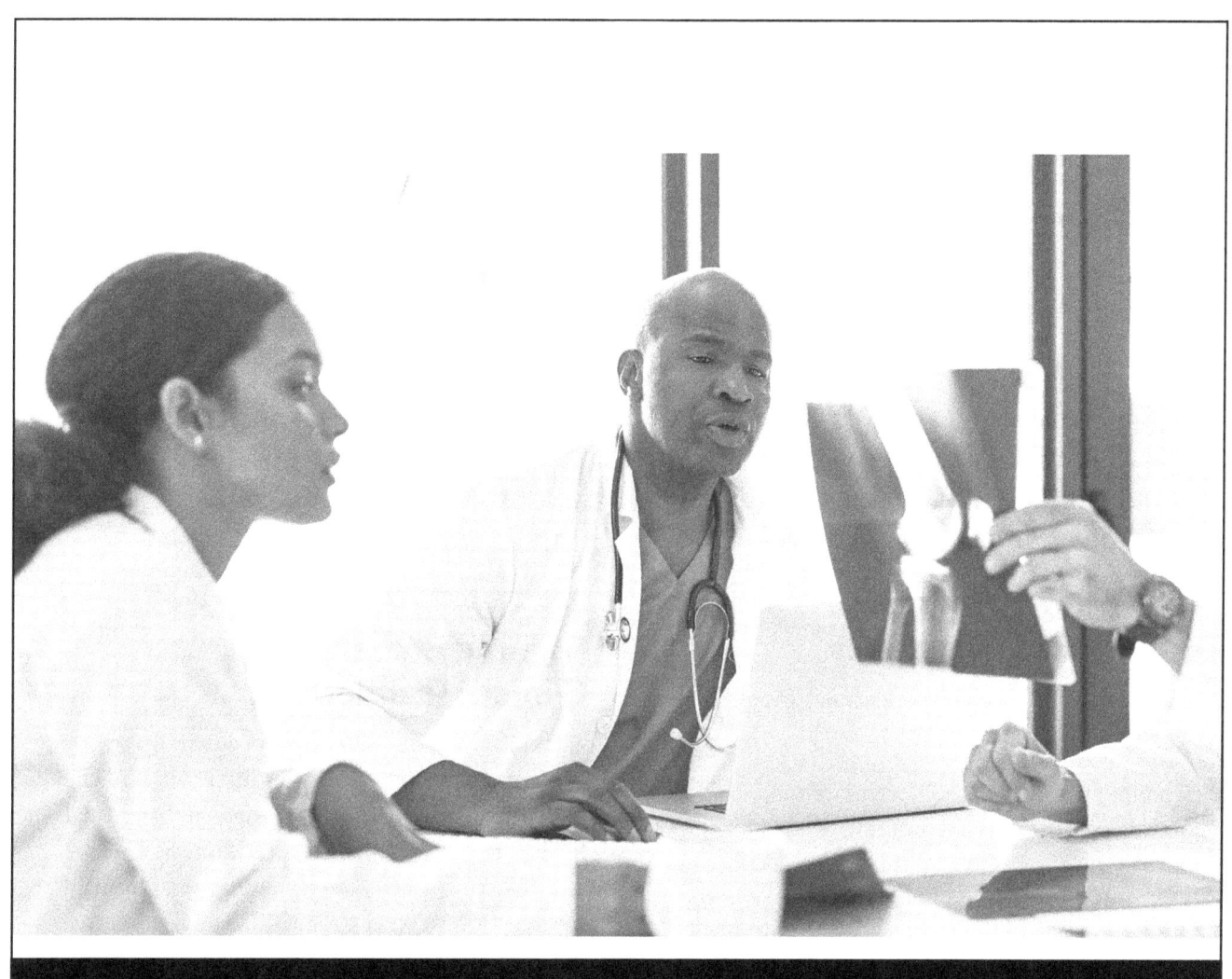

REPRODUCTIVE
ENDOCRINOLOGY

Approach to Thyroid and Parathyroid Disorders in Pregnancy: The Fetus is the Linchpin

Linda A. Barbour, MD, MSPH. Department of Medicine and Obstetrics and Gynecology, Divisions of Endocrinology Metabolism, and Diabetes and Maternal-Fetal Medicine, University of Colorado School of Medicine and Anschutz Medical Campus, Aurora, CO; Email: lynn.barbour@cuanschutz.edu

Educational Objectives

After reviewing this chapter, learners should be able to:

- Explain the difficulties in accurately interpretating thyroid function tests (TFTs) in pregnancy, not only due the dramatic effect of hCG and estrogen on total and free hormone levels, but also due to the limitations of the assays and absence of gestational normal ranges.

- Explain why there is no consensus on the diagnosis and treatment of subclinical hypothyroidism in pregnancy or isolated hypothyroxinemia and what may be a reasonable approach to their management based on potential benefits and risks.

- Distinguish Graves disease from gestational transient thyrotoxicosis (GTT) in the surveillance for fetal Graves disease and manage Graves disease to prevent overtreatment or undertreatment of the mother, which can result in significant morbidity to the fetus.

- Develop the skillsets to correctly interpret laboratory values that are affected by changes in calcium metabolism in pregnancy, diagnose and treat primary hyperparathyroidism (PHPT) and hypoparathyroidism, and determine when to recommend surgical treatment for PHPT.

Significance of the Clinical Problem

Thyroid hormone disorders occur in up to 10% of pregnancies when GTT is included, and they have major implications for maternal and fetal health. However, misinterpretation of TFTs and the confusion over what degree of thyroid dysfunction to treat to optimize fetal outcomes pose unique challenges in screening, diagnosis, and management. Common misinterpretation of TFTs is not only due to the marked metabolic changes in pregnancy that affect free and total hormone levels, but also to limitations of the available assays. Optimal treatment is substantially affected by confusion over what conditions should be treated, the lack of recognition that treatment goals are different from those outside of pregnancy, and the unappreciated consequences of overtreatment or undertreatment on fetal and newborn health. Adequate iodine intake is often not recognized or sufficiently addressed. Autoimmunity manifested by Graves or Hashimoto antibodies, often coexisting, have more compelling obstetric clinical implications than outside of pregnancy, especially on fetal and postpartum outcomes. Finally, due to limitations in randomized controlled trials that include heterogeneous populations, use of assays that are less accurate in pregnancy and without gestational normal ranges, the inability to initiate treatment early enough in pregnancy to affect fetal health, and poorly characterized outcomes that are difficult to measure, optimal management of some disorders remains highly contested.[1] This chapter reviews the essential maternal, placental, and fetal thyroid physiology; the appropriate considerations in accurately interpreting TFTs and their limitations; key areas that lack consensus; and approaches to the management of controversial areas that lack robust evidence-based data.[2] Specifically, the chapter will discuss management of overt hyperthyroidism from Graves disease and how it must be distinguished from GTT, as well as an approach to the treatment of subclinical hypothyroidism.

PHPT in pregnancy is often unappreciated because PTH levels are relatively lower in pregnancy, as are calcium levels, due to multiple pregnancy-related factors, including PTHrP. Symptoms are often nonspecific to pregnancy but, if unrecognized, maternal hypercalcemia can result in suppression of the fetal parathyroid leading to severe neonatal hypocalcemia and tetany.[3]

Practice Gaps

- Difficulties in the accurate interpretation of TFTs are not only due to marked metabolic changes in pregnancy that affect free and total levels, but also by the limitations of the assays available for measurement. Furthermore, the predictive value of newer assays on fetal outcomes, especially those measuring Graves and Hashimoto antibodies, have not been validated in large trials.

- The limitations in randomized controlled trials (population differences in ethnicity and geography, difficulties in initiating early treatment in pregnancy, inability to stratify outcomes according to various degrees of thyroid dysfunction, inclusion of healthy participants with thyroid autoimmunity, and the lack of precision in offspring neurocognitive testing and other outcomes)

result in a lack of consensus on the best practices for screening and treatment of subclinical hypothyroidism and isolated mild hypothyroxinemia.

- The lack of gestational-specific ranges for indices related to the changes in calcium metabolism in pregnancy that result in lower calcium concentrations unless corrected for albumin, a lower PTH level, and higher 24-hour calcium excretion, contributes to hypercalcemia caused by PHPT often being missed in pregnancy. As a result of the active transport of calcium by the placenta and suppression of the fetal parathyroid glands, the newborn may develop tetany, seizures, and be at risk for life-threatening hypocalcemia, and the mother may present with a hypercalcemic emergency immediately after delivery.

Discussion

Thyroid Disease in Pregnancy

Changes in Thyroid Hormone Physiology and Interpretation of TFTs in Pregnancy

Thyroid disease in pregnancy is one of the most common disorders with major implications for both maternal and offspring health. However, changes in physiology during pregnancy and major problems with test performance result in common misdiagnosis and mismanagement when interpreting TFT results.[4] Major physiologic changes include thyroid stimulation by hCG, estrogen-induced rise in thyroxine-binding globulin (TBG), changes in clearance of thyroid hormone, increased iodine metabolism, and placental activity of type 2 and 3 deiodinases. The thyroid gland increases in size by 10% to 15%, which is typically not appreciable by palpation. However, in iodine-deficient areas, gland size may increase 20% to 50%, also known as the thyroid goiter of pregnancy. Iodine requirements increase substantially in pregnancy (250 mg daily) and supplemental iodine is recommended in pregnancy (150 mcg daily). Insufficient iodine is common in pregnancy because the fetus also requires iodine for its own thyroid hormone synthesis. Pregnant persons with normal thyroid function can adapt appropriately to the increased demands of pregnancy, but those with inadequate iodine intake or with decreased thyroid reserve from Hashimoto thyroiditis, ablation, or partial thyroidectomy may not be able to adequately increase thyroid hormone production.

TSH levels are lower in pregnancy due to high hCG levels with thyrotropic activity, especially in the first and second trimesters. The American Thyroid Association recommends a downward shift in both the lower limit (by 0.4 mIU/L) and the upper limit (by 0.5 mIU/L) of the TSH reference range during pregnancy (usually a range near 0.1-4.0 mIU/L) if gestational-specific pregnancy ranges are not available.[1] Due to early effect of estrogen markedly stimulating TBG, total T_4 and total T_3 levels increase by 5% per week starting at 7 weeks' gestation up to approximately 50% by 16 weeks and they remain at that level.[1] Unfortunately, most free T_4 and free T_3 immunoassays are not reliable in pregnancy, especially in the late second trimester and third trimesters. This is due to both difficulties in accurate measurements (given free T_4 and free T_3 concentrations are less than 0.05% of total T_4 and total T_3 and due to a lack of gestational normal ranges due to free T_4 actually decreasing modestly in later pregnancy).[4] As a result, treatment decisions that involve free T_4 in the second half of pregnancy, especially in the titration of antithyroid drugs (ATDs), should be based on equilibrium dialysis assays with first, second, and third trimester gestational-specific normal ranges. Tandem mass spectrometry, also precise, is not readily available.[4] Alternatively, using the total T_4 and total T_3 levels and adjusting for the 50% increase in the upper limit of the normal range after 16 weeks' gestation is also an alternative method of assessing thyroid hormone levels.[1] Given that circulating free T_3 levels are even lower and hence more difficult to measure than free T_4 levels, the total T_3 assay (with adjustment) is preferred over free T_3 assays.

Treatment of Overt or Subclinical Hypothyroidism in Pregnancy

Patients with overt hypothyroidism (elevated TSH and low free T_4, or a TSH value >10.0 mIU/L irrespective of T_4) should be started on a levothyroxine dosage of 1.5 to 2.0 mcg/kg per day given that a full replacement levothyroxine dosage in pregnancy is approximately 2 to 2.2 mcg/kg per day compared with dosages in nonpregnant patients (~1.6 mcg/kg per day). At approximately 12 to 14 weeks' gestation, the fetal thyroid gland develops, and the hypothalamic-pituitary-thyroid axis begins to function. Before 16 weeks, the fetus relies solely on transplacental delivery of T_4, critical for neuronal migration, myelination, synaptogenesis, and connection.[5] Therefore, immediate treatment of overt hypothyroidism, especially before 16 to 18 weeks, should be with near-full replacement doses. TSH should be rechecked every 4 weeks until 18 weeks' gestation, every 4 to 6 weeks after dosage adjustments, and at least every 8 to 12 weeks later in pregnancy if stable. Because thyroid hormone requirements increase by 20% to 50% in pregnancy, especially for those who are athyreotic from ablation or thyroidectomy, a 25% increase in levothyroxine should be considered as soon as pregnancy is diagnosed.[5] This is due to the rapid increase in estrogen-stimulated TBG very early in pregnancy, in addition to increased volume of distribution, maternal weight gain, transplacental crossing of T_4, and placental deiodination of T_4 and T_3 (by type 3 deiodinase). This 25% increase can easily be done by adding 2 tablets per week to the patient's normal dose until TSH can be checked.

Subclinical hypothyroidism, especially with TPO antibodies, has been associated with preterm delivery and early miscarriage.[6] Pregnant persons with subclinical hypothyroidism, usually caused by Hashimoto thyroiditis in the United States and accompanied by TPO antibodies, have partial thyroid dysfunction and are usually effectively treated with lower dosages (50-75 mcg daily) depending on the degree of TSH elevation and the patient's weight. Although there is a lack of consensus in the treatment of subclinical hypothyroidism due to randomized controlled trials not clearly showing a benefit for maternal or infant outcomes,[7] trials were limited by their late start in treatment (usually at 15-16 weeks), recruitment of very mild subclinical hypothyroidism (mean TSH = 4-6 mIU/L), variable assessment of TPO antibodies (which alone may contribute to adverse outcomes from autoimmunity), and the myriad causes that influence childhood neurodevelopment at ages 3 to 5 years.[2] Therefore, the question of whether treatment of subclinical hypothyroidism with an elevated TSH concentration greater than 6.0 mIU/L (7.0-10.0 mIU/L) in early pregnancy improves outcomes remains unsettled. A meta-analysis of 9 randomized controlled trials and 13 cohort studies comprising 11,273 pregnant women with subclinical hypothyroidism showed no statistically significant differences between the levothyroxine group and control group in all primary and secondary outcomes, such as preterm delivery, miscarriage, gestational hypertension, preeclampsia, or gestational diabetes.[6] Given the potential benefit over the risk, lower TSH range in pregnancy, fetal dependence on maternal T_4 until 16 weeks, and minimal risk of low-dosage treatment, most experts elect to treat subclinical hypothyroidism (TSH >4.0 to <10.0 mIU/L) especially before 16 weeks' gestation, if the TSH concentration is greater than 6.0 mIU/L and if TPO antibodies are present.[1,2,8]

Causes of Hyperthyroidism in Pregnancy, When and How to Treat, and Surveillance for Fetal Graves Disease

Overt hyperthyroidism, unless due to hCG-mediated GTT, carries both maternal and fetal risks and should be treated, whereas subclinical hyperthyroidism (suppressed TSH alone without an increase in T_4 or T_3 adjusted for pregnancy) carries no risk and should NEVER be treated. GTT occurs in 3% to 11% of pregnancies and is caused by elevated levels of hCG, which binds to the TSH receptor and stimulates thyroid hormone release.

Posttranslational modification of the sialylation of hCG can change its affinity for the TSH receptor and half-life in the circulation, thus resulting in elevated thyroid hormone levels in the first half of pregnancy.[2] HCG concentrations greater than 100,000 IU/mL, which often cause severe nausea and vomiting of pregnancy and which can be seen in hyperemesis gravidarum, multifetal gestations, and especially molar pregnancies, can often cause a 30% to 60% increase in free T_4. Like GTT, Graves disease also may improve after the first trimester due to the immune suppression of pregnancy. Therefore, it may be challenging to determine the cause of hyperthyroidism in women who improve after 16 to 18 weeks' gestation, and Graves disease and GTT can simultaneously occur. A history of thyroid dysfunction symptoms predating pregnancy and the presence of a goiter, orbitopathy, or pretibial myxedema are highly suggestive of Graves disease. Elevated TSH receptor antibodies (TRAb) and thyroid-stimulating immunoglobulin (TSI) are useful both measures of Graves antibodies. T_3 levels are generally higher in Graves disease (typically total T_3-to-total T_4 ≥20:1) than in GTT because hyperemesis gravidarum results in a compromised nutritional state and decreased conversion of T_4 to T_3 in peripheral tissues. GTT should NOT be treated with ATDs since it improves or completely resolves by 16 to 18 weeks' gestation.[1,2,7,8]

Overt hyperthyroidism from Graves disease, toxic multinodular goiters, or toxic nodules should be treated. ATDs reduce thyroid hormone synthesis, and propylthiouracil (PTU) also inhibits deiodination of T_4 to T_3, which is why it is the preferred ATD for treatment of thyroid storm and primarily T_3 thyrotoxicosis.[2] ATDs should be avoided in the first trimester in cases of very mild overt hyperthyroidism, as both PTU and methimazole (MMI) are uncommonly associated with birth defects when given during organogenesis (5-10 weeks' gestation). PTU is preferred over MMI in the first trimester (less than 10 weeks' gestation) for moderate to severe overt hyperthyroidism given that MMI has been associated with a modest 2% to 3% increased risk of developing congenital malformations such as aplasia cutis, choanal or esophageal atresia, abdominal wall defects, ventricular septal defects, and eye and urinary abnormalities compared with risk in control participants. A recent study on PTU, which appears to be safer than MMI in the first trimester, demonstrated a 1% to 1.5% higher risk in the first trimester of usually more minor congenital malformations such as facial and neck cysts and urinary tract abnormalities.[8,9] If ATDs are required in the second and third trimester, MMI is often preferred over PTU due to less hepatotoxicity, unless the patient has mild Graves disease and it is anticipated that the ATD can be stopped. If MMI is substituted for PTU in the second trimester, a conversion of 20:1 PTU vs MMI is typically used.[2,8] The absolute lowest ATD dosage to maintain the free T_4 in the upper reference range or total T_4 at 1.5 times the upper nonpregnant range (corrected total T_4) is recommended. More aggressive treatment (normalization of free T_4 or corrected total T_4 to the midrange) greatly increases risk for fetal hypothyroidism given that ATDs, compared with thyroid hormone, cross the placenta better. TSH should NEVER be used to titrate ATDs since it can be suppressed for 6 to 12 months, and normalization of TSH often results in fetal overexposure of ATDs and fetal hypothyroidism.[1,2,7,8] The free T_4 or corrected total T_4 (and total T_3 if elevated) should be checked every 2 to 4 weeks during treatment since ATD requirements usually decrease with the immune suppression of pregnancy and overtreatment can cause fetal hypothyroidism.[1,2,8] Sometimes mild increases in T_3 (which crosses the placenta poorly) may need to be tolerated if increasing the ATD lowers the T_4 into the midnormal range, which can result in fetal hypothyroidism. Although overtreatment must be avoided, undertreatment of overt hyperthyroidism, especially in the second and third trimesters, can result in congenital newborn hypothyroidism due suppression of fetal thyrotropes and the newborn's inability to mount a critical TSH surge at birth.

In about 5% of cases, TSH-stimulating antibodies (TSI or TRAb) at levels 3 times the upper limit of the normal range after 18 weeks' gestation carry risks for fetal and newborn Graves disease. With very high levels of TRAb or TSI, fetal risk may be up to 30% for fetal or newborn Graves disease. Graves antibodies should also be checked in women with treated Graves disease from thyroidectomy or radioactive iodine, the latter resulting in high levels of TRAb or TSI for years after ablation. Due to the immune suppression of pregnancy, TRAb and TSI levels often decrease by approximately 18 weeks' gestation, when these IgG antibodies cross the placenta well. As a result, TRAb and TSI should be checked at 18 to 20 weeks' gestation, and if either is elevated 3 times or more times the upper normal limit, a maternal-fetal medicine provider should be consulted to monitor for evidence for fetal Graves disease by serial ultrasonography every 4 weeks.[1,2,8,10] Unfortunately, newer assays for TSI (functional assays or assays that measure the stimulating region of antibodies to the TSH receptor) or TRAb assays (competitive assays measuring antibodies that bind the TSH receptor whether stimulating or inhibiting) have not been studied in large trials to assess their performance in predicting fetal or newborn Graves, and the recommendations for monitoring if antibodies that are 3 or more times the upper normal limit are based on older assays. It is recommended that TRAb and TSI be checked at 34 weeks' gestation, and if values are 3 or more times the upper normal limit, the newborn should be screened for Graves antibodies. Infants born to mothers with Graves antibodies that are 3 or more times the upper normal limit or whose mothers received ATDs should have thyroid function checked after birth and the infant's neonatologist and/or pediatrician should be appropriately notified.

Thyroid Nodules, Thyroid Cancer, and Postpartum Thyroid Disease
Thyroid nodules are not uncommonly found in pregnancy and the indications for FNA are the same as outside of pregnancy and should be

guided by sonographic characteristics.[1,2,8] Thyroid cancer does not behave more aggressively during pregnancy with respect to long-term survival, and the second trimester of pregnancy is the best time to consider thyroidectomy if surgery is indicated or elected in pregnancy. Graves disease worsens in 70% of individual post partum, typically at 4 to 8 months. Dosages of up to 20 mg of MMI or 400 mg of PTU are considered compatible with breastfeeding. Rebound from Graves disease can usually be distinguished from the hyperthyroid phase of postpartum thyroiditis. The initial hyperthyroid phase of postpartum thyroiditis due to destruction of the gland and transient release of thyroid hormone tends to occur earlier post partum (1-3 months) than rebound from Graves disease, which tends to occur at 4 to 8 months post partum. Postpartum thyroiditis is associated with TPO antibodies (Hashimoto thyroiditis) rather than Graves antibodies, typically results in much less severe hyperthyroidism, and should only be managed with β-adrenergic blockers if necessary. Postpartum thyroiditis occurs in 5% of all pregnant women and is more common in women with type 1 diabetes (~20%) and in women with high TPO antibodies (up to 50%). Postpartum thyroiditis more commonly presents with hypothyroidism from further destruction of the thyroid gland that is often unrecognized at 3 to 8 months post partum.[1,2,8] Typically, the hypothyroidism from postpartum thyroiditis should be treated with levothyroxine until 1 year post partum if the woman is symptomatic or attempting another pregnancy. Alternatively, if asymptomatic, the TSH concentration is between 4.0 and 10.0 mIU/L, and there are no plans for pregnancy, it is reasonable to not treat and repeat TFTs 4 to 8 weeks later. Postpartum thyroiditis requires regular monitoring given that it usually recurs and results in permanent hypothyroidism in 30% to 70% of women at 10 years.

Parathyroid Disease in Pregnancy

During pregnancy, maternal calcium homeostasis must adapt to provide 25 to 30 g of calcium for fetal bone development and skeletal mineralization. These increased demands are achieved by increased maternal intestinal absorption of calcium due to estrogen, the 2- to 3-fold increase in 1,25-dihydroxyvitamin D production, and active transport across the placenta facilitated by PTHrP produced by both placental and breast tissue (stimulated by prolactin) such that cord levels of ionized calcium are higher than maternal levels. PTH levels are slightly lower in pregnancy due to the elevation of PTHrP, which peaks in the third trimester. As a result, PHPT in pregnancy may be associated with relatively lower PTH levels. Unlike PTH, 25-hydroxyvitamin D crosses the placenta well, such that maternal and cord levels of 25-hydroxyvitamin D correlate strongly, underscoring the need for adequate 25-hydroxyvitamin D levels in pregnancy. Given the increased absorption of vitamin D and the increase in glomerular filtration rate in pregnancy, 24-hour calcium excretion increases, especially postprandially (absorptive hypercalciuria).[3] In mothers with hyperparathyroidism and severe hypercalcemia, complications of preterm delivery, polyhydramnios, fetal growth restriction, miscarriage, and stillbirth are not uncommon; significant neonatal morbidities are as high as 80%.[11] Increased transport of calcium across the placental can suppress the fetal parathyroid glands, resulting in hypoparathyroidism at birth, severe hypocalcemia, tetany, seizures, and neonatal death if not recognized. The mother is at risk of a hypercalcemic crisis after birth due to the cessation of calcium delivery across the placenta, hemoconcentration after delivery, and the fall in glomerular filtration rate.

Only 20% of women with hypercalcemia are symptomatic and often their nonspecific symptoms of nausea, vomiting, fatigue, arthralgias, myalgias, constipation, and depression are thought to be due to pregnancy.[12] Unfortunately, hypercalcemia is often not recognized in pregnancy. Calcium levels are lower in pregnancy due to the fall in total calcium as a result of low albumin, active transport across the placenta, and hypercalciuria. Hyperparathyroidism in pregnancy is associated with hyperemesis gravidarum, nephrolithiasis (17%-36%), acute pancreatitis (7%-13%), peptic ulcer disease, and hypertensive disorders, including preeclampsia (25%-57%) (the latter is thought to be due to PTH stimulation of the renin-angiotensin-aldosterone system). As a result, anyone with any of these conditions should be screened for hypercalcemia.[3] A corrected calcium for the low albumin (corrected calcium) or ionized calcium is required for the diagnosis. It is always imperative to rule out familial hypocalciuric hypercalcemia (FHH) by a calcium-to-creatinine clearance ratio or 24-hour calcium excretion, given that this entity is associated with low calcium excretion, as opposed to PHPT which is associated with high urinary calcium excretion. 25-Hydroxyvitamin D should also be measured; although secondary hyperparathyroidism from vitamin D deficiency does not alone cause hypercalcemia, it can further increase PTH levels. Neck ultrasonography or neck MRI without contrast are preferred in locating an adenoma since sestamibi scans are avoided due to the potential risk of fetal radiation exposure. Infrequently, a ^{99m}Tc-MIBI scan could be considered if other modalities are not diagnostic since the exposure is lower than that associated with fetal harm.[3] A family history directed at multiple endocrine neoplasia (MEN) or FHH should be elicited and genetic testing of familial forms of PHPT such as MEN type 1 should be considered for women younger than 30 years, especially if multiglandular disease is discovered.[11]

If the corrected calcium (for albumin) is less than 1.0 mg/dL (<0.25 mmol/L) above the normal range (usually <11.4 mg/dL [<2.85 mmol/L]) or the ionized calcium is less than 5.8 mg/dL (<1.45 mmol/L), and especially if the patient is already in the third trimester, medical management may be appropriate for mild hypercalcemia.[3,12] Management includes vigorous hydration, a low-calcium diet, conservative replacement of vitamin D if low to prevent a

secondary rise in PTH. When calcium levels are above this range, parathyroidectomy by an experienced surgeon in the second trimester (after organogenesis is completed and before an increased risk of preterm labor) is recommended, especially if a single adenoma can be identified. Intraoperative PTH should be measured. Parathyroidectomy consistently results in the greatest benefit with lowest risk when the patient has severe hypercalcemia (corrected calcium >1.0 mg/dL [>2.85 mmol/L] above the normal range) or complications (eg, nephrolithiasis, peptic ulcer disease, pancreatitis). However, surgery is usually highly successful in all trimesters if hypercalcemia is severe and is likely safer than medical therapy, even in the third trimester.[13] Minimally invasive parathyroidectomy performed by an experienced surgeon has a success rate of 90% to 95% with a 1% to 3% risk of complications, and it usually results in better maternal-fetal outcomes than conservative treatment. If the patient declines surgery or is not a surgical candidate and conservative medical therapy is not successful, calcitonin can be considered (does not cross the placenta), but it is not effective long term and has a very short-lasting effect. Cinacalcet has been successfully used in a small number of patients, but it crosses the placenta. The placenta has a calcium-sensing receptor, and it is unclear whether it could inhibit transplacental calcium transport. Although there are case reports of neonatal hypocalcemia with cinacalcet, these instances may be due to fetal PTH suppression due to maternal hypercalcemia, and no other adverse outcomes were reported.[3] Bisphosphonates cross the placenta and potentially affect fetal bone formation. Their long-term effect on the fetal skeleton is unknown. Denosumab also crosses the placenta. Similar to bisphosphonates, denosumab has been associated with adverse fetal skeletal outcomes in animal studies.

Hypocalcemia, most often caused by hypoparathyroidism due to a complication of thyroid surgery, may also cause maternal and fetal complications. Maternal hypocalcemia may not result in fetal hypocalcemia until severe, because calcium is transferred by the placenta to the fetus at the expense of the maternal skeleton. However, severe prolonged maternal hypocalcemia could result in fetal hypocalcemia and lead to fetal hyperparathyroidism and demineralization of the fetal skeleton and increased risk of fractures and low birth weight.[3] Calcium and calcitriol should be used to keep the maternal calcium in the low-normal range (corrected for the low albumin) and magnesium deficiency should be corrected. More safety data are needed on the use of recombinant PTH for refractory hypocalcemia. Due to the activity of PTHrP in the placenta and especially the breast, calcitriol requirements may decrease later in pregnancy and especially post partum during lactation, which is also accompanied by increased bone resorption and renal calcium reabsorption. Abrupt cessation of breastfeeding can result in hypocalcemia, such that laboratory measurement every 4 weeks is indicated during breastfeeding and after it is stopped.[3]

Clinical Case Vignettes

Case 1

A 26-year-old woman (G3P2) has TFTs at 10 weeks' gestation because of a positive family history of Hashimoto thyroiditis and is found to have a TSH concentration of 6.0 mIU/L (0.1-4.0 mIU/L). Her weight is 176.4 lb (80 kg). She strongly prefers not starting medications unless this TSH value is critical.

Which of the following is the best recommendation?

A. Review options for management, defer treatment, recheck TSH in 4 weeks and assess TPO antibodies

B. Measure free T_4 to discern whether she has overt hypothyroidism and to determine optimal levothyroxine dosing

C. Recommend a levothyroxine dosage slightly less than a full replacement dosage of 150 mcg daily given that fetal dependence on maternal thyroid hormone before 16 weeks' gestation

and treating subclinical hypothyroidism improves infant cognitive outcomes

D. Assess TPO antibodies; if she is TPO antibody-positive, levothyroxine treatment will decrease both miscarriage rates and preterm delivery

E. Recommend levothyroxine, 50 to 75 mcg daily, because treatment, regardless of whether TPO antibodies are present, is likely to improve infant miscarriage rates, preterm delivery, and cognitive outcomes

Answer: A) Review options for management, defer treatment, recheck TSH in 4 weeks and assess TPO antibodies

This patient has mild subclinical hypothyroidism by her TSH alone (<10.0 mIU/L). Because TSH has a log linear relationship to the free T_4 and will rise long before the free T_4 decreases outside the normal range, this patient is highly unlikely to have overt hypothyroidism (Answer B). There is no consensus about treating subclinical hypothyroidism, but it can be useful to check TPO antibodies in patients with a borderline TSH value of 4.0 to 6.0 mIU/L to confirm that the patient has Hashimoto thyroiditis rather than laboratory error or diurnal TSH variation. Furthermore, elevated TPO antibodies supporting Hashimoto thyroiditis demonstrates that she is at risk for further increases in TSH with the increasing demand of thyroid hormone production in pregnancy.

Women with elevated TPO antibodies have up to a 20% risk of developing subclinical hypothyroidism or overt hypothyroidism in pregnancy. They are also at risk of developing postpartum thyroiditis. TSH should be rechecked again in 4 weeks and at least mid-trimester in TPO antibody–positive patients. Pregnant patients with elevated TPO antibodies are also at increased risk for miscarriage, although treatment with levothyroxine has not been conclusively demonstrated to prevent miscarriage if the patient has high TPO antibodies alone or positive TPO antibodies with subclinical hypothyroidism.[14] Treatment with levothyroxine (Answer D) has not been convincingly shown to decrease miscarriage associated with TPO antibodies.

There are no compelling data that treating a patient with a TSH concentration of 6.0 mIU/L (Answers C and E) will result in improved infant cognitive outcomes or preterm delivery, although the data clearly suffer from levothyroxine treatment that was often not initiated until an average of 16 weeks' gestation, when the fetus is already making its own thyroid hormone. Randomized controlled trial data are also limited when the TSH value is in the higher range of subclinical hypothyroidism (7.0-10.0 mIU/L) because the mean treated TSH value in most of the randomized controlled trials was 4.0 to 6.0 mIU/L, which did not show improved pregnancy outcomes with treatment.[2] However, treating a patient with a TSH value of 7.0 to 10.0 mIU/L with or without TPO antibodies may offer more potential benefit than risk, given inadequate data for withholding treatment when a patient has a TSH value in this higher subclinical range. Many experts would treat all TSH values above the normal pregnancy range, especially in those with positive TPO antibodies because the benefit of treating with a low levothyroxine dosage (50-75 mcg daily) likely outweighs any risk.[1,2,8] However, the American College of Obstetrics and Gynecology[7] provides the option of not treating subclinical hypothyroidism and rechecking TSH in 4 to 6 weeks to ensure it does not increase to greater than 10.0 mIU/L (considered overt hyperthyroidism).

Since the patient feels strongly about deferring levothyroxine unless clearly indicated, reviewing options for management, deferring treatment, and rechecking TSH in 4 weeks and assessing TPO antibodies (Answer A) is a reasonable choice.

Case 1 (continued)

The same patient is treated with levothyroxine, 50 mcg daily, in pregnancy. She is experiencing fatigue and excess weight gain at 32 weeks (she now weighs 225 lb [102 kg]) and has a TSH value of 2.4 mIU/L. She is taking no medications other than her prenatal vitamin and levothyroxine. She requests measurement of free T_4 and free T_3 to make sure her thyroid hormone levels are normal:

Free T_4 = 0.71 ng/dL (0.8-1.8 ng/dL)
(SI: 9.14 pmol/L [10.30-23.17 pmol/L])
Free T_3 = 1.8 pg/mL (2.0-4.4 pg/mL)
(SI: 2.77 pmol/L [3.07-6.76 pmol/L])

She believes she has isolated hypothyroxinemia and needs treatment with a higher levothyroxine dosage.

Which of the following is the best next step in this patient's management?

A. Increase her levothyroxine dosage to full replacement (200 mcg daily) given the low free T_4 (~2 mcg/kg)

B. Measure urinary iodine to ensure sure she does not have isolated hypothyroxinemia from iodine deficiency

C. Increase her levothyroxine dosage to 100 mcg daily

D. Measure free T_4 by equilibrium dialysis (send-out test that takes 5 to 7 days to return) or total T_4

E. Increase her levothyroxine dosage to 100 mcg daily and add a small dosage of triiodothyronine, 12.5 mcg daily, given both free T_4 and free T_3 are low

Answer: D) Measure free T_4 by equilibrium dialysis (send-out test that takes 5 to 7 days to return) or total T_4

Often isolated hypothyroxinemia is simply due to lab error in the late second and third trimesters since it is difficult to accurately measure free T_4 by commonly used immunoassays because greater than 99.5% of T_4 is bound to TBG. Free T_3 assays are even more inaccurate due to the even lower levels of circulating free T_3. Furthermore, it has been shown by equilibrium dialysis assays and tandem mass spectrometry that free T_4 levels actually do fall slightly in the later second and third trimesters of pregnancy. Immunoassays rarely report gestational-specific ranges, and an equilibrium dialysis method with gestational-specific ranges may be needed to confirm if the free T_4 is normal for gestation given that free T_4 levels are slightly lower in the second and third trimesters.[1,2,4] Alternatively, total T_4 can be measured recognizing that after 16 weeks, the total

T_4 and total T_3 ranges increase by 50%. Therefore, if the total T_4 nonpregnant normal range is 4.0 to 12.0 μg/dL (51.5-154.4 nmol/L), the normal range for pregnancy would be 6.0 to 16.0 μg/dL (77.2-205.9 nmol/L). Measuring this patient's free T_4 by equilibrium dialysis or her total T_4 (Answer D) is the best next step.

In individuals with severe iodine deficiency, typically only seen in iodine-deficient countries, T_3 is preferentially synthesized over T_4 and rarely, low free T_4 may occur without elevated TSH (isolated hypothyroxinemia). This is because T_3 will feedback on TSH, potentially causing TSH to be relatively normal. Patients with central hypothyroidism from a pituitary cause also often have a low free T_4 concentration but normal or slightly low TSH. However, this would be highly unusual to present for the first time in pregnancy if the patient spontaneously conceived since pituitary lesions typically affect LH/FSH secretion first, resulting in anovulation. This patient already demonstrated that her TSH was elevated early in pregnancy with a normal free T_4 value, so it is highly unlikely that this is anything other than lab error in the third trimester of pregnancy (from absence of gestational-specific ranges).

There is no reason to increase her levothyroxine dosage (Answers A and C) unless her total T_4 or free T_4 is low by equilibrium dialysis using gestational-specific ranges. If a patient does have central hypothyroidism from a pituitary deficiency or is thought to have iodine deficiency due to living in an iodine-deficient region as the cause of an isolated hypothyroxinemia, repletion with levothyroxine should be considered to raise the free T_4 or adjusted total T_4 into the normal range.

Supplementing with any amount of T_3 in pregnancy[1,2,8] (Answer E) is relatively contraindicated since it crosses the placenta poorly and the fetal brain primarily has T_4 receptors.

Urinary iodine measurement (Answer B) is useful in populations to ascertain regional iodine deficiency, but this has not been validated as an accurate indicator on an individual basis. However, it should be confirmed that she is getting 150 mcg of iodine in a prenatal vitamin or taking a supplement if not liberally using iodinated salt.

Case 2

A 32-year-old pregnant woman (G1P0) at 10 weeks' gestation is screened for hypothyroidism due to a positive family history and is found to have a TSH concentration of 30.0 mIU/L. Her free T_4 concentration is 0.55 ng/dL (7.08 pmol/L). She is fatigued and slightly anemic without symptoms or signs of overt hypothyroidism. Her current weight is 176.4 lb (80 kg).

Which of the following is the best next step?

A. Orally load her with 2 doses of 400 mcg of levothyroxine the first day followed by a full replacement dose the next day

B. Start levothyroxine, 162.5 mcg daily, and counsel her that her baby is likely to have significant developmental delays and should have neurodevelopmental testing immediately after birth

C. Given that levothyroxine will take some time to raise her T_4 and T_3 and that her hypothyroidism is so severe, recommend near-full replacement of levothyroxine (150 mcg daily) along with a small dosage of liothyronine (12.5 mcg twice daily) to more quickly replace her thyroid hormones; stop liothyronine after 1 week

D. Admit her to the hospital for several doses of intravenous T_4 given the severity of her hypothyroidism and early stage of pregnancy and discharge her on full levothyroxine replacement

E. Start levothyroxine, 162.5 mcg daily, and recheck in 2 weeks to see if TSH is trending downward

Answer: E) Start levothyroxine, 162.5 mcg daily, and recheck in 2 weeks to see if TSH is trending downward

A full levothyroxine replacement dosage in pregnancy is approximately 2.0 to 2.2 mcg/kg. A TSH value of 10.0 mIU/L or greater with a free T_4 or total T_4 value that is low should be immediately treated with a full replacement dose (~2 mcg/kg). However, a TSH value of 10.0 mIU/L or greater with a normal free T_4 or total T_4 for pregnancy could be treated with a midrange dosage (75-100 mcg) or slightly less than a full replacement dosage. Although aggressive replacement of levothyroxine should not be done in elderly patients due to concerns of ischemic heart disease, pregnant women with hypothyroidism are usually at low cardiac risk. Because the half-life of T_4 is about 5 to 7 days, full repletion of 2 mcg/kg may transiently cause mild hyperthyroidism for 1 week, but it is usually well tolerated. Because the fetus is dependent on maternal T_4 until 16 to 18 weeks' gestation, women with overt hypothyroidism before 16 to 18 weeks should be treated with a full replacement dosage to normalize T_4 levels as quickly as possible. TSH should be checked every 4 weeks before 18 weeks' gestation to target a concentration between 0.5 and 2.5 mIU/L while the fetus is dependent on maternal thyroid hormone. TSH should be rechecked every 4 to 6 weeks after dose adjustments and, if stable, after midgestation (at least every 8 to 12 weeks). In the setting of severe hypothyroidism early in pregnancy when the fetus is dependent on maternal thyroid hormone, it is reasonable to recheck TSH for trend in 2 weeks, especially if there is concern about adherence or absorption. Typically, TSH falls significantly within 2 weeks since the TSH half-life is only 1 hour, which can be helpful to confirm adherence and absorption (thus, Answer E is correct).

If there is no evidence of myxedema, loading with very high levothyroxine doses (Answer A) or admitting her to the hospital for intravenous levothyroxine (Answer D) is not indicated, although some would double the dose of levothyroxine for a couple days to partially "load" her.

Because T_3 crosses the placenta poorly and the fetal brain requires T_4, supplementing with liothyronine is relatively contraindicated. Although subtle cognitive delays in the infant have been associated with severe hypothyroidism in pregnancy, immediate replacement now is not likely to prevent significant neurodevelopmental issues.[15] Infants unable to make thyroid hormone are born with one-third the normal amount from maternal transport and usually demonstrate fairly normal cognitive outcomes if they are immediately replaced at birth (thus, Answer B is incorrect).

For women who are hypothyroid on levothyroxine before pregnancy, increasing their levothyroxine dose by adding 2 tablets a day to their current regimen as soon as pregnancy is confirmed is recommended, especially if they are athyreotic (status post ablation, thyroidectomy, or overtly hypothyroid from Hashimoto thyroiditis) until the patient can be appropriately monitored. If adherence is an issue, recommending a pill box with instructions that a missed dose can be made up the next day due to the half-life of levothyroxine of approximately 1 week can be helpful. Levothyroxine liquid gel caps (Tirosint) can be useful for patients with absorption problems.

Case 3

A 38-year-old pregnant woman (G1P0) at 13 weeks' gestation presents to the emergency department with nausea, vomiting, pulse rate of 120 beats/min, heat intolerance, and 5-lb (2.3-kg) weight loss.

Thyroid function test results:

> TSH, undetectable
> Free T_4 = 3.0 ng/dL (0.8-1.8 ng/dL)
>   (SI: 38.61 pmol/L [10.30-23.17 pmol/L])
> Total T_3 = 250 ng/dL (90-180 ng/dL [nonpregnancy range]) (SI: 3.85 nmol/L [1.39-2.77 nmol/L])

On physical examination, her thyroid gland is borderline enlarged, and she has a stare but no exophthalmos. She has a fine tremor, has increased reflexes, and is diaphoretic.

Which of the following is the most appropriate approach?

A. Obtain a hepatic panel and begin treatment with PTU, 100 mg 3 times daily, given she is still within the first trimester and overtly hyperthyroid

B. Recommend ultrasonography, measurement of TRAb and TSI antibodies (which will take a week to return), and starting a low-dosage β-adrenergic blocker if intravenous fluids do not improve her tachycardia

C. Obtain a hepatic panel and begin treatment with MMI, 10 mg twice daily, given she is ≥13 weeks pregnant, there is a risk of hepatotoxicity with PTU, and low-dosage β-adrenergic blockers have been shown to cause fetal growth restriction

D. Obtain hepatic panel and treat with MMI, 10 mg daily, and a β-adrenergic blocker given she ≥13 weeks pregnant

E. Obtain hepatic panel and begin PTU, 150 mg twice daily, with a low-dosage β-adrenergic blocker given her degree of hyperthyroidism and the fact that she is still within first trimester

Answer: B) Recommend ultrasonography, measurement of TRAb and TSI antibodies (which will take a week to return), and starting a low-dosage β-adrenergic blocker if intravenous fluids do not improve her tachycardia

Ultrasonography (Answer B) to confirm an intrauterine pregnancy, obtain accurate dating, and rule out a molar pregnancy should be done immediately. Generalized symptoms and signs of mild hyperthyroidism (tachycardia, heat intolerance, palpitations, diaphoresis, and hyperreflexia) are not specific and can be seen in both GTT and Graves disease. This patient's presentation is most consistent with hCG-induced hyperthyroidism (ie, hyperemesis gravidarum [nausea, vomiting, plus 5-lb (2.3-kg) weight loss]) with mild hyperthyroid signs and symptoms. Unlike Graves disease, GTT is not associated with a thyroid goiter or exophthalmos. In Graves disease, T_3 is typically proportionally higher

than T_4 due to increased peripheral conversion of T_4 to T_3.[2,8] However, in this case, the total T_3 value is what would be expected for this stage of pregnancy (total T_3 demonstrates a 5% increase per week starting at 7 weeks, up to a 50% increase at ≥16 weeks). At 14 weeks, her total T_3 would be estimated to be 40% increased (approximately 260 ng/dL [4.0 nmol/L]), so it is normal for this gestational age. Her tachycardia will most likely respond to intravenous fluids and a low-dosage β-adrenergic blocker may be considered if she remains tachycardic until her TRAb or TSI antibodies return.

Short-term use of low-dosage β-adrenergic blockers have not been shown to cause fetal growth restriction (thus, Answer C is incorrect).

GTT should not be treated with antithyroid drugs (Answers A, C, D, and E) given that it typically resolves by 16 to 18 weeks' gestation when hCG levels fall and treatment could cause unintended consequences such as fetal hypothyroidism or maternal liver toxicity. If her TRAb and TSI antibodies return positive, it is likely that she has Graves disease in addition to some degree of GTT (given her severe nausea and vomiting), and both can occur. Hyperthyroidism from mild Graves disease should be treated with a low-dosage of an ATD such as PTU, 50 mg 2 to 3 times daily, or MMI, 5 mg twice daily, to avoid overexposure to ATDs that are too high dosages. Because of the shorter half-life of ATDs in pregnancy, twice-daily dosing for MMI and 3 times daily dosing for PTU in the second and third trimesters is usually necessary, and a hepatic panel should be checked before starting treatment since hyperthyroidism may cause a mild elevation in aminotransferases. Organogenesis is completely by 8 to 10 weeks, so if ultrasonography confirms she is less than 10 to 12 weeks' gestation, PTU would be a better choice since it has been associated with a 1% to 1.5% increased risk of major malformations (likely less with low dosage) compared with 2% to 3% increased risk with MMI.[9] It is critical to avoid overtreating with ATDs and to titrate medication dosages every 2 to 4 weeks to maintain the free T_4 (or total T_4 corrected for gestation) at the upper limit of the normal range. The increasing immune suppression of pregnancy requires much lower dosage of ATDs in the second and third trimesters. In women with mild hyperthyroidism, ATDs can often be tapered and stopped. In the late second and third trimesters, if free T_4 is followed to titrate the ATD dosages (instead of total T_4), free T_4 should be measured by equilibrium dialysis that provides gestational ranges since free T_4 decreases in the second and third trimesters. An equivalent dose of PTU to MMI is about 20:1 if a patient with Graves is switched from PTU to MMI after 12 weeks' gestation. TRAb and TSI should be rechecked at 18 to 20 weeks and if 3 times greater than the upper normal limit, referral to a maternal-fetal medicine physician is indicated for fetal surveillance of Graves with ultrasonography every 4 weeks.

Case 4

A 32-year-old pregnant woman (G1P0) at 20 weeks' gestation continues to have persistent nausea and vomiting despite taking ondansetron, 4 mg every 8 hours; vitamin B_6; and prochlorperazine, 10 mg as needed every 8 hours. She has been taking calcium carbonate, 1 to 2 tablets twice daily, due to stomach discomfort and reflux, especially after she vomits. She has no pertinent medical history or family history of calcium disorders.

Laboratory test results:

> Serum calcium = 10.8 mg/dL (8.7-10.5 mg/dL) (SI: 2.7 mmol/L [2.13-2.55 mmol/L])
> Phosphate, normal
> Albumin = 3.0 g/dL (3.5-5.5 g/dL) (SI: 30 g/L [35-55 g/L])
> Hepatic function, normal
> Serum urea nitrogen, normal
> Creatinine, normal
> PTH = 60 pg/mL (10-55 pg/mL) (SI: 6.4 pmol/L [1.1 -5.8 pmol/L])
> 25-Hydroxyvitamin D = 22 ng/mL (20-50 ng/mL) (SI: 54.9 nmol/L [50-125 nmol/L])
> Urinary calcium = 370 mg/24 h (100-300 mg/24 h [nonpregnant range]) (SI: 9.3 mmol/d [2.5-7.5 mmol/d])

Which of the following is the best next step?

A. Neck ultrasonography; if parathyroid adenoma is identified, refer for parathyroidectomy

B. Neck MRI; if no parathyroid adenoma is identified, treat with hydration, stop calcium carbonate, and treat with vitamin D to achieve a 25-hydroxyvitamin D concentration in midnormal range to treat secondary hyperparathyroidism

C. Neck ultrasonography; if parathyroid adenoma is identified, treat with hydration, stop calcium carbonate, follow a low-calcium diet, start calcitonin, and check for genetic causes of MEN 1

D. Neck MRI; if parathyroid adenoma is identified, treat with hydration, stop calcium carbonate, follow a low-calcium diet, and start cinacalcet given her gestational age

E. Neck ultrasonography; if no parathyroid pathology is present, treat with hydration, stop calcium carbonate, follow a low-calcium diet, and treat with vitamin D to achieve a 25-hydroxyvitamin D concentration in the midnormal range to treat secondary hyperparathyroidism

Answer: A) Neck ultrasonography; if parathyroid adenoma is identified, refer for parathyroidectomy

Nausea and vomiting are common symptoms of hypercalcemia, and hCG-mediated causes of vomiting usually improve by the second trimester. Her dyspepsia may also be related to hypercalcemia because peptic ulcer disease is less common in pregnancy, although gastroesophageal reflux is very common due to progesterone's effect on smooth muscle. This patient has hypercalcemia to a degree that parathyroidectomy should be immediately considered given her corrected calcium for albumin is 11.6 mg/dL (2.9 mmol/L). Her 25-hydroxyvitamin D concentration is in the normal range, so there is no indication she has secondary hyperparathyroidism (which would not cause hypercalcemia) or that she should be further supplemented with vitamin D (thus, Answers B and E are incorrect).

Her calcium carbonate intake is not enough to cause hypercalcemia from milk-alkali syndrome, and in that case, her PTH would be expected to be suppressed. Her PTH value is substantially elevated for pregnancy (given PTHrP decreases PTH modestly in pregnancy) and is clearly inappropriate for her elevated calcium. Rarely, very high PTHrP from the placenta or enlarged breasts during lactation results in hypercalcemia, but PTH would be expected to be suppressed. Although her urinary calcium excretion is at or only slightly above the upper normal limit for pregnancy (given the increased glomerular filtration rate of pregnancy and postabsorptive hypercalciuria), her value argues against FHH. Also, there is no family history of this, and if neck ultrasonography suggests an adenoma, PHPT is overwhelmingly the diagnosis. The calcium-to-creatinine clearance ratio can be useful in distinguishing PHPT (>0.02) from FHH (<0.01), but calcium excretion increases in pregnancy and this approximation is not as accurate in pregnancy. Neck ultrasonography is recommended first as an imaging modality and has a sensitivity of 75% to 85% in identifying abnormal parathyroid tissue with a specificity of approximately 95%, although it is less sensitive if the patient has multiglandular disease.

Neck MRI may be helpful if neck ultrasonography is normal, but MRI has less sensitivity (thus, Answer B is incorrect). MRI with gadolinium, CT, and sestamibi scans should be avoided in pregnancy due to radiation risks.[3,11] Calcitonin does not cross the placenta and may be useful in patients near term or in preparation for surgery, but it is very short lasting (thus, Answer C is incorrect).

Cinacalcet has been used in a limited number of patients in whom surgery is not possible or is declined. However, cinacalcet does cross the placenta, there are calcium-sensing receptors in the placenta, and it is reserved for patients with moderate to severe hypercalcemia who are not surgical candidates or who are near term (thus, Answer D is incorrect).

Genetic causes of hyperparathyroidism such as MEN 1 should be considered, especially in patients with a relevant family history or who are younger than 30 years or if multiple parathyroid glands are involved. Although mild cases of hypercalcemia, especially near term, could be treated conservatively, this patient has a corrected calcium value more than 1 mg/dL above the upper normal limit. A systematic review including 382 pregnant women with PHPT showed a significantly lower infant complication rates for surgery compared with complication rates with conventional therapy (9.1% vs 38.9%), especially when surgery was performed by an experienced surgeon and in the second trimester.[13] Preterm labor risks are very low. Infants born to mothers with PHPT are at risk of severe neonatal hypocalcemia with major complications from the suppression of fetal PTH. Given the degree of this pregnant patient's hypercalcemia and her gestational age, she should be offered parathyroid surgery as the treatment of choice (Answer A).

Key Learning Points

- TSH is normally lower in pregnancy, total T_4 and total T_3 are higher in pregnancy, and free T_4 by immunoassay is often slightly lower in the second and third trimesters, underscoring the importance of interpreting TFT results correctly.

- Although treatment of subclinical hypothyroidism in pregnancy is controversial, treatment with levothyroxine, 50 mcg daily, for TSH values greater than 4.0 mIU/L (or upper level corrected by a 0.5 mIU/L decrease from nonpregnant normal range), especially when TPO antibodies are positive or the patient is less than 18 weeks' gestation, is more likely to confer benefit than risk. Overt hypothyroidism should be treated with near-replacement dosages of levothyroxine (2.0 mcg/kg). T_3 is relatively contraindicated in pregnancy due to poor placental crossing and predominant fetal brain T_4 receptors.

- Graves disease must be distinguished from GTT and treated with a minimum ATD dosage to maintain the total T_4 at the upper limit of the normal pregnancy range (adding 50% at 16 weeks) or the free T_4 in the upper range, recognizing that free T_4 falls modestly in the later second and third trimesters and gestational-specific ranges should be used, typically only offered with equilibrium dialysis assays.

- Women with a history of Graves disease, even when previously cured by radioactive iodine or near-total thyroidectomy, and all women with active Graves disease should have Graves antibody testing. If either TRAb or TSI antibody levels are 3 or more times the upper normal limit at 20 weeks' gestation, fetal surveillance with serial ultrasonography should be performed every 4 weeks until delivery.

- Calcium metabolism in pregnancy changes such that total calcium levels are lower (unless corrected for albumin), PTH levels are lower (due to PTHrP), and 24-hour urine calcium excretion is higher (due to elevated glomerular filtration rate and postabsorptive hypercalciuria). Women with PHPT and corrected total calcium levels greater than 11.4 mg/dL (>2.85 mmol/L) or ionized calcium greater than 5.8 mg/dL (>1.45 mmol/L) have better maternal and fetal outcomes if treated with parathyroidectomy, especially in the second trimester, if noninvasive testing is suggestive of an adenoma, and if surgery is performed by an experienced parathyroid surgeon.

References

1. American Thyroid Association Taskforce, Alexander EK, Pearce EN, Brent GA et al. Guidelines of the American Thyroid Association for the diagnosis and management of thyroid disease during pregnancy and the postpartum 2017. *Thyroid.* 2017;27(3):315-389. PMID: 28056690

2. Valent A, Barbour LA. Thyroid disease in pregnancy. In: Lockwood CJ, Moore TR, Copel JA, eds. *Creasy and Resnik's Maternal-Fetal Medicine: Principles and Practice.* 9th ed. Elsevier; 2023.

3. Appelman-Dikstra NM, Pilz S. Approach to the patient: management of parathyroid diseases across pregnancy. *J Clin Endocrinol Metab.* 2020;108(6):1505-1513. PMID: 36546344

4. Osinga JAJ, Derakhshan A, Palomaki GE et al. TSH and FT4 reference intervals in pregnancy: A systematic review and individual participant data meta-analysis. *J Clin Endocrinol Metab.* 2022;107(10);2925-2933. PMID: 36546344

5. Korevaar T, Tiemeier H, et al. Clinical associations of maternal thyroid function with foetal brain development: Epidemiological interpretation and overview of available evidence. *Clin Endocrinol (Oxf).* 2018;89(2):129-138. PMID: 29693263

6. Jiao XF, Zhang M, Chen J, et al. The impact of levothyroxine therapy on the pregnancy, neonatal and childhood outcomes of subclinical hypothyroidism during pregnancy: an updated systematic review, meta-analysis and trial sequential analysis. *Front Endocrinol (Lausanne).* 2022;13:964084. PMID: 36034430

7. ACOG Practice Bulletin. Thyroid disease in pregnancy: ACOG Practice Bulletin Number 223. *Obstet Gynecol.* 2020;135(6):e261-e274. PMID: 32443080

8. Lee SY, Pearce EN. Assessment and treatment of thyroid disorders in pregnancy and the postpartum period. *Nat Rev Endocrinol.* 2022;18(3);158-171. PMID: 34983968

9. Liu Y, Li Q, Xu Y, Chen Y, Men Y. Comparison of the safety between propylthiouracil and methimazole with hyperthyroidism in pregnancy: a systematic review and meta-analysis. *PLoS One.* 2023;18(5):e286097. PMID: 37205692

10. Cui Y, Rijhsinghani A. Role of maternal thyroid-stimulating immunoglobulin in Graves' disease for predicting perinatal thyroid dysfunction. *AJP Rep.* 2019;9(4):e341-e345. PMID: 31723454

11. Ali DS, Dandurand K, Khan AA. Primary hyperparathyroidism in pregnancy: literature review of the diagnosis and management. *J Clin Med.* 2021;10(13):2956. PMID: 34209340

12. Eremkina A, Bibik E, Mirnaya S, et al. Different treatment strategies in primary hyperparathyroidism during pregnancy. *Endocrine.* 2022;77(3):556-560. PMID: 35821184

13. Sandler ML, Ho R, Xing MH, et al. Primary hyperparathyroidism during pregnancy treated with parathyroidectomy: a systematic review. *Laryngoscope.* 2021;131(8):1915-1921. PMID: 33751589

14. Lau L, Benham JL, Lemieux P, Yamamoto J, Donovan LE. Impact of levothyroxine in women with positive thyroid antibodies on pregnancy outcomes: a systematic review and meta-analysis of randomised controlled trials. *BMJ Open.* 2021;11(2):e043751. PMID: 33622947

15. Eng L, Lam L. Thyroid function during the fetal and neonatal periods. *Neoreviews.* 2020;21(1):e30-e36. PMID: 31894080

Transgender and Gender-Diverse Adults: Challenging Cases

Sean J. Iwamoto, MD. Division of Endocrinology, Metabolism, and Diabetes, Department of Medicine, University of Colorado School of Medicine, Anschutz Medical Campus; Endocrinology Service, Medicine Service, Rocky Mountain Regional Veterans Affairs Medical Center; and UCHealth Integrated Transgender Program, Aurora, CO; Email: sean.iwamoto@cuanschutz.edu

Tamar Reisman, MD. Division of Endocrinology, Diabetes, and Metabolism, Department of Medicine, Weill Cornell Medicine, New York, NY; Email: tar4015@med.cornell.edu

Educational Objectives

After reviewing this chapter, learners should be able to:

- Recommend ways to reduce risks in transgender and gender-diverse (TGD) patients who desire to take estrogen for gender-affirming hormone therapy (GAHT).

- Manage testosterone use in TGD patients who would like to continue GAHT after experiencing a myocardial infarction (MI).

- Identify breast cancer risk and screening recommendations in TGD adults taking GAHT.

- Explain important considerations when initiating GAHT in older TGD adults that balance patient goals and safety.

Significance of the Clinical Problem

TGD individuals experience a gender identity that differs from their sex assigned at birth. If it fits within an individual's goals, appropriate medical care for TGD patients may include the use of GAHT to align their physical expression with their experienced gender. GAHT has been established to increase well-being in select TGD patients.[1,2] However, it can also be associated with adverse health effects. When TGD patients present with underlying medical conditions or complex medical histories, it can complicate the management of GAHT.

The 2017 Endocrine Society's Clinical Practice Guideline for Endocrine Treatment of Gender-Dysphoric/Gender-Incongruent Persons and the 2022 World Professional Association for Transgender Health's Standards of Care, Version 8 (WPATH SOC8), are examples of published guidelines written to assist endocrinologists and other clinicians in initiating and managing GAHT in TGD individuals.[1,2] While these guidelines provide a general overview and recommendations for routine management, they do not provide specific considerations for more challenging cases such as how to manage GAHT in TGD patients who experience venous thromboembolism (VTE), MI, or breast cancer before or during GAHT use. Guidelines also do not discuss specific guidance for how to manage gender affirmation in older TGD patients who would like to initiate GAHT at an older age. In this chapter, we specifically look at GAHT management in the setting of 4 common and complex circumstances: thromboembolism, cardiovascular disease, breast cancer, and aging.

Practice Gaps

- Data for TGD patients are largely extrapolated from cisgender data, which may or may not be applicable.
- Data addressing aging TGD patients are lacking.

Discussion

VTE and Estrogen

Typical feminizing GAHT regimens include the combination of an estrogen and an antiandrogen. Estrogen has been established as a risk factor for thromboembolism, particularly VTE, following early studies of combined oral contraceptives (COCs) in cisgender women.[3] Because exogenous estradiol is a risk factor for thromboembolism, a TGD patient's underlying risk factors for VTE must be considered before initiating an estrogen-containing GAHT regimen. Risk factors for VTE include heritable thrombophilias, a personal history of VTE, cigarette smoking, advanced age (in COC studies this is defined as women older than 35 years), history of systemic lupus erythematosus with positive antiphospholipid antibodies, and history of surgery with prolonged immobilization.[4] Migraines with aura have also been identified as a risk factor for ischemic stroke.

Having risk factors for VTE or even a history of VTE need not be an absolute contraindication to GAHT as steps can be taken to make GAHT a safe and feasible option for patients who need it. Patients with heritable risk factors for VTE should be referred to hematology for further evaluation and started on anticoagulation if appropriate. Smoking cessation should be encouraged and can be aided with the use of medication, nicotine replacement products, and support groups. Lower-risk estrogen preparations (eg, transdermal) should be substituted for higher-risk formulations whenever possible, particularly in older patients and patients with independent VTE risk factors.

Most COCs contain ethinyl estradiol, which is a higher-risk estrogen preparation when it comes to VTE,[5] and ethinyl estradiol is not recommended for GAHT in current guidelines. Guidelines also do not recommend conjugated equine estrogens (CEEs) due to the inability to measure serum estrogens with this formulation and an increase in VTE risk. Oral 17β-estradiol is relatively safer, while transdermal formulations (eg, patches and topical gels) are regarded as the safest.[6] In a study of 162 TGD women who were prescribed transdermal 17β-estradiol for an average of 4.4 years, no episodes of VTE occurred despite 18 of the study participants testing positive for a thrombophilic genetic pathogenic variant.[6] Unfortunately, there are minimal data available regarding the safety of injectable estradiol valerate and estradiol cypionate.

At this time, the use of coagulation assays and/or fibrinolysis assays in asymptomatic patients is not recommended for blood clot screening.

MI and Testosterone

Most studies have concluded that GAHT with testosterone does not increase TGD persons' risk of MI compared with their baseline risk or with the risk of reference populations, but it depends on the population to which transgender men are compared.[7] In a study of 1358 transgender men on GAHT in the Netherlands between 1972 and 2015 (median age, 23 years; median follow-up, 4.10 years [range 0.02-44.66]), transgender men had a higher incidence of MI compared with incidence in reference women (standardized incidence ratio [SIR], 3.60; 95% CI, 1.94-6.42) but a comparable incidence to that of reference men (SIR, 1.00; 95% CI, 0.53-1.74).[8] The Study of Transition, Outcomes, and Gender (STRONG) cohort included 2118 transgender men in the United States (15.7% older than 45 years; mean follow-up, 3.6 years [SD, 2.7]) and did not reveal a higher rate of MI among transgender men compared with that in either reference men or women.[9] Among the 585 transgender men who initiated testosterone between 2006 and 2016, there were no reported MI events. A 2017 meta-analysis of 20 studies with 1500 transgender men (mean ages per study ranged from 21.7 to 37.5 years) identified only one MI event after study follow-up ranging from 3 months to 41 years.[10] In most of these studies, the relatively young ages of transgender men taking testosterone may have contributed to the low MI rate. Survey data from the United States also have not shown increases in MI risk among transgender men compared with risk in cisgender men and women, but the impact of GAHT use is not analyzed in these studies.[11,12]

We continue to lack data to inform TGD-specific cardiovascular screening tools (eg, how to capture the influence of resilience factors, gender minority stress, and other stressors on cardiovascular disease risk). WPATH SOC8 recommends tailoring sex-based risk calculators to the needs of TGD people, taking into consideration GAHT duration, dosing, serum hormone levels, current age, and age at GAHT initiation.[1] As with any patient, optimizing cardiometabolic health guided by patient-centered discussions is important to reducing an individual's cardiovascular risk.

Breast Cancer

Breast cancer is the most common cancer in American (cisgender) women and the second leading cause of death. Male breast cancer is much less common and represents only 1% of all breast cancers. According to the most recent available data, the risk of breast cancer in transgender women is many times higher than that of cisgender men but still less than that found in cisgender women.[13,14] The risk of breast cancer in transgender men with breast tissue is about that of cisgender women, but the risk after chest masculinization surgery has not been well-defined.

Individuals can be considered to be at "high risk" for cancer if they have a personal history of breast cancer, a personal history of chest irradiation performed between 10 and 30 years of age, *BRCA1* or *BRCA2* pathogenic variants, Li-Fraumeni syndrome, Cowden syndrome, Bannayan-Riley-Ruvalcaba syndrome, or a first-degree relative with a genetic predisposition to cancer.[15] Additional factors that increase breast cancer risk may include

ethnic background (eg, Ashkenazi descent), length of GAHT treatment, hormone regimen, and chest surgery status. An individual's breast cancer risk can be stratified as high, intermediate, or low risk using one of several breast cancer risk models. These include the BRCAPRO, Gail, Claus, Breast Cancer Surveillance Consortium, and International Breast Intervention Study, or Tyrer-Cuzick models. However, none of these tools has been validated in TGD patients.

The American College of Radiology, University of California San Francisco, Fenway Health, and the Endocrine Society have each put forth breast cancer screening recommendations for the TGD population. The guidelines for transgender women vary as outlined in the *Table* (*following page*). For transgender men, the recommendations vary based on the presence of breast tissue (ie, whether patients have undergone chest masculinization). Although chest masculinization surgery significantly lowers the risk of cancer, the remaining risk of cancer is nonnegligible. Regardless, the above organizations do not recommend mammography screening for patients who have undergone surgery. Transgender men who have not had chest masculinization surgery are encouraged to follow the guidelines for cisgender women. The length of GAHT treatment with testosterone does not have a role in screening recommendations.

Older Adults

Most data informing management of GAHT in adults come from cohorts with small proportions of older adults. Calls have been made for more rigorous studies in older TGD adults to better understand if and how GAHT recommendations may need to be tailored to this population.[16] At this time, there is no literature to suggest that older adults should not initiate or continue GAHT if that aligns with their goals. This may entail starting or switching to transdermal routes of administration for better safety compared with safety of oral and parenteral routes. Whether transdermal routes lead to differential gender-affirming physical

Table. Screening Mammography Guidelines for Transgender Women[15]

Guiding organization	Length of hormone therapy	Risk level	Recommendation
American College of Radiology	≥5 years	"Higher than average"	Mammography/digital breast tomosynthesis "usually appropriate" at age 25-30 years
		Average	Mammography/digital breast tomosynthesis "may be appropriate" at age >40 years
	<5 years	"Higher than average"	Mammography/digital breast tomosynthesis "may be appropriate" at age 25-30 years
		Average	Mammography/digital breast tomosynthesis screening "usually not appropriate"
Endocrine Society	≥5 years	Any	Follow cisgender recommendations
University of California San Francisco	5-10 years	Any	Biennial mammography screening starting at age 50 years
Fenway	≥5 years	Any	Annual mammography screening starting at age 50 years

Adapted from Hayward JH. *Seminars in Ultrasound, CT, and MRI*, 2023; 44(1): 23-34. © Elsevier Inc.[15]

effects compared with other routes has yet to be determined. We also lack studies that demonstrate whether older TGD adults have differential gender-affirming physical effects compared to younger TGD adults with similarly achieved serum hormone levels. Important health concerns of aging such as cardiovascular disease, dementia, and osteoporosis need to be balanced with untreated gender dysphoria or gender incongruence. Potential hypogonadism of aging may also be alleviated in older TGD patients who initiate or continue GAHT, with sex hormone benefits to bone health. As with younger TGD adults, endocrinologists can be affirming and patient-centered when it comes to developing a safe and individualized plan for GAHT in older adults.

Clinical Case Vignettes

Case 1

A 22-year-old transgender woman in excellent health presents for initiation of feminizing GAHT. She reports identifying as female since childhood and she has not wavered in her thinking. She socially transitioned 1 year ago and is known to her friends, family, and colleagues as a woman. She does not take any medication and has no pertinent personal medical history. Her BMI is 24 kg/m². She does not smoke cigarettes or use illicit substances, and she drinks 1 to 2 alcoholic drinks weekly. She does, however, report a family history of inherited thrombophilia. Her mother has a history of homozygous factor V Leiden variant but has never had a blood clot. Her maternal grandmother is also homozygous for factor V Leiden variant and had recurrent DVT. The patient and her brother have not been tested. Her father has history of hypertension but no history of thromboembolism. There is no family history of early MI, atherosclerotic disease, or diabetes.

Which of the following statements is most accurate?

A. Factor V Leiden variants are considered an absolute contraindication for feminizing GAHT

B. She would likely benefit from a hematology referral for further testing and possible initiation of anticoagulation before GAHT

C. She is at high risk for VTE and should start oral ethinyl estradiol to reduce her risk

D. She is at high risk for VTE and should start an estrogen-sparing (ie, antiandrogen-only) regimen to reduce her risk

E. She is at high risk for VTE and should be encouraged to use CEEs to reduce risk

Answer: B) She would likely benefit from a hematology referral for further testing and possible initiation of anticoagulation before GAHT

This patient would likely benefit from a hematology referral for further testing and possible initiation of anticoagulation before GAHT (Answer B).

Inherited thrombophilias are not an absolute contraindication to GAHT (thus, Answer A is incorrect). Steps can be taken to reduce a patient's risk of VTE while they are treated with feminizing GAHT. CEEs (Answer E) and ethinyl estradiol (Answer C) are not the lowest-risk estrogen preparations. Had either answer mentioned transdermal estradiol, that would also be correct. Suppressing testosterone without replacing estrogen (Answer D) in a young patient is inadvisable, as this is likely to result in bone loss.

The patient chose to delay GAHT until she was evaluated by a hematologist. She was determined to be homozygous for both factor V Leiden and *MTHFR2* pathogenic variants. The hematologist advised empiric initiation of prophylactic dosing of rivaroxaban, 10 mg daily. She was eventually started on a transdermal estradiol patch (along with an antiandrogen).

Case 2

A 58-year-old transgender man with a history of hypertension, hyperlipidemia, obesity, and 22 pack-year cigarette smoking history (quit 5 years ago) is referred to the endocrinology outpatient clinic for management of GAHT following an MI 6 months ago. He has no family history of cardiovascular disease. His surgical history includes bilateral mastectomy 25 years ago and hysterectomy with bilateral oophorectomy 20 years ago. At the time of the MI, he had been on injectable testosterone for 26 years and was injecting testosterone cypionate, 100 mg intramuscularly weekly. He has never tried other testosterone routes of administration. A couple

weeks before the MI, his serum total testosterone concentration was 1058 ng/dL (36.71 nmol/L) (unclear timing of the venipuncture relative to the last testosterone injection), and his hematocrit was 49% (0.49). The cardiology team discontinued testosterone injections and suggested outpatient endocrinology consultation for management of testosterone in the setting of postacute MI. The patient has had increasing gender dysphoria since his testosterone was held and would like to consider restarting GAHT in a safe manner.

After discussing the risks and benefits of restarting testosterone after an MI, the informed patient decides to restart testosterone for GAHT.

Which of the following regimens should be recommended first based on available guidelines?

A. Switch to testosterone enanthate, 75 mg intramuscularly weekly

B. Switch to testosterone pellets, 150 mg inserted every 3 to 4 months

C. Switch to testosterone gel, 25 mg daily

D. Switch to testosterone undecanoate, 2000 mg intramuscularly every 12 weeks

E. Refuse to restart testosterone for GAHT

Answer: C) Switch to testosterone gel, 25 mg daily

For GAHT with testosterone, guidelines include testosterone injections (with cypionate, enanthate, or long-acting undecanoate), gels, or patches. (At the time of this writing, transdermal patches are no longer manufactured or available.) Insufficient data exist to support guideline recommendations for testosterone pellets for GAHT (Answer B). From a cardiovascular standpoint, transdermal route of administration with testosterone gel (Answer C) is thought to be safer than parenteral injections (Answers A and D), owing to more uniform levels with gel, although it may also be more difficult to achieve guideline-recommended target testosterone concentrations between 400 and 700 ng/dL (13.88-24.29 nmol/L) with gel. It is important to balance patient preference, availability of various routes of administration (eg, country, cost, or insurance coverage), and safety when making informed patient-centered decisions. Given the patient's hope to restart GAHT and the risks associated with the lack of endogenous sex hormone production (status post hysterectomy and oophorectomy, so at risk for decreasing bone mineral density) and increasing gender dysphoria, withholding testosterone (Answer E) does not seem to be the safest option now.

Case 3

A 34-year-old transgender woman presents for follow-up. She started GAHT 12 years ago and is currently taking oral 17β-estradiol and spironolactone. She is up-to-date with all her age-appropriate health screening. Today in clinic, the patient is anxious because her grandmother was recently diagnosed with breast cancer at 90 years old. Her grandmother has no known pathogenic variants. The patient does not have any other family members with breast or ovarian cancer. She wants to know if she needs to take any special precautions considering her grandmother's recent diagnosis.

How should this patient be advised?

A. Counsel the patient to stop taking GAHT immediately; it is contraindicated given her family history of breast cancer

B. Counsel the patient that she should start yearly mammography and MRI as she is considered to be at high risk for breast cancer

C. Provide reassurance only; the risk of breast cancer in transgender women is low

D. Discuss risks with the patient; start annual or biennial mammography at age 40 to 50 years

E. Counsel the patient to begin self-breast exams now, and then start biennial mammography at age 35 years

Answer: D) Discuss risks with the patient; start annual or biennial mammography at age 40 to 50 years

The patient does not meet the criteria for a high risk of breast cancer (Answer B) according to the American College of Radiology or the American

Cancer Society. However, even if she were at high risk, it would not be considered an absolute contraindication to GAHT (Answer A). Although the incidence of breast cancer in transgender women is lower than that in cisgender women, several organizations (including the Endocrine Society, American College of Radiology, Fenway, and University of California San Francisco) recommend routine breast cancer screening for transgender women. Accordingly, a reassurance-only response (Answer C) is not the best answer. Self-exams (Answer E) are not recommended for breast cancer screening, and 35 years is younger than recommended to begin mammography.

Breast cancer risk should be discussed with the patient, and annual or biennial mammography should be started at age 40 to 50 years (Answer D).

Case 4

A 68-year-old nonbinary patient is seen in the endocrinology outpatient clinic to discuss GAHT to "feel more like me with feminine features and more alignment with physical and emotional well-being." They have a history of obesity, type 2 diabetes, hyperlipidemia, and hypertension. Since age 6 years, they felt they were different but did not have the words to describe how they felt. They married their first wife who was not very supportive, and they divorced after 10 years. They married their current wife who is extremely supportive, and they also feel supported by their daughter and friends. They are not "out" as nonbinary at work because the company is very conservative, and they are concerned about their employment and potential discrimination. Despite these stressors, they have tried over-the-counter "female" vitamins for many years but did not see any feminizing effects. A previous clinician said they might be "too old" to start GAHT. They have never felt more ready to begin their hormonal transition and lost 40 lb (18.1 kg) in the last 2 years to improve their health. They have no preference on estrogen route of administration but want to start estrogen via the safest formulation. Blood pressure, lipids, and hemoglobin A_{1c} are well-controlled with medications.

Based on the patient's goals and available guidelines, which option is the best recommendation for GAHT initiation?

A. Oral estradiol, 6 mg daily

B. Injectable estradiol cypionate, 10 mg intramuscularly weekly

C. Advise against starting GAHT because of their age

D. Antiandrogen-alone therapy with spironolactone

E. Transdermal estradiol patch, 0.05 mg/day weekly or twice weekly

Answer: E) Transdermal estradiol patch, 0.05 mg/day weekly or twice weekly

The Endocrine Society Clinical Practice Guideline suggests that transdermal estradiol patches or injectable estradiol may confer an advantage over oral estradiol in older TGD adults who may have higher risk of VTE. The WPATH SOC8 goes further to suggest that transdermal estrogen (Answer E) be prescribed to TGD adults older than 45 years or those who have VTE history.

While oral estradiol (Answer A) and injectable estradiol cypionate (Answer B) may be options for this patient depending on availability, cost, insurance coverage, or patient preference, the listed dosages are at the highest end of guideline-recommended doses. If using oral or injectable estradiol, starting with lower recommended doses to monitor safety and adverse effects seems more prudent. We do not have data to suggest that there is an upper age limit for the initiation of GAHT (Answer C). Lastly, while some nonbinary patients may opt for antiandrogen-alone therapy for GAHT (Answer D), this patient is interested in taking estrogen, and clinician support is warranted to create a patient-centered GAHT management plan.

Key Learning Points

- Risk factors for VTE include inherited thrombophilias, a personal history of VTE, cigarette smoking, advanced age, history of systemic lupus erythematosus with positive antiphospholipid antibodies, and history of surgery with prolonged immobilization.

- Choose the lowest-risk estrogen in patients with VTE risk (currently understood to be transdermal 17β-estradiol).

- Age-appropriate screening mammography is recommended for TGD patients taking estrogen-containing GAHT. TGD patients treated with testosterone who have NOT undergone chest masculinization surgery also require age-appropriate screening mammography.

- Testosterone does not appear to increase MI risk in TGD adults, but it is important to consider the reference population to which risk is compared. While TGD-specific cardiovascular risk calculators have not yet been developed, a patient-centered approach to risk calculation can take into consideration GAHT duration, dosing, serum hormone levels, current age, and age at GAHT initiation.

- Data currently do not support any upper age limit after which GAHT cannot be initiated or continued. It is important to have patient-centered discussions about potential risks and benefits of GAHT with aging TGD patients.

References

1. Coleman E, Radix AE, Bouman WP, et al. Standards of care for the health of transgender and gender diverse people, version 8. *Int J Transgend Health.* 2022;23(Suppl):S1-S259. PMID: 36238954

2. Hembree WC, Cohen-Kettenis PT, et al. Endocrine treatment of gender-dysphoric/gender-incongruent persons: an Endocrine Society clinical practice guideline. *J Clin Endocrinol Metab.* 2017;102(11):3869-3903. PMID: 28945902

3. Gomes MP, Deitcher SR. Risk of venous thromboembolic disease associated with hormonal contraceptives and hormone replacement therapy: a clinical review. *Arch Intern Med.* 2004;164(18):1965-1976. PMID: 15477430

4. Martinez F, Avecilla A. Combined hormonal contraception and venous thromboembolism. *Eur J Contracept Reprod Health Care.* 2007;12(2):97-106. PMID: 17559006

5. Zucker R, Reisman T, Safer JD. Minimizing venous thromboembolism in feminizing hormone therapy: applying lessons from cisgender women and previous data. *Endocr Pract.* 2021;27(6):621-625. PMID: 33819637

6. Ott J, Kaufmann U, Bentz E-K, Huber JC, Tempfer CB. Incidence of thrombophilia and venous thrombosis in transsexuals under cross-sex hormone therapy. *Fertil Steril.* 2010;93(4):1267-1272. PMID: 19200981

7. Connelly PJ, Freel EM, Perry C, et al. Gender-affirming hormone therapy, vascular health and cardiovascular disease in transgender adults. *Hypertension.* 2019;74(6):1266-1274. PMID: 31656099

8. Nota NM, Wiepjes CM, de Blok CJM, Gooren LJG, Kreukels BPC, den Heijer M. Occurrence of acute cardiovascular events in transgender individuals receiving hormone therapy. *Circulation.* 2019;139(11):1461-1462. PMID: 30776252

9. Getahun D, Nash R, Flanders WD, et al. Cross-sex hormones and acute cardiovascular events in transgender persons: a cohort study. *Ann Intern Med.* 2018;169(4):205-213. PMID: 29987313

10. Maraka S, Singh Ospina N, Rodriguez-Gutierrez R, et al. Sex steroids and cardiovascular outcomes in transgender individuals: a systematic review and meta-analysis. *J Clin Endocrinol Metab.* 2017;102(11):3914-3923. PMID: 28945852

11. Alzahrani T, Nguyen T, Ryan A, et al. Cardiovascular disease risk factors and myocardial infarction in the transgender population. *Circ Cardiovasc Qual Outcomes.* 2019;12(4):e005597. PMID: 30950651

12. Nokoff NJ, Scarbro S, Juarez-Colunga E, Moreau KL, Kempe A. Health and cardiometabolic disease in transgender adults in the United States: behavioral risk factor surveillance system 2015. *J Endocr Soc.* 2018;2(4):349-360. PMID: 29577110

13. Leone AG, Trapani D, Schabath MB, et al. Cancer in transgender and gender-diverse persons: a review. *JAMA Oncol.* 2023;9(4):556-563. PMID: 36757703

14. Ly D, Hoyt AC, Weimer A, Chang EH, Capiro N, Xie C, Chow L. Breast cancer among transgender and nonbinary patients: paradigms for improving data collection and inclusion in breast imaging settings. *J Breast Imaging.* 2022;5(1):73-79. PMID: 38416956

15. Hayward JH. Updates in transgender breast imaging. *Semin Ultrasound CT MR.* 2023;44(1):23-34. PMID: 36792271

16. Iwamoto SJ, Defreyne J, Kaoutzanis C, Davies RD, Moreau KL, Rothman MS. Gender-affirming hormone therapy, mental health, and surgical considerations for aging transgender and gender diverse adults. *Ther Adv Endocrinol Metab.* 2023;14:20420188231166494. PMID: 37113210

Menopausal Hormone Therapy and Estrogen-Sensitive Cancers

JoAnn V. Pinkerton, MD. Department Obstetrics and Gynecology, University of Virginia Health, Charlottesville, Virginia; Email: Jvp9u@uvahealth.org

Malavika Kesavan, MD. Department Obstetrics and Gynecology, University of Virginia Health, Charlottesville, Virginia; Email: MK8HM@uvahealth.org

Educational Objectives

After reviewing this chapter, learners should be able to:

- Explain the risks of systemic estrogen therapy compared with those of vaginal estrogen for women with estrogen-sensitive breast cancer.

- Explain the benefits and risks of giving hormone therapy to women with *BRCA* pathogenic variants who are at high risk of breast cancer after premature menopause following risk-reducing oophorectomy (surgical menopause).

- Describe the therapeutic nonhormonal options for relief of vasomotor symptoms (VMS) and genitourinary syndrome of menopause (GSM) for women with estrogen-sensitive cancers.

Significance of the Clinical Problem

Cancer treatment and prevention recommendations may result in the loss of estrogen either through surgical removal of both ovaries, effects of chemotherapy or radiation, or the use of prolonged antiestrogen therapies. Menopausal symptoms, including VMS of hot flashes or night sweats, may be extremely bothersome and affect not only quality of life but workplace absenteeism, health care costs, and overall health.[1] For women who go through induced menopause, the symptoms are often more sudden and severe.[2] For those who have premature induced menopause, there are additional cardiovascular and osteoporosis health risks.[3] The decision to start hormone therapy is complex for many women, even without the additional concern for additional oncogenic risk. Thus, endocrinologists need to understand both the current landscape of risks and benefits of hormone therapy vs alternative and nonhormonal therapies to allow evidence-based individualized treatment options for menopausal women. Some cancer survivors with estrogen-sensitive cancers may be candidates for low-dosage vaginal hormone therapy to treat dyspareunia and progressive GSM, with the involvement of their oncologist. For survivors of epithelial ovarian, vaginal, and cervical cancer, systemic or vaginal hormone therapy may be considered unless the histologic subtypes are estrogen-sensitive histologic subtypes.[4]

Initiation of hormone replacement therapy in women with menopausal symptoms in the setting of estrogen-sensitive cancers (breast/endometrium) or those who have high risk of breast cancer depends on several factors, including the severity of menopausal symptoms, bone density, age, type of cancer, other medications such as aromatase inhibitors, and comorbidities.[4]

Practice Gaps

- Fear of systemic and vaginal estrogen for those at increased risk of breast cancer.

- Lack of recognition of the increased health risks of premature oophorectomy if estrogen is not taken until the age of natural menopause.

- Unmet need for relief of VMS in women who cannot or will not take hormone therapy.

- Understanding that systemic or even vaginal estrogen could potentially lower the effectiveness of aromatase inhibitors in women with breast cancer.

Discussion

Vasomotor Symptoms

For symptomatic menopausal women with bothersome VMS, administration of systemic hormone therapy has a favorable benefit-to-risk ratio if initiated under age 60 years or within 10 years of menopause.[5] During perimenopause, ethnic variations in VMS have been shown[6] in Black and Hispanic women who have VMS for an average of 8 to 10 years; White women with VMS for an average of 7 years; and Asian, Japanese, and Chinese women with VMS for an average of 5 to 6 years. Following premature surgical menopause after risk-reducing bilateral salpingo-oophorectomy (RRSO), VMS are more frequent and severe. Similarly, the adverse effects of abruptly lowering estradiol in premenopausal women with suppression of ovarian function can lead to more severe VMS in premenopausal patients.[2]

Breast Cancer Risk and Menopausal Hormone Therapy

Estrogen alone is used for symptomatic menopausal women who have had hysterectomy, with data suggesting more safety and less breast cancer risk. In the Women's Health Initiative, there were 7 fewer breast cancers per 1000 after almost 7 years of conjugated estrogen 625 mcg daily. However, for women with a uterus, either progestogens (progesterone or synthetic progestins) or the combination of conjugated estrogen/bazedoxifene are used to protect against endometrial hyperplasia and cancer seen with unopposed estrogen.[7] The combination of estrogen with progestogens for menopausal hormone therapy (MHT) has shown an increase in breast cancer, with a higher risk seen with the more potent synthetic progestins such as medroxyprogesterone compared to progesterone.[1,8]

In the long-term follow-up of the Women's Health Initiative randomized controlled trials (median of 20.3 years after randomization), previous randomization to conjugated equine estrogens alone for postmenopausal women with previous hysterectomy was associated with a significantly lowered risk of breast cancer incidence and mortality. In contrast, previous randomization to conjugated equine estrogens plus medroxyprogesterone acetate (estrogen-progestogen therapy) for women with an intact uterus was associated with a small but significantly increased incidence of breast cancer but no significant difference in breast cancer mortality.[7]

In some countries, oral tibolone is available, which has estrogenic, progestational, and androgenic actions, thus improving hot flashes, preventing bone loss, and possibly improving libido without the need for a progestational agent for women with a uterus. Placebo-controlled randomized trials have not shown that tibolone changes breast cancer rates in healthy women. However, in women with a history of breast cancer, tibolone is associated with increased risk and thus is considered contraindicated, similar to hormone therapy for women with previous breast cancer. Moderate-quality evidence reviewed in the Cochrane Database Review[9] suggests that tibolone is more effective than placebo but is less effective than MHT in reducing VMS. Higher incidence of unscheduled bleeding was seen with tibolone compared with placebo, but less unscheduled bleeding than with combined hormone therapy.[9]

MHT (estrogen alone or combined with a progestogen) is the most effective therapy for reducing hot flashes.[1,5,8] However, MHT is not recommended for use in breast cancer survivors, given the increased risk of breast cancer recurrence.[10,11] There are no data to prove that MHT is safe for patients with estrogen receptor–negative breast cancer in terms of cancer recurrence, and thus, systemic hormone therapy is not recommended for these women either.[10] Due to insufficient safety data, conjugated estrogen combined with bazedoxifene and tibolone are not recommended for use in breast cancer survivors. Nonhormonal options for treatment of menopausal symptoms are advised for these women.[11] High-dosage progestational agents have been used in the past for metastatic breast cancer, but their safety and efficacy are not known for women with early breast cancer.[10]

Premature Surgical Menopause

In healthy women with early or premature menopause, systemic estrogen–based MHT is recommended at least until the natural age of menopause.[3] However, in women taking antiestrogenic therapies such as aromatase inhibitors, estrogen-based therapies are contraindicated because of evidence of decreased efficacy of aromatase inhibitors.[12]

Observational trials reviewed by Marchetti and colleagues[13] assessed breast cancer events in 1100 participants with a *BRCA* pathogenic variant who had intact breasts and underwent RRSO. No elevated breast cancer risk was seen for carriers of *BRCA1* and *BRCA2* pathogenic variants who received MHT after RRSO (hazard ratio, 0.98 [95% CI, 0.63-1.52]). A nonsignificant reduction in breast cancer risk was seen for the estrogen-alone users compared with risk in participants taking estrogen-progestogen therapy (odds ratio, 0.53 [95% CI, 0.25-1.15]). Thus, the short-term use of hormone therapy, estrogen alone, or estrogen combined with a progestogen does not appear to elevate the risk of breast cancer after RRSO in these women at high risk,[5,8,13] allowing the benefits of estrogen to both decrease VMS and reduce the risks of cardiovascular and bone loss.

MHT and Cancer

Available data suggest that short-term use of MHT in patients with gynecologic cancer who do not have an estrogen-dependent malignancy does not adversely impact oncologic outcomes while improving VSM and GSM and preventing bone loss.[4] Candidates for hormone therapy include women with bothersome menopausal symptoms who have low-grade, early-stage endometrial cancer; cervical, vulvar, or vaginal cancer; and ovarian cancer. In a cross-sectional study, 137 of 199 women reported moderate or severe symptoms on the menopause rating scale (69%) a mean of 7.9 years after RRSO. Ninety-four of 137 women (57%) reported severe urogenital symptoms, and about 25% reported severe psychological and/or somato-vegetative symptoms.[4]

GSM in Women With Estrogen-Sensitive Cancers

For women with estrogen-sensitive cancers, nonhormonal options are initially recommended for GSM, which include lubricants and vaginal moisturizers containing hyaluronic acid.[8,12] Low-dosage vaginal estrogen is absorbed systemically in small amounts, with blood levels remaining within the normal postmenopausal range, but it could potentially stimulate occult breast cancer cells. Although low-dosage vaginal estrogen is poorly studied, it is not generally advised, particularly for those on aromatase inhibitors.[12] Intravaginal dehydroepiandrosterone and oral ospemifene have been approved to treat dyspareunia, although safety after breast cancer has not been established. Some are using vaginal laser therapy for GSM, but efficacy from sham-controlled studies is lacking. Therapies undergoing clinical trials include vaginal testosterone and estetrol.[12]

Nonhormonal Therapies for VMS

Off-label use of medications shown in randomized clinical trials to relieve hot flashes but approved by the FDA for other indications include low-dose antidepressants (venlafaxine, paroxetine), anticonvulsants (gabapentin), hypertension drugs (clonidine), and bladder relaxants (oxybutynin).[1,8,12] Two FDA-approved options for hot flash relief are the low-dosage antidepressant paroxetine salt 7.5 mg and the neurokinin 3 receptor antagonist fezolinetant, 45 mg.

Low-dosage paroxetine salt (7.5 mg) reduces hot flash frequency and severity. A systematic review of 5 randomized controlled clinical trials that included 1482 postmenopausal women confirmed a significant reduction of hot flashes compared with placebo, with a mean difference of 7.97 fewer (−10.51, −5.92) hot flash episodes per week.[14]

In phase 3 clinical trials, fezolinetant has been shown to reduce the frequency of VMS by about 65%, significantly more than placebo, and similar to the 75% reduction seen with MHT, with rapid onset within 1 week.[15] Both frequency and severity of hot flashes were reduced with maintenance of effect and safety at 52 weeks. Of the menopausal women participating in clinical trials, 1% to 2% reported adverse events, including headaches, abdominal pain, diarrhea, insomnia, back pain, hot flushes, and reversible elevated hepatic transaminases with infrequent serious adverse events.[15] Endometrial adverse effects were neither seen nor expected, as fezolinetant is a centrally acting, non–estrogen-containing medication. In addition, no loss of bone density was seen at 52 weeks.[15] Previous trials of neurokinin receptor antagonists raised concern about the potential for hepatotoxicity, but this was not seen in the fezolinetant trials. Increases in hepatic transaminases were described as asymptomatic, isolated, intermittent, or transient, with return to baseline either during treatment or after discontinuation.[15] However, the US FDA has placed a warning about liver injury potential with a recommendation of baseline liver function tests before starting fezolinetant and again at 3, 6, and 9 months after initiation. In addition, concomitant use of moderate CYP1A2 (cytochrome P450) inhibitors, including many antidepressants and antipsychotics, tamoxifen, warfarin, and cimetidine, should be avoided.

FDA-approved therapies for other indications tested in randomized controlled trials have shown reductions in VMS and, as such, have been used off-label due to a lack of adequate FDA-approved therapies.[8,12] These include venlafaxine, which has been shown to reduce hot flashes by up to 60%. Others with positive improvements in relief of hot flashes in women with a history of breast cancer include duloxetine, escitalopram, paroxetine, and sertraline. The selective serotonin reuptake inhibitors are potent inhibitors of CYP2D6, which could reduce the bioavailability of tamoxifen. Stellate ganglion block has shown efficacy, but pharmacologic interventions are usually recommended due to its invasiveness. Cognitive behavioral therapy (psychoeducation, paced breathing, and relaxation) reduced the perceived burden of hot flashes. Both hypnosis and some trials of acupuncture suggest benefit, but availability is limited. Over-the-counter supplements that have not been found to be more effective than placebo include black cohosh, most trials on phytoestrogens, magnesium, and vitamin E. Similarly, randomized controlled trials using magnet therapy and homeopathy did not show an effect greater than that of placebo.

Choosing a nonhormonal therapy should be a shared decision-making process and include consideration of concomitant medications, comorbidities, and safety profiles. Treatment should start with low dosages to evaluate response and tolerability.[10]

Clinical Case Vignettes

Case 1

A 49-year-old postmenopausal woman with a family history of breast cancer presents for routine examination. Breast examination shows thickened breast tissue but no masses. Because her breasts are extremely dense on mammography, she is enrolled in a clinical trial, and contrast-enhanced mammography is performed. An irregular 20-mm mass with indistinct margins is seen in the right breast. She chooses to undergo bilateral mastectomy and sentinel node biopsy. Right breast pathology shows a 2.5-cm grade 3 intraductal cancer, which invades skeletal muscle. The margins and sentinel lymph node are negative. Because of her high-risk oncotype score, she undergoes adjuvant chemotherapy and begins the aromatase inhibitor letrozole. In addition, she undergoes RRSO to reduce any ovarian stimulation. Adverse effects of the aromatase inhibitor include severe joint pain and hot flashes (day and night with sweating).

Which of the following statements is true?

A. Since she has undergone bilateral mastectomy, controlled clinical trials have shown that she can take estrogen for her hot flashes as long as she continues taking an aromatase inhibitor

B. No health risks, such as cardiovascular or bone loss, have been found for women taking aromatase inhibitors

C. There are no FDA-approved nonhormonal medications to relieve hot flashes

D. There are 2 FDA-approved nonhormonal medications to relieve hot flashes

E. Both escitalopram and gabapentin are FDA approved to relieve hot flashes

Answer: D) There are 2 FDA-approved nonhormonal medications to relieve hot flashes

Estrogen therapy is not recommended for women with estrogen-sensitive breast cancer on aromatase inhibitors.[4,10,11] Due to this patient's early surgical menopause, she is at increased risk of cardiovascular disease and bone loss,[3] which are both worsened by being on the aromatase inhibitor. Two FDA-approved medications shown to relieve moderate to severe hot flashes are low-dosage paroxetine salt, 7.5 mg, and fezolinetant, 45 mg, a neurokinin 3 inhibitor (Answer D). Extended-release gabapentin was tested in phase 3 clinical trials in women with 7 to 10 moderate to severe hot flashes per day with reduced hot

flash frequency and severity. However, it did not meet all FDA-required end points or receive FDA approval. Gabapentin is often used off-label for night sweats at dosages of 300 to 600 mg or up to 900 mg total per day.[12] Escitalopram, 10 and 20 mg, has been tested in randomized controlled trials for hot flashes, and benefits are similar to those of low-dosage 0.5-mg oral estradiol but it has not been tested in women with 7 to 10 moderate to severe hot flashes per day.

Case 1 (continued)

The patient tried multiple nonhormonal treatment options for hot flashes, including pollen extract and herbal remedies. Low-dosage gabapentin taken at night significantly improved her symptoms but led to leg swelling after 4 to 5 days. Both FDA-approved paroxetine salt, 7.5 mg, and off-label use of escitalopram, 10 mg, were declined by the patient, as she did not want to be on mood-altering medications. She continued to have severe hot flashes for 2 years.

Once fezolinetant became available, she was started on it after normal liver function was confirmed and while not taking any moderate CYP1A2 inhibitors. Within 2 weeks, her hot flashes and night sweats significantly resolved.

By 3 months, she feels like she has her life back; she is sleeping at night, has resumed working, and describes dramatic quality of life improvement.

Which of the following is true?

A. Fezolinetant has been shown to relieve hot flashes, but the benefit only lasts 3 months

B. The US FDA recommends that users of fezolinetant have liver function tests at baseline and every 3 months for 9 months after initiation

C. After 2 years, while continuing on the aromatase inhibitor, this patient should have been prescribed systemic hormone therapy for her hot flashes and her health risks of early menopause

D. In randomized controlled trials, escitalopram works only as well as placebo and thus should not be offered to women with hot flashes

E. If this patient has osteopenia, fezolinetant will provide not only relief of her hot flashes but has been shown to prevent bone loss

Answer: B) The US FDA recommends that users of fezolinetant have liver function tests at baseline and every 3 months for 9 months after initiation

In phase 3 randomized clinical trials and a 52-week safety trial, fezolinetant has been shown to effectively relieve hot flashes and night sweats, with rapid onset of benefit at 1 to 2 weeks and continued efficacy through 52 weeks.[15] As expected, no significant increase in bone loss has been documented with fezolinetant, as it works centrally in the brain. Despite rare reports of abnormal liver function test results that return to normal during or after treatment, concern about liver safety led the FDA to recommend baseline liver function tests and repeated testing every 3 months for 9 months (Answer B). Moderate CYP1A2 inhibitors should be avoided because they can interact negatively with fezolinetant. Aromatase inhibitors are often used for 5 to 7 years for women with estrogen-sensitive breast cancer, and they lower patients' estrogen levels to undetectable. Taking systemic estrogen could negatively affect the aromatase inhibitor's ability to reduce the risk of recurrent breast cancer. At a dosage of 10 to 20 mg, escitalopram was shown in randomized controlled trials to work as effectively as oral estradiol 0.5 mg, in reducing hot flashes and can be offered to women with estrogen-sensitive breast cancer.[1,8] However, the study participants enrolled did not need to meet the FDA requirement of 7 to 10 moderate to severe hot flashes per day. Escitalopram is less likely to work as well in women with frequent moderate to severe hot flashes.

Case 2

A 38-year-old woman (G2P2) with a *BRCA1* pathogenic variant has a history of acne and takes an oral contraceptive pill. Her older sister, mother, and maternal aunt have all had breast cancer. Her father and paternal grandfather died in their 50s of myocardial infarction. She is a marathon runner and is concerned about how removing her ovaries will affect her overall health. She has had a bilateral salpingectomy and is recently divorced. She does not smoke cigarettes and has no history of migraines.

Which of the following statements is true?

A. Women with a *BRCA1* pathogenic variant have a 45% lifetime risk of developing ovarian cancer

B. Bilateral salpingectomy significantly reduces the risk of developing ovarian cancer, and she does not necessarily need to undergo oophorectomy

C. Women are more likely to develop bothersome VMS in the pre- and perimenopausal period if they undergo RRSO

D. Risk of cardiovascular disease is not significantly increased with premature menopause

E. Risk of bone loss is not significantly increased with premature menopause

Answer: C) Women are more likely to develop bothersome VMS in the pre- and perimenopausal period if they undergo RRSO

The *BRCA1* and *BRCA2* genes produce proteins that help repair damaged DNA. Women who inherit a pathogenic variant in either of these genes have an increased risk of breast and ovarian cancer. Approximately 55% to 72% of women with a *BRCA1* variant and 45% to 69% of women with a *BRCA2* variant develop breast cancer by age 70 to 80 years. Approximately 39% to 44% of women with a *BRCA1* variant and 11% to 17% of women with a *BRCA2* variant develop ovarian cancer by age 70 to 80 years.[16] Women are more likely to develop VMS if they undergo RRSO, as they will be in surgical menopause (Answer C).[2] There is evidence that the most common type of ovarian cancer (epithelial) originates in the fallopian tube as serous tubal intraepithelial carcinoma lesions. In one Swedish study, bilateral salpingectomy appeared to reduce the risk of ovarian cancer by 65%, and there is ongoing research to evaluate the full effect of risk reduction in population studies.[17] RRSO reduces the risk of ovarian or fallopian tube cancers by 80%.[18] With premature menopause without estrogen supplementation to the natural age of menopause, risks of both cardiovascular disease and osteoporosis are increased.[3]

Case 2 (continued)

The patient's younger 28-year-old sister is also *BRCA1*-positive and has no known medical conditions.

Which of the following is the appropriate counseling regarding breast cancer prevention in the patient?

A. Mammography should have started annually at age 25 years

B. Breast MRI should have started annually at age 25 years; then alternating mammography and MRI beginning at age 30 years

C. No screening is indicated until age 40 years

D. Breast self-examination every 6 months until age 40 years, then discontinue self-examination

E. Tamoxifen for chemoprevention starting now

Answer: B) Breast MRI should have started annually at age 25 years; then alternating mammography and MRI beginning at age 30 years

This patient has a high risk of developing breast cancer, and early screening is indicated. Annual breast MRI is indicated for patients aged 25 to 29 years who have a known pathogenic *BRCA* variant. Beginning at age 30 years, alternating breast MRI and mammography are recommended annually (Answer B).[19] She should meet with a genetic counselor and breast surgeon to discuss the

possibility of risk-reducing surgery mastectomy in the future. Tamoxifen is a selective estrogen receptor modulator that can decrease the development of breast cancer by about one-third. However, it is associated with adverse effects such as hot flashes, uterine cancer, and increased risk of venous thromboembolism.

Case 2 (continued)

The patient ultimately decides to have a hysterectomy and RRSO.

Which of the following is the most appropriate therapy after hysterectomy and RRSO to recommend and discuss with the patient?

A. Oral estrogen supplementation

B. Continuation of the oral contraceptive pill

C. Transdermal estrogen patch

D. Venlafaxine

E. Only treat if she presents with bothersome VMS

Answer: C) Transdermal estrogen patch

Given her young age, increased risk of cardiovascular disease, and risk of bone loss, it is reasonable to offer and discuss appropriate hormone therapy. Observational data have not shown an increase in breast cancer with hormone therapy used in those with *BRCA* pathogenic variants to the average age of menopause (51 years).[13] Ultimately, if the patient does not desire any hormone therapy and is having hot flashes, venlafaxine (serotonin-norepinephrine reuptake inhibitor) is an appropriate choice. Compared with transdermal estrogen, oral estrogen is associated with increased rates of venous thromboembolism events. Oral contraceptive pills contain progestin, which is inappropriate in the setting of a patient with no uterus, as the use of menopausal estrogen combined with synthetic progestin has been associated with an increased breast cancer risk. The best answer for her overall health is to recommend transdermal estrogen (Answer C) to age 51 years and then re-evaluate.

Case 2 (continued)

Five years later, the patient has a provoked deep vein thrombosis in the setting of orthopedic surgery, and her hormone therapy is discontinued. She presents with uncomfortable vaginal dryness, dyspareunia, 20-lb (9.1-kg) weight gain, and worsening hot flashes occurring 7 to 10 times per day with sweating.

Which of the following therapies is most appropriate?

A. Vaginal estrogen alone

B. Vaginal estrogen and venlafaxine

C. Vaginal moisturizer and fezolinetant

D. Black cohosh as a bridge for 1 year, and then she can go back on hormone therapy

E. Progesterone-only pills

Answer: C) Vaginal moisturizer and fezolinetant

In this scenario, the patient has moderate to severe symptoms of menopause, including significant hot flashes with sweating, weight gain, and vaginal dryness, likely leading to dyspareunia. Given recent deep vein thrombosis, hormone therapy is not indicated. Vaginal estrogen (Answers A and B), although acting locally, could cause a slight increase in blood estrogen levels.[12] Black cohosh (Answer D) is a supplement with poor-quality evidence supporting its use as a therapy for bothersome hot flashes. It carries a risk of liver damage and should not be recommended for this patient. Progesterone-alone therapy (Answer E) is not indicated for this patient who has had hysterectomy. Vaginal moisturizer and fezolinetant, a neurokinin 3 receptor antagonist (Answer C), would manage her symptoms with minimal adverse effects and no increased risk of venous thromboembolism. There is no official recommendation for the length of time after the venous thromboembolism event before restarting hormone therapy.

Case 2 (continued)

Which of the following statements regarding estrogen is FALSE?

A. Later use of transdermal estrogen after a provoked deep vein thrombosis is associated with minimal to no increase in repeat venous thromboembolism

B. Oophorectomy before age 35 years increases the risk of cardiovascular disease by 7 times

C. Estrogen receptors are found only in the urogenital tract

D. Soy isolates may be agonists of estrogen receptors

E. Estrogen is not an anabolic (bone-building) therapy

Answer: C) Estrogen receptors are found only in the urogenital tract

Estrogen receptors are located throughout the body, including the temperature control center in the brain (thus, Answer C is correct). There is a growing body of research about the effect of estrogen on mental health, the cardiovascular system, and temperature control (perhaps explaining increased rates of cognitive decline, mood changes, and hot flashes associated with menopause). Oophorectomy before age 35 years without hormone replacement therapy is associated with a significant increase in cardiovascular disease without the protective effects of estrogen on the system.[3] However, data are mixed regarding the use of estrogen and/or progesterone as primary prevention at menopause for cardiovascular disease. Transdermal low-dosage estrogen is overall associated with minimal or low rates of venous thromboembolism, even in patients with previous venous thromboembolism.[19] Soy contains isoflavones with an estrogenlike structure and has been shown to bind weakly to estrogen receptors as agonists, partial agonists, or even antagonists. Estrogen has been shown to prevent bone loss and fractures through inhibition of bone resorption, mainly by direct actions on osteoclasts, and it is not an anabolic therapy.

Case 3

A 58-year-old woman with a history of type 2 diabetes (hemoglobin A_{1c} = 6.0% [42 mmol/mol]), BMI of 45 kg/m^2, and history of stage 1A well-differentiated endometrial cancer 6 years ago now has bothersome vaginal dryness and recurrent urinary tract infections (UTIs). She was recently hospitalized with pyelonephritis with a highly resistant klebsiella. There is a history of endometrial cancer in her maternal grandmother, but no other cancer or venous thromboembolism reported in her family history. She has tried over-the-counter lubricant and vaginal moisturizer with some improvement but notes dyspareunia.

Examination reveals vaginal narrowing, loss of the labia, vaginal petechiae, well-healed vaginal cuff without lesions, and a vaginal pH of 7.0.

Which of the following is the best therapy to minimize this patient's risk of future UTIs?

A. Vaginal estrogen

B. Vaginal laser

C. Venlafaxine and pelvic physical therapy

D. Ciprofloxacin prophylaxis after intercourse

E. Transdermal systemic estrogen

Answer: A) Vaginal estrogen

In the setting of low-risk cancer and now more than 5 years out from treatment in a patient with recurrent UTI and vaginal dryness, vagina estrogen (Answer A) is the most ideal option to alleviate her symptoms, restore the anatomy, and prevent future hospitalizations from sequelae of UTI.[20] Although there are some promising data for vaginal laser (Answer B) to treat vaginal dryness, this therapy was recently not shown to be better than sham for treatment of dyspareunia. No high-quality evidence demonstrates that vaginal laser treatment can prevent UTIs. Venlafaxine (Answer C) has not been shown to have benefits in improving vaginal dryness or UTI. Although antibiotic prophylaxis after intercourse (Answer D) may decrease her overall risk of UTI, ciprofloxacin is not an appropriate choice given its adverse effect profile. Nitrofurantoin daily would be more appropriate,

but it would not restore the anatomy. Lubricants and vaginal moisturizers may be helpful, but they will not restore the normal anatomy nor rebuild the missing top layer of epithelial cells, which can lead to increased glycogen and improvement in both the vaginal pH and the presence of lactobacilli.[1,8] Transdermal systemic estrogen (Answer E) would improve her symptoms, but local estrogen (Answer A) would more effectively restore anatomy and reduce risk of recurrent UTI with less risk of venous thromboembolism and less overall systemic absorption.[20] Vaginal estrogen, intravaginal dehydroepiandrosterone, or oral ospemifene would all treat vaginal atrophy. Due to the dyspareunia, she might have levator spasm and thus might need vaginal dilators or pelvic floor therapy to regain the ability to have sex without pain, even after her anatomy is restored with treatment.

Case 3 (continued)

Which of the following is NOT a way in which vaginal estrogen can help improve and prevent GSM in this patient?

A. Increase in vaginal pH

B. Lead to maturation of vaginal epithelial cells

C. Promote ovarian function (if present) to restart production of endogenous estrogen

D. Shift vaginal flora away from being dominated by enterobacter species

E. Improve sensitivity of α-adrenergic receptors in the urogenital tract

Answer: C) Promote ovarian function (if present) to restart production of endogenous estrogen

Vaginal estrogen has a host of benefits for the urogenital tract, including improving vaginal atrophy by helping the vaginal epithelial cells mature.[1,5] Improving the overall vaginal microenvironment by promoting average lactobacilli growth restores normal vaginal pH. This reduces the risk of aberrant bacterial growth and risk of developing UTI. Studies have shown that when vaginal flora are dominated by enterobacter species, patients are at higher risk of UTI. In a double-blinded, randomized control trial of 93 women with recurrent UTIs, those who received vaginal estrogen had a decrease in the number of UTIs from 5.9 to 0.5 infections per year. Similarly, a small randomized trial (n = 35) showed that fewer participants with recurrent UTI treated with vaginal estrogen had a UTI at 6 months.[20] There is no evidence that transvaginal estrogen can "activate" previous quiescent aging ovaries. High estrogen receptor β expression levels are detected in the epithelial cells of the urogenital tract, whereas the estrogen receptor α expression level is much lower.[21]

Case 3 (continued)

The patient would like to know if there is additional screening for endometrial cancer recurrence that she needs to complete if she starts vaginal estrogen.

Which of the following is the best recommendation?

A. No additional screening is needed
B. Monitoring for recurrence with vaginal cytology every 6 months
C. CT every 3 to 6 months
D. MRI of chest/abdomen/pelvis
E. PET annually

Answer: A) No additional screening is needed

In the setting of her low-risk endometrial cancer, now more than 5 years out, vaginal estrogen use by itself would not be an indication for further screening (thus, Answer A is correct). Recurrence of endometrial cancer is most likely to occur within 5 years of the initial diagnosis and is most likely to be at the vaginal cuff. Vaginal cytology (Answer B) has been shown to be effective in earlier diagnosis of recurrence, but in practice, has a low sensitivity and is not currently recommended for screening.[22] Pelvic examination is performed to identify vaginal lesions and pelvic masses and to assess for GSM. Additional imaging, such as CT (Answer C), PET (Answer E), or MRI (Answer D), help identify recurrence in women

with high-risk gynecological cancers or with recurrent or metastatic cancer but imaging is not indicated for this patient.

Key Learning Points

- For women at high risk of breast cancer who undergo RRSO, taking estrogen therapy until the age of natural menopause can be considered.

- For women with estrogen-sensitive cancer, systemic MHT is not recommended.

- For women with estrogen-sensitive cancer, nonhormonal therapies for VMS are recommended.

- The 2 FDA-approved nonhormonal options for VMS are low-dosage paroxetine salt (7.5 mg) and fezolinetant (45 mg).

- Non–FDA-approved therapies for VMS tested in controlled trials and used off-label include low-dosage antidepressants, gabapentin, oxybutynin, and clonidine.

- For women with GSM for whom lubricants and moisturizers fail, low-dosage vaginal hormone therapy may be considered with the involvement of the patient's oncologist.

- Vaginal estrogen should not be used as a first-line treatment in women on aromatase inhibitors, as it could potentially lessen the effectiveness of the aromatase inhibitors.

- For estrogen receptor-positive endometrial cancer survivors, low-dosage vaginal hormone therapy may be considered for low-risk cancers, particularly after 5 years, but it should be avoided in patients with high-risk subtypes.

References

1. Davis SR, Pinkerton J, Santoro N, Simoncini T. Menopause-biology, consequences, supportive care, and therapeutic options. *Cell.* 2023;186(19):4038-4058. PMID: 37678251

2. Stuursma A, van Driel CMG, Wessels NJ, de Bock GH, Mourits MJE. Severity and duration of menopausal symptoms after risk-reducing salpingo-oophorectomy. *Maturitas.* 2018;111:69-76. PMID: 29673834

3. Faubion SS, Kuhle CL, Shuster LT, Rocca WA. Long-term health consequences of premature or early menopause and considerations for management. *Climacteric.* 2015;18(4):483-491. PMID: 25845383

4. Del Carmen MG, Rice LW. Management of menopausal symptoms in women with gynecologic cancers. *Gynecol Oncol.* 2017;146(2):427-435. PMID: 28625396

5. The 2022 Hormone Therapy Position Statement of the North American Menopause Society Advisory Panel. The 2022 hormone therapy position statement of the North American Menopause Society. *Menopause.* 2022;29(7):767-794. PMID: 35797481

6. Avis NE, Crawford SL, Greendale G, et al; Duration of menopausal vasomotor symptoms over the menopause transition. *JAMA Intern Med.* 2015;175(4):531-539. PMID: 25686030

7. Chlebowski RT, Rohan TE, Manson JE, et al. Breast cancer after use of estrogen plus progestin and estrogen alone: analyses of data from 2 Women's Health Initiative Randomized Clinical Trials. *JAMA Oncol.* 2015;1(3):296-305. PMID: 26181174

8. Pinkerton JV. Hormone therapy for postmenopausal women. *N Engl J Med.* 2020;382(5):446-455. PMID: 31995690

9. Formoso G, Perrone E, Maltoni S, et al. Short-term and long-term effects of tibolone in postmenopausal women. *Cochrane Database Syst Rev.* 2016;10(10):CD008536. PMID: 27733017

10. Franzoi MA, Agostinetto E, Perachino M, et al. Evidence-based approaches for the management of side-effects of adjuvant endocrine therapy in patients with breast cancer. *Lancet Oncol.* 2021;22(7):e303-e313. PMID: 33891888

11. Harris BS, Bishop KC, Kuller JA, et al. Hormonal management of menopausal symptoms in women with a history of gynecologic malignancy. *Menopause.* 2020;27(2):243-248. PMID: 31738735

12. Santen RJ, Stuenkel CA, Davis SR, Pinkerton JV, Gompel A, Lumsden MA. Managing menopausal symptoms and associated clinical issues in breast cancer survivors. *J Clin Endocrinol Metab.* 2017;102(10):3647-3661. PMID: 28934376

13. Marchetti C, De Felice F, Boccia S, et al. Hormone replacement therapy after prophylactic risk-reducing salpingo-oophorectomy and breast cancer risk in BRCA1 and BRCA2 mutation carriers: a meta-analysis. *Crit Rev Oncol Hematol.* 2018;132:111-115. PMID: 30447915

14. Riemma G, Schiattarella A, La Verde M et al. Efficacy of low-dose paroxetine for the treatment of hot flushes in surgical and physiological postmenopausal women: systematic review and meta-analysis of randomized trials. *Medicina (Kaunas).* 2019;55(9):554. PMID: 31480427

15. Pinkerton JV, Redick DL, Homewood LN, Kaunitz AM. Neurokinin receptor antagonist, fezolinetant, for treatment of menopausal vasomotor symptoms. *J Clin Endocrinol Metab.* 2023;108(11):e1448-e1449. PMID: 37097747

16. Kuchenbaecker KB, Hopper JL, Barnes DR, et al. Risks of breast, ovarian, and contralateral breast cancer for BRCA1 and BRCA2 mutation carriers. *JAMA.* 2017;317(23):2402-2416. PMID: 28632866

17. Falconer H, Yin L, Gronberg H, Altman D. Ovarian cancer risk after salpingectomy: a nationwide population-based study. *J Natl Cancer Inst.* 2015;107(2):dju410. PMID: 25628372

18. American College of Obstetricians and Gynecologists. BRCA1 and BRCA2 Mutations: Frequently Asked Questions. Last updated December 2022. Accessed December 9, 2023. https://www.acog.org/womens-health/faqs/brca1-and-brca2-mutations.

19. Sobel TH, Shen W. Transdermal estrogen therapy in menopausal women at increased risk for thrombotic events: a scoping review. *Menopause.* 2022;29(4):483-490. PMID: 35357370

20. Ferrante KL, Wasenda EJ, Jung CE, Adams-Piper ER, Lukacz ES. Vaginal estrogen for the prevention of recurrent urinary tract infection in postmenopausal women: a randomized clinical trial. *Female Pelvic Med Reconstr Surg.* 2021;27(2):112-117. PMID: 31232721

21. Mäkelä S, Strauss L, Kuiper G, et al. Differential expression of estrogen receptors alpha and beta in adult rat accessory sex glands and lower urinary tract. *Mol Cell Endocrinol.* 2000;164(1-2):109-116. PMID: 11026563

22. Zhao C, Karunamurthy A, Jain S, Austin RM. Vaginal cytology results in follow-up of endometrial carcinoma after hysterectomy. *Am J Clin Pathol.* 2016;146(2):244-247. PMID: 27371362

Managing Menopause

Margaret E. Wierman, MD. Endocrinology, Diabetes, and Metabolism, Department of Medicine, University of Colorado Anschutz Medical Center, Aurora, CO; Email: Margaret.wierman@cuanschutz.edu

Educational Objectives

After reviewing this chapter, learners should be able to:

- Identify the signs and symptoms of menopause.

- Outline the benefits and risks of menopausal hormone therapy (MHT).

- Discuss MHT treatment options and alternatives.

Significance of the Clinical Problem

All women undergo reproductive senescence of the hypothalamic-pituitary-ovarian axis. The average age of menopause in the United States is 51 to 52 years, and premature menopause is defined as before age 40.[1] In some cultures menopause may occur earlier.[1] Loss of ovarian steroid production can be abrupt (surgical menopause) or gradual (natural menopause). The symptoms and signs have been well delineated and vary based on ethnicity and culture globally. After the initial report of the Women's Health Initiative (WHI) in 2002, which showed increased cardiovascular disease in older women on hormone replacement therapy, there has been a systematic lack of teaching providers about MHT in residencies and fellowships and therefore decreased use by many practitioners.[2] This has led to many women not being offered short-term MHT for signs and symptoms that are easily and safely treated with physiologic MHT and has prompted some women to seek alternative therapies without proven efficacy or safety. Many providers are not familiar with more recent data modulating the initial concern about absolute risk and demonstrating short-term benefit for many women.[1] Education of endocrinologists is critical to providing optimal care by selecting the appropriate type and dosage of MHT for personalized therapy and understanding the pros and cons of alternative therapies.

Practice Gaps

- A lack of understanding by practitioners on the benefits vs risks of MHT.

- Many providers have little clinical experience in using and optimizing MHT.

- A lack of understanding of the data on the benefits vs risks of alternative therapies.

Discussion

Menopause is a time of transition, and estrogen deficiency impacts all cells in the body. Estrogen deficiency is associated with vasomotor symptoms, which can alter sleep, concentration, cognition, and mood, leading to diminished quality of life. Additionally genitourinary symptoms occur as the bladder has estrogen receptors, and loss of bone mass leads to osteoporosis.[1,3,4] MHT has gotten a bad rap after the WHI 2002 publication.[5] It is important to realize that the study focused on secondary cardiac prevention by recruiting most of the participants more than 10 years after menopause and who had no symptoms.[4] Those are not the patients we are faced with in our clinic. There are no adequately powered clinical trials in younger symptomatic women aged 50 to 59 years. The risks and benefits of MHT in women after menopause has more recently been reassessed (*Figure*).[3,6] The reanalysis points out the consistent benefit for many outcomes with estrogen therapy and small risks of estrogen/ progestin therapy, especially in the subset of participants aged of 50 to 59 years, which is when women are typically symptomatic and desire treatment. This report included the 18-year cumulative data on risks of MHT,[3,6] and risk could be subdivided based on age of entry into the study. Importantly, the investigators documented no overall mortality risk with either estrogen/ progestin or estrogen over the 18-year cumulative follow-up.[1,3,6] These reports led the Endocrine society,[4] North American Menopause Society, and others[1] to redefine who should be considered for MHT. These recommendations for the practitioner are reassuring. The major take-home themes for each of the guidelines now include treating only symptomatic women and emphasize an individualized approach based on patient symptoms, personal preferences, and health status. Most suggest a baseline risk assessment in each patient to include any contraindications to MHT and assessment of cardiovascular and breast cancer risks. Contraindications to MHT include the potential for pregnancy, undiagnosed vaginal bleeding, estrogen-sensitive cancers such as breast or endometrial, history of myocardial infarction or stroke, and some consideration of the history of deep vein thrombosis or pulmonary embolism without prophylaxis and liver disease.[1] In a woman aged 50 to 59 years with vasomotor symptoms who is considering MHT, high cardiovascular disease risk is less common, but screening for coronary heart disease, cerebral vascular disease, and peripheral vascular disease should be performed.[1,4] If MHT is to be considered, most guidelines recommend transdermal therapy as the first-line option. However, other options should be considered based on availability, cost, and patient preference. In symptomatic women considering MHT, a breast cancer risk assessment includes family history and use of a risk

calculator (NCI Breast Cancer Risk Assessment Tool [5-year risk][7] or IBIS Breast Cancer Risk Evaluation Tool[8]), and if high (ie, >5%), alternative approaches and even risk-reducing medications would be considered.

Figure. Intergroup Difference in the Number of Events per 5 Years of Women Aged 50 to 59 Years Enrolled in the WHI Trials

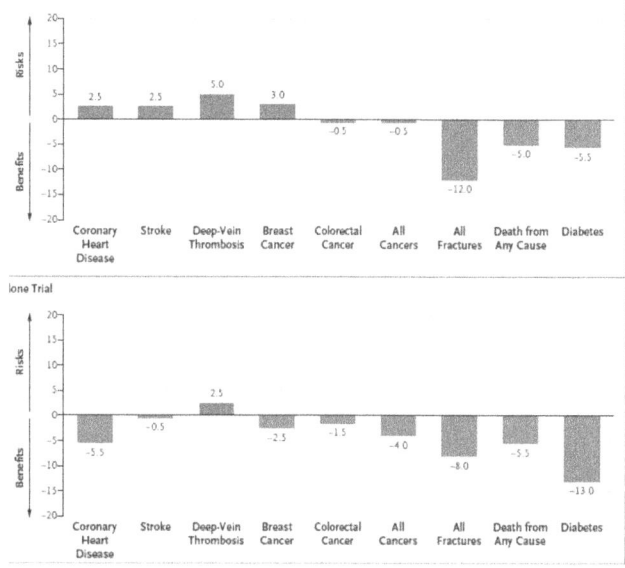

Reprinted with permission from Mason JE and Kaunitz AM. N Engl J Med, 2016; 374(9): 803-806. © Massachusetts Medical Society.[3]

[Color—Print (Color Gallery page CG35) or web & ePub editions]

Treatment Options for MHT

Based on the WHI and other studies, if a patient does not have a uterus, estrogen alone should be used.[1,3,9] If a uterus is present, then either progestin cyclically or continuously is prescribed to ensure prevention of endometrial cancer. Data concerning safety are available for medroxyprogesterone, 5 mg at night days 1 to 12 of each month or 2.5 mg daily, or micronized progesterone, 200 mg daily days 1 to 12 each month or 100 mg daily. In the United States, estrogen combined with basedoxifene—a selective estrogen receptor modulator that is an agonist in the bone and an antagonist in the breast and uterus—may be tried if a patient is intolerant to a progestin.[1] In other countries, tibolone has been used for menopausal symptoms. It is converted into metabolites with mixed estrogenic, androgenic, and progestogenic actions. Concern regarding breast and cardiovascular risk resulted in denial by the US FDA.

When deciding to initiate MHT, the following questions should be addressed: (1) type of estrogen, (2) route of administration (ie, oral vs transdermal vs vaginal); (3) dosage (ie, use lowest dosage to control symptoms), and (4) the type of progestin and timing (ie, cyclic or continuous). *Table 1* demonstrates the types of estrogens commonly used in MHT. These include oral options such as micronized estradiol, estradiol valerate used in Europe, and conjugated estrogens. Transdermal preparations include the estradiol patch weekly or biweekly, estradiol gel, and estradiol spray. A vaginal ring preparation is also available. Decision on type should be made with patient personal preference and comfort of prescribers. Cost and cultural acceptance are also considerations. In making decisions, we know that oral conjugated estrogens have extensive risk/benefit data and dosing, but risks initially published in the WHI trial decreased enthusiasm to prescribe them.[5,9] In addition, the inability to measure hormone levels is a potential disadvantage. After the WHI, conjugated estrogen formulations with lower dosing (ie, 0.45 and 0.3 mg and lower) were made available. Oral estradiol has extensive data concerning risk/benefit, and hormone levels can be measured.[1] Some women rapidly metabolize oral estradiol and do better when the dose is split twice daily (personal observation). There are concerns regarding the oral route having increased risk of venous thromboembolism and pulmonary embolism, as well as alterations in lipids (ie, better HDL-cholesterol and worse triglyceride levels). Transdermal routes have the advantage of avoiding the first-pass effects on lipids and perhaps less clotting risk. The vaginal ring provides steady dose delivery, and topical estradiol is used primarily for local symptoms and has variable absorption. In picking an estrogen, the goal is to provide the lowest dosage to adequately treat symptoms.

Many progestins are available commercially (*Table 2*). Based on the WHI and previous studies, most data are with medroxyprogesterone at various doses or with micronized progesterone which is made in peanut oil.[1,3] Because of reports of drowsiness or mood issues, progestins are usually taken at bedtime. More recently, some have suggested use of an intrauterine device (IUD), which releases an androgenic progestin levonorgestrel to protect the endometrium, and pairing it with an estrogen of choice. Long-term safety is unknown. Vaginal gel progesterone is available, although absorption and information on long-term safety and efficacy are not available. Cost, convenience, and availability may have a role in decision-making in the individual patient. There are also standardized combination oral and transdermal preparations of estrogens and various progestins available on the market (*Table 3, following page*), but they do not have extensive long-term safety information.

Table 1. Commonly Prescribed Estrogens Used in MHT

Type of estrogen	Route	Dose	Frequency
17β-estradiol	Oral Patch Gel Spray	0.5-2 mg 0.014-0.1 mg 0.25-1.25 mg 1.5 mg/spray	Daily or twice daily Weekly or biweekly Daily Daily
Conjugated estrogen	Oral	0.3-1.25 mg	Daily
Ethinyl estradiol	Oral	0.01-0.03 mg	Daily
Estradiol acetate	Vaginal ring	0.05-0.10 mg	90 days
Estropipate	Oral	0.625-5 mg	Daily

Adapted from Duralde ER et al. BMJ, 2023; 382: e072612. © BMJ Publishing Group Ltd.[1]

Table 2. Commonly Prescribed Progestins Used in MHT

Type of progestin	Route	Dose	Frequency
Medroxyprogesterone acctate	Oral	2.5 mg 5 mg	Daily Days 1-12 cycled
Micronizable progesterone	Oral	100 mg 200 mg	Daily Days 1-12 cycled
Norethindrone	Oral	0.35-0.7 mg	Daily, cycled
Norethindrone acetate	Oral	0.5 mg	Daily, cycled

Adapted from Duralde ER et al. BMJ, 2023; 382: e072612. © BMJ Publishing Group Ltd.[1]

Table 3. Combinations of Estrogens and Progestins Used in MHT

Type	Route	Dose	Frequency
17β-Estradiol/NETA	Patch Oral	0.05-0.25 mg 0.5 + 0.1 mg	Twice weekly Daily
17β-Estradiol + levonorgestrel	Patch	0.045 + 0.015 mg	Weekly
CEE + MPA	Oral	0.45-0.625 mg 5 mg	Daily Days 1-12, cyclic
17β-Estradiol + norgestimate	Oral	1 mg + 0.09 mg	Cyclic
17β-Estradiol + micronized progesterone	Oral	0.5-1.0 mg +100 mg	Daily
17β-Estradiol + drospirenone	Oral	0.5-1.0 mg + 0.25-1.0mg	Daily
BZA +CE	Oral	2.5-5 mg + 0.5-1.0 mg	Daily

Abbreviations: BZA, bazedoxifene acetate; CE, conjugated estrogen; CEE, conjugated equine estrogen.

Adapted from Duralde ER et al. BMJ, 2023; 382: e072612. © BMJ Publishing Group Ltd.[1]

Take-home: there are many different types of estrogens and progestins, doses, and routes of administration. Recently there has been more use of topical estradiol rather than oral, which is related to steady state levels and avoiding the first-pass effects in the liver. Many prescribers are using micronizable progestin because of some concern regarding medroxyprogesterone's effects on other steroid receptors or effects on the breast and cardiovascular system. However, most data showing effectiveness to prevent endometrial hyperplasia or cancer are with medroxyprogesterone. Continuous progestin has been shown in a meta-analysis to increase breast cancer risk compared with risk associated with cyclic progestin or no progestin.[10] However, the convenience of having no cycles after up to a year of cycling is preferred by many women. Clinically, as the dosage of estrogen is tapered, the need for progestin withdrawal when using cyclic progestin is decreased and it can be used every month or every third month to ensure endometrial shedding. There are many new estrogens and progestins in the pipeline, but research is needed to determine whether they are as effective and safe as the options we use today.

Duration of Therapy

The current recommendations are to discuss MHT yearly and to trial dose tapering to control symptoms. The medications should be continued considering the patient's treatment goals and individual risk evaluation. Data support minimal risk in many women up to 5 years.[1] With longer use, transdermal and lower dosages are recommended. Although some studies have shown no difference in abrupt stopping and taper, many patients and providers use a taper strategy. Importantly, women with premature ovarian insufficiency may receive MHT at least to the time of natural menopause (age 51). The American College of Obstetricians and Gynecologists and the North American Menopause Society have recommended that in the small number of women who have vasomotor symptoms after age 65 years, shared decision-making should be implemented, discussing risk-benefit and using the lowest dosage to control symptoms.[1] Evaluation for other causes of symptoms is also important.

What About Alternatives to MHT?

Compounded Hormones

Many women seek alternatives if their provider is unwilling to prescribe MHT. The internet and social media claim that bioidentical hormones that are compounded are safer and more effective. Importantly, we have bioidentical compounds with oral and transdermal and vaginal estradiol and micronizable progestin that are FDA approved and tested. Many compounding pharmacies combine E1, E2, and E3 in creams or troches and various progestin formulations. There are scant data showing safety and efficacy of these products and studies have shown that often they do not contain the labeled dose and the pharmacology is not established. Thus, patients who desire bioidentical MHT should be reassured that it is available through FDA-approved options.

Herbals, Soy, and Supplements

Most recent meta-analyses do not show short- or long-term benefits of soy products.[11] When consumed in a diet, several kilograms of soy are needed to have an estrogenic effect. However, now that soy is available in powders, there may be potential estrogenic effects that have not been carefully evaluated and would need to be considered in a woman with vasomotor symptoms after breast cancer. All herbal preparations to date have not shown long-term beneficial effects in controlled studies.[11] Concern with alternatives is the potential of drug-drug interactions with other medications the patient has been taking. Practically, a provider can use lipids and bone biomarkers to acutely monitor a "supplement" that a patient is taking (personal observation).

Selective Estrogen Receptor Modulators

Tamoxifen is FDA approved for prevention of breast cancer. It worsens hot flashes, has somewhat positive effects on bone, and has adverse endometrial effects and increased risk of venous thromboembolism.[3] Raloxifene is FDA approved for prevention of breast cancer in women at high risk, and it lacks endometrial adverse effects. It has beneficial effects to prevent spinal but not hip fractures. It was not shown to have cardiovascular protection in randomized controlled trials. Again, it worsens hot flashes in early menopause and has the same venous thromboembolism and stroke risk as MHT.[3] Bazedoxifene in combination with conjugated estrogen has been shown to decrease vasomotor symptoms. It does not cause endometrial hyperplasia and has smaller effects on the skeleton, which are dependent on the estrogen dosage.[1] Ospemifene is a selective estrogen receptor modulator approved for treatment of vulvar and vaginal atrophy and dyspareunia.[1] Long-term studies are not available.

Testosterone

The most recent international guidelines recommend against the use of testosterone in postmenopausal women.[12,13] Studies to define the role of testosterone in women have been limited by the lack of a clear-cut "androgen deficiency syndrome" (ie, signs and symptoms associated with low testosterone levels that are improved with physiologic testosterone therapy. Androgens have been described to be associated with sexual function; however, female sexual dysfunction does not rise at menopause and symptoms and signs of hypoactive sexual desire disorder do not correlate with a specific testosterone concentration. Until recently, we were unable to accurately measure testosterone in children and postmenopausal women. Mass spectrometry measurements have shown a decline with age rather than hormonal status and then a rebound in levels with advancing age. Studies with a testosterone patch showed that high physiologic levels were effective in improving sexual health in the subset of women with hypoactive sexual desire disorder.[13] The patch was denied by the US FDA because of concerns regarding risk of breast cancer and cardiovascular disease. A testosterone gel product for women is available in Australia. The most recent international guidelines suggest if testosterone is to be tried off label in postmenopausal women for sexual dysfunction, it should be trialed for 3 to 6 months and discontinued if not effective. Patients should be monitored for overuse and signs of hyperandrogenism. Practitioners have used compounded preparations or off-label parts of testosterone gel packets approved for men. There is concern about pharmacologic dosing, which can affect male-pattern balding, hirsutism, adverse lipid profiles and unknown long-term effects. The guidelines reported that there are insufficient data to recommend testosterone for premenopausal women and that there are no beneficial effects of physiologic testosterone on cognition, well-being, depression, bone mineral density, fracture, or musculoskeletal strength.[12]

Injectable MHT

Many clinics in the United States and globally are administering pharmacologic levels of estrogen, progestin, and testosterone to premenopausal and postmenopausal women. The Endocrine

Society, North American Menopause Society and FDA caution against these practices because of unknown efficacy and potential risk.

Clinical Case Vignettes

Case 1

A 51-year-old woman presents to discuss pros and cons of MHT. Menarche was at age 12, and she is G2P2. Her last menstrual period was 12 months ago. Her main symptoms are dyspareunia, mood issues, and 7 to 8 hot flashes per day causing sleep disturbance. She is otherwise healthy. She has heard that MHT is dangerous.

On physical examination, her vital signs are normal. Her BMI is 31 kg/m^2, and she has no notable abnormalities on examination.

A history of which of the following would be a contraindication to MHT prescription in this patient?

A. Colon cancer

B. Osteoporosis

C. Deep venous thrombosis

D. Breast cancer

E. Hypertension

Answer: D) Breast cancer

Importantly, we consider treating symptomatic women with MHT at the time of menopause, and this patient is symptomatic. Breast cancer (Answer D) is a contraindication to MHT. Estrogen therapy of any kind is not recommended in women with a history of breast cancer. Standard therapy for estrogen-receptor positive breast cancer includes administration of a selective estrogen modulator or, more recently, an aromatase inhibitor to block estrogen action or production.

Colon cancer (Answer A) is not a contraindication to MHT. In the WHI combined estrogen/progestin arm, the incidence of colon cancer was lower in women who took MHT.[5]

Osteoporosis (Answer B) is not a contraindication; it could be an indication: both arms of the WHI proved that MHT prevented and treated osteoporosis.[5,9] However, there are many other drugs available to treat osteoporosis in women with contraindications to MHT.

A pulmonary embolus is a relative contraindication to MHT; however, if a patient is on long-term anticoagulation for a previous clotting event, MHT can be considered.[14] Similarly, depending on the cause and the resolution of a remote deep venous thrombosis (Answer C), MHT can be considered.

A history of high blood pressure (Answer E) is not a contraindication but should be controlled. However, a history of stroke or myocardial infarction are contraindications.

Liver dysfunction or disease is listed by some authors, but the risk profile with appropriate choice of MHT is unclear. Additional considerations are the possibility of pregnancy, which would be unusual in this patient, as the average age of menopause in developed countries is 51 to 52 years and she has experienced 12 months of amenorrhea. Additionally, any undiagnosed vaginal bleeding must be evaluated before considering therapy. Endometrial cancer is listed as a contraindication; however, if a patient is cured of the cancer (ie, low stage and appropriate therapy), there are not strong data to support risk from MHT.

Case 1 (continued)

What if the patient were 60 years old and symptomatic (11 years after the onset of menopause)? Should you consider prescribing MHT?

A. Yes

B. No

Answer: B) No

Most guidelines suggest the risk/benefit for MHT is exceeded when the patient is 10 years beyond menopause. Data from the WHI, in which most women recruited were more than 10 years out from menopause, showed that women who received conjugated estrogen and daily progestin had increased clotting and cardiovascular risk, as well as increased risk of breast cancer.[5] In the analysis of women aged 50 to 59 years, the benefits were greater and the risks were not significantly increased.[1,3] Data suggest that MHT should be given to symptomatic women at the time of menopause and can be safely administered for up to 5 to 10 years. Yearly visits are needed, and the dosage should be decreased accordingly to control symptoms and decrease risk. Few women continue to have vasomotor symptoms after 10 years, and a personalized approach is recommended outlining the pros and cons of MHT.[1]

Case 2

A 48-year-old menopausal woman with symptomatic vasomotor flushes presents to discuss MHT. She is otherwise healthy and has no family history of early breast cancer.

Which of the following regimens is the best recommendation?

A. Ethinyl estradiol, 35 mcg, and levonorgestrel, 1 mg daily

B. Levonorgestrel IUD and progesterone, 100 mg daily

C. Transdermal estradiol, 0.5 mg daily, and medroxyprogesterone, 5 mg days 1 to 12 monthly

D. Estradiol, 2 mg twice daily, and progesterone, 100 mg daily

E. Depot medroxyprogesterone acetate, 150 mg monthly

Answer: C) Transdermal estradiol, 0.5 mg daily, and medroxyprogesterone, 5 mg days 1 to 12 monthly

There are myriad choices for MHT available across the globe (*Tables 1, 2,* and *3*). Providers must ask: which regimen has the most efficacy and safety in preclinical and clinical studies and what are the patient preferences? In a patient with a uterus, a combination of some form of estrogen and either cyclic or daily progesterone or a progestin IUD is needed. Based on results of the WHI, which used a standard conjugated

estrogen, and results of some preclinical studies suggesting benefit from estradiol, many providers have increased the use of oral estradiol and now more frequently transdermal estradiol in patch or gel form. The dosages of estrogens have decreased since the WHI with conjugated estrogen, 0.45 mg, equivalent to 1 mg twice daily of oral estradiol and 0.5 mg of the biweekly or weekly estradiol patches. The transdermal route is suggested by most guidelines to avoid first-pass effects of oral estrogen on clotting factors.[1] The type of progestin and pattern of administration are being actively discussed. Most safety and efficacy data to prevent endometrial hyperplasia or cancer are with medroxyprogesterone. Medroxyprogesterone was given at a dosage of 5 mg daily in the WHI.[5] Because of concerns regarding breast cancer and cardiovascular disease risk, many propose the use of micronizable progesterone. Micronizable progesterone can be administered at 200 mg days 1 to 12 or at 100 mg daily with some irregular bleeding for 6 to 9 months, followed by amenorrhea. A recent meta-analysis of breast cancer risk with MHT suggests that risk increases with daily compared with intermittent progestin exposure.[10] Thus, I tend to prescribe cyclic progestin with low-dosage estradiol (Answer C). Bleeding is reliable and decreases with time as the dosage of estradiol is tapered. Any unexplained vaginal bleeding while using MHT must be evaluated.

Ethinyl estradiol, 35 mcg, and levonorgestrel, 1 mg daily (Answer A), are the ingredients in a standard combined oral contraceptive, which is not indicated for MHT.

Some have suggested that a progestin IUD may be used with transdermal estradiol to avoid oral progestin and bleeding. However, a levonorgestrel IUD would not be combined with micronized progesterone (Answer B).

Estradiol, 2 mg twice daily, with progesterone, 100 mg daily (Answer D), is an excessive estradiol dosage, and the progestin dosage would be inadequate to prevent breakthrough bleeding.

Depot medroxyprogesterone acetate (Answer E)) is a long-acting progestin used as a contraceptive and is not appropriate for MHT.

As an aside, there has been a rash of clinics offering injectable and pellets of estrogen, progestin, and testosterone to women. These are pharmacologic dosing and have unknown risks and are not recommended.

Case 2 (continued)

The patient now returns at age 53 years and wants to discuss when and how to stop MHT. Her current regimen consists of an estradiol patch, 0.037 mg biweekly, and intermittent progestin withdrawal every other month days 1 to 12, with light menses lasting 1 to 2 days. Her vasomotor symptoms are intermittent but less severe.

Which of the following is the best recommendation?

A. Stop MHT abruptly

B. Taper estradiol to 0.25 mg and continue with intermittent progestin for a month and then discontinue MHT

C. Increase estradiol to 0.5 mg and continue with intermittent progestin as she is still symptomatic

D. Continue MHT

E. Any of the above

Answer: E) Any of the above

The patient is currently 5 years past menopause. Her MHT has been tapered, and she is still symptomatic. Studies have not shown a dramatic difference in short- or long-term results on the pattern of MHT taper. Some would favor abrupt cessation (Answer A) if she were not symptomatic or desired to discontinue after discussing the risks and benefits. Many would favor a slower taper to the lowest dosage of estradiol and then discontinue (Answer B). Individual patient preference would guide decision-making, and if other signs of estrogen deficiency were noted on further questioning (eg, sleep disturbance, urinary frequency, mood disturbance), a short trial of a higher dose of estradiol (Answer C) or not stopping MHT (Answer D) could be considered. Thus, discussion with the patient is needed to individualize the length of MHT and the taper regimen.

Case 3

A 52-year-old woman who has been menopausal for 2 years presents with vasomotor symptoms. She does not want conventional MHT but has read extensively on the internet and would like to discuss the risks and benefits of yam progesterone, compounded bioidentical estrogens, and testosterone troches.

Which of the following statements best describes what we know about compounded hormone therapy?

A. Compounded hormone therapy has been tested to ensure equivalence to FDA-approved MHT products

B. Compounded hormone therapy has been tested for safety in human trials

C. Compounded hormone therapy is easier to use than conventional MHT

D. Compounded hormone therapy is recommended by most guidelines

E. Compounded hormone therapy is not recommended by the Endocrine Society

Answer: E) Compounded hormone therapy is not recommended by the Endocrine Society

The Endocrine Society, North American Menopause Society, and other societies recommend against compounded hormone preparations (Answer E). Whether in troches, gels, or creams, the pharmacology of delivery has not been adequately evaluated. The dose is often unreliable, and the efficacy and safety have not been studied to the extent required by the FDA or other national drug agencies globally.

Case 3 (continued)

Which of the following alternative therapies has shown benefit for symptoms of menopause?

A. Neurokinin B antagonists for vasomotor flushes in menopause

B. Yam progesterone for mood changes in menopause

C. Soy and isoflavones for sleep disruption in menopause

D. Testosterone for urinary frequency in menopause

E. DHEA for improved sexual function

Answer: A) Neurokinin B antagonists for vasomotor flushes in menopause

Many supplements and herbals have been trialed for hot flashes. Initial studies showed the benefit of selective serotonin reuptake inhibitors and serotonin-norepinephrine reuptake inhibitors to a modest effect about one-half that of MHT.[15] Over the last 10 years, researchers have discovered the control of vasomotor symptoms as related to changes in the KnDy neurons in the hypothalamus that produce kisspeptin, neurokinin B, and dynorphin.[16] With estrogen deficiency at menopause, there is an increase in the neurokinin B secretion, which affects temperature control and the vascular system to induce a hot flash. Researchers have developed neurokinin B antagonists to test in humans. Several have failed due to adverse effects, but fezolinetant is the first FDA-approved agent for vasomotor flushes and is being used for women with contraindications to MHT (Answer A).

Yam progesterone (Answer B) is a widely touted product without safety or efficacy data.

Soy and isoflavones (Answer C) have mild estrogenic effects. In the natural state, one would need to ingest more than 2 kg to detect an estrogenic action. However, with the production of potent soy powders, there may be some effects. This would be of concern with women with history of breast cancer. Meta-analyses show little effects of these products, and no long-term safety data are available.

Testosterone (Answer D) to treat sexual dysfunction has been studied extensively in pre- and postmenopausal women. Early studies were conducted with pharmacologic dosing and showed some anabolic effects. A detailed review of clinical trials with a testosterone patch showed that in women with hypoactive sexual desire disorder a high physiologic dose improved desire and satisfying sexual relations one/month. The latest international guidelines on the role of androgens in women recommend against the routine use of testosterone for women,[12] as does the Endocrine Society Clinical Guidelines on Androgens in Women.[13] There are currently no approved testosterone doses for women except in Australia. Some have suggested off-label testosterone for women with hypoactive sexual desire disorder, with monitoring for overuse and effectiveness for symptoms for 6 months.

DHEA (Answer E) is a prohormone that is converted to testosterone and then to estrogen. Extensive studies have been performed in healthy women and in those with adrenal insufficiency. The guidelines recommend against the use of DHEA in either population.[12,13]

Key Learning Points

- Understanding the real risks vs benefits of MHT is important for all endocrinologists.

- Low-dosage MHT is effective and safe for short-term management of the signs and symptoms of menopause.

- Optimizing the type and duration of MHT is easily understood and practiced.

- Many alternatives exist to manage symptoms of menopause. As practitioners, we need to know which ones are scientifically sound.

References

1. Duralde ER, Sobel TH, Manson JE. Management of perimenopausal and menopausal symptoms. *BMJ*. 2023;382:e072612. PMID: 37553173

2. Kling JM, MacLaughlin KL, Schnatz PF, et al. Menopause management knowledge in postgraduate family medicine, internal medicine, and obstetrics and gynecology residents: a cross-sectional survey. *Mayo Clin Proc*. 2019;94(2):242-253. PMID: 30711122

3. Manson JE, Kaunitz AM. Menopause management--getting clinical care back on track. *N Engl J Med*. 2016;374(9):803-806. PMID: 26962899

4. Stuenkel CA, Davis SR, Gompel A, et al. Treatment of symptoms of the menopause: an Endocrine Society clinical practice guideline. *J Clin Endocrinol Metab*. 2015;100(11):3975-4011. PMID: 26444994

5. Rossouw JE, Anderson GL, Prentice RL, et al; Writing Group for the Women's Health Initiative Investigators. Risks and benefits of estrogen plus progestin in healthy postmenopausal women: principal results from the Women's Health Initiative randomized controlled trial. *JAMA*. 2002;288(3):321-333. PMID: 12117397

6. Manson JE, Chlebowski RT, Stefanick ML, et al. Menopausal hormone therapy and health outcomes during the intervention and extended poststopping phases of the Women's Health Initiative randomized trials. *JAMA*. 2013;310(13):1353-1368. PMID: 24084921

7. Nickson C, Procopio P, Velentzis LS, et al. Prospective validation of the NCI Breast Cancer Risk Assessment Tool (Gail Model) on 40,000 Australian women. *Breast Cancer Res*. 2018;20(1):155. PMID: 30572910

8. Kurian AW, Hughes E, Simmons T, et al. Performance of the IBIS/Tyrer-Cuzick model of breast cancer risk by race and ethnicity in the Women's Health Initiative. *Cancer*. 2021;127(20):3742-3750. PMID: 34228814

9. Anderson GL, Limacher M, Assaf AR, et al; Women's Health Initiative Steering Committee. Effects of conjugated equine estrogen in postmenopausal women with hysterectomy: the Women's Health Initiative randomized controlled trial. *JAMA*. 2004;291:1701-1712. PMID: 15082697

10. Collaborative Group on Hormonal Factors in Breast Cancer. Type and timing of menopausal hormone therapy and breast cancer risk: individual participant meta-analysis of the worldwide epidemiological evidence. *Lancet*. 2019;394(10204):1159-1168. PMID: 31474332

11. Franco OH, Chowdhury R, Troup J, et al. Use of plant-based therapies and menopausal symptoms: a systematic review and meta-analysis. *JAMA*. 2016;315:2554-2563. PMID: 27327802

12. Davis SR, Baber R, Panay N, et al. Global consensus position statement on the use of testosterone therapy for women. *J Clin Endocrinol Metab*. 2019;104:4660-4666. PMID: 31498871

13. Wierman ME, Arlt W, Basson R, et al. Androgen therapy in women: a reappraisal: an Endocrine Society clinical practice guideline. *J Clin Endocrinol Metab*. 2014;99:3489-3510. PMID: 25279570

14. Morris G, Talaulikar V. Hormone replacement therapy in women with history of thrombosis or a thrombophilia. *Post Reprod Health*. 2023;29(1):33-41. PMID: 36573625

15. Shams T, Firwana B, Habib F, et al. SSRIs for hot flashes: a systematic review and meta-analysis of randomized trials. *J Gen Intern Med*. 2014;29(1):204-213. PMID: 23888328

16. St Onge E, Phillips B, Miller L. Fezolinetant: a new nonhormonal treatment for vasomotor symptoms. *J Pharm Technol*. 2023;39(6):291-297. PMID: 37974591

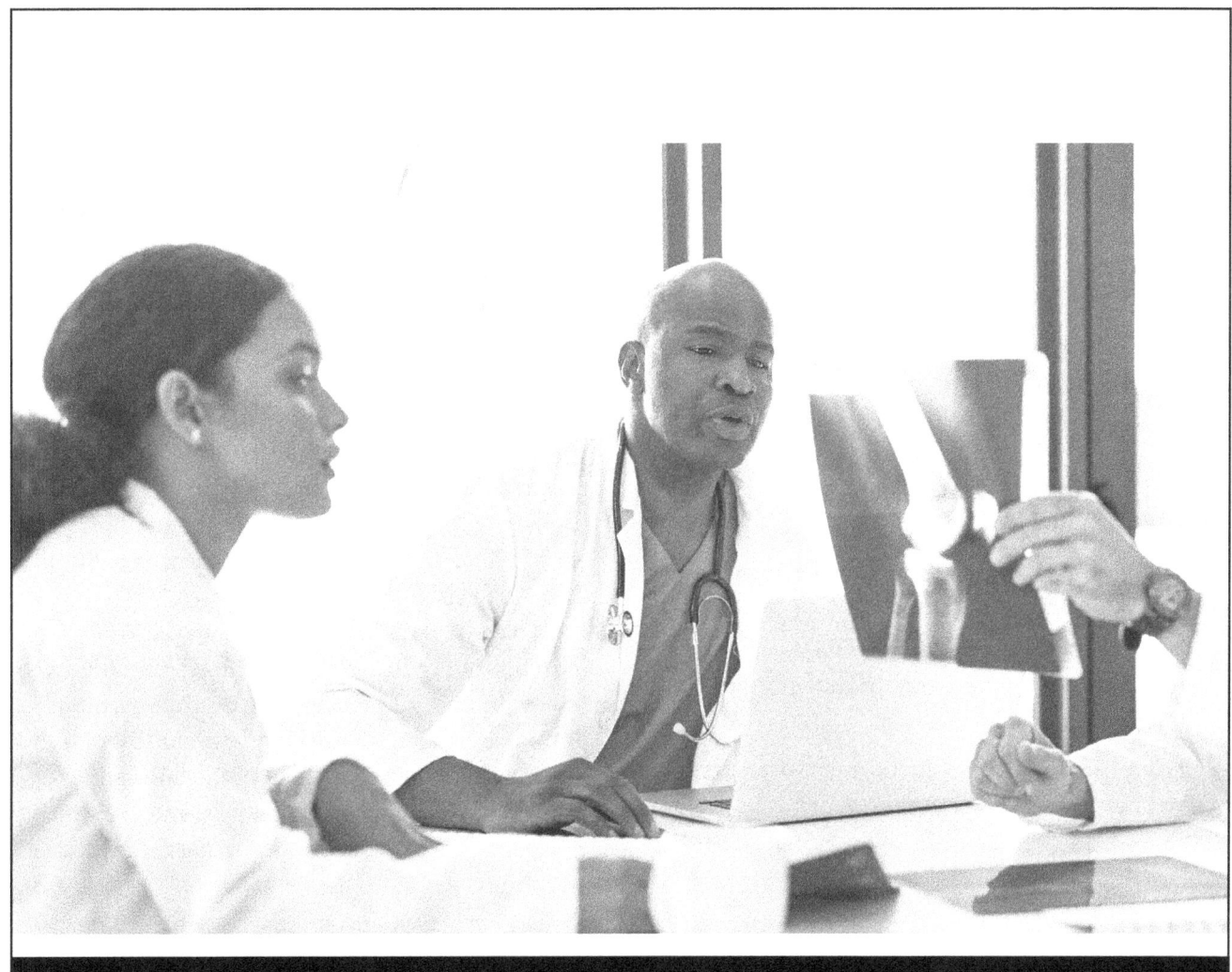

THYROID

Weird Thyroid Function Test Results

Trevor E. Angell, MD. Thyroid Center and Division of Endocrinology and Diabetes, Keck School of Medicine of USC, Los Angeles, CA; Email: Trevor.angell@med.usc.edu

Educational Objectives

After reviewing this chapter, learners should be able to:

- Explain which aspects of thyroid hormone physiology are assessed with different thyroid function tests (TFTs).

- Identify causes of discordant TFT results in the absence of underlying thyroid disease, including assay interference.

- Diagnose thyroid dysfunction that presents with unusual TFT patterns.

- Identify common patterns of discordant or unusual TFT results.

- Develop systematic approaches to manage patients with unusual TFT patterns.

Significance of the Clinical Problem

The assessment of thyroid function is among the most common evaluations performed by endocrinologists and primary care providers. Current assays for determining serum concentrations of TSH and peripheral thyroid hormones have been well developed and generally have a high degree of accuracy. Despite the frequency of thyroid evaluation, knowledge of thyroid physiology, and accuracy of testing, there are still numerous scenarios in which thyroid function tests may be confusing or difficult to interpret.

A strong understanding of thyroid testing is necessary to provide optimal patient care with respect to arriving at a correct diagnosis, excluding thyroid disease when it is not present, and selecting appropriate management. Doing so requires an understanding of the breath of potential thyroid conditions, recognizing limitations and pitfalls that exist in TFTs, and a systematic approach to "weird" TFT patterns when they arise.

To address the most relevant scenarios representing challenging TFT interpretations, we review important principles of thyroid hormone physiology, describe the most relevant thyroid function disorders to include in the differential diagnosis while interpreting TFTs, and explore case examples to broaden the learners' knowledge and ability.

Practice Gaps

- Distinguishing when anomalous TFTs do not represent underlying thyroid hormone abnormality can be challenging.

- Systematic approaches should be implemented to identify causes of anomalous TFT findings.

- Appropriate additional thyroid evaluation should be pursued when initial TFTs are "weird."

Discussion

Thyroid Physiology[1]

Fundamental aspects of thyroid hormone secretion, circulation, and metabolism are shown in the *Figure (following page)*. Most endocrinologists are familiar with the canonical endocrine feedback loop that predominantly governs thyroid function. To start at the hypothalamus, thyrotropin-releasing hormone stimulates TSH secretion from the anterior pituitary, which in turn signals the thyroid to increase thyroid hormone production. Under normal physiologic conditions, the thyroid produces predominantly T_4, with a small, but not negligible, amount of T_3. Free T_4 provides the strongest signal at the level of the pituitary to modulate TSH secretion, thereby completing the feedback loop.

In the circulation, T_4 is bound to thyroid-binding globulin (TBG), as well as albumin and other carrier proteins. Thyroid hormone acts on essentially every metabolically active cell in the body. Thyroid hormones cross the cell membrane through transporters such has MCT8, and can undergo further metabolism intracellularly. Intracellular conversion of T_4 to T_3 confers tight regulation on thyroid hormone action. Once trafficked to the nucleus, T_3 binds to thyroid hormone receptor, and along with transcription factors, induces expression of thyroid hormone–dependent genes.

Thyroid hormone is metabolized through modification by deiodinase enzymes. These enzymes are responsible for not only conversion of T_4 to T_3, which we commonly think of when considering thyroid hormone action and persistently symptomatic patients with hypothyroidism whom we see in the clinic, but they also convert thyroid hormones to other inactive metabolites, such as reverse T_3 and T_2. Other enzymes responsible for thyroid hormone disposal result in sulfation or glucuronidation of thyroid hormone.

Initial Assessment of Causes[1-5]

When confronted with abnormal TFT results of any variety, it is necessary to reflect on various causes. Patterns that are physiologically consistent and those that appear incongruous may result from true thyroid disorders, whether common or uncommon, or more esoteric etiologies, be they physiologic, iatrogenic, or spurious in nature. Key patterns of TSH, free T_4, and free T_3 and possible etiologies are summarized in the *Table 1 (following page)*.

Figure. Cartoon Schema of Thyroid Hormone Physiology

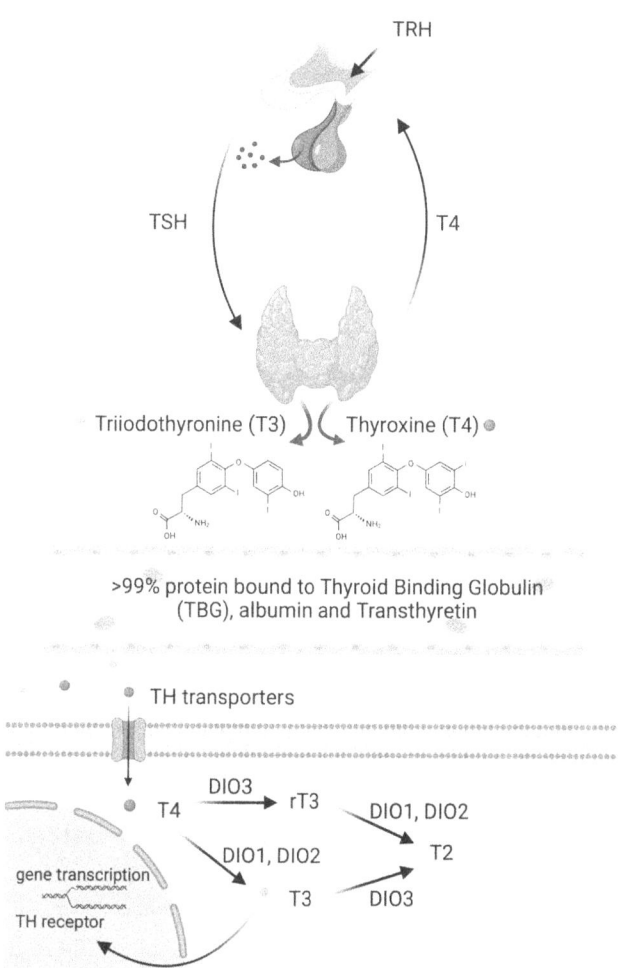

>99% protein bound to Thyroid Binding Globulin (TBG), albumin and Transthyretin

Abbreviations: DIO1, deiodinase type 1; DIO2, deiodinase type 2; DIO3, deiodinase type 3; TH, thyroid hormone; TSH, thyroid stimulating hormone; TRH, thyrotropin releasing hormone.

[Color—Print (Color Gallery page CG36) or web & ePub editions]

Identify Laboratory Assay Interference[6-8]

The possibility of spurious laboratory values should always be kept in mind, particularly for discordant TFT results, or when follow-up testing after initiation of management does not result in expected changes in TFT values.

Biotin (vitamin B_7) supplementation effects the results of TFT and has been much reported recently. Many current assays for TSH measurement involve a biotinylated monoclonal anti-TSH antibody that engages in biotin–streptavidin interaction to ultimately result in TSH detection. High concentrations of free biotin in

Table 1. TFT Patterns and Potential Etiologies

TFT			Causes
TSH	**Free T$_4$**	**Free T$_3$**	
↑ or ↔	↑	↑ or ↔	Central hyperthyroidism (TSHoma), RTH, meds (phenytoin, heparin), disorders of thyroid transport, Low adherence to LT$_4$ with recent administration (high TSH, normal free T$_3$)
↑	↔	↔	Subclinical hypothyroidism, inadequate TH replacement, recovery from NTI, RTH, obesity, advanced age
↑ or ↔	↔	↓	LT$_4$ treatment, NTI, physiologic (fasting, stress), assay inaccuracy (isolated low free T$_3$)
↑	↓	↓	Primary hypothyroidism,[a] iodine deficiency (often normal free T$_3$)
↔	↔	↓	LT$_4$ treatment, NTI, physiologic (fasting, stress), assay inaccuracy
↔	↓	↔	Exogenous T$_3$, treated T$_3$-toxicosis, late pregnancy
↔	↓	↓	Central hypothyroidism, NTI
↓	↑	↑ or ↔	Primary hyperthyroidism[b], LT$_4$ treatment (normal T$_3$), struma ovarii[c]
↓	↔	↔ or ↑	Subclinical hyperthyroidism, early pregnancy, NTI, meds (steroids, dopamine), T$_3$-toxicosis (high free T$_3$, and may include low FT$_4$)
↓	↓	↓ or ↔	Central hypothyroidism, treated hyperthyroidism

Abbreviations: NTI, nonthyroidal illness; TH, thyroid hormone; RTH, resistance to thyroid hormone; LT$_4$, levothyroxine.

[a] Causes of primary hypothyroidism: chronic lymphocytic thyroiditis (ie, Hashimoto thyroiditis), iodine deficiency, post thyroidectomy, post radiation (radioactive iodine or eternal beam therapy), infiltrative (amyloidosis, sarcoidosis, tuberculosis, chronic invasive fibrous thyroiditis), post thyroiditis (post partum, subacute, medication-induced).

[b] Causes of primary hyperthyroidism: Graves disease, autonomous nodularity (toxic nodule or toxic multinodular goiter), RTH, destructive thyroiditis, recent iodine exposure (including amiodarone, CT contrast).

[c] Low thyroid uptake but high ovarian uptake seen if radioiodine whole-body scan is used.

the serum at the time of measurement can disrupt this interaction, spuriously altering test results. For TSH, this spuriously lowers the value, but the direction of the inaccurate results depends on the type of assay used. Because this, biotin results in elevated free T$_4$ and free T$_3$. While typical dosages of over-the-counter biotin supplements, such as 1 mg, 5 mg, and 10 mg, are sufficient to result in values outside of the reference range, lab results consistent with severe hyperthyroidism have been observed in patients taking 100 mg daily or more of biotin, including undetectable TSH, high free T$_4$, and even positive TSH-receptor antibodies!

Interference causing high TSH is observed in the presence of HAMA (human antimouse antibodies), which bind antibody components of the TSH assay and result in a greater detection signal. This should be excluded during the evaluation of any patient for whom the diagnosis of central hyperthyroidism or resistance to thyroid hormone is being considered. Interference causing high TSH may also be due to "macro TSH," or antibodies to ruthenium-labeled test components.

Measurement of free T$_4$ or free T$_3$ can be affected by HAMA or antibodies against thyroid hormones themselves. Unfractionated heparin and low–molecular weight heparin can both cause an increase in measured free T$_4$ due to displacement of T$_4$ from TBG. T$_4$ is also displaced from TBG by loading doses of the antiseizure medication diphenylhydantoin. The most relevant causes of high or low total T$_4$ concentration are summarized in the *Table 2 (following page)*. Although abnormal binding of thyroid hormone to serum binding proteins typically does not affect free thyroid hormone levels, measurement of free T$_4$ or free T$_3$ can be falsely high when there is abnormal protein binding as seen in familial dysalbuminemic hyperthyroxinemia or transthyretin (transthyretin-associated hyperthyroxinemia).

Table 2. Causes of Abnormal Total Thyroid Hormone Concentrations

Hyperthyroxinemia	Hypothyroxinemia
TBG excess	**Reduced TBG**
Exogenous estrogen or pregnancy	Genetic TBG deficiency
Genetic TBG excess	Malnutrition
Active hepatitis C infection	Nephrotic syndrome
	Androgens
Increased binding	**Decreased TBG binding**
Mitotane	Salicylates
Methadone	Furosemide
Familial dysalbuminemic hyperthyroxinemia	Heparin
	Phenytoin

Abbreviation: TBG, thyroid-binding globulin.

Key Situations to Consider[1,3,6]

Patients Taking Thyroid Hormone Medications

Given the number of patients on levothyroxine replacement therapy, interpreting TFTs in treated patients is incredibly common. Although assessing TSH alone to guide dosage titration is straightforward in most cases, it can be useful to consider confusing results that occur in patients taking thyroid medication. In patients whose condition was previously stable on levothyroxine who present with abnormal TFT results, every step along the path of administration and metabolism should be considered. First, one should consider a prescription error or any change in the formulation, including from brand to generic or vice versa, or a change in generic manufacture with different bioequivalence. Second, one should determine whether the patient has been adherent to the regimen, or if there have been any intentional or unintentional gaps in therapy. Third, any issues with absorption should be identified, including the timing of food consumption, vitamins, other medications in relation to when thyroid medication is taken; reduction in gastric acid induced by proton-pump inhibitors or *Helicobacter pylori* infection; and intrinsic gastrointestinal conditions, such as celiac

disease. Finally, any change in metabolism that has possibly affected thyroid hormone availability should be identified (the most notable example being exogenous estrogen, which results in more T_4 and T_3 bound to TBG). Through a similar mechanism, pregnancy can result in TSH elevation in someone on a previously stable dosage of thyroid hormone replacement.

If free T_4 and/or free T_3 has been measured in a patient on thyroid medication, additional interpretation may be required. A high free T_4 value in the setting of normal TSH should not, in isolation, raise concern for overtreatment or the presence of another disorder. The distribution of levothyroxine for approximately 4 to 8 hours after administration causes serum levels to rise but is unlikely to have clinical significance. Free T_4 can be reassessed after the patient delays taking the medication until after testing on that day. When patients are taking proportionally more T_3 (eg, T_4-T_3 combination therapy, or natural desiccated thyroid preparations), low-normal or low free T_4 may be measured and free T_3 may be high, normal, or low because of the short serum half-life. Because free T_3 levels vary more widely and measurement is less accurate at the lower range, a slightly low free T_3 value in levothyroxine-treated patients cannot be used to assess adequacy of treatment or requirement for additional T_3 supplementation.

Lagging Behind

Patients with thyrotoxicosis that results in fully suppressed TSH may experience a lag in TSH rise when thyroid hormone levels return to the euthyroid range or even become low. This occurs in Graves hyperthyroidism after antithyroid drug treatment has been initiated or as a sequela of previous thyroiditis. The resulting TFT pattern can thus be low free T_4 and low free T_3 with concurrent low TSH. This does not represent pituitary pathology, nor is it permanent. In this clinical setting, evaluation of central hypothyroidism should be deferred and appropriate treatment initiated, either a decrease in the dosage of the antithyroid drug in Graves disease or possible initiation of levothyroxine in the post-thyroiditis setting. If only TSH is assessed, the true thyroid status may be missed, making it imperative to check both TSH and free T_4 in the initial phase of resolving hyperthyroidism.

Interpreting the "Other" TFTs

Checking the serum concentration of thyroid hormone by other methods or measuring other thyroid hormone metabolites is rarely indicated. Assessment of total T_4 may be used during pregnancy, with a reference range of 1.5 times that of the nonpregnant reference range used by the assay. In other circumstances, total thyroid hormone concentrations are less likely to reflect biologically relevant thyroid hormone status and may be high or low in a number of circumstances (*Table 1*).

Clinical Case Vignettes

Case 1

A 44-year-old woman presents for evaluation of abnormal TFTs. Her chief concerns are weight gain, fatigue, intermittent constipation, palpitations, and insomnia. She remembers a recent febrile illness with upper respiratory symptoms 1 to 2 months ago and does not recall any specific neck pain. She is not taking any prescription medications, but she does take over-the-counter vitamins. She has regular menses.

On physical examination, she is calm and appears well. Temperature is 97.9°F (36.6°C), pulse rate is 105 beats/min, and blood pressure is 125/76 mm Hg. Her weight is 194 lb (88 kg) (BMI = 34.4 kg/m²). Physical examination findings, including those from visual, orbital, cardiac, pulmonary, skin, and gastrointestinal evaluations, are normal. The thyroid gland is not palpable.

Laboratory test results:

> TSH = 0.03 mIU/L (0.4-4.0 mIU/L)
> Free T_4 = 0.67 ng/dL (0.8-1.6 ng/dL) (SI: 8.6 pmol/L [10.3-20.6 pmol/L])

Which of the following is the best next evaluation in this patient's workup?

A. Measure serum α-subunit level

B. Perform ^{123}I uptake and scan

C. Measure free T_3

D. Measure serum biotin

E. Perform MRI of the sella

Answer: C) Measure free T_3

This patient presents with low TSH and free T_4 concentrations. Her symptoms, some suggestive of hypothyroidism and others of hyperthyroidism, and physical examination findings are unrevealing. The preceding viral infection suggests possible thyroiditis, which has progressed to the hypothyroid phase with a "lagging" TSH response that is still low. Alternatively, a cause of excess T_3 may account for the biochemical findings. Therefore, measurement of free T_3 (Answer C) could be illuminating.

A radioiodine scan (Answer B) would not differentiate among several possible etiologies.

Measurement of serum biotin (Answer D) would not be a useful test to detect whether biotin interference is present, and the observed pattern of TSH and free T_4 would be less expected if it were related to the effects of biotin.

Central hypothyroidism (ie, TSH deficiency) certainly should be considered, but normal menses and the absence of other symptoms makes a sellar tumor causing hypopituitarism less likely. Sellar MRI (Answer E) to evaluate the pituitary would be warranted to exclude anatomic reasons for central hypothyroidism, but this has not yet been biochemically confirmed.

Measurement of α-subunit (Answer A) is used to evaluate potential excess TSH production (ie, TSHoma), rather than deficiency.

Case 1 (continued)

The patient returns after further TFTs:

> TSH = 0.07 mIU/L (0.4-4.0 mIU/L)
> Free T_4 = 0.56 ng/dL (0.8-1.6 ng/dL) (SI: 7.2 pmol/L [10.3-20.6 pmol/L])

Free T_3 = 7.5 pg/mL (2.3-4.2 pg/mL)
(SI: 11.5 pmol/L [3.5-6.5 pmol/L])

Which of the following is the best recommendation for this patient?

A. Perform thyroid ultrasonography

B. Perform ^{123}I uptake and scan

C. Measure TSH-receptor antibodies

D. Start methimazole therapy

E. Check for HAMA

Answer: B) Perform ^{123}I uptake and scan

Testing has now demonstrated the presence of an elevated free T_3 concentration, suggesting a state of excess T_3 leading to low TSH, but with low free T_4. This pattern, referred to as "T_3-toxicosis," can be found in autonomously functioning (ie, "toxic") nodules, occasionally in Graves disease, and with exposure to exogenous T_3. Therefore, a radioiodine uptake and scan (Answer B) would be useful to differentiate all of these etiologies from the others.

Thyroid ultrasonography (Answer A) may identify a nodule but would not yield functional information.

TSH-receptor antibody assessment (Answer C) would not distinguish between all 3 of the potential etiologies.

Initiation of an antithyroid drug (Answer D) would be premature now.

Interference by HAMA (Answer E) would be expected to raise, rather than lower, TSH.

Case 1 (continued)

The patient performs the addition requested evaluations. Iodine 123 diagnostic imaging show uptake of 1.1% at 4 hours (normal, 5%-15% at 4 hours) and 2.9% at 23 hours (normal, 10%-30% at 24 hours), with a diffuse homogeneous pattern.

Which of the following is the best next step?

A. Start prednisone

B. Start methimazole

C. Start iodine supplementation

D. Stop vitamins

E. Repeat TFTs in 3 months

Answer: D) Stop vitamins

The combination of T_3 toxicosis and low iodine uptake on radionucleotide testing suggests an exogenous source of T_3. Upon questioning, the patient's regimen included "vitamins" marketed for energy and weight loss. Some over-the-counter (or over-the-internet) products sold for these reasons contain thyroid hormones, which may not be included on the labeling. Other treatment for thyroiditis (Answer A), Graves disease (Answer B), or iodine deficiency (Answer C) would not address the cause of her thyroid hormone imbalance. Repeating TFTs (Answer E) without addressing the underlying cause would not be the best option.

Case 2

A 67-year-old man on levothyroxine replacement therapy presents for evaluation of difficult-to-treat hypothyroidism. He has a history of papillary thyroid carcinoma 20 years ago, treated with total thyroidectomy and radioactive iodine ablation. Thyroglobulin has been undetectable for many years and TSH has been maintained in the low-normal range for the past 5 years. During the past year, TSH has remained persistently elevated despite increasing his levothyroxine dosage. He is currently undergoing treatment for an advanced gastrointestinal stromal tumor.

He has experienced 6 months of fatigue, dry skin, cold intolerance, and constipation.

On physical examination, he appears tired and is in no acute distress. His temperature is 97.7°F (35.5°C), pulse rate is 55 beats/min, blood pressure is 132/89 mm Hg, and respiratory rate is 10 breaths/min. He has a well-healed thyroidectomy scar with no masses or other abnormalities in the neck. Cardiovascular examination documents sinus bradycardia. The skin is dry and slightly sallow. Deep tendon reflexes are delayed during the relaxation phase. No other abnormalities are noted.

Previous TFT results:

Assessment	TSH (0.4-4.0 mIU/L)	Free T$_4$ (0.8-1.6 ng/dL [SI, 10.3-20.6 pmol/L])	Levothyroxine dosage
1	23.4 mIU/L	0.81 ng/dL (SI: 10.4 pmol/L)	88 mcg daily
2	32.0 mIU/L	0.54 ng/dL (SI: 7.0 pmol/L)	100 mcg daily
3	55.3 mIU/L	0.33 ng/dL (SI: 4.2 pmol/L)	125 mcg daily
4	76.8 mIU/L	0.18 ng/dL (SI: 2.3 pmol/L)	175 mcg daily

Which of the following should be performed next?

A. Observed administration of oral levothyroxine, 1000 mcg, and recheck TSH and free T$_4$

B. Measure reverse T$_3$

C. Assess for heterophile antibody interference (ie, HAMA)

D. Administer intravenous levothyroxine, 175 mcg

E. Assess for tissue transglutaminase antibodies

Answer: B) Measure reverse T$_3$

This is an athyreotic patient on levothyroxine therapy who presents with refractory hypothyroidism despite greater than physiologic levothyroxine dosages. This is due to high expression of deiodinase type 3 (DIO3) by the gastrointestinal stromal tumor leading to inactivation of levothyroxine. A high reverse T$_3$ concentration (Answer B) would confirm this.

The patient is clinically hypothyroid but not in acute distress; therefore, urgent administration of levothyroxine (Answer D) is not necessary. Inability to absorb levothyroxine is another possible cause of refractory TSH elevation. In that scenario, free T$_4$ would also remain low, but the serum reverse T$_3$ concentration would be low rather than high. Observed administration of oral levothyroxine (Answer A) is not necessary.

Although celiac disease (Answer E) is common, there is no clinical suggestion of this condition.

Interference by heterophile antibodies, or HAMA (Answer C), can also cause persistent TSH elevation and result in unnecessary dosage escalations of levothyroxine. Free T$_4$ levels rise appropriately with dosage increases, and the patient would not be clinically hypothyroid, potentially even showing symptoms of excess thyroid hormone administration.

Case 2 (continued)

In addition to treating the gastrointestinal stromal tumor, which of the following would be the most effective intervention for this patient's hypothyroidism?

A. Double the levothyroxine dosage

B. Start a deiodinase inhibitor

C. Stop levothyroxine and start liothyronine

D. Change to levothyroxine gel capsules

Answer: C) Stop levothyroxine and start liothyronine

The treatment for "consumptive hypothyroidism," when T$_4$ is rapidly inactivated to reverse T$_3$, is treatment with T$_3$.[9,10] On liothyronine (Answer C), euthyroidism will be restored after dosage titration to normalize TSH. After discontinuation of levothyroxine, reverse T$_3$ rapidly declines. No effective type 3 deiodinase inhibitor (Answer B) is available and shown to be effective for treatment of this condition. The remaining options (Answers A and D) would not be effective.

Case 3

A 30-year-old woman is referred from primary care for evaluation of abnormal TFT results:

TSH = 2.4 mIU/L (0.4-4.0 mIU/L)
Free T$_4$ = 2.6 ng/dL (0.8-1.6 ng/dL) (SI: 33.5 pmol/L [10.3-20.6 pmol/L])

On physical evaluation, she has a palpable thyroid gland without detectable nodules. Examination findings are normal with the exception of elevated heart rate (105 beats/min) and a diffuse goiter approximately 2 to 3 times normal size.

She reports a history of situational anxiety and palpitations and describes a pressure-like sensation that affects her swallowing. She has no other medical problems.

Which of the following is the best initial assessment to perform?

A. Check for TSH assay interference

B. Measure TSH-receptor antibodies

C. Measure TPO antibodies

D. Perform MRI of the sella

E. Perform genetic testing for pathogenic variants in the thyroid hormone receptor gene

Answer: A) Check for TSH assay interference

The findings of high free T_4 with nonsuppressed TSH should be carefully assessed. Numerous uncommon and difficult-to-diagnosis conditions may be represented in this weird pattern of TFTs, including resistance to thyroid hormone, TSH-secreting pituitary adenoma (TSHoma), and assay interference. To avoid unnecessary testing, as well as unnecessary treatments such as surgery, a systematic approach to evaluation should be adopted. Early determinations should be performed to exclude the possibility of assay interference (Answer A). Testing for interference can be done by measuring TSH with serial dilutions of the patient sample or by directly measuring heterophile antibodies that falsely elevate TSH (in a patient who has primary hyperthyroidism). Measuring free T_4 by equilibrium dialysis can confirm a truly elevated concentration. The other answer choices would not be directly relevant to this evaluation (Answers B and C) or would be premature at this stage (Answers D and E).

Case 3 (continued)

After further testing, the patient returns for management recommendations. Tests for assay inaccuracy and free T_4 by equilibrium dialysis do not result in changes. She is not taking any medications that could alter TFT results. She has

had no recent illnesses. Upon further questioning, she recalls a family member who also had "thyroid problems," but she does not know the details.

Her α-subunit molar ratio is normal. Pituitary MRI shows no abnormalities. A trial of liothyronine administration results in a normal TSH response. After these tests, thyroid hormone receptor β gene analysis is performed, and a known pathologic variant is discovered.

Which of the following is the best recommendation for this patient?

A. No further treatment

B. Thyroidectomy

C. β-Adrenergic blocker and liothyronine

D. β-Adrenergic blocker

E. Hypophysectomy

Answer: C) β-Adrenergic blocker and liothyronine

Resistance to thyroid hormone (RTH) is a syndrome of impaired thyroid hormone sensitivity, usually caused by germline pathogenic variants in the thyroid hormone receptor gene that produce a thyroid hormone receptor with lower thyroid hormone affinity.[1,11] Pathogenic variants in the thyroid hormone receptor β gene (*THRB*) cause RTH-β and account for most cases of RTH, but up to 15% of persons with RTH do not have an identifiable thyroid hormone receptor pathogenic variant. Manifestations of RTH-β include goiter and tachycardia. As illustrated in this vignette, comprehensive testing and systematic exclusion of other causes should be performed (thus, Answer A is incorrect). Another possible study that could be performed is the thyrotropin-releasing hormone test, which can detect TSHoma via a blunted TSH response in 80% to 90% of cases.[12]

Treatment for thyrotoxic symptoms with a β-adrenergic blocker can palliate symptoms, and administration of liothyronine can reduce TSH and reduce goiter size (Answer C), both of which are problems for this patient. Although some tissues, such as the pituitary, experience relative hypothyroidism, higher dosages of levothyroxine can worsen sinus tachycardia due to preserved thyroid hormone sensitivity in THRα-expressing cardiac tissue. A β-adrenergic blocker alone (Answer D) is not unreasonable management, but additional therapy to address the symptomatic goiter would be ideal. Surgical treatments (Answers B and E) are not necessary. Thyroidectomy would address the goiter but has unfavorable risks of complications.

Key Learning Points

- A careful approach to incongruous (aka, "weird") TFT patterns should be used to avoid an incorrect diagnosis.

- An incongruous nonsuppressed TSH value demands a systematic workup to correctly differentiate real thyroid conditions and spurious findings.

- A low TSH value with discordant TFT values or without a compatible clinical presentation should be assessed further to detect other etiologies before typical hyperthyroidism is assumed.

References

1. Braverman LE Cooper DS Werner SC Ingbar SH. *Werner & Ingbar's the Thyroid: A Fundamental and Clinical Text.* 10th ed. Wolters Kluwer/Lippincott Williams & Wilkins; 2013.

2. Gurnell M, Halsall DJ, Chatterjee VK. What should be done when thyroid function tests do not make sense. *Clin Endocrinol (Oxf).* 2011;74(6):673-678. PMID: 21521292

3. Praw SS, Brent GA. Approach to the patient with a suppressed TSH. *J Clin Endocrinol Metab.* 2023;108(2):472-482. PMID: 36329632

4. Knudsen N, Laurberg P, Rasmussen LB, et al. Small differences in thyroid function may be important for body mass index and the occurrence of obesity in the population. *J Clin Endocrinol Metab.* 2005;90(7):4019-4024. PMID: 15870128

5. Surks MI, Hollowell JG. Age-specific distribution of serum thyrotropin and antithyroid antibodies in the US population: implications for the prevalence of subclinical hypothyroidism. *J Clin Endocrinol Metab.* 2007;92(12):4575-4582. PMID: 17911171

6. Van Uytfanghe K, Ehrenkranz J, et al. Thyroid stimulating hormone and thyroid hormones (triiodothyronine and thyroxine): an American Thyroid Association-commissioned review of current clinical and laboratory status. *Thyroid.* 2023;33(9):1013-1028. PMID: 37655789

7. Minkovsky A, Lee MN, Dowlatshahi M, et al. High-dose biotin treatment for secondary progressive multiple sclerosis may interfere with thyroid assays. *AACE Clin Case Rep.* 2016;2(4):e370-e373. PMID: 27917400

8. Favresse J, Burlacu MC, Maiter D, Gruson D. Interferences with thyroid function immunoassays: clinical implications and detection algorithm. *Endocr Rev.* 2018;39(5):830-850. PMID: 29982406

9. Maynard MA, Marino-Enriquez A, Fletcher JA, et al. Thyroid hormone inactivation in gastrointestinal stromal tumors. *N Engl J Med.* 2014;370(14):1327-1334. PMID: 24693892

10. Huang SA, Tu HM, Harney JW, et al. Severe hypothyroidism caused by type 3 iodothyronine deiodinase in infantile hemangiomas. *N Engl J Med.* 2000;343(3):185-189. PMID: 10900278

11. Ortiga-Carvalho TM, Sidhaye AR, Wondisford FE. Thyroid hormone receptors and resistance to thyroid hormone disorders. *Nat Rev Endocrinol.* 2014;10(10):582-591. PMID: 25135573

12. Beck-Peccoz P, Persani L, Mannavola D, Campi I. Pituitary tumours: TSH-secreting adenomas. *Best Pract Res Clin Endocrinol Metab.* 2009;23(5):597-606. PMID: 19945025

Challenging Thyroid Nodules

Amanda La Greca, MD. Division of Endocrinology, Metabolism, and Diabetes, University of Colorado School of Medicine, Aurora, CO; Email: amanda.lagreca@cuanschutz.edu

Sarah E. Mayson, MD. Division of Endocrinology, Metabolism, and Diabetes, University of Colorado School of Medicine, Aurora, CO; Email: sarah.mayson@cuanschutz.edu

Educational Objectives

After reviewing this chapter, learners should be able to:

- Recognize common and uncommon thyroid nodule presentations.

- Evaluate the strengths and limitations of thyroid nodule sonographic risk stratification systems (RSSs).

- Identify pitfalls in the cytologic diagnosis of medullary thyroid carcinoma (MTC).

- Determine when it is appropriate to consider molecular testing in the evaluation of thyroid nodules with indeterminate cytopathologic results.

Significance of the Clinical Problem

Thyroid nodules can be detected on neck ultrasonography in approximately 40% of adults. Most thyroid nodules are benign, either hyperplastic nodules, inflammatory lesions, or cysts, while a small percentage are of nonthyroidal origin (eg, parathyroid adenoma) and 5% to 10% are malignant. Although the clinical evaluation of a thyroid nodule is typically straightforward, unusual thyroid nodule presentations may occur, and the interpretation of findings on imaging, pathology, and molecular testing can be complex. Given the high prevalence of thyroid nodules in the adult population, all endocrinologists and collaborating specialists must be armed with the knowledge and skills to contend with "challenging" thyroid nodules in clinical practice.

Practice Gaps

- Several different thyroid nodule sonographic RSSs are currently in use in clinical practice, each with their own strengths and limitations.

- Molecular testing has become an important tool in the evaluation of thyroid nodules with indeterminate cytopathology; however, there is still much to learn regarding the prognostic and therapeutic consequences of such testing.

Discussion

The initial evaluation of a thyroid nodule begins with the history and physical examination, measuring serum TSH, and performing ultrasonography of the thyroid gland and cervical lymph nodes. A low serum TSH value may indicate the presence of an autonomously functioning (toxic) thyroid nodule and should prompt thyroid scintigraphy (preferably with ^{123}I or ^{131}I). In general, FNA is not recommended for a thyroid nodule confirmed to be autonomously functioning on scintigraphy in a hyperthyroid patient. Historically, the malignancy rate for autonomously functioning thyroid nodules has been quoted to be less than 1%. Although the rate of malignancy is lower for autonomously functioning thyroid nodules than for nonfunctioning nodules, the true incidence of malignancy in toxic nodules is uncertain, as no high-quality prospective study has been conducted. Retrospective surgical series of autonomously functioning thyroid nodules have reported malignancy rates of up to 10% to 34%, but such studies are limited by selection bias.[1] Autonomously functioning follicular, papillary, and oncocytic carcinomas of the thyroid have all been reported. Autonomously functioning thyroid nodules demonstrating suspicious clinical and/or ultrasonographic findings should prompt further diagnostic testing to exclude thyroid malignancy.

The management of a nonfunctioning thyroid nodule is largely dictated by the ultrasonographic findings, while taking into account a patient's risk factors for thyroid cancer, personal preferences, and potential clinical manifestations (eg, compressive symptoms). The 5 categories of ultrasonographic findings that should be determined for all thyroid nodules are (1) composition (cystic, solid, or mixed); (2) echogenicity; (3) shape (measured in the transverse plane); (4) margins; and (5) the presence of echogenic foci. All of the current thyroid nodule sonographic RSSs, including those from the American Thyroid Association (ATA) and the American College of Radiology (ACR), incorporate these same grayscale findings.[2,3]

The ACR's Thyroid Imaging Reporting and Data System (TI-RADS) was designed to be used in the evaluation of incidentally noted thyroid nodules. A point value is assigned for each sonographic feature, and the points from each of the 5 categories are tallied to yield an overall TI-RADS score for the nodule.[3] Unlike the ATA's system, TI-RADS does not incorporate patient clinical risk factors into its recommendations for FNA or ultrasound follow-up. In addition, TI-RADS is not applicable to the follow-up of thyroid nodules that have previously been biopsied. The ATA's RSS is qualitative; it was developed based on the concept that certain constellations of grayscale features tend to occur together (to yield distinct sonographic patterns) in benign vs malignant thyroid nodules.[2] However, approximately 8% of thyroid nodules cannot be classified into any of the specified sonographic patterns using the ATA's 2015 system.[4] The updated ATA RSS, which is expected to be published some time in 2024, plans to address this gap.

The assigned ATA sonographic pattern or overall TI-RADS score can help to predict a thyroid nodule's risk of malignancy and guide patient management decisions, including FNA. It is important to note that these sonographic RSSs propose different thresholds for FNA, which influences their diagnostic accuracy and the number of thyroid nodules that are ultimately recommended for biopsy.

With the goal of optimizing diagnostic yield, thyroid nodule FNA should always be performed under ultrasound guidance and should incorporate rapid on-site evaluation of cytology specimens, when available. The Bethesda System for Reporting Thyroid Cytopathology (TBSRTC) is the standard reporting system for thyroid cytopathology in the United States. This system was first proposed in 2007 and was most recently updated in 2023.[5] The TBSRTC has 6 reporting categories in total, including 3 for indeterminate cytology: atypia of undetermined significance (AUS), follicular neoplasm (FN), and suspicious for malignancy. Molecular diagnostic testing can be used to further risk stratify thyroid nodules with indeterminate cytopathology. When negative, molecular tests (eg, Afirma Genomic Sequencing Classifier [GSC], ThyGeNEXT/ThyraMIR, and ThyroSeq Genomic Classifier v3) can help to identify thyroid nodules that are likely benign, allowing them to be triaged to clinical rather than operative management. However, it is important to recognize that the negative predictive value and positive predictive value of any clinical diagnostic test are affected by disease prevalence. The likelihood that a thyroid nodule with indeterminate cytopathology is malignant may also be influenced by the patient's clinical risk factors, the specific TBSRTC reporting category, and findings on ultrasonography or other diagnostic testing (eg, elevated uptake on ^{18}F-fluorodeoxyglucose PET-CT). A prospective cohort study of 375 thyroid nodules with Bethesda III/IV cytopathology subclassified them based on sonographic characteristics as either ATA high-suspicion pattern or ATA intermediate/low-suspicion pattern.[6] For the ATA high-suspicion

subgroup, the malignancy rate was 78% to 80% based on sonographic and cytopathologic findings alone and was not significantly affected by the results of molecular diagnostic testing, whether positive or negative. In contrast, the molecular test results significantly modified the risk of malignancy within the ATA low/intermediate-suspicion subgroup. The malignancy rate was 21% to 24% overall, 56% to 67% if the molecular results were positive, and 2.1% to 3.8% if the results were negative. This study nicely demonstrates how sonographic findings can influence the clinical utility of molecular testing. When clinical or radiographic findings suggest a high risk of thyroid malignancy in the context of indeterminate cytopathologic results, definitive management with surgery is generally recommended.

Molecular testing may also reveal specific genetic alterations that are associated with more aggressive tumor behavior, while the prognostic and therapeutic implications of other findings on molecular testing remain uncertain. Pathogenic variants in the telomerase reverse transcriptase (*TERT*) promoter are associated with both distant metastases and decreased survival in papillary thyroid carcinoma (PTC), especially when coexistent with a second pathogenic variant in *RAS* or *BRAF* V600E. Pathogenic variants in *TERT* are also associated with decreased survival in follicular thyroid carcinoma (FTC) and have been proposed as a criterion to modify the decision for completion thyroidectomy in both minimally invasive and encapsulated angioinvasive FTC.[7] Although *TERT* variants have been reported in both minimally invasive and aggressive oncocytic carcinoma of the thyroid (OCA), further research is needed to understand the clinical implications of these genetic findings in OCA. Fortunately, only approximately 5% of thyroid nodules with indeterminate cytopathologic findings harbor *TERT* promoter variants.

Clinical Case Vignettes

Case 1

A 70-year-old man with a recent diagnosis of Parkinson disease presents for evaluation of a 4.5-cm right thyroid nodule. The patient reports no history of radiation exposure or family history of thyroid cancer. He describes intermittent dysphagia with both solids and liquids, which has been attributed to Parkinson disease. Barium esophagography showed no extrinsic compression of the esophagus. He has no dysphonia, cough, or shortness of breath. Examination of the patient's neck is notable for a 4-cm firm nodule in the right thyroid lobe without clinical evidence of substernal extension. There is no adenopathy. His serum TSH concentration is 2.0 mIU/L.

Neck ultrasonography demonstrates a right 4.4 × 4.1 × 3.5-cm thyroid nodule (*Figure 1*). There are no contralateral thyroid nodules or suspicious lymph nodes in the central or bilateral lateral neck.

Figure 1. Ultrasound Image of the Right Thyroid Nodule

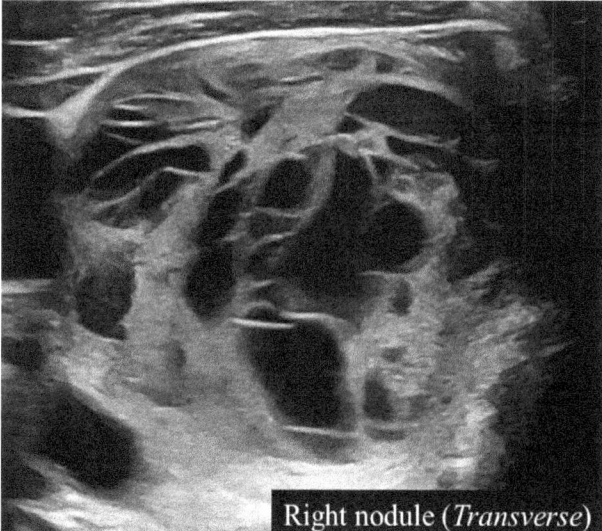

Right nodule (*Transverse*)

Which of the following is the best next step in the evaluation of this patient's thyroid nodule?

A. Counsel the patient that neither FNA nor follow-up ultrasonography is needed

B. Repeat neck ultrasonography in 2 years

C. Refer for ultrasound-guided FNA

D. Refer for right hemithyroidectomy

E. Review cine images provided by the radiology technician

Answer: E) Review cine images provided by the radiology technician

Review of cine images provided by the radiology technician demonstrates the findings shown in *Figure 2*.

Figure 2. Additional Ultrasound Images of Right Thyroid Nodule

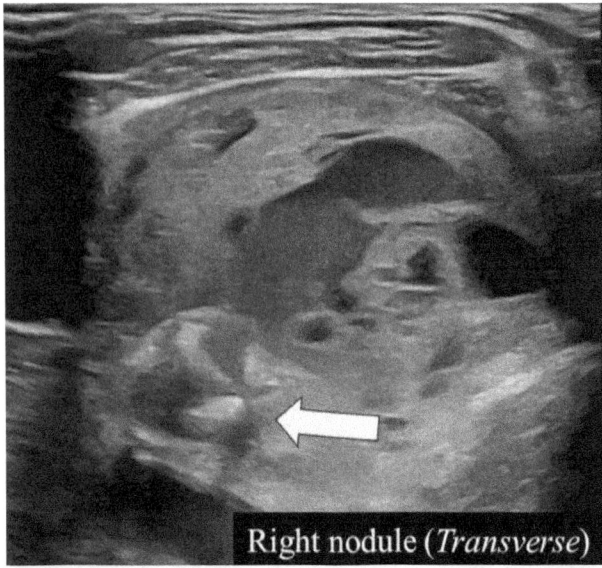

Right nodule (*Transverse*)

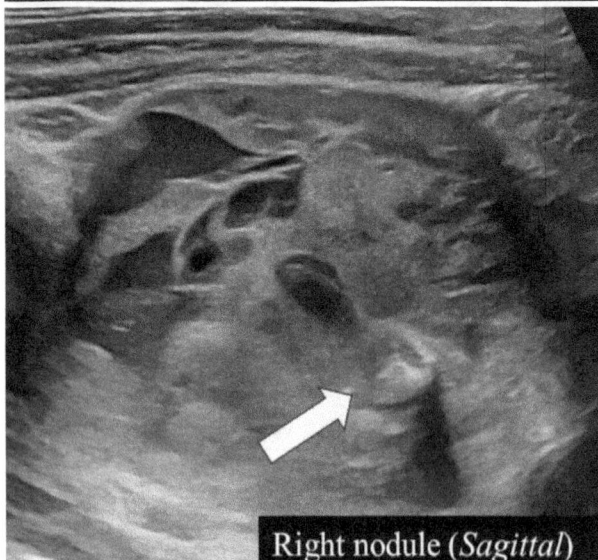

Right nodule (*Sagittal*)

Yellow arrows indicate macrocalcifications inferiorly and posteriorly within the nodule.

[Color—Print (Color Gallery page CG37) or web & ePub editions]

Case 1 (continued)

Ultrasound-guided FNA of the right thyroid is subsequently performed, yielding cytologic specimens that are deemed adequate for diagnosis. The cytologic findings are interpreted as AUS (Bethesda III) due to the sample being moderately cellular and composed almost exclusively of oncocytic cells (*Figure 3*). No microfollicles, nuclear crowding, or other architectural atypia is seen. No nuclear atypia is noted.

Figure 3. Cytologic Specimen Composed of Oncocytic Cells Forming Macrofollicular Groups

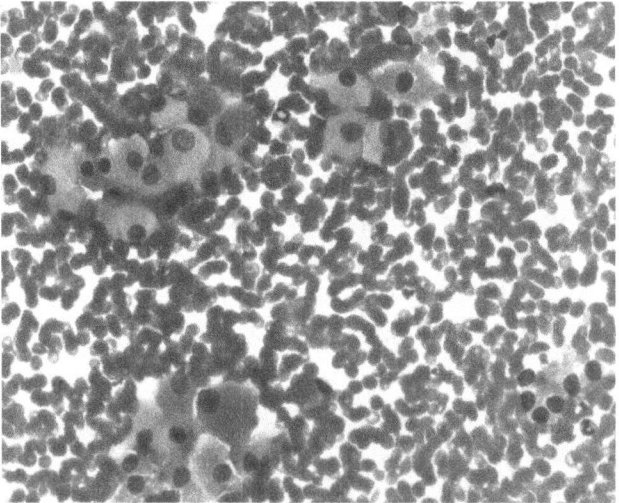

[Color—Print (Color Gallery page CG37) or web & ePub editions]

Which of the following is the most appropriate next step in this patient's management?

A. Measure serum TPO antibodies

B. Send FNA specimen for molecular analysis

C. Repeat neck ultrasonography in 12 months

D. Refer for right hemithyroidectomy

E. Refer for total thyroidectomy

Answer: B) Send FNA specimen for molecular analysis

The first step in the evaluation of a thyroid nodule using the ACR TI-RADS RSS is to determine its composition. At first glance, the nodule shown in Case 1 may appear to be spongiform. Spongiform composition means that at least 50% of a nodule's volume is composed of microcystic areas. This definition can be expanded to include nodules with larger cystic spaces if the interposed solid areas are all microcystic. However, the nodule in Case 1 does not fulfill these criteria and is more accurately classified as mixed cystic and solid (1 point) and isoechoic (1 point). Based on review of only the static ultrasound image that was provided initially, this nodule would be assigned no additional points and would be scored as TI-RADS 2, and neither FNA nor ultrasound follow-up would be indicated per ACR TI-RADS.

One goal of this case, however, was to demonstrate a shortcoming of static ultrasound images: they do not always tell the whole story. On review of the cine images (ie, video clip) taken by the radiology technician as a part of the same ultrasound exam, this nodule was noted to contain macrocalcifications at its inferior posterior aspect (*Figure 2*). The published literature on macrocalcifications is somewhat limited by heterogeneity and because most studies do not evaluate macrocalcifications as an independent variable. However, a recent large series of 3603 consecutive nodules 1 cm or larger demonstrated that macrocalcifications were an independent predictor of malignancy across different nodule compositions, including subgroups of partially cystic nodules.[8] The presence of macrocalcifications can thus be said to modestly elevate malignancy risk when documented in either solid or partially cystic nodules. If another point is awarded to this nodule for macrocalcifications, it would be classified overall as TI-RADS 3 (3 total points), and ultrasound-guided FNA would be recommended (FNA if ≥2.5 cm). It is important to note that application of the ATA's 2015 sonographic RSS would yield a "nonclassifiable" result for this nodule.

The second part of Case 1 is focused on the management of thyroid nodules with indeterminate cytopathology. Based on the results of this patient's evaluation leading up to the second question, there is no strong indication for diagnostic surgery (no compressive symptoms, clinical risk factors for malignancy, or high-suspicion ultrasound findings). Preferred next steps in this patient's management include repeating the FNA for cytologic evaluation (not a given answer choice) and/or proceeding with molecular testing. As previously mentioned, when the cytopathologic results are indeterminate (AUS or FN) and the findings on ultrasonography are low to intermediate risk, molecular testing may be used to further refine the risk of malignancy. Molecular testing in Case 1 demonstrated both a pathogenic variant in the *TERT* promoter and genome haploidization-type chromosomal copy number alterations (CNAs). Together, these findings indicate a high (~80%) risk of malignancy. A series of 111 thyroid nodules with CNAs on molecular testing found that among nodules demonstrating the genome haploidization-type CNAs that are characteristic of oncocytic tumors, the probability of malignancy increased by 1.9 for every centimeter increase in size.[9] The authors performed a separate analysis of 58 resected oncocytic thyroid nodules and found that the co-occurrence of chromosomal CNAs with a second pathogenic variant was documented only in the malignant nodules. Given the high risk of malignancy based on the molecular findings and the large nodule size (>4 cm), this patient chose to undergo total thyroidectomy for definitive diagnosis and management. His surgical pathology ultimately demonstrated a minimally invasive OCA without angioinvasion, and postoperative serum thyroglobulin measured 0.1 ng/mL with negative thyroglobulin antibodies.

Case 2

A 90-year-old woman was first diagnosed with a toxic multinodular goiter at age 73 years. She was treated with 29 mCI of ^{131}I the same year as her diagnosis. Thereafter, she remained euthyroid for 18 years, but was subsequently diagnosed with recurrent hyperthyroidism with the following laboratory test results:

TSH = <0.01 mIU/L (0.45-5.33 mIU/L)
Free T$_4$ = 2.07 ng/dL (0.89-1.76 ng/dL)
(SI: 26.6 pmol/L [11.5-22.6 pmol/L])
Total T$_3$ = 245 ng/dL (60-181 ng/dL) (SI: 3.8 nmol/L
[0.9-2.8 nmol/L])

Physical examination reveals a firm and fixed 2- to 3-cm left thyroid nodule, with no palpable cervical lymphadenopathy. She has no dysphonia, dysphagia, cough, or shortness of breath.

Given her remote history of toxic multinodular goiter treated with radioiodine and the recent thyroid function tests demonstrating hyperthyroidism, thyroid scintigraphy is performed. This reveals heterogeneous uptake in a hyperfunctioning left thyroid nodule with suppression of the contralateral lobe (*Figure 4*).

Neck ultrasonography is also performed, which demonstrates a left thyroid nodule (*Figure 5*).

In addition to initiation of a β-adrenergic blocker, which of the following is the best next step in the evaluation of this patient's thyroid nodule?

A. Monitor thyroid function tests periodically

B. Repeat neck ultrasonography in 1 year

C. Refer for ultrasound-guided FNA biopsy

D. Refer for radioiodine therapy

E. Refer for radiofrequency ablation

Answer: C) Refer for ultrasound-guided FNA biopsy

Ultrasound-guided FNA of the left thyroid nodule is subsequently performed, yielding cytologic specimens that are deemed adequate for diagnosis. The cytologic findings are interpreted as AUS. In a few of the slides, background colloid is abundant. In other slides, the sample is predominantly blood, representing the vascularity of this lesion. The

Figure 4. Thyroid Scintigraphy

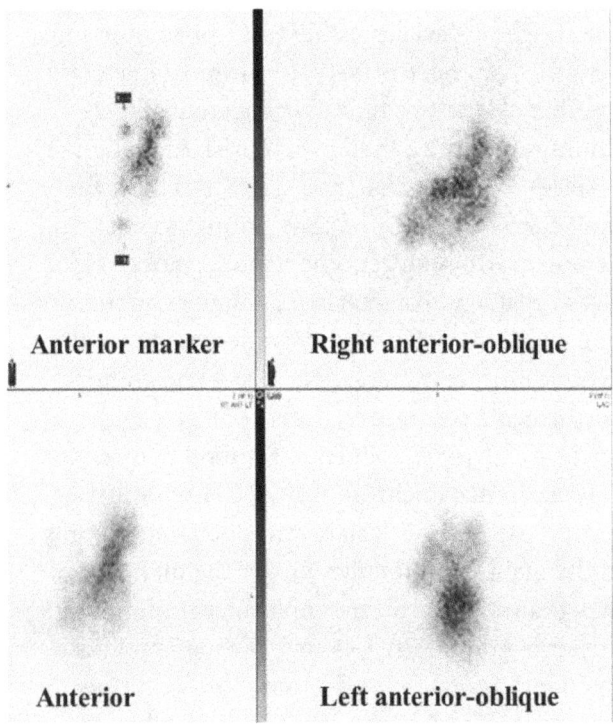

Anterior marker   Right anterior-oblique

Anterior   Left anterior-oblique

Figure 5. Ultrasound Image of the Left Thyroid Nodule

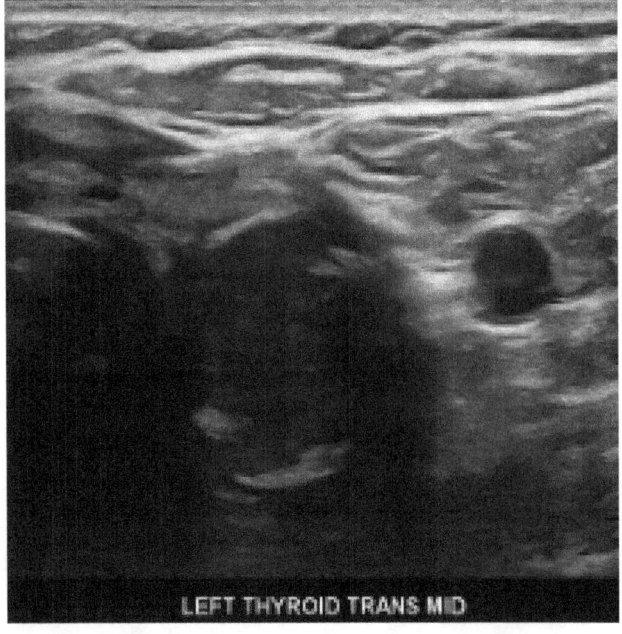

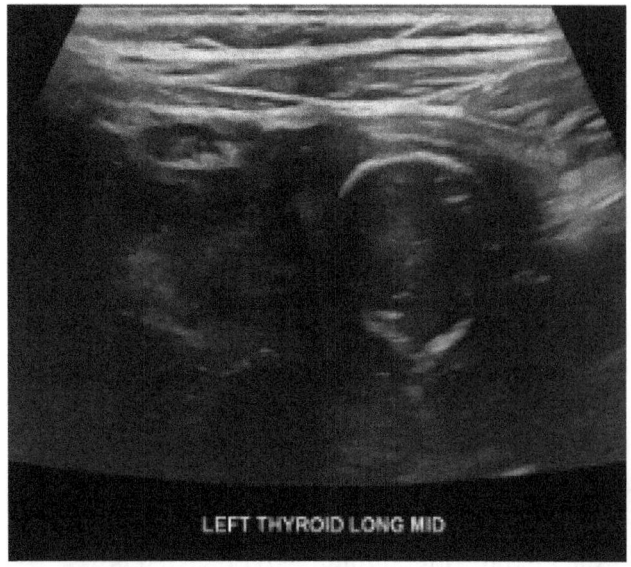

hypercellularity and the monotony of the follicular cells are concerning for a population of atypical follicular cells. No cytologic features of PTC are identified. A sample is sent for molecular testing (ThyroSeq v3). Results are "negative," indicating a low (<3%) probability of cancer.

Given the negative molecular test results and the patient's preference for a less-invasive management approach, treatment of hyperthyroidism is initiated with methimazole, and she is recommended to complete repeat neck ultrasonography in 1 year.

Repeated neck ultrasonography 1 year later demonstrates both a slight enlargement of the left thyroid nodule and a 1 × 0.7 × 1.8-cm, isoechoic, soft-tissue nodule along the left internal jugular vein in level 3, consistent with tumor invasion into vein (tumor thrombus) (*Figure 6*).

As detailed in this chapter, the initial evaluation of a thyroid nodule begins with the history and physical exam, measuring serum TSH, and performing ultrasonography of the thyroid gland and cervical lymph nodes. In Case 2, thyroid scintigraphy was first ordered to evaluate the patient's hyperthyroidism. Although the left thyroid nodule was found to be autonomously functioning and would be expected to have a low risk of malignancy, the patient's clinical findings (hard, fixed thyroid nodule) and the nodule's highly suspicious sonographic appearance (hypoechoic solid mass in the left thyroid lobe with infiltrative margins and macrocalcifications) prompted further evaluation with ultrasound-guided FNA.

The second part of Case 2 is focused on the management of thyroid nodules with indeterminate cytology and highly suspicious sonographic findings. A retrospective study evaluating the 2015 ATA and ACR TI-RADS RSSs found that thyroid nodules classified as ATA high-suspicion pattern or TI-RADS 5 had a 100% rate of malignancy for Bethesda III cytology, and malignancy rates of 67% and 50%, respectively, for Bethesda IV cytology.[10] As mentioned previously, negative molecular testing has an insufficient negative predictive value to rule out malignancy in nodules with indeterminate cytology and highly suspicious sonographic findings. However,

Figure 6. Ultrasound Image Showing Tumor Thrombus in the Left Internal Jugular Vein

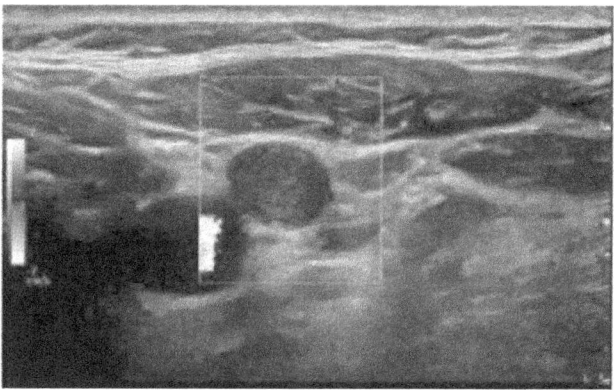

Left neck zone III trans

[Color—Print (Color Gallery page CG38) or web & ePub editions]

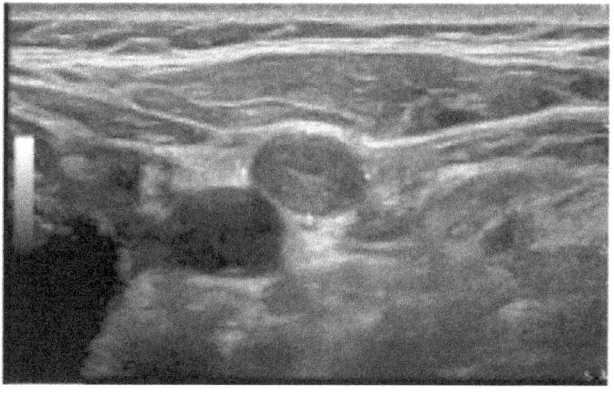

Left neck zone III trans

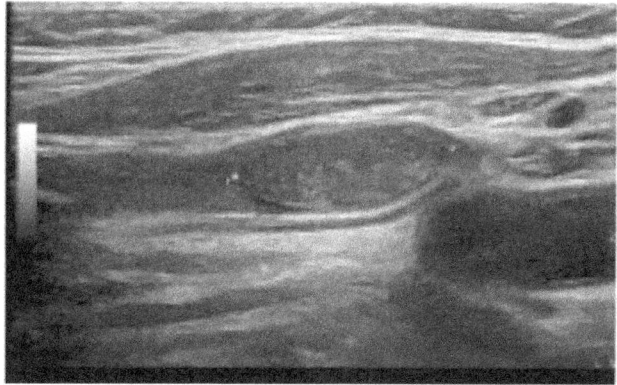

Left neck zone III long

this patient initially chose to pursue clinical and ultrasound follow-up because of her advanced age. Follow-up neck ultrasonography 1 year later demonstrated tumor thrombus in the left internal jugular vein (*Figure 6*) and prompted neck CT, which confirmed this finding. The patient elected to undergo left thyroid lobectomy, and surgical pathology demonstrated OCA with angioinvasion and tumor thrombus within a vessel. Retrospective studies indicate that both FTC and OCA may be overrepresented among malignant autonomously functioning thyroid nodules.[11] Intraluminal tumor thrombus in the great cervical veins as a result of thyroid carcinoma is extremely rare and only case reports are found in the literature.[12]

Case 3

A 57-year-old woman is seen for a thyroid nodule that was found during evaluation of an inferior vena cava (IVC) mass. She initially presented with bilateral lower-extremity edema. Her evaluation included transthoracic echocardiography, which suggested a poorly defined echogenic structure visualized in the IVC. Chest CT was obtained to better define the IVC mass, and it incidentally revealed a 2.3-cm, solid-appearing right thyroid nodule. No IVC mass was visualized.

Examination findings of the patient's neck are notable for a prominent right thyroid lobe (with no discrete thyroid nodule palpated). There is no adenopathy.

Her serum TSH concentration is 2.7 mIU/L.

Neck ultrasonography demonstrates a right 3.6 × 3.3 × 2.2-cm nodule (*Figure 7*). There are no contralateral thyroid nodules or suspicious lymph nodes in the central or bilateral lateral neck.

Ultrasound-guided FNA of the right thyroid nodule is subsequently performed, yielding cytologic specimens that are deemed adequate for diagnosis. The cytologic findings are interpreted as positive for "neoplastic cells" (*Figure 8*).

Figure 8. Cytologic Specimens From FNA of the Right Thyroid Nodule

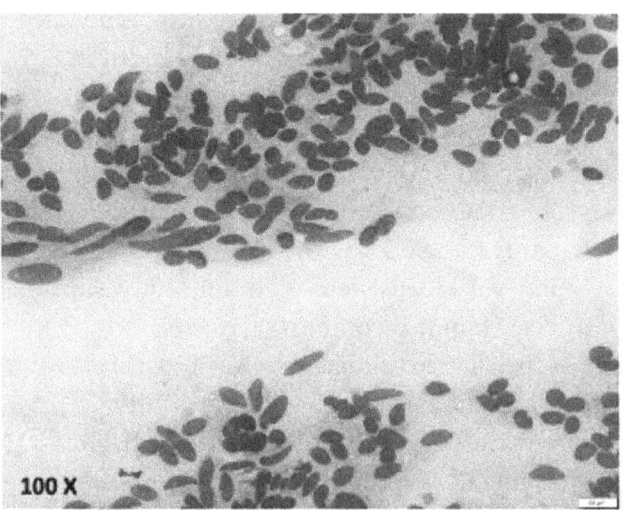

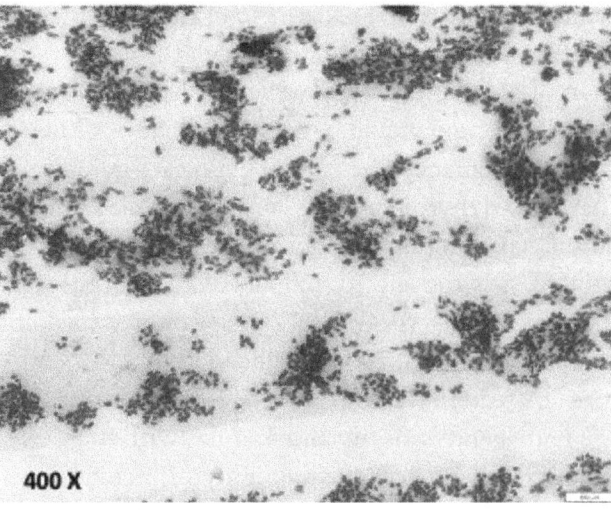

Hypercellular aspirate with numerous noncohesive spindle-shaped cells. The nuclei are elongated with granular chromatin and inconspicuous nucleoli.

[Color—Print (Color Gallery page CG38) or web & ePub editions]

Figure 7. Ultrasound Image of the Right Thyroid Nodule

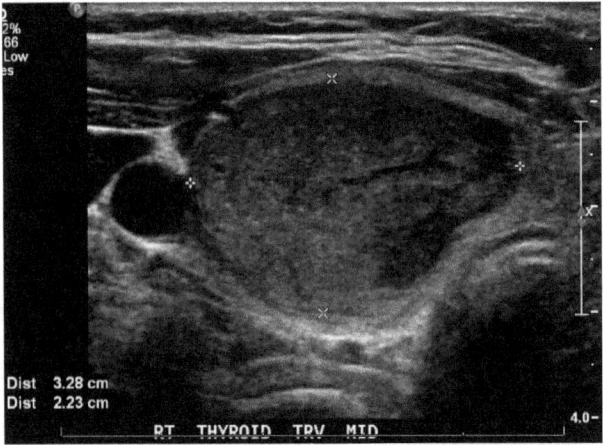

Which of the following is the best next step in the evaluation of this patient's thyroid nodule?

A. Repeat ultrasound-guided FNA biopsy

B. Counsel the patient that neither FNA nor follow-up ultrasonography is needed

C. Send sample for molecular analysis

D. Refer for right hemithyroidectomy

E. Repeat neck ultrasonography in 1 year

Answer: C) Send sample for molecular analysis

This sample was sent for molecular testing and the result was reported as "positive" for MTC. MTC is sometimes called the "great masquerader" of the thyroid gland. The case illustrates the difficulties of diagnosing MTC in both the sonographic and cytologic aspects. The ultrasound features of MTC are not as distinctive as those of PTC, and MTC nodules may not be flagged as suspicious. While hypoechogenicity and macrocalcifications are common sonographic features of MTC nodules, MTC is less likely than PTC to demonstrate microcalcifications, irregular margins, and taller-than-wide shape. A study that evaluated both the sonographic features of MTC and the performance of ultrasound-based RSSs to identify MTC found that 45.4% to 47.4% MTCs were classified as high risk based on ultrasonography, and that FNA was recommended in only 48.7% to 63.8% of all nodules that ultimately were diagnosed as MTC.[13]

The second part of this case illustrates that diagnosing MTC on FNA can be challenging. MTC can have a variety of appearances on cytology and may be misinterpreted as other tumors, especially OCAs or FNs. Common features include plasmacytoid/spindled cells, reduced cell cohesion, binucleation, "salt and pepper" chromatin, intranuclear pseudoinclusions, and extracellular amyloid deposition. A meta-analysis by Trimboli et al reported that the sensitivity of cytology alone (with no calcitonin wash) for diagnosing MTC ranged from 12.5% to 88.2% (mean 56.4%).[14] With the addition of calcitonin needle rinse from the FNA specimen ("calcitonin washout"), the sensitivity increased to greater than 95% for all studies. Although the sensitivity of serum calcitonin for MTC is also high, it is not routinely recommended as part of the standard evaluation of a thyroid nodule due to the lack of pentagastrin-stimulation testing in some countries. Lastly, high sensitivity and specificity for the diagnosis of MTC has been documented for some commercially available molecular tests.[15]

Key Learning Points

•   Incorporation of bedside ultrasonography and/or review of cine clips may allow for more accurate sonographic risk stratification of thyroid nodules, especially when large.

•   Although uncommon, autonomously functioning thyroid cancer does occur; suspicious clinical and/or sonographic findings should prompt this consideration.

•   MTC should be branded the "great masquerader" of the thyroid gland and must always be considered during the diagnostic evaluation of thyroid nodules.

References

1. Lau LW, Ghaznavi S, Frolkis AD, et al. Malignancy risk of hyperfunctioning thyroid nodules compared with non-toxic nodules: systematic review and a meta-analysis. *Thyroid Res.* 2021;14(1):3. PMID: 33632297

2. Haugen BR, Alexander EK, Bible KC, et al. 2015 American Thyroid Association management guidelines for adult patients with thyroid nodules and differentiated thyroid cancer: the American Thyroid Association Guidelines Task Force on Thyroid Nodules and Differentiated Thyroid Cancer. *Thyroid.* 2016;26(1):1-133. PMID: 26462967

3. Tessler FN, Middleton WD, Grant EG, et al. ACR thyroid imaging, reporting and data system (TI-RADS): white paper of the ACR TI-RADS Committee. *J Am Coll Radiol.* 2017;14(5):587-595. PMID: 28372962

4. Kwon D, Kulich M, Mack WJ, Monedero RM, Joyo E, Angell TE. Malignancy risk of thyroid nodules that are not classifiable by the American Thyroid Association ultrasound risk stratification system: a systematic review and meta-analysis. *Thyroid.* 2023;33(5):593-602. PMID: 36855336

5. Ali SZ, Baloch ZW, Cochand-Priollet B, Schmitt FC, Vielh P, VanderLaan PA. The 2023 Bethesda system for reporting thyroid cytopathology. *Thyroid.* 2023;33(9):1039-1044. PMID: 37427847

6. Hu TX, Nguyen DT, Patel M, et al. The effect modification of ultrasound risk classification on molecular testing in predicting the risk of malignancy in cytologically indeterminate thyroid nodules. *Thyroid.* 2022;32(8):905-916. PMID: 35611970

7. Park H, Shin HC, Yang H, et al. Molecular classification of follicular thyroid carcinoma based on TERT promoter mutations. *Mod Pathol.* 2022;35(2):186-192. PMID: 34497362

8. Shin HS, Na DG, Paik W, et al. Malignancy risk stratification of thyroid nodules with macrocalcification and rim calcification based on ultrasound patterns. *Korean J Radiol.* 2021;22(4):663-671. PMID: 33660454

9. Doerfler WR, Nikitski AV, Morariu EM, et al. Molecular alterations in Hurthle cell nodules and preoperative cancer risk. *Endocr Relat Cancer.* 2021;28(5):301-309. PMID: 33792557

10. Ahmadi S, Herbst R, Oyekunle T, et al. Using the ATA and ACR TI-RADS sonographic classifications as adjunctive predictors of malignancy for indeterminate thyroid nodules. *Endocr Pract.* 2019;25(9):908-917. PMID: 31170369

11. Mirfakhraee S, Mathews D, Peng L, Woodruff S, Zigman JM. A solitary hyperfunctioning thyroid nodule harboring thyroid carcinoma: review of the literature. *Thyroid Res.* 2013;6(1):7. PMID: 23641736

12. Onaran Y, Terzioglu T, Oguz H, Kapran Y, Tezelman S. Great cervical vein invasion of thyroid carcinoma. *Thyroid.* 1998;8(1):59-61. PMID: 9492155

13. Matrone A, Gambale C, Biagini M, Prete A, Vitti P, Elisei R. Ultrasound features and risk stratification systems to identify medullary thyroid carcinoma. *Eur J Endocrinol.* 2021;185(2):193-200. PMID: 34010144

14. Trimboli P, Treglia G, Guidobaldi L, et al. Detection rate of FNA cytology in medullary thyroid carcinoma: a meta-analysis. *Clin Endocrinol (Oxf).* 2015;82(2):280-285. PMID: 25047365

15. Randolph GW, Sosa JA, Hao Y, et al. Preoperative identification of medullary thyroid carcinoma (MTC): clinical validation of the Afirma MTC RNA-sequencing classifier. *Thyroid.* 2022;32(9):1069-1076. PMID: 35793115

Complex Hyperthyroidism Cases

Layal Chaker, MD, PhD. Department of Internal Medicine, Academic Center for Thyroid Disease, Erasmus MC, Rotterdam, The Netherlands; Email: l.chaker@erasmusmc.nl

Robin Peeters, MD, PhD. Department of Internal Medicine, Academic Center for Thyroid Disease, Erasmus MC, Rotterdam, The Netherlands; Email: r.peeters@erasmusmc.nl

Educational Objectives

After reviewing this chapter, learners should be able to:

- Explain the diagnostic steps and pitfalls in the diagnosis of various types of thyrotoxicosis.

- Present the benefits and risks of different treatment modalities for thyrotoxicosis.

- Formulate the optimal treatment (options) for patients with thyrotoxicosis who would like to become pregnant.

- Diagnose rare causes of thyrotoxicosis.

- Discuss novel potential treatment modalities.

Significance of the Clinical Problem

Untreated thyrotoxicosis is associated with decreased quality of life and increased risk of cardiovascular events and mortality. Optimal treatment depends on the underlying etiology, with Graves disease, toxic nodular goiter, and thyroiditis being the most common causes of overt thyrotoxicosis. The incidence of drug-induced thyrotoxicosis has increased with relatively new drug classes such as immune checkpoint inhibitors, tyrosine kinase inhibitors, and specific monoclonal antibodies.[1] Strictly speaking, thyrotoxicosis is the clinical manifestations of excess thyroid hormone action at the tissue level, whereas the term hyperthyroidism refers to conditions of increased synthesis and secretion of thyroid hormones by the thyroid gland. However, in clinical practice, these terms are often used interchangeably.

The preferred therapeutic choice for thyrotoxicosis with hyperthyroidism depends on the underlying pathophysiology, but the most common options are antithyroid drugs (ATDs), radioactive iodine treatment (RAI), and thyroidectomy. The preferred first-line treatment option for Graves disease in Europe and the Asia-Pacific region is usually ATDs. Over the last 2 decades in the United States, there has a been a shift in treatment choices in favor of ATDs vs RAI use.[2] More recent evidence on efficacy and safety of long-term, low-dosage ATD administration in patients with Graves disease will likely affect future treatment preferences.[1]

Although the laboratory diagnosis is usually straightforward, there are circumstances where analytical interference can cause confusion. Furthermore, less frequent causes of thyrotoxicosis such as TSHoma or iatrogenic hyperthyroidism can pose a diagnostic challenge. Once the diagnosis has been established, optimal treatment is not only dependent on the underlying etiology, but also on severity and stage of disease and patient-specific factors such as age, sex, and comorbidities.

Practice Gaps

- Lack of awareness of the diagnostic pitfalls, including detailed knowledge of the strengths and weaknesses of various laboratory assays.

- Lack of large randomized controlled trials comparing clinical outcomes of the different treatment modalities in patients with different disease categories.

- Uncertainty about the optimal treatment of hyperthyroidism in patients who would like to become pregnant and taking into account maternal and fetal thyroid physiology.

- Differences in physician preference across the globe.

Discussion

Strategies for Diagnosis

Overt thyrotoxicosis is characterized by suppressed serum TSH concentrations (usually <0.01 mIU/L) in combination with elevated serum free T_4 and/or total or free T_3. Please see Chaker et al[3] for a more detailed review on the diagnosis and treatment of hyperthyroidism. The free fraction of T_4, reflecting the freely available hormone, is the preferred measurement over total T_4. Due to limitations of currently available free T_3 assays, either total or free T_3 can be measured. Laboratory diagnosis of thyrotoxicosis is usually straightforward, although there are several causes of diagnostic confusion.

Discordant thyroid function tests (eg, elevated thyroid hormone levels with unsuppressed TSH) can be the result of circulating heterophilic antibodies that cause analytical interference with TSH measurements. Amiodarone use can also result in discordant thyroid function tests with elevated T_4 levels in euthyroidism due to its effect on T_4 clearance, intracellular T_4 transport, and deiodinase activity. Spuriously elevated immunoreactive free T_4 concentrations can be the result of variant thyroid hormone-binding proteins (familial dysalbuminemic

hyperthyroxinemia [FDH]), whereas in rare instances, patients with thyroid autoimmunity may have circulating autoantibodies to T_4 or T_3 that cause analytical interference.

Falsely elevated thyroid hormone levels combined with falsely suppressed TSH levels, leading to the erroneous diagnosis of thyrotoxicosis, can occur in patients ingesting biotin supplements when assays are used that use streptavidin-biotin detection systems. Two rare conditions present with elevated serum thyroid hormone levels and unsuppressed serum TSH: TSH-secreting pituitary tumors causing central thyrotoxicosis and resistance to thyroid hormone β (RTHβ), caused by pathogenic variants in the gene encoding thyroid hormone receptor β. Finally, severe nonthyroidal illness, central hypothyroidism, and high-dosage glucocorticoid therapy are associated with subnormal serum TSH levels but normal or low levels of thyroid hormones. Suppressed TSH with normal free T_4 and free T_3 can also be seen in early pregnancy. See Koulouri et al[4] for a more detailed discussion of various causes of discordant thyroid function tests.

Measurement of antibodies to the TSH receptor (TRAb) is the key diagnostic assessment in all patients suspected of having Graves disease. TRAb can be measured with immunoassays, which do not distinguish between thyroid-stimulating antibodies (TSI) and thyroid-blocking antibodies (TBI). This can cause diagnostic challenges in specific cases because both antibodies can coexist in patients with Graves disease. Novel automated bridge-based binding assays have become commercially available to more selectively, but not exclusively, measure TSI.[5] Both assay methods provide excellent diagnostic sensitivity and specificity in general patient populations.

When the cause of thyrotoxicosis is not readily apparent, thyroid scintigraphy is a useful tool in determining the etiology. Diffuse accumulation of the radiotracers iodine 123, iodine 131, or technetium 99 is seen throughout the thyroid gland, with elevated or high-normal uptake in patients with Graves disease but also in patients with rarer causes of thyrotoxicosis such as

TSHoma and RTHβ, whereas uptake is usually very low or absent in all causes of thyroiditis and in patients with iodine-induced hyperthyroidism due to competition for uptake with the administered radiotracer. In patients with toxic nodular goiter, scintigraphy usually shows areas of hyperfunction and hypofunction within the thyroid gland ("hot" and "cold" nodules).

When thyroid nodules are detected on physical examination or on scintigraphy in the case of cold nodules, thyroid ultrasonography is indicated. In some centers where thyroid scintigraphy is not available, ultrasonography with color-flow Doppler is used to assess thyroidal vascularity to differentiate Graves disease from other causes of thyrotoxicosis. Thyroidal blood flow is increased in Graves disease but is normal or low in various forms of thyroiditis. The disadvantage of this approach is the high risk of identifying thyroid incidentalomas with subsequent overdiagnosis of thyroid nodules and microcarcinomas.[6]

Strategies for Therapy and/or Management

The preferred choice of therapy in patients with hyperthyroidism depends on underlying pathophysiology, but the most common options are ATDs, RAI, and thyroidectomy. In case of cardiac concerns, mainly palpitations, β-adrenergic blockers can be considered regardless of the etiology of hyperthyroidism. In patients with toxic adenoma or multinodular goiter, RAI and surgery are usually the preferred treatments, although more recent studies show that long-term low-dosage treatment with ATDs is effective, especially in older patients or in those who are poor candidates for RAI or surgery. In Graves disease, all 3 treatment modalities are effective, but ATDs seem to be the patient-preferred approach.[7] Patients with Graves disease who receive RAI report lower quality of life 10 years after treatment compared with the quality of life reported by patients treated with ATDs or surgery.

Carbimazole and its metabolite methimazole are generally preferred over propylthiouracil because of superior efficacy and tolerability. According to American and European Guidelines,[7,8] patients with newly diagnosed Graves hyperthyroidism can be treated for 12 to 18 months with carbimazole or methimazole after which carbimazole or methimazole can be discontinued in the setting of normal TSH serum levels and negative TRAb. When high TRAb persists while on treatment or when there is relapse after treatment withdrawal, patients can choose to reinitiate carbimazole or methimazole for another 12 months (or longer) or opt for more definitive treatment with RAI or thyroidectomy. Although a single course of ATDs has relatively high relapse rates (~50%), a second course of ATD therapy can achieve long-term remission in more than 75% of patients.[9] Long-term or even lifelong treatment with low-dosage carbimazole or methimazole also seems to be a safe and effective option as suggested by recent studies.[1] Agranulocytosis occurs in less than 0.5% of patients, typically within the first 3 months of treatment. Treating physicians should inform patients to be on the alert for the occurrence of fever and/or sore throat. If agranulocytosis is confirmed, ATDs should be discontinued permanently.

ATDs can be titrated to the lowest dosage needed to maintain euthyroidism (monotherapy) or a "block and replace" regimen can be used, with ATDs in a higher dosage to fully block thyroid function accompanied by levothyroxine replacement to avoid hypothyroidism. Overtreatment resulting in hypothyroidism should be avoided, as this may provoke or exacerbate thyroid eye disease in patients with Graves disease.

RAI is first-line treatment in most cases of toxic adenoma and toxic multinodular goiter, especially for older patients with comorbidities incurring higher surgery risk. Permanent hypothyroidism occurs in 50% to 85% of patients with RAI-treated Graves disease and is more common with higher administered RAI activities. Development of thyroid eye disease or worsening of preexisting thyroid eye disease is the most severe adverse effect, especially in patients who smoke cigarettes. For this reason, RAI is contraindicated in patients with Graves disease who have severe orbitopathy. In those with mild orbitopathy or those at risk of de novo thyroid eye disease (persons who smoke cigarettes, have severe orunstable hyperthyroidism, or have high serum TRAb), glucocorticoid prophylaxis is recommended when RAI therapy is initiated. Although several studies have shown no difference in cancer incidence or mortality with RAI, there may be some evidence of a dose-dependent association between RAI and increased risk in any solid cancer mortality, but findings are controversial.[10] Based on patient preference or when other treatments are ineffective, not tolerated, or contraindicated (eg, RAI in severe orbitopathy), thyroidectomy can also be considered as first-line treatment.

Treatment modalities have remained similar for decades and have important limitations, such as the high relapse rates after withdrawal of ATDs and permanent hypothyroidism after RAI or surgery. In recent years, drugs with novel potential treatment targets for Graves disease have been tested in small and mainly open-label phase I and II clinical studies. Their mechanisms of action include: (1) restoration of immune tolerance (immunomodulatory TSHR peptides), (2) counteracting TSH-receptor signaling (TRAb blockers, small molecular TSHR antagonists), (3) modulating B-cell function and activation (rituximab, iscalimab, belimumab), and (4) inhibition of IgG recycling by neonatal Fc receptor blockade (rozanolixizumab, efgartigimod). Results of large, randomized multicenter trials are expected in the coming years to establish or refute these promising but still preliminary results.[3]

Thyrotoxicosis and Pregnancy

Overt hyperthyroidism during pregnancy is associated with adverse pregnancy and neonatal outcomes, including increased risk of miscarriage, stillbirth, preeclampsia, preterm birth, and low birth weight. Available evidence suggests that women who receive adequate antenatal care do not have these increased risks.[11] However, ATD treatment in early pregnancy, especially weeks 5 through 11, carries a small but significant risk of teratogenic adverse effects with differences in pattern and severity generally in favor of propylthiouracil over carbimazole or methimazole. Therefore, women with hyperthyroidism who are planning pregnancy would ideally receive definitive therapy before pregnancy. When RAI therapy is chosen as definitive therapy, women are generally advised to avoid pregnancy for 6 to 12 months due to radiation-related risks. Additionally, it is also important to realize that TRAb can temporarily increase and remain high for up to 1 year after RAI therapy. TRAb can cross the placenta and stimulate the fetal thyroid during pregnancy, potentially resulting in fetal hyperthyroidism.

Clinical Case Vignettes
Case 1

A 34-year-old woman with thyrotoxicosis is referred because she would like to become pregnant. She has nervousness, tachycardia, and weight loss. On physical examination, she has an obvious goiter.

Laboratory test results:

TSH = <0.001 mIU/L (0.5-5.0 mIU/L)
Free T_4 = 4.82 ng/dL (0.85-1.94 ng/dL)
    (SI: 62.0 pmol/L [11.0-25.0 pmol/L])
TRAb = 35 IU/L (<1.9 IU/L)

Given that the patient would like to become pregnant as soon as possible, which of the following is the best recommendation?

A. Medical therapy with methimazole and levothyroxine (block and replace); tell her she can become pregnant once euthyroidism has been achieved

B. Medical therapy with methimazole at the lowest possible dosage (monotherapy); tell her she can become pregnant once euthyroidism has been achieved

C. Medical therapy with propylthiouracil at the lowest possible dosage (monotherapy); tell her she can become pregnant once euthyroidism has been achieved

D. Definitive therapy with RAI; tell her she should wait 6 months after RAI before becoming pregnant

E. Definitive therapy with thyroidectomy; she can become pregnant once euthyroidism has been achieved after surgery

Answer: E) Definitive therapy with thyroidectomy; she can become pregnant once euthyroidism has been achieved after surgery

In a case like this, there is not a single correct answer. Shared decision-making based on the patient's preference and individual risk factors has an important role. However, block and replace therapy in patients who would like to become pregnant is NOT an option. ATDs cross the placenta and can cause fetal hypothyroidism. Therefore, pregnant patients and patients desiring pregnancy should always be treated with the lowest possible dosage. In addition, ATD treatment, particularly in early pregnancy, results in an increased risk of teratogenic effects. Therefore, this patient would ideally receive definitive therapy before pregnancy, especially because of the very small recurrence risk of Graves disease based on the severity of the hyperthyroidism, goiter, and high TRAb concentration.

This patient already has clearly elevated TRAb levels (>15 times the upper normal limit) and she wants to become pregnant as soon as possible. Her TRAb will likely temporarily increase and remain high for up to 1 year after RAI therapy, placing her child at risk of fetal orneonatal hyperthyroidism when she becomes pregnant. For that reason, thyroidectomy (Answer E) at a high-volume center (with known low complication rates) would be the preferred choice. If she insists on medical therapy, propylthiouracil would be the correct option because the teratogenic profile is generally more favorable than that of carbimazole or methimazole.

Case 2

A 32-year-old man presents to his primary care provider because he has had sudden onset of palpitations that persist for minutes for the last 3 weeks. He has no relevant medical history, but he broke up with his girlfriend 6 weeks ago after a relationship of 10 years. His family history is positive for autoimmune disease (mother with rheumatoid arthritis and sister with systemic lupus erythematosus) but negative for thyroid disease. He has no other relevant concerns, no heat intolerance, and no weight loss. Physical examination findings are normal, including normal thyroid gland on palpitation.

As part of the diagnostic workup, his primary care provider orders laboratory testing:

TSH = 0.5 mIU/L (0.4-4.3 mIU/L)
Free T_4 = 1.98 ng/dL (0.70-1.48 ng/dL)
(SI: 25.5 pmol/L [9.0-19.0 pmol/L])

Repeat testing at a different laboratory with a different platform shows similar results:

TSH = 0.45 mIU/L
Free T_4 = 2.13 ng/dL (SI: 27.4 pmol/L)

Which of the following is this patient's most likely diagnosis?

A. Graves disease

B. Toxic nodule

C. Thyroiditis

D. Pituitary adenoma

E. Something else

Answer: E) Something else

In patients with overt thyroid disease, TSH is the most sensitive marker. A normal TSH value makes Graves disease (Answer A), toxic nodule (Answer B), and thyroiditis (Answer C) highly unlikely. Pituitary adenoma (Answer D) could be an option; however, the lack of clear symptoms and the rarity of this diagnosis makes other causes (Answer E) such as an assay artifact much more likely at this stage.

Case 2 (continued)

TRAb is negative and total T_3 is normal. A serum sample is sent to a reference laboratory, where repeated testing shows a TSH value of 0.51 mIU/L and a free T_4 value of 0.73 ng/dL (0.85-1.94 ng/dL) (SI: 9.4 pmol/L [11.0-25.0 pmol/L]).

Which of the following is the most likely diagnosis?

A. Pituitary adenoma

B. Resistance to thyroid hormone β (RTHβ)

C. Familial dysalbuminemic hyperthyroxinemia

D. Use of kelp

E. Use of biotin-containing supplements

Answer: C) Familial dysalbuminemic hyperthyroxinemia

The normal T_3 value makes a pituitary adenoma (Answer A) and RTHβ (Answer B) highly unikely. Kelp (Answer D) can affect thyroid function tests, but this is consistent across laboratories. The discrepancy in free T_4 measurement between different platforms suggests an artifact, with falsely high free T_4 in 2 assays and falsely low free T_4 in the third assay. In case of biotin interference (Answer E), a normal free T_4 value would be expected in the third assay. This patient had familial dysalbuminemic hyperthyroxinemia (Answer C) due to a pathogenic Arg218His variant in the albumin gene. Typically, 70% of T_4 is bound to thyroxine-binding globulin, 20% to transthyretin, and 10% to albumin. In patients with familial dysalbuminemic hyperthyroxinemia, roughly 30% of T_4 is bound to albumin (with 60% bound to thyroxine-binding globulin and 10% to transthyretin). This altered albumin binding causes a falsely high free T_4 value in most but not all assays. In some assays, free T_4 is falsely low.

Case 3

A 66-year-old woman with metastatic renal cell carcinoma to bone is started on the immune checkpoint inhibitors ipilimumab/nivolumab. Before starting therapy, her TSH value was 0.4 mIU/L (0.4-4.3 mIU/L) and free T_4 value was 1.6 ng/dL (0.85-1.94 ng/dL) (SI: 20.0 pmol/L [11.0-25.0 pmol/L]). She takes vitamin D supplementation. After 4 cycles of immunotherapy, CT shows almost complete remission. One week later, she comes to the outpatient clinic because of agitation and fatigue. Physical examination findings are unremarkable.

Thyroid function test results:

> TSH = <0.001 mIU/L
> Free T_4 = ng/dL (SI: 36.0 pmol/L)
> TRAb = 1.0 IU/L (<1.9 IU/L)

Which 2 of the following explanations could be a likely cause of this patient's current biochemical thyrotoxicosis?

A. Iodine-induced hyperthyroidism

B. Graves disease induced by immune checkpoint inhibitor therapy

C. Thyroiditis induced by immune checkpoint inhibitor therapy

D. Assay interference

E. Toxic multinodular goiter

Answer: A and C) Iodine-induced hyperthyroidism and Graves disease induced by immune checkpoint inhibitor therapy

There are several possible explanations for thyrotoxicosis in this patient. Her pretherapy TSH value was relatively low, and in combination with her free T_4 value, she could be classified as having subclinical hyperthyroidism. At her age, multinodular goiter (Answer E) is a common cause of subclinical hyperthyroidism, and this may be aggravated by iodine-containing contrast media (Answer A) that is used for CT. Immune checkpoint inhibitor–induced thyroiditis (Answer C) is common, especially with anti-PD1/PDL-1 therapy, and it can occur in up to 10% of patients with anti-PD1/PDL-1 and CTLA4 combination therapy (eg, nivolumab/ipilimumab). Although Graves disease after initiation of immune checkpoint inhibitors (Answer B) has been described, it is far less likely, especially because the TRAb is negative. Assay interference (Answer D) has not been described, and it is unlikely in a patient only using vitamin D supplementation in addition to her anticancer therapy.

Case 3 (continued)

She continues to experience fatigue and agitation, but these symptoms are stable throughout the next weeks. Follow-up CT 2 months later shows a stable response to therapy. Her thyroid function tests over the next few weeks develop as shown in the *Figure*.

Figure. Patient's Free T$_4$ Concentration Over 4 Months

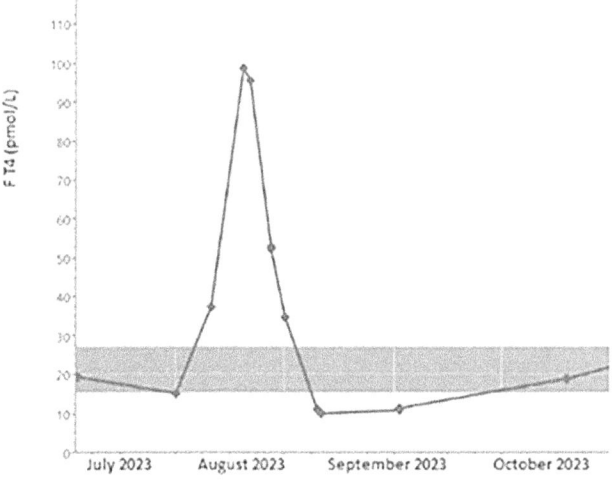

[Color—Print (Color Gallery page CG38) or web & ePub editions]

Which of the following is the most likely explanation for the thyrotoxicosis now?

A. Iodine-induced hyperthyroidism

B. Graves disease induced by immune checkpoint inhibitor therapy

C. Thyroiditis induced by immune checkpoint inhibitor therapy

D. Assay interference

E. Toxic multinodular goiter

Answer: C) Thyroiditis induced by immune checkpoint inhibitor therapy

The course of thyroid function in this patient suggests she has an immune checkpoint inhibitor–induced thyroiditis (Answer C). Thyrotoxicosis induced by immune checkpoint inhibitor therapy is thought to be due to a silent destructive thyroiditis that is usually transient and self-limiting.[12] Thyrotoxicosis can quickly evolve either to hypothyroidism or euthyroidism. It is therefore reasonable to monitor patients and manage them symptomatically, with β-adrenergic blockers if needed and levothyroxine therapy if they are rendered hypothyroid after documenting normal adrenal function. There is rarely a need to discontinue the immune checkpoint inhibitor therapy, and glucocorticoid treatment is indicated only in severe cases (eg, severe pain).

Key Learning Points

- In case of incongruent thyroid function tests, always consider an assay artifact as a possible cause.

- ATDs, RAI, and thyroidectomy are all effective treatment modalities for hyperthyroidism. The preferred choice of therapy in patients with hyperthyroidism depends on the underlying pathophysiology, as well as individual patient characteristics and patient preference.

- In patients with thyrotoxicosis who desire to become pregnant, the risks and benefits of definitive therapy (eg, RAI or thyroidectomy) should be balanced against the use of ATDs.

- Thyroiditis due to immune checkpoint inhibitor therapy is fulminant biochemically and develops within weeks or months after treatment initiation. It can present insidiously with mild symptomatology and rarely needs treatment with glucocorticoids and rarely requires discontinuation of anticancer treatment.

References

1. Azizi F, Amouzegar A, Tohidi M, et al. Increased remission rates after long-term methimazole therapy in patients with Graves' disease: results of a randomized clinical trial. *Thyroid.* 2019;29(9):1192-1200. PMID: 31310160

2. Brito JP, Schilz S, Singh Ospina N, et al. Antithyroid drugs-the most common treatment for Graves' disease in the United States: a nationwide population-based study. *Thyroid.* 2016;26(8):1144-1145. PMID: 27267495

3. Chaker L, Cooper D, Walsh J, Peeter RP. Hyperthyroidism. *Lancet.* 2024;403(10428):768-780. PMID: 38278171.

4. Koulouri O, Moran C, Halsall D, Chatterjee K, Gurnell M. Pitfalls in the measurement and interpretation of thyroid function tests. *Best Pract Res Clin Endocrinol Metab.* 2013;27(6):745-762. PMID: 24275187

5. Diana T, Wuster C, Olivo PD, et al. Performance and specificity of 6 immunoassays for TSH receptor antibodies: a multicenter study. *Eur Thyroid J.* 2017;6(5):243-249. PMID: 29071236

6. Ahn HS, Kim HJ, Kim KH, et al. Thyroid cancer screening in South Korea increases detection of papillary cancers with no impact on other subtypes or thyroid cancer mortality. *Thyroid.* 2016;26(11):1535-1540. PMID: 27627550

7. Kahaly GJ, Bartalena L, Hegedus L, Leenhardt L, Poppe K, Pearce SH. 2018 European Thyroid Association guideline for the management of Graves' hyperthyroidism. *Eur Thyroid J.* 2018;7(4):167-186. PMID: 30283735

8. Ross DS, Burch HB, Cooper DS, Greenlee MC, Laurberg P, Maia AL, et al. 2016 American Thyroid Association guidelines for diagnosis and management of hyperthyroidism and other causes of thyrotoxicosis. *Thyroid.* 2016;26(10):1343-1421. PMID: 27521067

9. Liu X, Qiang W, Liu X, et al. A second course of antithyroid drug therapy for recurrent Graves' disease: an experience in endocrine practice. *Eur J Endocrinol.* 2015;172(3):321-326. PMID: 25468954

10. Kitahara CM, Preston DL, Sosa JA, Berrington de Gonzalez A. Association of radioactive iodine, antithyroid drug, and surgical treatments with solid cancer mortality in patients with hyperthyroidism. *JAMA Netw Open.* 2020;3(7):e209660. PMID: 32701159

11. Pillar N, Levy A, Holcberg G, Sheiner E. Pregnancy and perinatal outcome in women with hyperthyroidism. *Int J Gynaecol Obstet.* 2010;108(1):61-64. PMID: 19766207

12. de Filette J, Jansen Y, Schreuer M, et al. Incidence of thyroid-related adverse events in melanoma patients treated with pembrolizumab. *J Clin Endocrinol Metab.* 2016;101(11):4431-4439. PMID: 27571185

Management of Hereditary Medullary Thyroid Carcinoma

Saumya Agrawal, MD. Department of Surgery, Creighton University School of Medicine, Omaha, NE; Email: saumyaagrawal@creighton.edu

Uriel Clemente-Gutierrez, MD. Department of Surgical Oncology, Section of Surgical Endocrinology, University of Texas MD Anderson Cancer Center, Houston, TX; Email: ueclemente@mdanderson.org

Bernice L. Huang, MD. Department of Surgical Oncology, Section of Surgical Endocrinology, University of Texas MD Anderson Cancer Center, Houston, TX; Email: bhuang2@mdanderson.org

Danica M. Vodopivec, MD. Department of Endocrine Neoplasia and Hormonal Disorders, University of Texas MD Anderson Cancer Center, Houston, TX; Email: dmvodopivec@mdanderson.org

Nancy D. Perrier, MD. Department of surgical Oncology, Section of Surgical Endocrinology, University of Texas MD Anderson Cancer Center, Houston, TX; Email: nperrier@mdanderson.org

Educational Objectives

After reviewing this chapter, learners should be able to:

- Recognize the clinical manifestations of and define the appropriate workup for hereditary medullary thyroid carcinoma (MTC).

- Explain the prognostic implications of specific *RET* pathogenic variants regarding the role and timing of risk-reducing thyroidectomy (previously known as prophylactic thyroidectomy) based on the American Thyroid Association risk categories.

- Summarize the recommended follow-up for patients with MTC.

- Describe the surgical management of hereditary MTC, including the indications for therapeutic and prophylactic cervical lymph node dissection.

- Determine the indications of targeted therapies in advanced and recurrent MTC.

Significance of the Clinical Problem

MTC is a rare neuroendocrine tumor arising from parafollicular or C cells of the thyroid, and it accounts for 1% to 2% of all thyroid cancers. MTC may occur sporadically (75%) or in hereditary form (25%) as a component of multiple endocrine neoplasia type 2 (MEN 2) and familial MTC.

Although MTC has a wide range of clinical behaviors, varying from indolent to aggressive tumors with a reported 10-year survival of 69% to 89%, it has the potential to be treated early based on genetic testing. Risk-reducing thyroidectomy in patients with inherited disease and an associated *RET* pathogenic variant, who are at 100% risk of developing this cancer, is highly preventive as well as curative. Lymph node metastases in MTC depend on the size of the primary lesion in the thyroid; thus, timely prophylactic intervention could prevent extrathyroidal spread of the disease. The secretory products of C cells, including calcitonin and carcinoembryonic antigen (CEA), are important tumor markers used for diagnostic and prognostic purposes.

Practice Gaps

- Difficulty in diagnosing hereditary MTC due to heterogeneity of clinical presentation.

- Establishing a correlation between genotype and phenotype in hereditary MTC.

- Defining the optimal timing and extent of risk-reducing surgery for pediatric patients.

- Complexity of the disease requires treatment and follow-up in referral centers.

- Targeted therapies have specific indications.

Discussion

Clinical Presentation and Diagnostic Workup

MTC is either diagnosed as a result of screening patients with a family history of MTC or during workup of a thyroid nodule. Hereditary MTC is the most consistent feature of MEN 2A and 2B, where it may present as a palpable thyroid nodule with or without calcitonin excess or as a nonpalpable, asymptomatic nodule on screening.

Important differences to note in the presentation of sporadic and hereditary MTCs is younger age of presentation for hereditary cases, even after the genetically screened ones are excluded. Some studies have noted more microscopic disease (≤1 cm), multifocality, C-cell hyperplasia, and smaller tumor size for hereditary MTC as compared with findings in sporadic MTC. Sporadic disease has more capsular invasion,

soft-tissue invasion, and distant metastases with stage IV disease showing greater progression.

In both inherited and sporadic types, disease recurrence and survival correlate with extent of disease at presentation.

MEN 2 can present with different phenotypes and thus different clinical manifestations. MEN 2A represents 95% of MEN 2 cases and it is characterized by the development of MTC, primary hyperparathyroidism, and pheochromocytoma. Nonendocrine manifestations, such as cutaneous lichen amyloidosis and Hirschsprung disease, are rare. The other variant, MEN 2B, accounts for 5% of all MEN 2 cases and its clinical manifestations are early-onset MTC, pheochromocytoma, and nonendocrine physical features such as marfanoid body habitus and ganglioneuromas affecting the aerodigestive tract, lacrimal duct, and eye lids. These clinical manifestations should prompt workup for MEN 2 in the pediatric population.

Up to 50% of MEN 2A cases are familial. These are defined as families or single individuals with germline *RET* pathogenic variants and MTC alone in the absence of pheochromocytoma or parathyroid adenoma/hyperplasia. Previously, familial MTC was a separate diagnosis but this led to misclassification of families as having familial MTC (because of too-small family size or later onset of other manifestations of MEN 2A), therefore overlooking the risk of associated conditions. Hence, familial MTC is now a subtype of MEN 2A in which there is a lack of or delay in the onset of the other (nonthyroidal) manifestations of MEN 2A. Current management guidelines recommend that patients thought to have pure familial MTC also be screened for pheochromocytoma and hyperparathyroidism.

Initial workup should be the same as with any thyroid nodule, including thyroid function tests, cervical ultrasonography, and FNA. Signs and symptoms indicating excess calcitonin secretion or metastatic disease should be addressed, especially flushing, diarrhea, and bone pain. Hyperparathyroidism and pheochromocytoma biochemical evaluation should be performed in all patients without exception. The biochemical workup of suspected MTC nodules includes measuring serum concentrations of secretory products of parafollicular C cells, which are used as tumor markers, particularly calcitonin and CEA. Some pathologic conditions can lead to falsely elevated calcitonin, including chronic kidney disease, hypercalcemia, some neuroendocrine tumors (ie, gastrinomas), the presence of heterophilic antibodies to calcitonin, and the use of certain medications (glucocorticoids, β-adrenergic blockers, and proton-pump inhibitors). Basal serum calcitonin concentrations in MTC often correlate with tumor burden; nonetheless, normal calcitonin levels in the presence of high CEA levels could reflect tumor dedifferentiation.

Staging of MTC

TNM staging of MTC according to American Joint Committee on Cancer guidelines is shown in *Table 1*. This has prognostic significance, and an analysis of patients with MTC using the National Cancer Database and the SEER data set (Surveillance, Epidemiology, and End Results) demonstrated that the seventh and eighth editions of the AJCC staging system were associated with 5-year overall survival rates of 95% in stage I, 91% in stage II, 89% in stage III, and 68% in stage IV. Furthermore, disease-specific survival rates were 100% in stage I, 99% in stage II, 97% in stage III, and 82% in stage IV.

Genetics

The RET protooncogene is expressed in cells derived from the neural crest. The type of variant in the gene dictates the clinical aggressiveness of the disease, hence the prognosis. While almost

Table 1. MTC TNM Staging AJCC UICC 8th Edition[a]

Primary tumor (T)	
T category	T criteria
TX	Primary tumor cannot be assessed
T0	No evidence of primary tumor
T1	Tumor ≤2 cm in greatest dimension limited to the thyroid
T1a	Tumor ≤1 cm in greatest dimension limited to the thyroid
T1b	Tumor >1 cm but ≤2 cm in greatest dimension limited to the thyroid
T2	Tumor >2 cm but <4 cm in greatest dimension limited to the thyroid
T3	Tumor ≥4 cm or with extrathyroidal extension
T3a	Tumor ≥4 cm in greatest dimension limited to the thyroid
T3b	Tumor of any size with gross extrathyroidal extension invading only strap muscles (sternohyoid, sternothyroid, thyrohyoid or omohyoid muscles)
T4	Advanced disease
T4a	Moderately advanced disease: Tumor of any size with gross extrathyroidal extension into the nearby tissues of the neck, including subcutaneous soft tissue, larynx, trachea, esophagus, or recurrent laryngeal nerve.
T4b	Very advanced disease: Tumor of any size with extension toward the spine or into nearby large blood vessels, gross extrathyroidal extension invading the prevertebral fascia, or encasing the carotid artery or mediastinal vessels.

Regional lymph nodes (N)	
N category	**N criteria**
NX	Regional lymph nodes cannot be assessed
N0	No evidence of locoregional lymph node metastasis
N0a	One or more cytologically or histologically confirmed benign lymph nodes
N0b	No radiologic or clinical evidence of locoregional lymph node metastasis
N1	Metastasis to regional nodes
N1a	Metastasis to level VI or VII (pretracheal, paratracheal, or prelaryngeal/Delphian, or upper mediastinal) lymph nodes; this can be unilateral or bilateral disease
N1b	Metastasis to unilateral, bilateral, or contralateral lateral neck lymph nodes (levels I, II, III, IV, or V) or retropharyngeal lymph nodes

Distant metastasis (M)	
M category	**M criteria**
M0	No distant metastasis
M1	Distant metastasis

Prognostic stage groups			
When T is...	**And N is...**	**And M is...**	**Then the stage group is...**
T1	N0	M0	I
T2	N0	M0	II
T3	N0	M0	II
T1-3	N1a	M0	III
T4a	Any N	M0	IVA
T1-3	N1b	M0	IVA
T4b	Any N	M0	IVB
Any T	Any N	M1	IVC

ᵃ Abbreviations: TNM, tumor, node metastasis; UICC, Union for International Cancer Control.

Reprinted from Chapter 54, "Thyroid- medullary," pages 896-97 in Amin MB et al., eds. *AJCC Cancer Staging Manual, Eighth Edition*, 2017. Published by Springer International Publishing. Corrected at 4th printing, 2018.

all patients with MEN 2A and MEN 2B have a *RET* germline variant, about 50% of patients with sporadic MTC have a somatic *RET* variant. Up to 7% of patients with presumed sporadic MTCs have hereditary disease on testing. Hence, genetic counseling and testing should be offered to all new patients. Very specifically, the MEN 2B and somatic *RET* codon pathogenic variant M918T is associated with poor prognosis due to an aggressive disease course. The relationship of common *RET* variants to risk of aggressive MTC

in MEN 2A and 2B and other associated conditions in MEN 2A is shown in *Table 2 (following page)*.[1]

American Thyroid Association (ATA) guidelines on MTC management suggest that patients with suspected hereditary MTC undergo genetic testing via a tiered approach, beginning with the most commonly mutated "hotspots" and then proceeding to analysis of other exons if needed. However, with increasing availability and decreasing cost of next-generation sequencing technology, some commercial genetic testing labs are able to offer sequencing of the entire coding (and certain intronic and noncoding) region of the gene.[2] More than 100 *RET* pathogenic variants have been identified in patients with hereditary MTC; the most commonly described variants in persons with MEN 2A are those affecting the cysteine codons in exons 10 and 11. Ninety-five percent of patients with MEN 2B have a pathogenic variant in exon 16, codon 918 (M918T), and the remaining 5% have a pathogenic variants in exon 15, codon 883 (A883F). Since *RET* pathogenic variants are inherited in autosomal dominant manner and are associated with varied age of disease onset, presentation, and degree of penetrance, if identified in a patient, genetic counseling should be offered to all at-risk family members (first-degree relatives, including siblings and children) and a detailed pedigree analysis completed based on the genetic status of parents.

Risk-Reducing thyroidectomy: Timing, Indications, and Follow-Up

The aggressiveness of MTC and, hence, the recommended timing of risk-reducing thyroidectomy (now the preferred term over *prophylactic thyroidectomy*) in individuals with MEN 2 is largely dependent on the specific *RET* pathogenic variant. The ATA has designated a classification system for common *RET* variants to predict risk of aggressive MTC.[1] The M918T variant is considered highest risk, variants in

Table 2. Common *RET* Pathogenic Variants and Risk of Aggressive MTC in MEN 2A and 2B and Incidence of Pheochromocytoma, Hyperparathyroidism, and Hirschsprung Disease in MEN 2A

RET pathogenic variant	Exon	Risk of aggressive MTC	Approximate incidence of pheochromocytoma	Approximate incidence of hyperparathyroidism	Presence of cutaneous lichen amyloidosis	Hirschsprung disease
G533C	8	Moderate	10%	-	N	N
C609F/G/R/S/Y	10	Moderate	10%-30%	10%	N	Y
C611F/G/S/Y/W	10	Moderate	10%-30%	10%	N	Y
C618F/R/S	10	Moderate	10%-30%	10%	N	Y
C620F/R/S	10	Moderate	10%-30%	10%	N	Y
C630R/Y	11	Moderate	10%-30%	10%	N	N
D631Y	11	Moderate	50%	-	N	N
C634F/G/R/S/W/Y	11	High	50%	20%-30%	Y	N
K666E	11	Moderate	10%	-	N	N
E768D	13	Moderate	-	-	N	N
L790F	13	Moderate	10%	-	N	N
V804L	14	Moderate	10%	10%	N	N
V804M	14	Moderate	10%	10%	Y	N
A883F	15	High	50%	-	N	N
S891A	15	Moderate	10%	10%	N	N
R912P	16	Moderate	-	-	N	N
M918T	16	Highest	50%	-	N	N

Reprinted with permission from Wells SA, Jr. et al. Thyroid, 2015; 25(6): 567-610. © American Thyroid Association. Published by Mary Ann Liebert, Inc.[1]

codons 634 and 883 (eg, C634X and A883F) are considered high risk, and all other variants are classified as moderate risk. Patients in the ATA highest-risk category should undergo thyroidectomy during the first year of life. Patients in the ATA high-risk category are recommended to have risk-reducing thyroidectomy with consideration of age, pathogenic variant status, calcitonin levels, and family preference. Thyroidectomy should be offered around age 5 or 6 years. Factors such as school and family dynamics are important for psychologic welfare, and therefore surgical procedures are usually scheduled during summer or school breaks. If calcitonin levels are found to be elevated or there is evidence of a rising trend before age 5 years, thyroidectomy should be performed earlier. Patients in the ATA moderate-risk category must be screened on a 6-month to annual basis, starting at age 5 years. Physical examination, neck ultrasonography, and calcitonin measurement serve as the screening tools. Thyroidectomy is indicated based on a proven rising trend of calcitonin or identification of any thyroid abnormalities on ultrasonography. Long-term screening can be a concerning topic for some parents; if this is the case, prophylactic thyroidectomy could be considered based on timing that is appropriate for the family with input from the endocrinologist and endocrine surgeon.

Studies have demonstrated that lymph node metastases are rare in patients younger than 11 years and in patients with a preoperative calcitonin concentration below 40 pg/mL (<11.7 pmol/L). Therefore, for patients in all ATA risk categories, prophylactic central neck dissection, which would place the recurrent laryngeal nerve and parathyroid at significantly increased risk, is not indicated unless worrisome lymph nodes are encountered during preoperative assessment or intraoperatively. MTC generally presents before parathyroid disease in patients with MEN 2A and likewise before pheochromocytoma in either MEN syndromes. Hence, calcium, PTH, and metanephrines should always be measured during preoperative workup of any patient with MTC to rule out an association. If detected,

pheochromocytoma should be medically blocked and surgically removed before the thyroid gland. Pheochromocytomas can develop as early as age 8 years in individuals with MEN 2A who have codon 634 variants.[3] In general, screening for pheochromocytoma in these individuals is recommended to start at age 11 years.

After risk-reducing thyroidectomy has been performed in patients with hereditary MTC, the suggested follow-up strategy is to evaluate with physical exam, neck ultrasonography, and biochemical tests (calcitonin and CEA measurement) every 6 months for the first postoperative year and then annually. If the serum calcitonin concentration is elevated but less than 150 pg/mL (<43.8 pmol/L), doubling times are evaluated with measurement of calcitonin and CEA every 3 to 6 months; if the doubling time is less than 6 months or the calcitonin concentration is greater than 150 pg/mL (>43.8 pmol/L), imaging studies should be used to evaluate for recurrent and metastatic disease.

How Extensive Should Thyroidectomy and Lymph Node Dissection Be?

When the index family member with hereditary MTC presents for medical evaluation, they usually have a palpable thyroid nodule. Lymph node involvement is found in more than 70% of these patients (this presentation is much more similar to that seen in patients with sporadic MTC). In this case, the standard treatment for MTC is total thyroidectomy and, depending on preoperative serum calcitonin levels, neck ultrasound findings, and intraoperative evaluation, possibly compartmental cervical lymph node dissection. More than 70% of patients with MTC show central compartment involvement,[4] and involvement of the compartment ipsilateral to the thyroid lesion is frequently observed. Contralateral lymphadenopathy has been documented when preoperative calcitonin levels are greater than 200 pg/mL (>58.4 pmol/L). For this reason, prophylactic central compartment lymphadenectomy (level VI) is recommended in all patients, lateral compartment dissection (levels II, III, IV, and V) is indicated when abnormal lymphadenopathy is documented in the preoperative ultrasonography, and contralateral prophylactic lymphadenectomy can be considered if calcitonin levels are above 200 pg/mL (>58.4 pmol/L).[1,5]

Factors different from the presence or absence of cervical lymphadenopathy or calcitonin levels have been studied to potentially omit or recommend prophylactic lymphadenectomy in specific population subgroups. The absence of desmoplastic stromal reaction has demonstrated to be a favorable prognostic factor, and prophylactic lymphadenectomy could be of poor utility in this group.[6] Interestingly, specific *RET* pathogenic variants, such as those occurring in exons 11 and 13, are associated with an elevated risk of cervical lymph node metastases.[7]

Adjuvant Therapy

Since MTC is not driven by TSH, there is no role of postoperative TSH suppression. Hence, the dosage of thyroid hormone replacement after total thyroidectomy should be tailored to age- and weight-specific requirements. On similar grounds, ^{131}I has no role in adjuvant treatment of locally advanced or metastatic disease.

External beam radiotherapy has a role in palliative treatment of metastatic MTC such as bone, brain, or lung metastases. External beam radiation is also considered for patients with gross residual disease after surgery, although the optimal dose is controversial.

Recurrent Disease: Indications for When to Start Systemic Therapy

Many patients with distant metastases have indolent disease—with stable to slow-growing lesions and tumor markers increasing at a slow pace—that requires active surveillance without the need of systemic therapy for years. Systemic therapy is reserved for metastatic disease with at least 1 of the following characteristics: (1)

progressive (by RECIST) within 12 to 14 months, (2) symptomatic and not treatable with local or symptom-specific therapies, (3) compromises nearby structures not treatable with localized therapies, (4) calcitonin or CEA doubling time less than 6 months with structural evidence of clinically significant disease, and (5) severe, intractable MTC-related diarrhea or Cushing syndrome with lack of an alternative effective treatment.

The US FDA has approved tyrosine kinase inhibitors for the treatment of MTC, and they are divided into 2 different categories: (1) multikinase inhibitors[8]: vandetanib[9] and cabozantinib,[10,11] and (2) selective RET-inhibitors: selpercatinib and pralsetinib. Selpercatinib[12] and pralsetinib[13] are considered first choice because they are receptor specific and hence better tolerated (fewer adverse events).

In general, if metastatic disease is stable in all but one area, systemic therapy should be avoided and localized treatment in the form of external beam radiation, surgical resection, embolization, or cryoablation is preferred. Starting systemic therapy should not be taken lightly, as it confers toxicities, is not curative, requires long-term use for disease control, and loses efficacy over time due to acquired resistance. The take-home message is that the use of systemic treatment for advanced MTC should remain reserved for patients with structurally progressive disease not amenable to other treatments.

Clinical Case Vignettes
Case 1

A 6-year-old boy with no family history of endocrinopathies and who is otherwise healthy presents for evaluation of lesions in his lips and tongue, which the mother notes have been present since early life. She points out that peculiarly, similar lesions have appeared in his eyelids, causing corneal irritation. Physical examination confirms what the mother has described and reveals a 2-cm anterior cervical mass. After appropriate workup with cervical ultrasonography, FNA, and biochemical laboratory tests, MTC is diagnosed.

Which of the following statements is correct?

A. Genetic testing with a tiered approach will probably identify a *RET* pathogenic variant in exon 10 or 11

B. The most common pathogenic variant affecting persons with MEN 2B is found in exon 15

C. The M918T pathogenic variant is the most probable cause of this patient's condition

D. The patient does not have family history indicating a hereditary condition, hence, genetic testing is not indicated

Answer: C) The M918T pathogenic variant is the most probable cause of this patient's condition

All patients with newly diagnosed MTC should be referred for genetic counseling and undergo genetic testing, especially when syndromic characteristics are identified such as the ganglioneuromas described in this patient (thus, Answer D is incorrect). This patient's phenotype is consistent with MEN 2B. He has ganglioneuromas of the oral cavity and the eyelid, and these nonendocrine manifestations are not seen in MEN 2A (thus, Answer B is incorrect). The M918T pathogenic variant is identified in 95% of patients with MEN 2B, while the A883F pathogenic variant in exon 15 is found in the remaining 5% of patients with MEN 2B (thus, Answer C is correct and Answer B is incorrect).

Case 2

A 10-year-old girl who is otherwise healthy presents to clinic for evaluation. Her mother was recently diagnosed with MEN 2A and she has also tested positive for a *RET* pathogenic variant in codon 634. Cervical ultrasonography does not reveal abnormalities of the thyroid gland or concerning lymph nodes.

Laboratory test results:

TSH, normal
Free T$_4$, normal
Basal calcitonin = 17 pg/mL (SI: 5.0 pmol/L)
Calcium = 9.3 mg/dL (SI: 2.3 mmol/L)

Which of the following is the most appropriate next step in this patient's management?

A. Surveillance

B. Total thyroidectomy

C. Total thyroidectomy with bilateral central neck dissection

D. Total thyroidectomy with bilateral central neck dissection and bilateral lateral neck dissection

E. Total thyroidectomy with subtotal parathyroidectomy

Answer: B) Total thyroidectomy

For patients with a high-risk pathogenic variant (C634X and A883F), MTC often develops early in life and annual screening with physical exam, cervical ultrasonography, and biochemical evaluation is recommended to start at age 3 years, with the timing of risk-reducing thyroidectomy generally considered around age 5 to 6 years. For these reasons, total thyroidectomy (Answer B) is the best answer. If calcitonin levels are noted to be elevated or rising prior to this age, thyroidectomy should be performed earlier. Surveillance (Answer A) in patients with hereditary MTC after age 5 to 6 years would be indicated only in individuals with a moderate-risk variant. Prophylactic lymph node dissection in pediatric patients with hereditary MTC is not routinely performed, and lymphadenectomy is only indicated when there are clearly affected lymph nodes (thus, Answers C and D are incorrect). Subtotal parathyroidectomy (Answer E) is not correct because parathyroidectomy will only be indicated in case of confirmed hyperparathyroidism.

Case 2 (continued)

The patient's surgical pathology demonstrates a medullary microcarcinoma, 0.15 cm in largest dimension, with 2 lymph nodes that are negative for carcinoma. Her calcitonin level 3 months after surgery is undetectable.

What further treatment and surveillance for persistent or recurrent disease is recommended for this patient moving forward?

A. TSH suppression with levothyroxine

B. Biochemical studies (thyroid function, calcitonin, CEA) every 3 months

C. Physical examination, cervical ultrasonography, and biochemical studies every 6 months for 1 year, then annually

D. Cervical ultrasonography and biochemical studies every 6 months indefinitely

E. No further treatment or surveillance indicated

Answer: C) Physical exam, cervical ultrasonography, and biochemical studies every 6 months for 1 year, then annually

Since MTC is not a follicular neoplasm, postoperative replacement therapy with levothyroxine should be administered with the objective of maintaining serum TSH levels in the normal range (thus, Answer A is incorrect). The suggested follow-up dictated by the ATA for patients with a high-risk pathogenic variant, which this patient has, is to continue postoperative surveillance with physical exam, ultrasonography of the cervical region, and measurement of serum levels of calcitonin and CEA every 6 months for the first year and annually thereafter (Answer C). Answers B, D, and E do not meet these recommendations.

Case 3

A 34-year-old woman with a personal and family history of a germline exon 10 *RET* pathogenic variant (C620R) leading to MEN 2A (ATA moderate-risk category) presents to clinic for active surveillance.

One and a half years ago, she was diagnosed with metastatic MTC and a pheochromocytoma in the right adrenal gland. Preoperative calcitonin and CEA values are shown (*Table 3*). Preoperative staging scans showed metastatic disease in lateral cervical lymph nodes, bilateral subcentimeter lung nodules, and a single small liver metastasis (biopsy-proven MTC). Surgical resection of the pheochromocytoma was addressed first through a posterior retroperitoneoscopic approach. Three months after adrenalectomy, in the absence of biochemical and structural evidence of pheochromocytoma, as well as re-staging scans showing stable distant metastatic disease, the patient underwent total thyroidectomy with bilateral central and lateral neck dissection.

At today's clinic visit (12 months after neck surgery), she has no concerns and specifically has no flushing or diarrhea. Her calcitonin and CEA are both rising (*Table 3*). Imaging shows stable metastatic lesions in the lungs and a 3-mm increase of the liver lesion over a 12-month interval (1.1 to 1.4 cm). Liver enzymes are within normal limits, the liver lesion is not causing any

Table 3. Patient's Preoperative and Postoperative Calcitonin and CEA Values

Measurement	Preoperative Time of initial diagnosis	Preoperative 3 months after pheochromocytoma resection	Postoperative 6 months after neck surgery	Postoperative 12 months after neck surgery (today's clinic visit)
Calcitonin (reference range ≤7.6 pg/mL [≤2.2 pmol/L])	4968 pg/mL (SI: 1451 pmol/L)	4972 pg/mL (SI: 1452 pmol/L)	1145 pg/mL (SI: 334 pmol/L)	1202 pg/mL (SI: 351 pmol/L)
CEA (reference range ≤3.8 ng/mL [≤3.8 µg/L])	47.6 ng/mL (SI: 47.6 µg/L)	50.9 ng/mL (SI: 50.9 µg/L)	25.5 ng/mL (SI: 25.5 µg/L)	30.2 ng/mL (SI: 30.2 µg/L)

bile duct obstruction, and the lesion is not located close to the Glisson capsule.

Which of the following is the best next step in this patient's management?

A. Start intravenous chemotherapy

B. Start a tyrosine kinase inhibitor

C. Start immune checkpoint inhibitor therapy

D. Continue to observe

E. Give external beam radiotherapy targeting the liver metastasis

Answer: D) Continue to observe

In patients with MEN 2, pheochromocytoma must be resected first to avoid cardiovascular complications in future operative interventions. In this patient who had known distant metastatic disease at the time of initial diagnosis, the intent of neck surgery was not curative but to control disease burden in the neck to prevent tumor invasion into the trachea and esophagus or wrapping around major neck vessels. If the 3-month restaging scans after adrenalectomy had shown rapid metastatic disease progression, a selective RET inhibitor would have been started and the neck surgery deferred. Even though this patient has metastatic disease, the lesions are not rapidly growing and she is asymptomatic. Thus, continuing to observe (Answer D) is the most appropriate. Not only does the patient not meet indications to start systemic treatment (Answer A), but tyrosine kinase inhibitors have completely replaced cytotoxic chemotherapy with the advent of precision oncology. Immunotherapy (Answer C) is not effective treatment of MTC.

External beam radiotherapy (Answer E) would have been appropriate if, in the presence of stable metastatic disease in all other areas, the single liver lesion was continued to rapidly grow or cause biliary obstruction or pain due to its proximity to the Glisson capsule.

Key Learning Points

- MTC is a rare neuroendocrine cancer, arising from parafollicular/C cells of the thyroid.

- Clinical evaluation includes neck inspection and imaging with ultrasonography, evaluating for signs and symptoms indicating excess calcitonin secretion, and evaluating for nonendocrine manifestations (cutaneous lichen amyloidosis, Hirschsprung disease, and oral/eyelid ganglioneuromas).

- Genetic counseling and germline testing is necessary for all patients newly diagnosed with MTC; if a *RET* pathogenic variant is identified, patients can undergo risk-reducing or therapeutic thyroidectomy, depending on the clinical context.

- The timing of and indications for risk-reducing thyroidectomy are based on the aggressiveness of MTC, which depends on the patient's genotype.

- Therapeutic thyroidectomy should include unilateral central neck dissection.

- Follow-up after thyroidectomy consists of clinical, radiological, and laboratory evaluation every 6 months for the first year and yearly thereafter.

References

1. Wells SA, Jr., Asa SL, Dralle H, et al; American Thyroid Association Guidelines Task Force on Medullary Thyroid Carcinoma. Revised American Thyroid Association guidelines for the management of medullary thyroid carcinoma. *Thyroid.* 2015;25(6):567-610. PMID: 25810047

2. Hyde SM, Cote GJ, Grubbs EG. Genetics of multiple endocrine neoplasia type 1/multiple endocrine neoplasia type 2 syndromes. *Endocrinol Metab Clin North Am.* 2017;46(2):491-502. PMID: 28476233

3. Rowland KJ, Chernock RD, Moley JF. Pheochromocytoma in an 8-year-old patient with multiple endocrine neoplasia type 2A: implications for screening. *J Surg Oncol.* 2013;108(4):203-206. PMID: 23868299

4. Moley JF, DeBenedetti MK. Patterns of nodal metastases in palpable medullary thyroid carcinoma: recommendations for extent of node dissection. *Ann Surg.* 1999;229(6):880-887. PMID: 10363903

5. Machens A, Dralle H. Biomarker-based risk stratification for previously untreated medullary thyroid cancer. *J Clin Endocrinol Metab.* 2010;95(6):2655-2663. PMID: 20339026

6. Niederle MB, Riss P, Selberherr A, et al. Omission of lateral lymph node dissection in medullary thyroid cancer without a desmoplastic stromal reaction. *Br J Surg.* 2021;108(2):174-181. PMID: 33704404

7. Wang S, Wang B, Xie C, Ye D. RET proto-oncogene gene mutation is related to cervical lymph node metastasis in medullary thyroid carcinoma. *Endocr Pathol.* 2019;30(4):297-304. PMID: 31494787

8. Cabanillas ME, Hu MI, Jimenez C. Medullary thyroid cancer in the era of tyrosine kinase inhibitors: to treat or not to treat--and with which drug--those are the questions. *J Clin Endocrinol Metab.* 2014;99(12):4390-4396. PMID: 25238206

9. Wells SA Jr, Robinson BG, Gagel RF, et al. Vandetanib in patients with locally advanced or metastatic medullary thyroid cancer: a randomized, double-blind phase III trial. *J Clin Oncol.* 2012;30(2):134-141. PMID: 22025146

10. Elisei R, Schlumberger MJ, Müller SP, et al. Cabozantinib in progressive medullary thyroid cancer. *J Clin Oncol.* 2013;31(29):3639-3646. PMID: 24002501

11. Schlumberger M, Elisei R, Müller S, et al. Overall survival analysis of EXAM, a phase III trial of cabozantinib in patients with radiographically progressive medullary thyroid carcinoma. *Ann Oncol.* 2017;28(11):2813-2819. PMID: 29045520

12. Wirth LJ, Sherman E, Robinson B, et al. Efficacy of selpercatinib in *RET*-altered thyroid cancers. *N Engl J Med.* 2020;383(9):825-835. PMID: 32846061

13. Subbiah V, Hu MI, Wirth LJ, et al. Pralsetinib for patients with advanced or metastatic RET-altered thyroid cancer (ARROW): a multi-cohort, open-label, registrational, phase 1/2 study. *Lancet Diabetes Endocrinol.* 2021;9(8):491-501. PMID: 34118198

Lobectomy for Thyroid Cancer: Update on Indications, Risk Assessment, and Follow-up Strategy

Eyal Robenshtok, MD. Institute of Endocrinology and Davidoff Cancer Center, Rabin Medical Center, Petah-Tikva, Israel; Email: robensht@gmail.com

Educational Objectives

After reviewing this chapter, learners should be able to:

- Communicate to patients the benefits and risks of thyroid lobectomy compared with other treatment options.

- Improve patient selection for thyroid lobectomy.

- Explain the impact of patients' and treating physicians' attitudes and beliefs on the extent of surgery.

- Quantify the risk associated with histological "high-risk" features described on pathology reports.

- Assess the risk associated with follicular thyroid carcinoma (FTC) and determine which patients require completion thyroidectomy.

- Implement follow-up strategies for patients after thyroid lobectomy.

Significance of the Clinical Problem

The incidence of thyroid cancer has increased dramatically during the past 3 decades, mostly due to the diagnosis of small thyroid cancers on neck ultrasonography. In fact, autopsy studies demonstrate thyroid cancer presence in 4% to 11% of the adult population, of whom only a small minority is diagnosed in clinical practice (0.3% of the US adult population according to SEER database).[1] Tailoring treatment according to individual risk assessment is therefore important, with most patients at low risk being suitable candidates for a less aggressive approach, including lobectomy or active surveillance. Multiple studies in recent years demonstrate lobectomy to be a safe and effective treatment for low-risk differentiated thyroid cancer (DTC), with similar survival rates to those of total thyroidectomy. Locoregional recurrence rates are less than 5% and less than 10% with lobectomy and completion thyroidectomy, respectively, in properly selected patients.[2]

With the increased popularity of lobectomy, many challenges have emerged in clinical practice. First, while the 2015 American Thyroid Association (ATA) guidelines included a general recommendation to consider lobectomy for DTC up to 4 cm, many factors should be considered for this selection, including patient age, preferences, tumor characteristics (such as multifocality, location [eg, near the recurrent laryngeal nerve]), and more. Second, the pathology report following lobectomy often includes histological features not known before surgery, including minimal extrathyroidal extension, multifocality, microscopic lymph nodes, and tumor variants. In this chapter, we discuss how to assess these features and how to determine when completion thyroidectomy is required. Third, while the long-term follow-up strategy after total thyroidectomy is well established, in patients undergoing lobectomy there are questions regarding the value of thyroglobulin measurement, proper follow-up for patients with positive thyroglobulin antibodies, and management of nodules in the remaining contralateral lobe.

Practice Gaps

- Lack of knowledge or experience leads to underuse of thyroid lobectomy.

- Good-quality ultrasonography, which is required to properly select patients, is not universally available.

- Patients must be engaged in choosing the extent of surgery according to personal preferences.

- Some of the indications for completion thyroidectomy are controversial. For example, minimal extrathyroidal extension used to be an indication for completion surgery, but recent studies question this indication and support continued surveillance.

Discussion
Lobectomy Outcome and Complication Rate

Assessing oncological outcomes of lobectomy for low-risk DTC requires long-term follow-up and a large sample size, as these patients have low recurrence rates and very low risk of mortality from the disease. It is safe to say that with lobectomy, most patients will be cured of their disease, with a recurrence risk ranging from 4% to 9%, depending on the inclusion criteria, the population evaluated, and how recurrence is defined.[3] When providing information for patients who are considering lobectomy vs other treatment options, we usually quote a 5% recurrence risk, with a slightly higher risk of 9% in young patients.

In patients with low- or low-intermediate risk disease, treatment with either lobectomy or total thyroidectomy, with or without radioiodine (RAI) ablation, is effective with a low recurrence rate. Several recent meta-analyses compared these strategies and reported heterogeneous results, mostly due to low-quality data. While some demonstrated similar outcomes in patients with low- to intermediate-risk disease undergoing lobectomy vs total thyroidectomy + RAI, others found a slightly elevated risk or recurrence with lobectomy (in a recent study 3.8% vs 1% recurrence rate), with most recurrences detected in the remaining contralateral lobe.[4] Overall, these studies demonstrate a small difference in oncological outcome between lobectomy and total thyroidectomy, emphasizing the importance of patient preference and complication risk when selecting the optimal surgical approach.

Complication rates, as expected, are lower with lobectomy that with total thyroidectomy.[4] Patients undergoing lobectomy have significantly lower risk of temporary vocal cord paralysis (3.3% vs 4.5%), temporary hypoparathyroidism (2.2% vs 21.3%), and permanent hypoparathyroidism (0% vs 1.8%).[4] In terms of quality-of-life assessment, several studies have used standardized questionnaires or interviews and reported conflicting results. It seems that quality of life is mostly related to hypothyroidism and the requirement for levothyroxine therapy, rather than to the extent of surgery. Therefore, patients who have a normal TSH concentration before surgery and normal contralateral lobe on ultrasonography are expected to do best after lobectomy, as most will not require levothyroxine therapy.

Selecting Patients for Thyroid Lobectomy

The rate of patients with DTC who are treated with lobectomy (compared with active surveillance or total thyroidectomy) varies significantly among centers and countries, even among high-volume centers of excellence. This is due to the nature of the disease, which is slow-growing with excellent outcomes (in low-risk disease), the type of studies available in the field (mostly retrospective and often with conflicting results), and the various definitions of outcomes (eg, biochemical vs clinical recurrence). Despite these limitations, a growing consensus has developed over recent years on how to select patients for lobectomy. This chapter covers the proper selection of patients, looking at the "lower" threshold of lobectomy vs active surveillance in patients with microscopic papillary thyroid carcinoma (PTC), and the "upper" limits of lobectomy vs total thyroidectomy for larger tumors.

In patients with PTC smaller than 1 cm (microPTC), treatment options generally include active surveillance or thyroid lobectomy. The selection for one approach or the other is based on several factors and not on size alone. A useful framework for decision-making was suggest by Brito et al,[5] which includes ultrasonography features, patient characteristics, and medical team characteristics. This framework was designed for patients with microPTC but is also valuable for deciding the extent of surgery in patients with larger tumors.

Ultrasonography Features

On the basis of sonographic features, patients can be classified as ideal, appropriate, or inappropriate candidates for active surveillance. Patients with tumors suspicious for minimal extrathyroidal extension, adjacent to the recurrent laryngeal nerve, with wide base on the trachea, or with documented growth during follow-up, are inappropriate candidates for active surveillance and should be referred for lobectomy (*Figure 1c*). Patients with tumors with subcapsular locations (not adjacent to the recurrent laryngeal nerve and without extrathyroidal extension), ill-defined margins, multifocal, or fluorodeoxyglucose (FDG)-avid are defined as appropriate candidates for active surveillance, although many patients choose lobectomy (*Figure 1b*). Patients with tumors that are solitary with well-defined margins, surrounded by 2 mm or more of normal thyroid parenchyma are sonographically ideal candidates for active surveillance (*Figure 1a*). In this case, patients or the medical team could choose lobectomy or active surveillance, based on their preferences.

Figure 1. Tumor Suitability for Active Surveillance

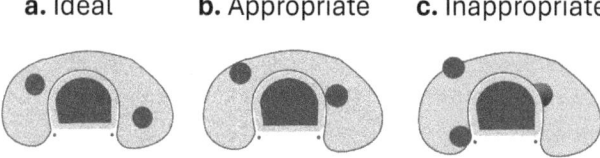

a. Ideal   **b.** Appropriate   **c.** Inappropriate

Tumor location: (a) surrounded by normal tissue; (b) adjacent to the thyroid capsule, without evidence of extrathyroidal extension; and (c) suspicious for extrathyroidal extension, wide base on the trachea, adjacent to the recurrent laryngeal nerve.

Patient Characteristics

A diagnosis of cancer, even a small PTC, is a stressful life event and many patients prefer lobectomy, which offers very high cure rates, rather than active surveillance. This approach is also preferred in patients younger than 18 years and in patients who are unlikely to be adherent to follow-up recommendations. However, in patients who prefer a nonsurgical approach, in older patients (especially those older than 60 years who have a lower risk of growth), and in those who are adherent to follow-up, an active surveillance approach can be chosen.

Medical Team Characteristics

Much of the variability in lobectomy rates among hospitals and countries is related to the medical team beliefs regarding thyroid cancer management. For example, in 2016, the European Association of Nuclear Medicine declined to endorse the ATA guidelines, claiming that most patients with thyroid cancer would benefit from RAI and thus would require total thyroidectomy. Such an approach has led to less use of lobectomy in some European countries compared with the United States. However, since then many studies have demonstrated an excellent outcome with thyroid lobectomy in patients at low risk and even in select patients at intermediate risk.[2,3,6-8] Better knowledge of current literature, which is the goal of this Meet the Professor chapter, could help to tailor the extent of surgery according to tumor characteristics and patient preferences.

In patients with PTC of 1 to 4 cm for whom the ATA guidelines recommend either lobectomy or total thyroidectomy, similar considerations can be used as described above: assessing the tumor characteristics, patient preferences and characteristics, and opinions of the treating team. As long as the tumor is unilateral and confined to the thyroid, lobectomy is a safe and effective treatment option. Tumors surrounded by normal tissue are the best candidates for lobectomy, but subcapsular tumors are eligible since even if minimal extrathyroidal extension is detected in the pathology report, it has little influence on the risk of recurrence.[6] Also, several recent studies demonstrated lobectomy is safe in the presence of contralateral benign nodules, provided that regular ultrasonography follow-up is available to detect the small proportion of patients (~5%) who may need completion surgery.[9] In the few patients who require completion thyroidectomy, treatment with surgery and RAI is effective, and there is no effect on overall survival. Of note, with increasing size of PTC, more patients will have extrathyroidal extension and/or lymph node involvement on ultrasonography, so lobectomy is less common for larger tumors approaching 4 cm.

Importantly, patients who are referred for thyroid lobectomy may end up undergoing total thyroidectomy based on intraoperative findings detected by the surgeon. These findings include gross extrathyroidal extension or macroscopic lymph node involvement not identified on preoperative ultrasonography. While uncommon, patients should be counseled about this possibility before surgery, and the intraoperative findings should be communicated to the treating team to guide further management.

The Pathology Report and Postoperative Risk Stratification: PTC

While lobectomy is performed for tumors presumed to be low risk preoperatively, the pathology report may add new information,

including the presence of minimal extrathyroidal extension, small metastatic lymph nodes, or multifocality. As these histological high-risk features are common (30%-50% of cases), some authors advocate against the widespread use of lobectomy for the treatment of PTC, assuming many would require completion thyroidectomy. However, studies from recent years have demonstrated that as long as these high-risk features are small in size, they have little effect on recurrence risk.[6-9]

- **Minimal extrathyroidal extension:** Multiple studies have evaluated the impact of minimal extrathyroidal extension on disease recurrence and have reported conflicting results due to inclusion of various patient groups (N0 or N1 disease, multifocal or not, different age groups) and various treatments (lobectomy, total thyroidectomy, with or without RAI). In a meta-analysis of patients without lymph node involvement (N0 disease), minimal extrathyroidal extension alone had little effect on recurrence risk after total thyroidectomy (3.5% with extrathyroidal extension vs 2.2% without extrathyroidal extension).[6] This difference was significant due to the large sample size but is not clinically significant as such small differences are not likely to change treatment preferences. While most of these studies evaluated patients following total thyroidectomy, a few studies have evaluated the effect of minimal extrathyroidal extension following lobectomy and reported no significant impact on recurrence risk in tumors up to 2 cm.[6] Of note, some consider posterior extension toward the trachea or the recurrent laryngeal nerve to pose higher recurrence risk (based on limited data), which may be considered an indication for further treatment.

- **Multifocality:** In the 2015 ATA risk stratification system, multifocality was not regarded as a high-risk feature and did not upstage patients from low to intermediate risk, as it has a small effect on recurrence risk.[7] In the uncommon case of numerous tumor foci in the gland, recurrence risk would be higher, but in the common scenario of a few distinct foci, multifocality alone (in the presence of a normal contralateral lobe) should not be an indication for completion thyroidectomy.

- **Small metastatic lymph nodes:** "Subclinical" small central neck metastatic lymph nodes are very common. When prophylactic central neck dissection is performed in patients with PTC with clinically node-negative disease, small metastatic lymph nodes are detected in up to 50%.[10] In the past, these data led many centers to perform prophylactic central neck dissection for most patients with clinically node-negative disease. However, in recent years, several studies have demonstrated similar recurrence rates with or without prophylactic central neck dissection in patients with low-risk disease, but with slightly higher complication rates with lymph node dissection.[10] Therefore, this procedure is less common today in low-risk disease. With this in mind, microscopic "subclinical" lymph nodes detected in pathological specimens seem to have little effect on recurrence risk in patients who have no other high-risk features. This notion is supported by the 2015 ATA guidelines, in which lymph nodes smaller than 2 mm were included in the low-risk category, and it is reasonable to also include in the group slightly larger lymph nodes not seen on preoperative ultrasonography or during surgery.

- **Tall cell variant:** Recent changes in the World Health Organization criteria for the diagnosis of tall cell variant, lowering the threshold to 30% or more tall cells of the tumor cells (from the previous ≥50%), has led to an increase in the diagnosis of this subtype. Typically, these tumors present at a more advanced age and T stage and have higher rates of nodal disease and extrathyroidal extension, leading to higher rates of recurrence. Therefore, the ATA guidelines classify this variant as intermediate risk, which often leads to completion thyroidectomy

when detected after surgery. However, in cases where the tumor is small and limited to the thyroid without any other aggressive histological features, patients may not benefit from total thyroidectomy and RAI, because the recurrence risk is low and since these tumors are less responsive to RAI therapy. Indeed, a recent study from Memorial Sloan Kettering Cancer Center evaluated lobectomy for node-negative tall cell variant PTC up to 4 cm, with excellent results, similar to outcomes with classic PTC.[8] In this study, 93% of patients had T1 disease (up to 2 cm) and 31.4% had minimal extrathyroidal extension. The authors conclude that node-negative tall cell PTC 2 cm or smaller can be satisfactorily managed with thyroid lobectomy, with equivalent oncological outcomes to those of classic PTC. This conclusion is also supported by other studies demonstrating that tall cell variant alone that is smaller than 2 cm and confined to the thyroid without any other aggressive features has low recurrence risk, independent of tall cell percentage.

Overall, mounting evidence suggests that these high-risk histological features that are commonly found after lobectomy are not an indication for completion thyroidectomy or RAI in most cases (if minimal in size). This is reassuring when counseling patients with PTC about lobectomy, as less than 10% are expected to require completion thyroidectomy based on the pathology report.

The Pathology Report and Postoperative Risk Stratification: FTC

Most FTC is diagnosed after surgery that was performed for Bethesda III or IV cytology. Following surgery, and based on the pathology report, a decision must be made whether further treatment is required. Pathological risk stratification for FTC is based on the extent of tumor capsule invasion (minimally invasive or widely invasive) and extent of vascular invasion (minimal or extensive). In 2017, the World

Health Organization Classification of Endocrine Tumors grouped FTC into 3 categories: minimally invasive (capsular invasion only); encapsulated angioinvasive (presence of angioinvasion, regardless of the number of foci); and widely invasive. As widely invasive tumors will be usually evident on preoperative imaging and these patients will undergo total thyroidectomy, in the postlobectomy scenario, only minimally invasive and angioinvasive tumors will be evaluated. With minimally invasive disease (capsular invasion only), multiple studies have demonstrated excellent long-term outcome with lobectomy, and it is a well-accepted treatment even for large tumors. In patients with vascular invasion, decision-making is more complex. First, the number of vessels involved is dependent on the extent of tumor processing and how many slides are evaluated. If tumor processing is partial, vascular invasion might be missed or undervalued. Therefore, full tumor processing is required to assess the whole tumor capsule with its vessels. Second, the criteria of "true" angioinvasion is somewhat controversial. The presence of tumor cells in the vessel's lumen is insufficient to diagnose vascular invasion, and more rigid criteria of tumor tissue in the vessel covered with endothelium and with thrombus adherent to the tumor is much more predictive of distant metastases. Third, some authors have suggested subdivision into 2 groups: extensive vascular invasion (≥4 foci) with significant risk of distant metastases and requiring total thyroidectomy, and focal angioinvasion (<4 foci) with low risk of distant metastases and be managed with lobectomy. However, other authors found that even patients with 2 or more foci of vascular invasion, especially in patients older than 55 years with large tumors, might have worse clinical outcomes and require completion thyroidectomy.[11]

In summary, patients with FTC require detailed histological evaluation. Patients with minimal capsular invasion only and/or 1 focus of angioinvasion can be safely followed without completion thyroidectomy. Patients with 2 to 3 foci of vascular invasion should be evaluated based on age and tumor size, as older patients with larger tumors would probably benefit from completion thyroidectomy. Patients with extensive vascular invasion (≥4 foci) should routinely be referred for completion surgery.

TSH Target Following Lobectomy

TSH target in patients following lobectomy has changed since the 2015 ATA guidelines, which recommended a TSH concentration in the mid to lower reference range (0.5-2.0 mIU/L) based on low-quality evidence and with weak recommendation. The guidelines noted there was little evidence to guide TSH targets in this group and that more research was needed. This recommendation has led many patients to receive levothyroxine therapy, sometimes for life even with a TSH value within the upper normal range. Recently, a large study by Xu et al[12] published in *Thyroid* evaluated 2297 patients treated with lobectomy and found that the mean TSH concentration during follow-up was not associated with recurrence risk, and, therefore, a normal TSH reference range is recommended after lobectomy. These data are important, as they greatly decrease the need for levothyroxine after surgery, improving patients' quality of life. This should be noted in the preoperative counseling process, especially for patients who express their concern about levothyroxine therapy.

Postoperative Thyroglobulin Levels

The prognostic value of thyroglobulin following lobectomy has gained interest in recent years. In 2016, Momesso et al[13] proposed a new response to therapy assessment tool for patients treated with lobectomy, suggesting excellent response to therapy based on a nonstimulated thyroglobulin concentration less than 30 ng/mL together with undetectable thyroglobulin antibodies. While this was an attractive tool that could have potentially allowed better postoperative risk stratification, several later studies evaluated this threshold and found significant overlap between thyroglobulin levels in patients with or without recurrence, with no threshold that could distinguish between the 2 groups.[14] This is due to considerable interpatient variability in remaining lobe size, TSH levels, presence of lymphocytic thyroiditis, thyroid nodules, and other factors. This is also true for patients with positive thyroglobulin antibodies, which are not predictive of recurrence after lobectomy. Therefore, long-term follow-up after lobectomy is based mostly on neck ultrasonography, which is very effective in detecting locoregional recurrences. Of note, despite the thyroglobulin concentration not being useful in detecting local recurrence, it may be significant when extremely elevated (in the hundreds or thousands) to detect rare cases of unsuspected distant metastases.

Clinical Case Vignettes

Case 1

A 59-year-old woman is diagnosed with a 1.5 × 1.2 × 1.1-cm right thyroid nodule (*Figure 2*) with Bethesda VI cytology compatible with PTC. The rest of the thyroid is normal in size and texture, and there are no suspicious lymph nodes. Her TSH is normal, she has no relevant medical history, no family history of thyroid disorders, and no history of radiation exposure. She prefers minimal intervention to avoid levothyroxine therapy and asks about active surveillance or radiofrequency ablation.

Figure 2. Ultrasonography Image of the 1.5 × 1.2 × 1.1-cm Nodule

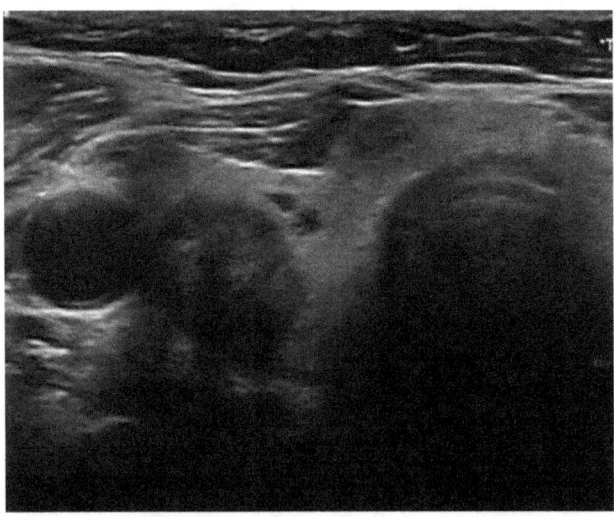

[Color—Print (Color Gallery page CG39) or web & ePub editions]

Which of the following treatments would be best?

A. Total thyroidectomy
B. Radiofrequency ablation
C. Active surveillance
D. Lobectomy
E. Total thyroidectomy and prophylactic level VI dissection

Answer: D) Lobectomy

The tumor is larger than 1 cm and is situated along the posterior aspect on the thyroid, and although there is no evidence of extrathyroidal extension on ultrasonography, minimal extension might be present. Therefore, this tumor is not suitable for active surveillance (Answer C) or radiofrequency ablation (Answer B).

While either lobectomy (Answer D) or total thyroidectomy (Answer A) may be considered, the patient's wish for limited intervention and avoidance of levothyroxine therapy makes lobectomy a preferable option for her. Prophylactic level VI dissection (Answer E) has not been proven to be sufficiently effective in this scenario in preventing recurrence. Total thyroidectomy would allow better follow-up with thyroglobulin and RAI therapy if required but is associated with higher risk of complications and lifelong levothyroxine therapy. Before surgery, she should be counseled about the unlikely scenario in which the surgeon might detect gross extrathyroidal extension or macroscopic lymph node involvement during surgery that was not detected on ultrasonography, which would require total thyroidectomy. If surgery goes as planned, she will likely not require levothyroxine treatment, given a normal baseline TSH, a normal-looking contralateral lobe, and a TSH target within the normal range (and not up to 2.0 mIU/L). If the pathology demonstrates PTC limited to the thyroid or even minimal extrathyroidal extension (not seen by the surgeon), she would be able to continue follow-up without completion thyroidectomy.

Case 2

A 56-year-old woman undergoes workup for 2 thyroid nodules, a large right hypoechoic 4.6-cm nodule with Bethesda IV cytology (follicular lesion) and a left isoechoic 1.1-cm nodule with a benign cytology. Neck ultrasonography does not show any abnormal lymph nodes. She has no local symptoms and no family history of thyroid disease. She has a diagnostic right lobectomy, which, on pathology, demonstrates a 4.1-cm FTC with 2 foci of tumor capsule invasion, no vascular invasion, and no extrathyroidal extension. One month after surgery, her TSH is 3.4 mIU/L and thyroglobulin is 25 ng/mL (25 µg/L) with normal thyroglobulin antibodies.

Which of the following is the best recommendation?

A. Continued surveillance

B. Completion thyroidectomy and radioiodine

C. Completion thyroidectomy alone

D. TSH suppression to less than 0.5 ng/mL

E. Genetic sequencing of the tumor

Answer: A) Continued surveillance

The initial surgery was diagnostic lobectomy, and presence of a small contralateral benign nodule does change the extent of surgery. On pathology, minimally invasive FTC is detected, with no vascular invasion. Careful attention is required to ensure sufficient slides were examined (usually 10 slides per 1 cm of tumor) and vascular invasion was specifically looked for. In this case, the entire capsule was processed, and no vascular invasion was detected. The risk of metastases from this tumor is extremely low, and therefore lobectomy alone is sufficient and continued surveillance can be recommended (Answer A). Completion thyroidectomy (Answer C) or radioiodine (Answer B) is not required.

It is important to note that in cases where quality pathologic examination is not available and the status of angioinvasion is not well documented, completion thyroidectomy may be considered to allow thyroglobulin assessment and/or RAI ablation (especially in the presence of thyroglobulin antibodies).

Genetic sequencing of the tumor (Answer E) would not change management, and TSH should be maintained within the normal range, not suppressed to less than 0.5 mIU/L (Answer D).

Case 3

A 36-year-old man had a left lobectomy 3 years ago for a 1.3-cm PTC confined to the thyroid, without lymph node involvement. He has no family history of thyroid disease. During follow-up, he is doing well without levothyroxine therapy and continues to work full time. On ultrasonography, the right lobe is normal in size and texture, and on the left side there is an isoechoic 0.5 × 0.7-cm thyroid bed nodule (seen on the first postoperative ultrasound, which has remained stable). On review of preoperative ultrasonography, the tumor was located in the anterior aspect of the lobe. His blood tests during the 3 years of follow-up are shown:

Measurement	First year	Second year	Third year
TSH	2.2 mIU/L	3.1 mIU/L	2.8 mIU/L
Thyroglobulin	44 ng/mL (SI: 44 µg/L)	50 ng/mL (SI: 50 µg/L)	59 ng/mL (SI: 59 µg/L)
Thyroglobulin antibodies	Negative	Negative	Negative

What is the significance of the findings detected during follow-up?

A. Thyroid bed nodule is an indication for completion thyroidectomy and RAI therapy

B. Thyroglobulin increase over time and the thyroid bed nodule are not an indication for further treatment

C. Thyroglobulin increase over time indicates disease progression and requires completion thyroidectomy and RAI therapy

D. Thyroglobulin increase over time is an indication for FDG PET-CT

E. Whole-body scan with RAI may help detect residual disease

Answer: B) Thyroglobulin increase over time and the thyroid bed nodule are not an indication for further treatment

Small discrete nodules are often found in the thyroid bed on postoperative ultrasonography, most of which are benign lesions due to residual thyroid tissue, postoperative fibrosis, or suture granulomas. However, a small fraction represent persistent thyroid cancer (<3%). In the absence of suspicious sonographic features (such as discrete hypoechoic nodule, microcalcifications) and without a history of positive lymph nodes at initial surgery, the malignancy rate is even lower.[15] Therefore, the presence of a small isoechoic thyroid bed nodule in this case does not require further treatment (Answer A), and continued follow-up is recommended (Answer B).

Thyroglobulin levels following lobectomy are not predictive of recurrence unless they are extremely high (in the hundreds or thousands). A study that evaluated the thyroglobulin-to-TSH ratio over time showed a gradual increase after lobectomy, even in patients without recurrence.[14] This may be due to compensatory hypertrophy of the remaining lobe over time. Therefore, a moderate increase in thyroglobulin levels, as demonstrated in this case, is common and is not an indication for further therapy (Answer C). In the unusual cases where thyroglobulin levels after lobectomy are in the hundreds, it may be prudent to consider further imaging or even completion thyroidectomy to avoid missing the rare cases of unsuspected distant metastases. However, thyroglobulin levels in the current patient are not unusually high, and there is no clear indication for FDG PET-CT (Answer D).

RAI whole-body scans (Answer E) have no role after lobectomy, as the normal lobe will take up RAI and residual disease, if present, will not be demonstrated.

Key Learning Points

- Lobectomy is a safe and effective treatment for low-risk disease, with lower complication rates compared with those of total thyroidectomy and without the need for levothyroxine therapy in most cases. Therefore, it is the preferable surgery for most patients with low-risk disease.

- Patient selection for lobectomy is based on sonographic characteristics (tumor location and sonographic features), patient characteristics (age, preference for minimal or maximal intervention, follow-up adherence), and medical team characteristics (treatment approach, availability of quality ultrasonography and high-volume surgeons).

- "High-risk" histological features in patients with PTC, including minimal extrathyroidal extension, small lymph node metastases or multifocality, when minimal in size, have little effect on the risk of recurrence and are not a clear indication for completion thyroidectomy.

- Patients with minimally invasive FTC should be treated with lobectomy alone. In patients with angioinvasion, the risk of metastases increases with the number of vessels involved, larger tumor size, and patient age.

- The TSH target following lobectomy for patients at low risk is within the reference range.

- Follow-up in patients who have had lobectomy is based on neck ultrasonography. The thyroglobulin concentration and trend over time have limited value in detecting recurrence.

References

1. Furuya-Kanamori L, Bell KJL, Clark J, Glasziou P, Doi SAR. Prevalence of differentiated thyroid cancer in autopsy studies over six decades: a meta-analysis. *J Clin Oncol.* 2016;34(30):3672–3679. PMID: 27601555
2. Bojoga A, Koot A, Bonenkamp J, et al. The impact of the extent of surgery on the long-term outcomes of patients with low-risk differentiated non-medullary thyroid cancer: a systematic meta-analysis. *J Clin Med.* 2020;9(7):2316. PMID: 32708218
3. Vaisman F, Shaha A, Fish S, Michael Tuttle R. Initial therapy with either thyroid lobectomy or total thyroidectomy without radioactive iodine remnant ablation is associated with very low rates of structural disease recurrence in

properly selected patients with differentiated thyroid cancer. *Clin Endocrinol (Oxf)*. 2011;75(1):112-119. PMID: 21521273

4. Hsiao V, Light TJ, Adil AA, et al. Complication rates of total thyroidectomy vs hemithyroidectomy for treatment of papillary thyroid microcarcinoma: a systematic review and meta-analysis. *JAMA Otolaryngol Head Neck Surg.* 2022;148(6):531-539. PMID: 35511129

5. Brito JP, Ito Y, Miyauchi A, Tuttle RM. A clinical framework to facilitate risk stratification when considering an active surveillance alternative to immediate biopsy and surgery in papillary microcarcinoma. *Thyroid.* 2016;26(1):144-149. PMID: 26414743

6. Diker-Cohen T, Hirsch D, Shimon I, et al. Impact of minimal extra-thyroid extension in differentiated thyroid cancer: systematic review and meta-analysis. *J Clin Endocrinol Metab.* 2018 [Online ahead of print] PMID: 29506045

7. Cho JS, Kim HK. Unilateral multifocality is not a risk factor for recurrence after thyroid lobectomy: a study of 1,684 patients with differentiated thyroid cancer. *In Vivo.* 2023;37(4):1802-1808. PMID: 37369469

8. Woods RSR, Fitzgerald CWR, Valero C, et al. Surgical management of T1/T2 node-negative papillary thyroid cancer with tall cell histology: is lobectomy enough? *Surgery.* 2023;173(1):246-251. PMID: 36257862

9. Ritter A, Bachar G, Hirsch D, et al. Natural history of contralateral nodules after lobectomy in patients with papillary thyroid carcinoma. *J Clin Endocrinol Metab.* 2017;103(2):407-414. PMID: 29240898

10. Alsubaie KM, Alsubaie HM, Alzahrani FR, et al. Prophylactic central neck dissection for clinically node-negative papillary thyroid carcinoma. *Laryngoscope.* 2022;132(6):1320-1328. PMID: 34708877

11. Yamazaki H, Sugino K, Katoh R, et al. Role of the degree of vascular invasion in predicting prognosis of follicular thyroid carcinoma. *J Clin Endocrinol Metab.* 2023 [Online ahead of print]

12. Xu S, Huang Y, Huang H, et al. Optimal serum thyrotropin level for patients with papillary thyroid carcinoma after lobectomy. *Thyroid.* 2022;32(2):138-144. PMID: 34617446

13. Momesso DP, Vaisman F, Yang SP, et al. Dynamic risk stratification in patients with differentiated thyroid cancer treated without radioactive iodine. *J Clin Endocrinol Metab.* 2016;101(7):2692-2700. PMID: 27023446

14. Park S, Jeon MJ, Oh H-S, et al. Changes in serum thyroglobulin levels after lobectomy in patients with low-risk papillary thyroid cancer. *Thyroid.* 2018;28(8):997-1003. PMID: 29845894

15. Frates MC, Parziale MP, Alexander EK, Barletta JA, Benson CB. Role of sonographic characteristics of thyroid bed lesions identified following thyroidectomy in the diagnosis or exclusion of recurrent cancer. *Radiology.* 2021;299(2):374-380. PMID: 33650902

Molecular Profiling as a Tool for Management of Thyroid Nodules

Jennifer A. Sipos, MD. Division of Endocrinology, The Ohio State University, Columbus, OH; Email: jennifer.sipos@osumc.edu

Educational Objectives

After reviewing the chapter, learners should be able to:

- Discuss the various types of indeterminate cytology with a particular emphasis on the recent changes in the Bethesda cytologic classification system.

- Review the most commonly used molecular tests in patients with thyroid nodules with a focus on the strengths/limitations of each.

- Outline the clinical indications for molecular testing for patients with thyroid nodules.

Significance of the Clinical Problem

Thyroid nodules are increasingly prevalent in an aging population. The distinction of benign and malignant neoplasms relies heavily on the sonographic appearance of the nodule and, when indicated, the cytologic evaluation. However, even with cytology, not all nodules are readily classifiable. Up to 30% of nodules are indeterminate on FNA, although a recent analysis suggests this number may be escalating, with rates as high as 60% or more.[1] For the purposes of this review, nodules with a cytologic diagnosis of atypia of undetermined significance (AUS) and follicular neoplasm are included in the indeterminate category because of their relatively low rate of malignancy (approximately 10%-30%).[2] Since most nodules in this category are benign, performing diagnostic surgery for all indeterminate cytology leads to a high rate of "unnecessary" procedures and associated risks of complications. Molecular testing of nodules to rule out malignancy offers the opportunity to enrich the surgical pool with a higher rate of therapeutic rather than diagnostic procedures. Worldwide, a number of commercially available tests have been developed to stratify indeterminate nodules. This chapter will review the most commonly used tests in the United States with a discussion of the strengths and limitations of each. Additionally, the clinical indications for molecular testing will be outlined. Finally, this chapter will identify the gaps in the current knowledge about the use of molecular testing with an emphasis on important areas for future research.

Practice Gaps

- Confusion about the appropriate clinical indications for use of molecular testing.

- Lack of data regarding optimal long-term surveillance strategy of cytologically indeterminate, molecularly benign nodules.

- Hesitation about the use of the molecular tests for oncocytic tumors.

Discussion

Introduction

The evaluation of a thyroid nodule should be holistic, considering the sonographic pattern, cytologic features, and patient factors to derive a malignancy risk assessment and thereby inform management decisions. The decision to perform FNA of a thyroid nodule is largely based on sonographic appearance, but other factors, including patient age and comorbidities, should be taken into account. FNA of nodules with a very low-, low-, or intermediate-risk sonographic pattern and a lack of other radiologic findings concerning for an aggressive thyroid malignancy may be eschewed in older patients, especially those with significant comorbidities that may shorten their life expectancy.[3] Considering FNA at a lower size threshold may be appropriate for patients with a high risk for malignancy, such as those with a family history of thyroid cancer or childhood radiation exposure. Existing sonographic risk stratification systems (SRSSs) do not account for such demographic factors in the determination of when to perform FNA. Nonetheless, it is important for the clinician to weigh these issues in the evaluation and management of thyroid nodules.

Ultrasound Risk Stratification Systems

Several SRSSs are available to aid in the determination of when to perform FNA. While each SRSS has its strengths and limitations, generally all systems categorize nodules similarly, particularly in the low- and high-risk categories.[4] The main difference in the performance parameters of these systems is derived from the size thresholds used for recommending FNA.[5] Specifically, the American Thyroid Association (ATA) SRSS, which uses a smaller size threshold for FNA, is associated with high sensitivity and lower specificity. The American College of Radiology (ACR) Thyroid Imaging Reporting and Data System (TIRADS), which uses a larger size threshold, has a higher

specificity and lower sensitivity. When the ACR-TIRADS size thresholds are imposed on ATA-classified nodules, the specificity increases and the sensitivity declines, similar to that seen with ACR-TIRADS classification. Similarly, when the size thresholds for FNA of the ATA SRSS are imposed on ACR-TIRADS–classified nodules, the sensitivity improves and specificity declines.[5] Thus, sensitivity and specificity of an individual SRSS are inextricably linked with the system's size thresholds used for recommendation of FNA.

All SRSSs are optimally designed to identify papillary thyroid cancers. Most studies evaluating the performance parameters of SRSSs exclude nodules with indeterminate cytology, which by default eliminates many follicular thyroid cancers (FTC) from the performance analysis. Indeed, a meta-analysis examining the performance of SRSSs, which included 9 studies with 19,494 nodules, found that only 1.5% of cancers were FTC.[6] As such, it is important to bear this significant limitation in mind when evaluating nodules and assigning malignancy risk based on the sonographic appearance. In general, nodules with a high-risk sonographic appearance represent papillary thyroid cancers, as these tumors are more likely to be solid and hypoechoic and have punctate echogenic foci, taller-than-wide shape, and/or infiltrative margins.[7] In contrast, follicular-patterned tumors are more likely to have a low- or intermediate-risk sonographic appearance.[7]

Epidemiology of Indeterminate Cytology

Historically, up to one-third of aspirated nodules were designated as cytologically indeterminate.[2] However, recent studies have demonstrated that an increasing proportion of nodules are being diagnosed as having a diagnosis of AUS. In one study, a diagnosis of AUS was seen in 21.3% of nodules in 2014, whereas in 2021, 51.5% of nodules were so categorized.[1] Several possibilities exist to explain the rise in indeterminate cytology, including increasing reliance on molecular testing by cytopathologists, lower rates of FNA for nodules with a clearly benign sonographic pattern, or an escalation in the incidence (or detection) of follicular-patterned tumors. Regardless of the cause, it is incumbent on the clinician to have a strong understanding of how to triage indeterminate thyroid nodules.

The Bethesda System for Reporting Thyroid Cytopathology

The Bethesda System for reporting thyroid cytopathology was recently updated.[2] This third edition made important changes in the classification of nodules, including the use of only one name for each of the 6 diagnostic categories (*Table 1*). The term "follicular lesion of undetermined significance" (FLUS) was dropped from the Bethesda III class to avoid confusion in reporting and management.[2] Additionally, the terms "suspicious for follicular neoplasm & SFN" were deleted to avoid confusion with Bethesda Class V, or "suspicious for malignancy" (SFM).[2] Further, the risk of malignancy (ROM) with each Bethesda class was updated, although it is important to recognize that these estimates may be artificially elevated by selection bias since benign nodules do not routinely undergo surgical excision.[2] Within the AUS diagnostic category, the authors acknowledged that there is a difference in malignancy risk based on the pattern of atypia seen, thus contributing to the wide reported ROM within this class. Specifically, nodules with predominantly nuclear atypia harbor a higher ROM than those with architectural atypia or oncocytic cell (previously called Hurthle cell) predominance.[2] Consequently, the authors recommend subcategorization of the AUS diagnosis into 2 groups: "nuclear" and "other" to further inform the management decisions.[2]

Table 1. Bethesda Class and Diagnostic Cytologic Category and Associated ROM With Management Recommendations

Diagnostic category (Bethesda class)	Risk of malignancy, mean (range)	Usual management
Nondiagnostic (I)	13% (5%-20%)	Repeat FNA under ultrasound guidance
Benign (II)	4% (2%-7%)	Clinical and ultrasonography follow-up
Atypia of undetermined significance (III)	22% (13%-30%)	Repeat FNA, molecular testing, lobectomy, or surveillance
Follicular neoplasm (IV)	30% (23%-34%)	Molecular testing or diagnostic lobectomy
Suspicious for malignancy (V)	74% (67%-83%)	Molecular testing, total thyroidectomy or lobectomy
Malignant (VI)	97% (97%-100%)	Total thyroidectomy or lobectomy

Adapted with permission from Ali SZ et al. Thyroid, 2023; 33(9): 1039-1044. © Mary Ann Liebert, Inc.[2]

Although most nodules with indeterminate cytology (AUS and follicular neoplasm) have a low ROM that renders surgery impractical for all, the malignancy risk is too high to overlook, necessitating further evaluation for most patients. It is in this context that molecular testing has taken such a prominent role.

Commercially Available Molecular Tests

The optimal molecular test provides insight into which nodules have a sufficiently low ROM to warrant observation alone (high negative predictive value), while also providing a relatively high specificity to indicate when a malignancy is present (high positive predictive value). Three main tests are commercially available in the United States and in many other countries: Afirma gene sequencing classifier (GSC), ThyGeNEXT/ ThyraMIR, and ThyroSeq version 3 (*Table 2, following page*). As our understanding of the molecular underpinnings of thyroid cancer has evolved, each of these tests has undergone modifications to further improve performance parameters since initial release.

Table 2. Comparison of 3 Commercially Available Molecular Tests

Comparisons	Afirma GSC	ThyroSeq version 3	ThyGeNEXT + ThyraMIR
Testing platform description	RNA sequencing	DNA and RNA sequencing	DNA sequencing & microRNA
Quality control classifier for identification of follicular cells, oncocytic cells, parathyroid cells, and C cells?	Yes	Yes	Yes
Result reporting	Benign/ suspicious	Negative/ currently negative/ positive	Negative/ moderate/ positive
Able to be performed on previously collected specimens/ slides?	No	Yes	Yes
Prospective validation study	No[a]	Yes	No

[a] Validation of the GSC was performed on samples collected during the initial prospective validation study of the gene expression classifier.

It is important to understand how these tests perform in a clinical setting. In particular, the key parameters of positive predictive value and negative predictive value are dependent on disease prevalence. Specifically, as disease prevalence declines, negative predictive value increases and positive predictive value decreases. And conversely, with a rise in disease incidence, the negative predictive value decreases and the positive predictive value increases. Consequently, when comparing the performance of 2 or more tests, it is important to make a note of the disease prevalence as this alters the negative predictive value and positive predictive value. Furthermore,

prior to ordering a molecular test, the clinician should be aware of the disease prevalence in that particular clinical setting. If the ROM is higher than what was seen in the validation study for the molecular test being used, the negative predictive value will be lower. Consequently, a negative result may not truly rule out cancer with the same degree of confidence.

Another important parameter in molecular testing is the benign call rate, which represents the percentage of molecular tests that are resulted as benign (negative). When disease prevalence is low and the negative predictive value is high, the benign call rate reflects those patients who will be managed similarly to those who have a benign cytologic diagnosis. By allowing for monitoring rather than diagnostic surgery, the benign call rate is an important parameter for assessing the clinical utility of a test. If a benign call rate is very low, the test is not effectively triaging most benign nodules.

Prospective validation studies are a critical component of the determination that a particular molecular test correctly identifies which indeterminate biopsies are benign compared with how the gold standard (surgical histopathology) identifies which are benign. It is important to understand how these tests perform in a wide range of patient populations and across practice types. Additionally, these tests should be analyzed in a blinded fashion, such that the pathologists are not aware of the molecular testing results when assessing the histopathology.

RNA-Based Testing
The Afirma GSC[8] (Veracyte, Inc) is an updated version of the initial gene expression classifier that was released in 2011. The GSC provides a dichotomous result of "benign" or "suspicious," using a proprietary algorithm with multiple classifiers and RNA sequencing to distinguish the expression patterns of more than 10,000 genes.[8] The initial quality control classifiers also identify parathyroid lesions, medullary thyroid carcinoma, *BRAF* V600E pathogenic variants, and *RET/PTC* fusions. Further, an oncocytic cell index was added that detects transcript levels of nuclear and

mitochondrial RNAs and identifies chromosomal-level loss events commonly seen in this tumor type.[8] The clinical validity of this test relied on samples obtained from the initial validation study of the gene expression classifier. This newer iteration improved the specificity by 36% while maintaining a high sensitivity (91%) and negative predictive value (96%).[8] Real-world experience studies have demonstrated that the revised test performs better than the original version (gene expression classifier) with a higher benign call rate and positive predictive value with persistently elevated sensitivity. Furthermore, with GSC, the benign call rate increased 2.5-fold for oncocytic neoplasms.[9]

The specific somatic alterations detected with the GSC are now available as a supplementary panel called the Xpression Atlas. This includes 593 genes with 905 variants and 235 fusions. Additionally, telomerase reverse transcriptase promoter pathogenic variants may be detected with a special request (this is a DNA-based analysis). Although these data are not validated to drive clinical decision-making, the information may be useful for patients with refractory or progressive thyroid cancer to aid in the identification of driver mutations that would alter therapy.

DNA-Based Testing
ThyroSeq version 3 is a DNA-based expanded analysis of 2 earlier versions that incorporates more recently discovered genomic alterations associated with thyroid cancer.[10] After determination of adequate cellularity, the sample is evaluated by the cellular composition classifier for detection of parathyroid cells, C cells, and nonthyroidal cells. Upon completion of the initial classifier phase, the sample is analyzed with next-generation sequencing of DNA and RNA to identify single nucleotide variants, indels (short insertions or deletions), fusions, gene expression, and copy number alterations in 112 genes.[10] The detected alterations are associated with a score based on the associated malignancy risk; the score from the sum of all identified alterations aids in the classification of the test result as "negative" (score of zero or 1) or "positive" (score

of 2 or more). The report includes the score and the specific genetic alterations for each nodule tested. This information may also be used in the identification of targetable driver mutations in iodine-refractory thyroid cancers.

A prospective, multicenter, blinded cohort study of 286 nodules with Bethesda III and IV cytology found ThyroSeq version 3 demonstrated a 94% sensitivity and 82% specificity with a negative predictive value of 97% and positive predictive value of 66% when cancer/noninvasive follicular thyroid neoplasm with papillarylike nuclear features prevalence was 28%.[10] Real-world validation studies have confirmed the high sensitivity and found a benign call rate of 80% with Bethesda III cytology and approximately 50% for nodules with Bethesda IV cytology.[11] Although few nodules with a negative result have been resected, the rate of missed malignancy appears to be low.[11,12]

Multiplatform Testing
ThyGeNEXT + ThyraMIR (Interpace Diagnostics) combines an initial expanded variant panel with a reflex 10 microRNA panel.[13] If the initial panel fails to identify an alteration, the microRNA testing is triggered. The test results are reported in 1 of 3 categories: negative, moderate, or positive based on the findings of the variant panel and the microRNA thresholds.

Prospective validation testing of this platform has not been undertaken. The performance parameters are based on a multicenter retrospective analysis of archived FNA cytology slides from 197 nonconsecutive patients with Bethesda III, IV, and V cytology who later underwent surgical resection.[13] With a cancer/noninvasive follicular thyroid neoplasm with papillarylike nuclear features prevalence of 36%, the test demonstrated 95% sensitivity and 90% specificity. An advantage of this platform is that it can be performed from previously collected FNA samples. Prospective, blinded validation studies are needed to confirm the performance characteristics of this molecular test.[13]

Head-to-Head Comparison of the Tests

There are very limited data directly comparing the performance characteristics of the molecular tests. A recent single-center, parallel, prospective, block-randomized clinical trial compared the performance characteristics of ThyroSeq v3 and the GSC in nodules with AUS and follicular neoplasm cytology.[14] They found the performance parameters were very similar and concluded that there was no significant difference between the 2 tests.

When to Use Molecular Testing

The sonographic appearance of a nodule may alter the malignancy risk prediction of a cytologically indeterminate nodule. Nodules with AUS cytology and a suspicious sonographic pattern have a higher ROM than nodules with low- or intermediate-risk sonographic patterns. Indeed, one prospective study[15] demonstrated that nodules with low- and intermediate-risk sonographic patterns had a ROM of 21% to 24% based on cytology alone. The addition of a suspicious molecular test increased the ROM to 56% to 66%, further enhancing the clinical decision-making in favor of surgical removal. In contrast, the ROM for high-risk sonographic-patterned nodules was 77.8% to 80% by cytology alone, and the addition of a suspicious molecular testing result increased the ROM to 87.5% to 100%. The authors propose that the higher-risk patterns have a sufficiently high ROM to justify proceeding directly to surgery and that molecular testing adds little to further enhance the diagnostic predictive value.

Patient preference should also be considered before ordering a molecular test. Molecular analysis should not be performed if the patient is inclined to pursue surgical removal regardless of the test result, as it only adds cost without a meaningful impact on clinical management. While some have advocated for the use of molecular testing to guide the extent of surgery (ie, lobectomy vs total thyroidectomy), a rigorous analysis of this approach in terms of cost and outcomes has not been undertaken. As such,

prior to ordering molecular testing, the provider should have a careful discussion with the patient regarding their symptoms, the long-term management plan, and the expected outcomes.

Long-Term Follow-Up of Benign Molecular Test Results

There are few studies regarding the long-term outcomes of nodules with a benign, newer-generation molecular test result. A single center analysis[12] found that 84% of nodules (67/80) with a benign GSC result that were nonoperatively followed up remained sonographically stable during a median surveillance of 34 months. There were no missed malignancies identified in the 9 nodules that went on to have a repeated FNA or surgery due to nodule growth. Similarly, 84% of nodules (69/82) with a negative ThyroSeq version 3 result remained stable on serial ultrasonography.[12] Eight nodules underwent either a repeated FNA and/or surgery; one malignancy was identified. Additional study is needed to determine the optimal surveillance intervals between ultrasonography and duration of follow-up for molecularly benign nodules.

Clinical Case Vignettes
Case 1

A 53-year-old woman presents with an incidentally detected thyroid nodule identified on chest CT during evaluation for pulmonary embolism. Her TSH value is 2.9 mIU/L. Ultrasonography reveals a sonographically high-risk nodule (ATA high risk/ACR-TR5) that measures 1.3 × 0.9 × 1.5 cm (*Figure 1, following page*).

FNA cytology is interpreted as AUS with identification of nuclear atypia.

Figure 1. 1.3 × 0.9 × 1.5-cm Thyroid Nodule

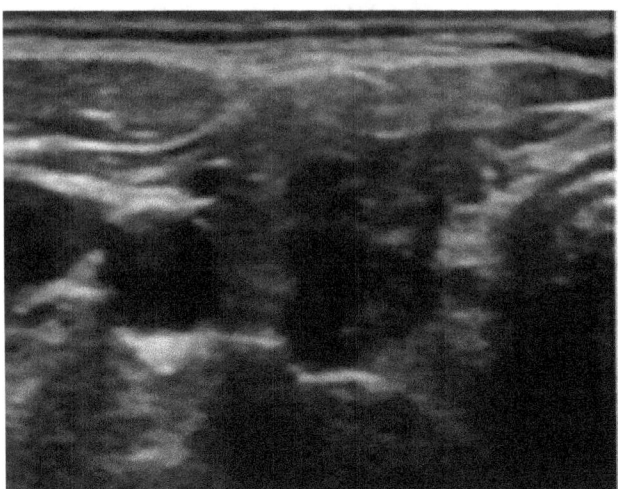

Which of the following is the best next step?

A. Observation

B. Lobectomy

C. Molecular testing

D. Radioactive iodine uptake/scan

Answer: B) Lobectomy

This nodule has a ROM of at least 50% based on its sonographic appearance alone. Additionally, the finding of nuclear atypia (as opposed to architectural atypia) increases the ROM on the higher end of the spectrum associated with an AUS diagnosis. Molecular testing (Answer C) is unlikely to further inform the ROM for this already high-risk lesion and is unnecessary in this clinical scenario. With a ROM greater than 50%, it is clinically reasonable to proceed with surgery (Answer B).

Observation (or active surveillance) (Answer A) is a reasonable option for some small cancers and, by extension, some cytologically indeterminate nodules. This is not the optimal choice for this patient because of the nodule's posterior location and possible extrathyroidal extension anteriorly.

An uptake scan (Answer D) is also not the correct option because the patient's TSH concentration is normal. Functional imaging is unlikely to reveal a toxic nodule. Demonstration of a warm or cold nodule would not be helpful.

Another option in this case would be to consider a repeated FNA, although this was not provided as an answer option. Given the highly suspicious sonographic appearance, a benign cytology diagnosis should raise the concern for a possible false-negative result and prompt another FNA.

Case 2

A 35-year-old woman is found to have a thyroid nodule on routine physical examination. She has no compressive symptoms. There is no relevant medical history (including no radiation exposure) and no family history of thyroid cancer. Her mother has hypothyroidism.

The patient's TSH value is 6.1 mIU/L. Neck ultrasonography reveals a 1.7 × 1.8 × 2.2-cm solid, isoechoic nodule with no suspicious sonographic features (ATA low risk/ACR-TR3) (*Figure 2, following page*).

FNA is performed and is interpreted as Bethesda IV with oncocytic cell predominance.

Which of the following is the best next step in management?

A. Lobectomy

B. Radiofrequency ablation

C. Observation

D. Molecular testing

Answer: D) Molecular testing

Early versions of molecular tests that relied primarily on genomic alterations associated with papillary and follicular thyroid cancers were of very low specificity and had a benign call rate of 16% to 26% with oncocytic cytology (the results were nearly always "suspicious" but most were benign). Consequently, early molecular testing did not significantly reduce the requirement for surgical interventions for patients with oncocytic lesions. Recognizing the unique genetic landscape of oncocytic tumors in comparison to other differentiated thyroid cancers, newer versions of Afirma and ThyroSeq used mitochondrial DNA

Figure 2. 1.7 × 1.8 × 2.2-cm Thyroid Nodule

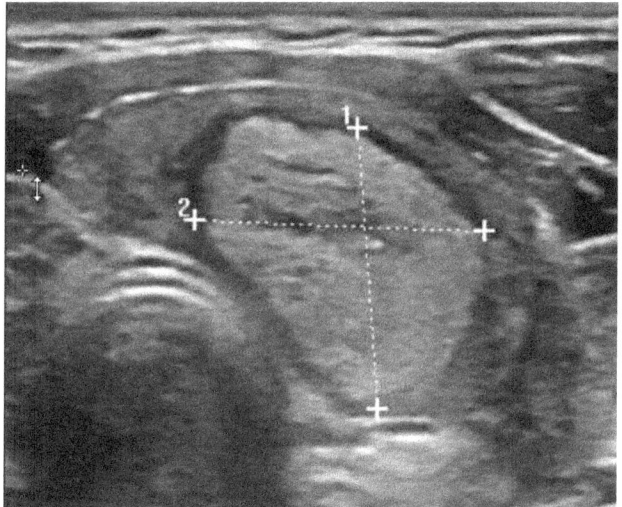

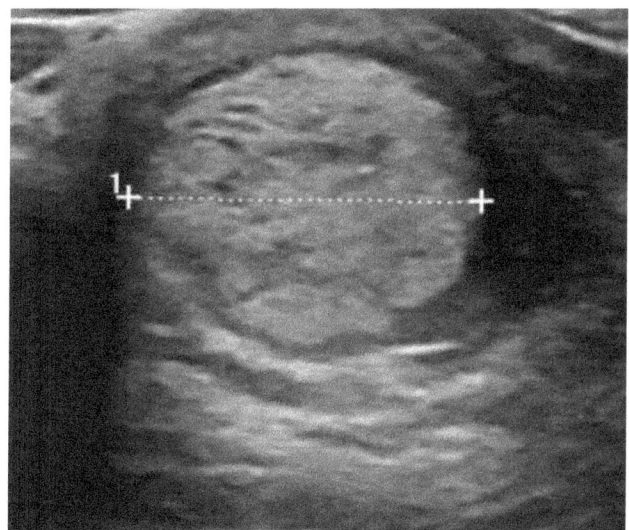

Figure 3. 2.7 × 2.6 × 3.5-cm Thyroid Nodule

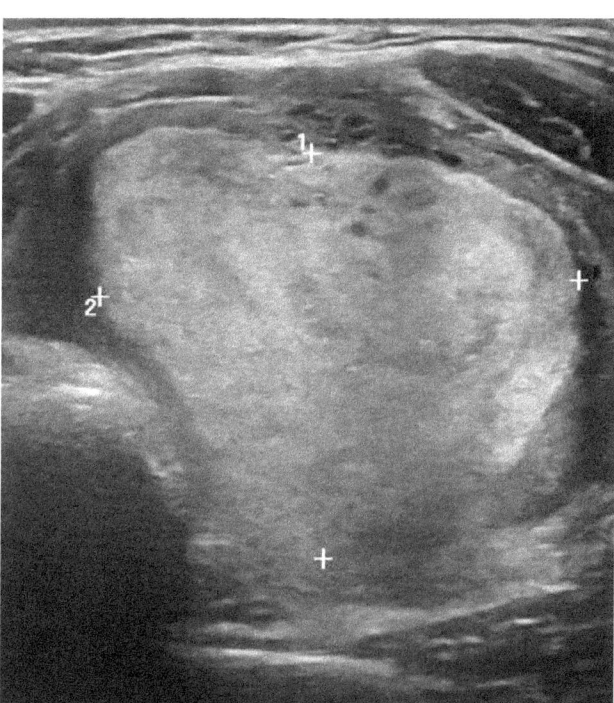

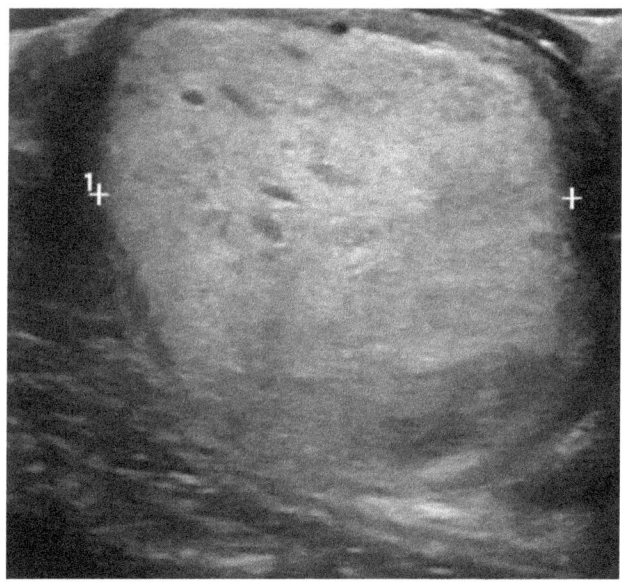

and chromosomal copy number alterations. As a result, the performance characteristics with an oncocytic diagnosis have significantly improved; the benign call rate has increased to 68% with the Afirma GSC and to 59% for ThyroSeq version 3.[16] Thus, the best next step in this patient's management is molecular testing (Answer D).

Radiofrequency ablation (Answer B) is not currently recommended for the management of nodules with indeterminate cytology.

Observation (Answer C) would not be appropriate for this nodule based on the size and lack of other comorbidities in this otherwise healthy patient.

While lobectomy (Answer A) may ultimately be required depending on the molecular test results, the patient is currently asymptomatic. Surgery, and its attendant risks, could potentially be avoided with the use of molecular testing.

Case 3

A 47-year-old man presents for evaluation of a neck mass. He has had increasing difficulty with swallowing and he found the nodule while shaving. On further questioning, the patient endorses difficulty with swallowing solid foods and is aware of the nodule with movement of his neck. It is becoming increasingly bothersome to him now that he has noticed it.

His medical history is notable only for well-controlled hypertension. He has no history of radiation exposure and no family history of thyroid cancer.

His TSH value is 2.0 mIU/L. Neck ultrasonography reveals a 2.7 × 2.6 × 3.5-cm isoechoic solid nodule with no suspicious sonographic features (*Figure 3, previous page*). Background thyroid parenchyma is heterogeneous. The nodule is aspirated and cytology is interpreted as Bethesda IV/follicular neoplasm.

Which of the following is the best next step in this patient's management?

A. Another FNA

B. Molecular testing

C. Diagnostic lobectomy

D. Observation

Answer: C) Diagnostic lobectomy

This patient has compressive symptoms that are attributable to the large nodule. Of the listed choices, only diagnostic lobectomy (Answer C) will address this clinical issue. While molecular testing (Answer B) would provide insight into the underlying diagnosis, if the patient desires removal of the nodule due to mass effect, surgical pathology will also provide the diagnosis.

A repeated FNA (Answer A) is not currently recommended as a management option for nodules that have a diagnosis of follicular neoplasm.

Similarly, observation (Answer D) would not be recommended in this case due to the size of the nodule and the compression symptoms. With a possibility of malignancy of 23% to 34%, not pursuing additional diagnostic evaluation would be inappropriate.

Key Learning Points

- Not all indeterminate nodules require reflexive molecular testing. Consideration should be given to sonographic risk stratification, patient preference, nodule size, and cytologic findings prior to performing a molecular analysis of an indeterminate nodule.

- When performed, molecular testing is a useful tool to reduce the rates of diagnostic lobectomy.

- Patients with a benign/negative molecular test should be followed up with serial ultrasonography.

- Afirma GSC and ThyroSeq version 3 have improved performance parameters for evaluation of oncocytic neoplasms.

References

1. Ramonell KM, Ohori NP, Liu JB, et al. Changes in thyroid nodule cytology rates after institutional implementation of the Thyroid Imaging Reporting and Data System. *Surgery*. 2023;173(1):232-238. PMID: 36244809

2. Ali SZ, Baloch ZW, Cochand-Priollet B, Schmitt FC, Vielh P, VanderLaan PA. The 2023 Bethesda System for reporting thyroid cytopathology. *J Am Soc Cytopathol*. 2023;12(5):319-325. PMID: 37438235

3. Wang Z, Vyas CM, Van Benschoten O, et al. Quantitative analysis of the benefits and risk of thyroid nodule evaluation in patients ≥70 years old. *Thyroid*. 2018;28(4):465-471. PMID: 29608439

4. Kim PH, Suh CH, Baek JH, Chung SR, Choi YJ, Lee JH. Diagnostic performance of four ultrasound risk stratification systems: a systematic review and meta-analysis. *Thyroid*. 2020;30(8):1159-1168. PMID: 32303153

5. Yim Y, Na DG, Ha EJ, et al. Concordance of three international guidelines for thyroid nodules classified by ultrasonography and diagnostic performance of biopsy criteria. *Korean J Radiol*. 2020;21(1):108-116. PMID: 31920034

6. Trimboli P, Castellana M, Piccardo A, et al. The ultrasound risk stratification systems for thyroid nodule have been evaluated against papillary carcinoma. A meta-analysis. *Rev Endocr Metab Disord*. 2021;22(2):453-460. PMID: 32959174

7. Jeh SK, Jung SL, Kim BS, Lee YS. Evaluating the degree of conformity of papillary carcinoma and follicular carcinoma to the reported ultrasonographic findings of malignant thyroid tumor. *Korean J Radiol.* 2007;8(3):192-197. PMID: 17554185

8. Patel KN, Angell TE, Babiarz J, et al. Performance of a genomic sequencing classifier for the preoperative diagnosis of cytologically indeterminate thyroid nodules. *JAMA Surg.* 2018;153(9):817-824. PMID: 29799911

9. Vuong HG, Nguyen TPX, Hassell LA, Jung CK. Diagnostic performances of the Afirma Gene Sequencing Classifier in comparison with the Gene Expression Classifier: a meta-analysis. *Cancer Cytopathol.* 2021;129(3):182-189. PMID: 32726885

10. Steward DL, Carty SE, Sippel RS, et al. Performance of a multigene genomic classifier in thyroid nodules with indeterminate cytology: a prospective blinded multicenter study. *JAMA Oncol.* 2019;5(2):204-212. PMID: 30419129

11. Desai D, Lepe M, Baloch ZW, Mandel SJ. ThyroSeq v3 for Bethesda III and IV: an institutional experience. *Cancer Cytopathol.* 2021;129(2):164-170. PMID: 33030808

12. Kim NE, Raghunathan RS, Hughes EG, et al. Bethesda III and IV thyroid nodules managed nonoperatively after molecular testing with Afirma GSC or Thyroseq v3. *J Clin Endocrinol Metab.* 2023;108(9):e698-e703. PMID: 36995878

13. Lupo MA, Walts AE, Sistrunk JW, et al. Multiplatform molecular test performance in indeterminate thyroid nodules. *Diagn Cytopathol.* 2020;48(12):1254-1264. PMID: 32767735

14. Livhits MJ, Zhu CY, Kuo EJ, et al. Effectiveness of molecular testing techniques for diagnosis of indeterminate thyroid nodules: a randomized clinical trial. *JAMA Oncol.* 2021;7(1):70-77. PMID: 33300952

15. Hu TX, Nguyen DT, Patel M, et al. The effect modification of ultrasound risk classification on molecular testing in predicting the risk of malignancy in cytologically indeterminate thyroid nodules. *Thyroid.* 2022;32(8):905-916. PMID: 35611970

16. Endo M, Nabhan F, Angell TE, et al. Letter to the editor: use of molecular diagnostic tests in thyroid nodules with Hurthle cell-dominant cytology. *Thyroid.* 2020;30(9):1390-1392. PMID: 32228149

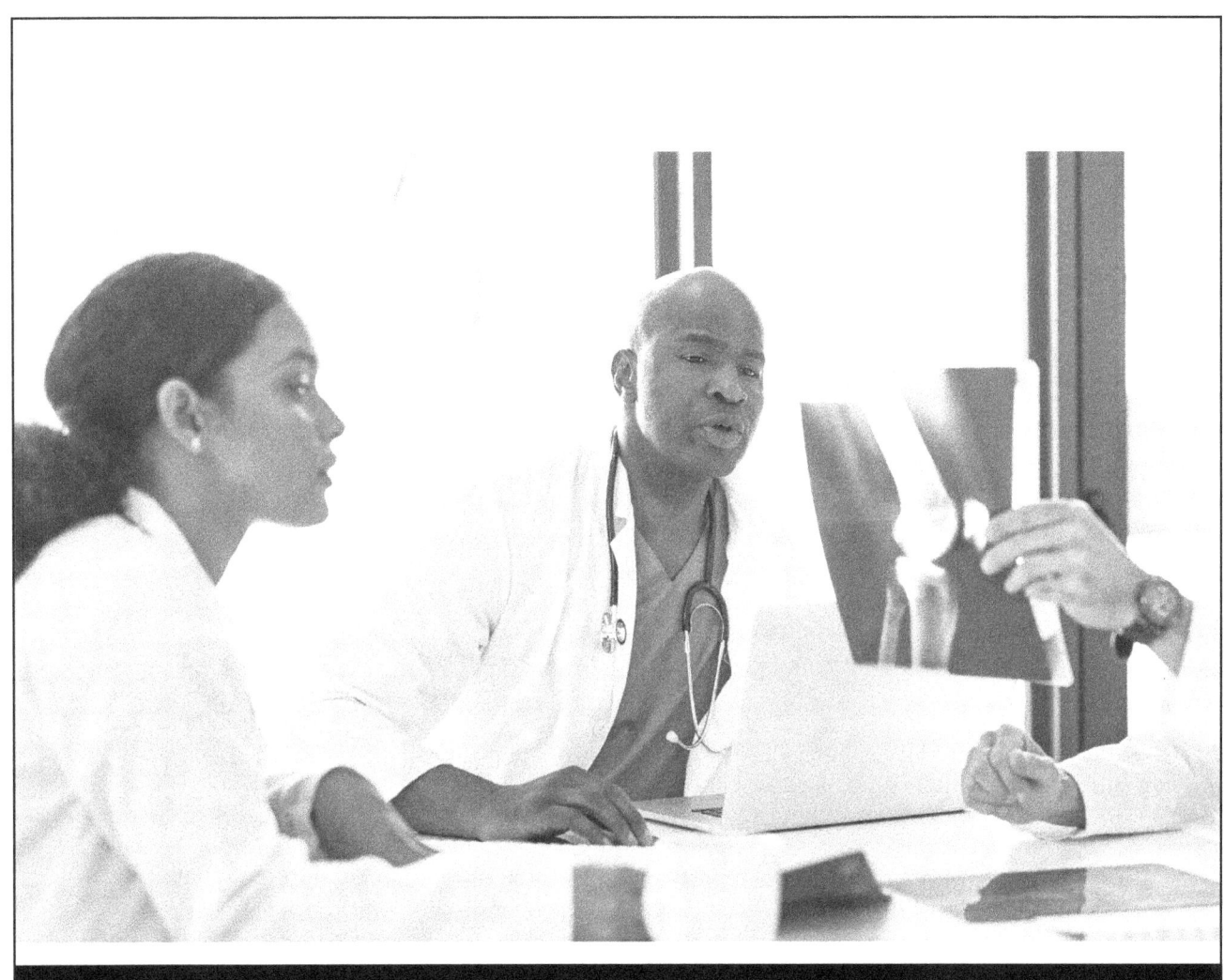

TUMOR BIOLOGY

Predisposition to Endocrine Tumors: Challenges and Dynamics of Genetic Testing

Tobias Else, MD. Department of Internal Medicine, MEND, Division of Genetic Medicine, University of Michigan, Ann Arbor, MI; Email: telse@umich.edu

Educational Objectives

After reviewing this chapter, learners should be able to:

- Deduce a clinical strategy for care based on personal history, family history, and genetic testing results.

- Interpret genetic testing results in a gene- and variant-specific fashion (eg, using guidelines, genetic databases).

- Manage hereditary endocrine tumor syndromes in a cost-effective and efficient manner.

Significance of the Clinical Problem

Genetic testing encompasses germline and somatic genetic testing. While somatic testing is the analysis of genetic changes in a tumor, which may identify variants that guide specific treatments (eg, somatic *RET* variants in sporadic medullary thyroid cancer [MTC] and use of *RET* tyrosine kinase inhibitors), germline genetic testing evaluates for genetic predisposition (eg, pathogenic germline variants in *MEN1* confirming the diagnosis of multiple endocrine neoplasia type 1 [MEN 1]).

The traditional implication of a germline genetic diagnosis of an inherited endocrine tumor syndrome is to define recommendations for future tumor surveillance, guided by published guidelines and expert opinions. Recently, the underlying germline diagnosis often also defines the suitability for certain syndrome-specific therapeutic considerations. In addition, there is accumulating evidence for differences in risk association with specific pathogenic variants, which require different approaches despite the same overall genetic diagnosis (eg, different *RET* variants vary regarding their MTC risk association). There is also a greater recognition of differences in tumor risk associated with pathogenic variants in different genes causing the overall same syndrome (eg, lifetime risk for paraganglioma or pheochromocytoma [PPGL] with *SDHB* of approximately 30% vs *SDHA* <5%). Furthermore, gene variant classifications should be regarded as dynamic. Variants are constantly reviewed and, in some cases, can even be reclassified from pathogenic (= disease-causing) to benign (= normal variant), requiring outreach to the patient or family and discussion of changes in care recommendations.

These considerations must be constantly integrated into genetic counseling, individual surveillance recommendations, and the care plan for patients with hereditary tumor predisposition.

Practice Gaps

- Awareness of changes in tumor risk estimates associated with different genes.

- Knowledge that not all pathogenic variants in a certain gene result in the same level of cancer risk.

- Routine review of databases classifying gene variants as pathogenic, likely pathogenic, variant of uncertain significance, likely benign, or benign.

- Individualization of surveillance for families with a phenotype suggestive of a hereditary predisposition, but without a disease-causing pathogenic variant.

Discussion

Somatic and Germline Genetic Testing

This chapter focuses on germline genetic testing and result interpretation, which is done to identify individuals at risk for development of syndromic tumors who may benefit screening for associated tumors. Germline genetic testing also serves as the basis for family cascade testing to identify unaffected at-risk family members who would also benefit from screening. In addition, germline genetic testing can inform therapeutic strategies for tumors arising in patients with an underlying hereditary tumor predisposition syndrome.

Genetic testing is separated into 2 types: somatic tumor testing and germline genetic testing. Somatic testing is commonly ordered by oncologists to identify genetic changes unique to the tumor that can be exploited using targeted therapies. It is important to carefully review somatic test results, as they can suggest the presence of germline variants. For example, the presence of a common founder *SDHD* variant (eg, *SDHD* pathogenic variant p.P81L) in a metastatic PPGL is likely a germline variant, albeit identified by somatic tumor testing. The germline presence of these variants must be confirmed by dedicated germline testing (eg, saliva or blood). Germline testing identifies tumor predisposition either in affected patients or at-risk family members through family cascade testing. Genetic testing for any patient with cancer or patients with a

significant family history of cancer is often done by using large next-generation sequencing (NGS) panels (often >50 genes), which bear the potential to identify incidental pathogenic variants in genes unrelated to the tumor spectrum observed in the patient or family.

Choice of Genes, Review of Methods, and Interpretation of Germline Genetic Test Results

When considering genetic testing for a certain condition, the core predisposing genes should be included in testing. For example, germline genetic testing for a patient with an abdominal PGL should, at minimum, include *SDHB* and *SDHD*. Genes associated with PPGL but rarely with abdominal PPGL (eg, *SDHA, SDHC, SDHAF2, VHL, RET, TMEM127, MAX*, and *FH*) are often included in NGS panels offered by commercial laboratories.[1] Some laboratories also (optionally) include preliminary evidence genes in their testing panels, which have only been suggested, but not confirmed, to be PPGL-predisposing genes (eg, *MDH2, MEN1, SLC25A11*). Based on family history and patient preferences, initial NGS testing panels might include a long list of additional genes, which are not related to the risk for PPGL but are worthwhile to analyze for patients with, for example, a significant personal or family history of breast, colon, or other cancers.

Genetic variants are classified as benign/likely benign (B/LB), variant of uncertain significance (VUS), or pathogenic/likely pathogenic (P/LP) using the ACMG (American College of Medical Genetics) criteria.[2] In general, the consensus is to only assign a definitive diagnosis and to recommend appropriate surveillance and family cascade testing to patients with P/LP variants. However, the ACMG criteria of variant classification (a new version will likely be published in 2024) are quite general and might not apply perfectly to all genes. In an effort to resolve this issue, ClinGen consortium (https://clinicalgenome.org/) is aiming to provide gene-specific interpretation criteria, including for those genes causing endocrine tumor predisposition syndromes. It is important to understand that variant interpretation is a dynamic concept that changes over time. For example, VUS will likely be reclassified in the future as either B/LB or P/LP, making a regular review of these variants at each patient's visit necessary. A detailed review of previous genetic testing results and the method by which they were ascertained is important, particularly for those patients diagnosed before the era of widespread use of NGS methods (roughly before 2016). For example, larger deletions often escaped traditional Sanger sequencing and appropriate methods, such as MLPA (multiplex ligation-dependent probe amplification) were not regularly used. Therefore, retesting may be indicated. Although germline genetic DNA does not change over time in an individual, analytical methods do!

All genetic variants should be reviewed using large disease-related variant interpretation databases (eg, ClinVar, https://www.ncbi.nlm.nih.gov/clinvar/) and "normal" population databases (eg, gnomAD (https://gnomad.broadinstitute.org/). ClinVar interpretation entries are helpful to update variant classification and, for example, reclassify a VUS to B/LB or P/LP. The presence of a variant in a significant number of patients in gnomAD (eg, exceeding the estimated incidence of the genetic syndrome) makes pathogenicity unlikely.

Incidental Genetic Findings

Incidental findings are increasingly common and have become a frequent reason for referral to a specialized cancer genetics clinic. Most genetic counselors and physicians ordering testing offer patients a targeted NGS gene panel, based on the patient's personal and family history. However, as mentioned above, they will often extend testing to larger NGS panels based on family history and patient preference. Regarding incidental findings in genes associated with endocrine hereditary cancer syndromes, the SDHA p.R31X and RET p.V804M pathogenic variants are the most common, but other genetic changes are also incidentally

observed (eg, in VHL and SDHB). The potential for incidentally identifying unrelated hereditary predisposition to tumor development should ideally be addressed in pretest genetic counseling. The incidental discovery of unrelated germline predisposition must be carefully reviewed to make the best recommendations for the patient and their family, keeping cost-effectiveness in mind. To this end, it is important to review resources for variant interpretation and take guidelines and expert opinions into consideration. As SDHA pathogenic variants are among the commonly observed incidental findings, a recent United Kingdom consensus put forth recommendations regarding further surveillance and family testing.[3] For example, due to the relatively low risk associated with SDHA pathogenic variants, no further surveillance or family testing is recommended in the absence of any personal or family history of associated tumors.

Individualized Surveillance Based on Genetic Diagnosis, Variant, and Family History

Careful review of the gene underlying a certain diagnosis, the specific variant observed, and considerations arising from the personal and family history of a patient are important when making decisions regarding future surveillance and family testing. For example, hereditary PPGL syndrome can be caused by pathogenic variants in SDHA, SDHB, SDHC, SDHD, or SDHAF2. Lifetime risks for tumor development vary depending on the causative gene: risk is highest for SDHD pathogenic variants (~50%-80%), followed by SDHB pathogenic variants (~30%). This contrasts with the risk associated with SDHA pathogenic variants (<5%). Therefore, the usual recommendation for annual biochemical surveillance with metanephrine measurement and whole-body imaging surveillance every 2 years should be individualized depending on the underlying syndrome.[4] In our practice, we continue to recommend whole-body MRI screening for patients with SDHD pathogenic variants every 2 years but decrease the frequency for patients with pathogenic variants in *SDHB* if the first 2 to 3 imaging surveillances did not show any pathological findings. For *SDHA* pathogenic variants, we discuss initial baseline imaging only, if there is a family or personal history of associated tumors, and we continue an individualized discussion regarding frequency of future surveillance imaging.

RET pathogenic variants causing MEN 2 are another example of the importance of detailed variant review. First, only oncogenic variants confer tumor risk, and second, variants differ significantly regarding their associated tumor risk. Oncogenic variants (gain-of-function variants) increase the risk for MEN 2–associated tumors with varying lifetime risk. Interestingly, however, both gain-of-function and loss-of-function variants can increase the risk for Hirschsprung disease. For example, Hirschsprung disease is commonly observed in patients with MEN 2B. The American Thyroid Association classifies MTC risk with pathogenic *RET* variants as moderate, high, and highest risk.[5] Patients with the highest-risk variants (MEN 2B) should undergo thyroidectomy before age 1 year and carriers of high-risk variants by age 5 years. Individuals with moderate-risk variants can be observed with annual biochemical screening. The p.V804M *RET* variant is commonly observed as an incidental finding in large NGS testing panels. As a moderate-risk variant with rather low penetrance (ie, how many gene carriers are affected with a certain associated manifestation) and an estimated lifetime risk of MTC of 4%, individuals with this variant can certainly be followed biochemically with annual measurement of calcitonin, carcinoembryonic antigen, metanephrines, and calcium.[6] Providers should always carefully review guidelines for surveillance of patients with hereditary tumor syndromes to prevent harm and practice cost saving. For example, individuals with MEN 2 do not need regular imaging[5,7]; biochemical surveillance is sufficient. On the contrary, MEN 1 surveillance for pancreatic neuroendocrine tumors (pNET) is largely based on imaging rather than biochemistry. Among other analytes, chromogranin A has been shown to be unreliable in screening for pNET.[8]

Targeted Therapy Based on the Underlying Syndrome

An important advancement in recent decades is the availability of drugs that specifically target pathomechanisms underlying tumors in hereditary conditions, such as Lynch syndrome or *BRCA1/2*-associated breast and ovarian cancer syndrome and endocrine tumor syndromes (eg, MEN 2, von Hippel-Lindau syndrome [VHL], and neurofibromatosis type 1). Probably most important for the endocrinologist are tyrosine kinase inhibitors targeting the RET tyrosine kinase that can be used to treat MTC arising in patients with germline pathogenic variants in *RET*, as well as belzutifan, a hypoxia-inducible factor 2a inhibitor that is approved for several VHL-associated tumors.[9-11] Furthermore, tumors arising in patients with Lynch syndrome, such as adrenal cancer, are often hypermutated and can be treated with immunotherapy. Several immunotherapy agents are approved in a tissue-agnostic fashion for hypermutated tumors.[12]

Clinical Case Vignettes

Case 1

A 60-year-old woman with MEN 1 presents for a follow-up visit. Her long-time endocrinologist has retired, and this her first visit to this clinic. She has a personal history of primary hyperparathyroidism (PHPT). Her daughter, mother, and niece have the same diagnosis. Her brother and one of her daughters have a diagnosis of an ileal carcinoid. Fifteen years ago, germline genetic testing revealed an *MEN1* variant (c.1618C>T, p.P540S). For the last 15 years, she has had regular surveillance for pituitary adenomas, PHPT, and pNETs with no pathologic findings.

Which of the following is the best next step in this patient's care?

A. Order annual surveillance with PTH, calcium, prolactin, and gastrin measurement and pituitary and pancreatic imaging

B. Recommend genetic testing for the familial variant in all other family members with PHPT

C. Recommend genetic testing for the familial variant in all first-degree relatives

D. Review databases, such as ClinVar, for information on the specific *MEN1* variant

E. Tell the patient that she needs to find a specialist to take over her care, as you do not see patients with rare endocrine conditions

Answer: D) Review databases, such as ClinVar, for information on the specific MEN1

This patient had germline genetic testing 15 years ago, which predates the most recent recommendation for genetic variant classification by the ACMG, as well as the availability of large databases of germline variants (eg, gnomAD) and variant classification (eg, ClinVar). Therefore, a thorough review of classification is necessary (Answer D). The *MEN1* variant c.1618C>T, p.P540S is categorized either as a VUS or LB. This variant is present in 114 of 806,787 individuals in the gnomAD database (including one individual homozygous for this variant), of which most can be assumed not to have MEN 1. This prevalence alone exceeds the estimated prevalence of MEN 1 in the population (~1:10,000-1:30,000).

Answer A describes the minimal surveillance for patients with MEN 1. Surveillance should ONLY be recommended if the patient/family carry a diagnosis of MEN 1. Current guidance on MEN 1 surveillance can be found as an expert opinion, but there will be new guidance documents published soon.[13,14] A careful review of current interpretation of the variant should precede any further testing (Answers B and C).

Case 1 (continued)

The following information is retrieved from ClinVar: 12 contributors comment on the classification of this variant (10 laboratories classify it as a VUS and the 2 laboratories most commonly used for genetic testing by your clinic call it an LB variant).

Based on these findings, which of the following is the best plan?

A. Stop all surveillance, there is no concern for MEN 1

B. Share your doubts that the variant is pathogenic, but continue all surveillance

C. Recommend testing for this variant in all other family members with PHPT to prove that this variant is truly causing MEN 1 in her family

D. Recommend repeat genetic testing for MEN 1 and other causes of familial PHPT

E. Continue screening for MEN 1–related manifestations as the family fulfills clinical diagnostic criteria for MEN 1

Answer: D) Recommend repeat genetic testing for MEN 1 and other causes of familial PHPT

Multiple family members in this pedigree are affected with PHPT and some have ileal carcinoid. There are no family members with known pituitary tumors. Ileal carcinoids are midgut tumors and are NOT a typical manifestation of MEN 1. Neuroendocrine tumors associated with MEN 1 are usually foregut neuroendocrine tumors, arising in the stomach, lung, duodenum, or pancreas. Neither the patient nor the family currently fulfills clinical criteria for a diagnosis of MEN 1, and continued surveillance should not be encouraged (thus, Answer E is incorrect). However, the strong history of PHPT suggests a familial form of PTH-driven hypercalcemia, including MEN 1. Genetic testing for MEN 1 and other associated conditions, such as familial hypocalciuric hypercalcemia, *CDKN1B*-related MEN and *CDC73*-related disorders is the best next step (Answer D). There is usually no use in repeating genetic testing for the same gene because the genetic makeup of an individual does

NOT change over time. However, when testing for alternative genes, it is reasonable to include *MEN1* because the methods of testing and the extent of gene coverage have changed over time (eg, in this case no multiplex ligation dependent probe amplification geared toward identification of larger deletions had been initially conducted). Repeat genetic testing should be done before recommending changes in further surveillance (Answers A and Answer B). Segregation analysis (Answer C) can be supportive of pathogenicity, but not by itself, and it is of limited value. Even in the absence of any pathogenic variants in repeat extended genetic testing, it is reasonable to recommend sporadic calcium testing for all family members based on the number of affected family members. In cases of negative genetic testing, family history is an important indicator for risk assessment used by providers in cancer genetics clinics.

Case 2

A 65-year-old woman recently underwent germline genetic testing with a large germline NGS panel, which revealed a pathogenic variant in *SDHA*, p.R31X. Genetic testing had been pursued due to a family history of multiple cancers, such as prostate cancer in her father and breast cancer in a paternal aunt and paternal grandmother. Of note, she has no family or personal history of PPGL. Posttest genetic counseling includes a discussion about the diagnosis of *SDHA*-related hereditary PPGL syndrome, and she is referred for further management.

Which of the following is the best next step in this patient's care?

A. Order DOTATATE-PET and metanephrine measurement

B. Recommend testing for the *SDHA* variant in all first-degree relatives

C. Reassure the patient that although she carries the diagnosis of *SDHA*-related hereditary PPGL syndrome, she does not require any dedicated surveillance

D. Order whole-body MRI and metanephrine measurement

E. Advise the patient to avoid moving to higher elevation, as this would significantly increase her risk of developing PPGL

Answer: C) Reassure the patient that although she carries the diagnosis of SDHA-related hereditary PPGL syndrome, she does not require any dedicated surveillance

While pathogenic variants in *SDHA*, *SDHB*, *SDHC*, *SDHD*, and *SDHAF2* all confer the diagnosis of hereditary PPGL syndrome, the lifetime risks for developing a tumor differ significantly (eg, 50%-80% for *SDHD*, 30% for *SDHB*). The lifetime risk associated with *SDHA* pathogenic variants is likely less than 5%. Moreover, there are some pathogenic variants, such as the *SDHA* p.R31X variant (which this patient has) that are present in approximately 1 in 4000 individuals in gnomAD, making it unlikely to be a high-penetrance variant. Indeed, these common variants are more often found as an incidental finding in patients who undergo genetic testing for other reasons than in affected individuals. A recent United Kingdom consensus recommends not conducting any dedicated screening for PPGLs *or* family testing in the absence of any family history of PPGL (thus, Answer C is correct, and Answer B is incorrect).[3]

If the patient had a pathogenic variant in *SDHB*, *SDHC*, or *SDHD* or a had family member with a PPGL, then DOTATATE-PET and metanephrine measurement (Answer A) or whole-body MRI and metanephrine measurement (Answer D) would be surveillance options.[4,15]

While there is some suggestion that the incidence of PPGL increases with less oxygen tension, the evidence is too poor to make a final recommendation regarding this issue (thus, Answer E is incorrect). Furthermore, it is important to be reasonable in terms of patient burden and presumed cost-effectiveness when making decisions regarding surveillance. Regular surveillance can be a psychological and socioeconomic burden.

Case 3

A 63-year-old man is referred after recent identification of a *RET* pathogenic variant, p.V804M, and he would like to establish care for MEN 2.

Which of the following is the best next step in this patient's care?

A. Refer to an endocrine surgeon for prophylactic thyroidectomy

B. Order adrenal CT and neck ultrasonography; measure calcitonin, carcinoembryonic antigen, calcium, and metanephrines

C. Review his family history and the American Thyroid Association guidelines regarding this variant

D. Educate the patient on the possibility that he might have Hirschsprung disease

E. Google "*RET* oncogene AND p.V804M"

Answer: C) Review his family history and the American Thyroid Association guidelines regarding this variant

MEN 2 is mainly caused by pathogenic variants in several hotspots in the *RET* gene.[5,7] The variants confer ligand-independent signaling by RET tyrosine kinase, which explains their oncogenicity and the existence of oncogenic hotspot variants. The American Thyroid Association classifies the associated MTC risk with different variants (thus, Answer C is correct).[5] The p.M918T variant is associated with the highest risk and an MEN 2B diagnosis. Persons with this pathogenic variant should undergo thyroidectomy before age 1 year. Several other classic variants, such as changes in the cysteine residue at codon 634, cause classic MEN 2A, and surgery is advised by age 5 years. The p.V804M variant is associated with moderate disease risk. Review of guidelines should happen before making any patient care recommendations (Answers A and B). Although persons with MEN 2, as well as patients with inactivating *RET* variants, are at risk for Hirschsprung disease, this risk counseling (Answer D) is less important

at this point, and the p.V804M variant is not particularly associated with neurocristopathies.

Case 3 (continued)

The patient had initially been tested because his daughter (age 27 years) underwent a large germline NGS genetic testing panel due to a maternal history of kidney cancer and melanoma, which incidentally revealed the *RET* p.V804M variant. No other pathogenic variant was identified on a 77-gene panel. Review of the American Thyroid Association guidelines reveals that the p.V804M variant is associated with moderate risk for MTC. His daughter accompanies him to his visit and would like to learn about further care for herself and her father.

Which of the following is the best recommendation?

A. Order biochemical screening for both the patient and his daughter (calcitonin, carcinoembryonic antigen, calcium, and metanephrine measurement)

B. Measure calcitonin, carcinoembryonic antigen, calcium, and metanephrine levels and refer the patient and his daughter to an endocrine surgeon for prophylactic thyroidectomy

C. Recommend preimplantation genetic diagnosis to minimize the risk for transmission of the pathogenic variant, in case the daughter plans a pregnancy

D. Reassure the patient and his daughter that they do not need any surveillance in the absence of any MEN 2 manifestations in their family

E. Explain that you can only make medical recommendations for the patient, but not his daughter, because she is not your patient

Answer: A) Order biochemical screening for both the patient and his daughter (calcitonin, carcinoembryonic antigen, calcium, and metanephrine measurement)

The p.V804M variant is a moderate-risk allele causing MEN 2 (thus, Answer D is incorrect) with a lifetime MTC risk of about 4%. Biochemical surveillance with calcitonin and carcinoembryonic antigen is the most appropriate approach for all carriers (thus, Answer A is correct, and Answer B is incorrect). They do not require risk-reducing thyroidectomy. It is always important to review risks of inheritance, and while options such as preimplantation genetic diagnosis can be discussed, this is a very personal patient decision and should never be a recommendation (thus, Answer C is incorrect). Caring for families is a common scenario in genetics clinics, and recommendations are made for families, as well as for individuals (thus, Answer E is incorrect).

Case 4

A 27-year-old man with a molecularly confirmed diagnosis of VHL comes for an annual visit. His history includes hemangioblastoma in the left eye treated at age 16 years, left pheochromocytoma at age 19 treated with left partial adrenalectomy, cerebellar hemangioblastoma surgery at age 22 years, and cervical spine hemangioblastoma surgery at age 24 years.

Recent screening shows a large hemangioblastoma of the thoracic spine. The neurosurgical team recommends therapy, but also comments on a high surgical risk for neurological deficits, including paraplegia. On abdominal imaging, there are multiple pancreatic cysts, a 1.2-cm, T2 bright lesion in the right adrenal gland, and a 2.1-cm, T2 bright lesion in the left adrenal gland. Recent plasma metanephrine levels are normal and normetanephrine levels are 2.2-times the upper normal limit. Blood pressure and physical examination findings are normal. He states that he has a mildly increased tendency to sweat over the last 6 months. Review of imaging 1 year ago shows a 0.9-cm lesion in the right adrenal gland and a 2.0-cm lesion in the left adrenal gland.

Which of the following is the best recommendation for this patient's care?

A. Refer to an endocrine surgeon to remove both adrenal nodules before any intervention for the hemangioblastoma of the spine

B. Start the patient on α-adrenergic blockade in anticipation of neurosurgery

C. Consider medical therapy with belzutifan now

D. Start α-adrenergic blockade and continue imaging surveillance of the CNS, pancreas, and kidney in 1 year

E. Refer to an endocrine surgeon for potential adrenal surgery, to a neurologist to monitor neurological function, to a urologist to monitor for kidney tumors, and to an interventional gastroenterologist for endoscopic ultrasonography and potential biopsy of the pancreatic cysts

Answer: C) Consider medical therapy with belzutifan now

Traditionally patients with VHL were treated with surgery for most of the manifestations. However, because this patient is asymptomatic, he does not need surgery for the pheochromocytoma now (thus, Answer A is incorrect). Simple surveillance (Answer D) is not a good choice for the hemangioblastoma because the neurosurgical team already recommends therapy. However, the high surgical risk means that neurosurgery (Answer B) is also not the preferred next step. VHL is one of the rare conditions for which a specific medication is available. Belzutifan (Answer C) has been shown to decrease the size of VHL-associated renal cell cancer, hemangioblastomas, and pancreatic neuroendocrine tumors.[10] Therefore, it is reasonable to initiate therapy with belzutifan, mainly for the hemangioblastoma, and to watch and wait regarding the asymptomatic PCC. Most endocrinologists would likely start α-adrenergic blockade (Answers B and D), but it is unclear if it is necessary in a largely asymptomatic, normotensive patient with only minimally elevated normetanephrine levels. Although surveillance for the different manifestations is necessary, one should try to minimize the number of health care appointments for these patients (thus, Answer E is incorrect). Appointments with multiple providers are difficult to sustain, and patients are best served with follow-up in a dedicated center with multidisciplinary clinics and expertise. Pancreatic cysts in patients with VHL never pose a risk regarding the development of malignant lesions, and biopsies are risk-bearing and unnecessary.

Key Learning Points

- Genetic testing increasingly affects care of patients with endocrine tumors.

- With increased of availability of genetic testing, incidental findings—particularly with low-penetrance alleles or "moderate-risk" genes—are regularly reported.

- While genetic test results do not change over time, methods of genetic testing and variant interpretation can change, and all genetic variants must be reviewed on a regular basis.

- Although different genes cause the same syndrome, the associated risk for tumors varies, resulting in different screening recommendations.

- Different variants in the same gene can confer varying levels of risk, and surveillance should be individualized.

- There is an increasing number of hereditary syndromes for which specific therapies are available.

References

1. Horton C, LaDuca H, Deckman A, et al. Universal germline panel testing for individuals with pheochromocytoma and paraganglioma produces high diagnostic yield. *J Clin Endocrinol Metab.* 2022;107(5):e1917-e1923. PMID: 35026032

2. Richards S, Aziz N, Bale S, et al. Standards and guidelines for the interpretation of sequence variants: a joint consensus recommendation of the American College of Medical Genetics and Genomics and the Association for Molecular Pathology. *Genet Med.* 2015;17(5):405-424. PMID: 25741868

3. Hanson H, Durkie M, Lalloo F, et al; UK Cancer Genetics Centres. UK recommendations for *SDHA* germline genetic testing and surveillance in clinical practice. *J Med Genet.* 2023;60(2):107-111. PMID: 35260474

4. Else T, Greenberg S, Fishbein L. Hereditary paraganglioma-pheochromocytoma syndromes. In: Adam MP, Feldmen J, Mirzaa GM, et al, eds. *GeneReviews.* University of Washington, Seattle; 1993-2024.

5. Wells SA Jr, Asa SL, Dralle H, et al; American Thyroid Association Guidelines Task Force on Medullary thyroid Carcinoma. Revised American Thyroid Association guidelines for the management of medullary thyroid carcinoma. *Thyroid.* 2015;25(6):567-610. PMID: 25810047

6. Loveday C, Josephs K, Chubb D, et al. p.Val804Met, the most frequent pathogenic mutation in RET, confers a very low lifetime risk of medullary thyroid cancer. *J Clin Endocrinol Metab.* 2018;103(11):4275-4282. PMID: 29590403

7. Eng C, Plitt G, Multiple endocrine neoplasia type 2. In: Adam MP, Feldmen J, Mirzaa GM, et al, eds. *GeneReviews.* University of Washington, Seattle; 1993-2024.

8. de Laat JM, Pieterman CRC, Weijmans M, et al. Low accuracy of tumor markers for diagnosing pancreatic neuroendocrine tumors in multiple endocrine neoplasia type 1 patients. *J Clin Endocrinol Metab.* 2013;98(10):4143-4151. PMID: 23956349

9. Fox E, Widemann BC, Chuck MK, et al. Vandetanib in children and adolescents with multiple endocrine neoplasia type 2B associated medullary thyroid carcinoma. *Clin Cancer Res.* 2013;19(15):4239-4248. PMID: 23766359

10. Jonasch E, Donskov F, Iliopoulos O, et al. Belzutifan for renal cell carcinoma in von Hippel-Lindau disease. *N Engl J Med.* 2021;385(22):2036-2046. PMID: 34818478

11. Shankar A, Kurzawinski T, Ross E, et al. Treatment outcome with a selective RET tyrosine kinase inhibitor selpercatinib in children with multiple endocrine neoplasia type 2 and advanced medullary thyroid carcinoma. *Eur J Cancer.* 2021;158:38-46. PMID: 34649088

12. Nebot-Bral L, Brandao D, Verlingue L, et al. Hypermutated tumours in the era of immunotherapy: the paradigm of personalised medicine. *Eur J Cancer.* 2017;84:290-303. PMID: 28846956

13. Thakker RV, Newey PJ, Walls GC, et al. Clinical practice guidelines for multiple endocrine neoplasia type 1 (MEN1). *J Clin Endocrinol Metab.* 2012;97(9):2990-3011. PMID: 22723327

14. Giusti F, Marini F, Brandi ML. Multiple endocrine neoplasia type 1. In: Adam MP, Feldmen J, Mirzaa GM, et al, eds. *GeneReviews.* University of Washington, Seattle; 1993-2024.

15. Amar L, Pacak K, Steichen O, et al. International consensus on initial screening and follow-up of asymptomatic SDHx mutation carriers. *Nat Rev Endocrinol.* 2021;17(7):435-444. PMID: 34021277

What's New in Diagnosis and Management of Multiple Endocrine Neoplasia Type 1?

Omair A. Shariq, MD, MS. Division of Endocrine Surgery, Department of Surgery, Mayo Clinic, Rochester, MN; Email: shariq.omair@mayo.edu

Educational Objectives

After reviewing this chapter, learners should be able to:

- Describe recent advances in the genetic diagnosis of multiple endocrine neoplasia type 1 (MEN 1), including differences in clinical course between genotype-positive and genotype-negative patients.

- Explain new modalities and technologies that have emerged for the diagnosis of MEN 1–related manifestations, and their implications for early detection and disease management.

- Evaluate recent developments in the therapeutic management of MEN 1–related primary hyperparathyroidism (PHPT), duodeno-pancreatic neuroendocrine tumors (DP-NETs), and pituitary adenomas, including updates in surgical and pharmacological therapies.

Significance of the Clinical Problem

MEN 1 is an inherited endocrine tumor syndrome that has an estimated prevalence of 1 to 3 per 100,000 individuals.[1] It is characterized by the occurrence of PHPT, NETs of the pancreas and duodenum, and anterior pituitary adenomas.[2] These manifestations are commonly referred to as the "3 Ps"; however, the spectrum of MEN 1–related tumors has been expanded since

patients may also develop, albeit less commonly, adrenocortical neoplasms, bronchial and thymic NETs, and other nonendocrine tumors (*Figure 1*).[2] Most patients with MEN 1 (80%-90%) harbor a detectable germline pathogenic variant affecting the coding region of the *MEN1* gene on chromosome 11q13, which encodes a ubiquitously expressed tumor suppressor protein, menin. In these patients, tumorigenesis is initiated in predisposed somatic cells due to inactivation (loss of heterozygosity) of the remaining wild-type *MEN1* allele. The syndrome is highly penetrant, such that greater than 95% of *MEN1* pathogenic variant carriers develop manifestations by age 50

Figure 1. Tumors Associated With MEN 1

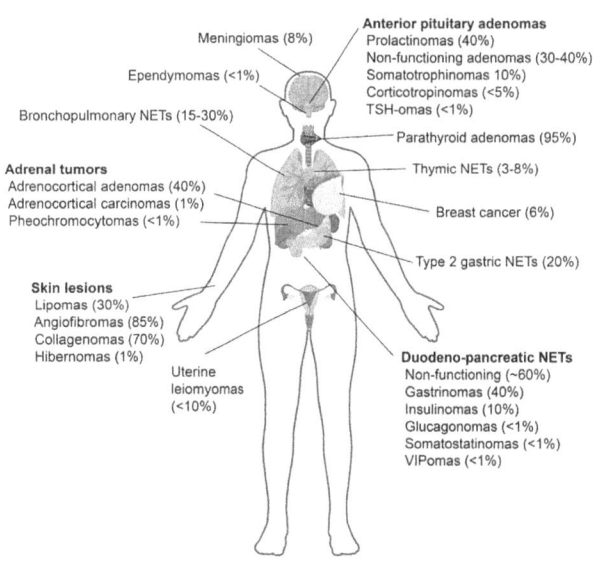

Percentages indicate estimated lifetime penetrance of each tumor type.

[Color—Print (Color Gallery page CG39) or web & ePub editions]

years.[2] MEN 1 follows an autosomal dominant pattern of inheritance. Thus, establishing the diagnosis in an individual patient has significant implications for family members, who have a 50% risk of inheriting the pathogenic variant depending on their relationship to the proband.

Patients with MEN 1 have a decreased life expectancy compared with that of the general population, predominantly due to malignant NETs. Furthermore, the development of synchronous or metachronous hormonally active tumors can lead to substantial morbidity. To address this, international clinical practice guidelines (first published in 2001[3] and subsequently updated in 2012[2]) recommend an intensive regimen of surveillance, encompassing clinical, biochemical, and radiological evaluations beginning in childhood to facilitate early detection and treatment. Owing to the rarity and complexity of MEN 1, such surveillance should be coordinated by dedicated multidisciplinary teams with expertise in managing this syndrome. In the decade that has elapsed since the most recent iteration of the guidelines, several multicenter (including population-based) and large single-center studies of patients with MEN 1 have been published. These cohorts have furthered our knowledge of the natural course and management of this syndrome and its manifestations, particularly in subgroups, such as children, adolescents, and so-called genotype-negative patients.[4-6] Concurrently, improvements in conventional and nuclear medicine imaging techniques have allowed for the earlier detection of tumors and occult metastases. The surgical management of MEN 1–related DP-NETs and PHPT has also evolved due to an increased understanding of the long-term outcomes of various operative strategies and the advent of minimally invasive surgical technologies. This chapter provides an update on advances in the diagnosis and management of MEN 1 and the 3 most commonly encountered manifestations in clinical practice—PHPT, DP-NETs, and pituitary adenomas—with an emphasis on data that have been published since the most recent clinical practice guidelines.

Practice Gaps

- Absence of defined surveillance protocols for patients with genotype-negative MEN 1.

- Controversies regarding timing and extent of surgery for MEN 1–related PHPT.

- Difficulties surrounding diagnosis and surgical management of Zollinger-Ellison syndrome (ZES).

- Lack of reliable biomarkers for predicting the aggressiveness of MEN 1–related nonfunctioning pancreatic NETs.

Discussion

Recent Advances in MEN 1 Genetic Testing and Diagnosis

Per the most recent guidelines, the diagnosis of MEN 1 can be made based on clinical, familial, and/or genetic criteria.[2] A clinical diagnosis requires the occurrence of 2 or more primary MEN 1 tumor types (ie, parathyroid, pituitary, and/or enteropancreatic). In family members of a patient with a clinical diagnosis, the development of one MEN 1–associated tumor is sufficient for familial diagnostic criteria to be fulfilled. A genetic diagnosis requires the identification of a germline pathogenic variant in the *MEN1* gene. In recent years, the value of definitively making a diagnosis of MEN 1 based on clinical or familial criteria in the absence of confirmatory genetic testing has been called into question. This is because 10% to 30% of patients diagnosed with clinical MEN 1 do not have an *MEN1* pathogenic variant, as classified by the American College of Medical Genetics, detectable on standard genetic testing, which should include DNA sequence analysis of coding exons and splice junctions, as well as multiplex ligation-dependent probe amplification for the analysis of larger deletions or duplications. Determining the germline variant status of a patient with clinical MEN 1 is of significant importance since emerging data show that those who do not have a detectable pathogenic variant in the *MEN1* gene (referred to as genotype-negative patients, excluding those with variants of undetermined significance or likely benign variants) exhibit a less aggressive disease phenotype. For example, a retrospective cohort study of the Dutch MEN 1 database found that genotype-negative patients had a median age of first tumor manifestation that was 13 years later than in genotype-positive patients.[6] Furthermore, no genotype-negative patients developed a third MEN 1 manifestation compared with approximately 50% of genotype-positive patients, and life expectancy in the former group was comparable to that of the general population.[6] These findings have been corroborated in an independent US cohort[5] and suggest that a less intensive screening program for genotype-negative patients could be used, although the optimal protocol remains to be defined.

There are several possible explanations for why an individual who fulfills clinical diagnostic criteria for MEN 1 may receive a negative result on standard genetic testing. The sensitivity of conventional genetic testing is less than 100% due to user errors, technical issues, and sequence characteristics leading to allelic dropout (a phenomenon that can occur when the variant *MEN1* allele is not properly amplified during polymerase chain reaction, leading to a false-negative homozygous genotyping result). Recent advances in *MEN1* molecular genetic studies have also highlighted the importance of screening noncoding regions (eg, promoters, introns, and untranslated regions) of the *MEN1* gene since these regions, while not directly coding for proteins, may still have crucial roles in gene regulation. Although individual case reports have been described, a recent study that involved targeted next-generation sequencing of the entire *MEN1* gene in 76 unrelated probands detected no point or short insertion-deletion (indel) pathogenic variants in these regions, suggesting that such variants are rare.[7] A small proportion of genotype-negative patients initially diagnosed with MEN 1 based on clinical criteria have actually been shown to harbor pathogenic variants in other monogenic disease genes that may mimic the MEN 1 phenotype. These are referred to as MEN 1 phenocopies and include the cyclin-dependent kinase inhibitor genes, *CDKN1B*, *CDKN2B*, *CDKN2C*, and *CDKN1A*.[2] Individuals harboring *CDKN1B* pathogenic variants are classified as having MEN 4, a condition characterized by later age of onset of parathyroid disease, absence of prolactinomas, and decreased prevalence of DP-NETs compared with findings in MEN 1. Additional gene variants that can present as MEN 1 phenocopies include those in *CDC73*, associated with hyperparathyroidism–jaw tumor syndrome; *CASR*, associated with familial hypocalciuric hypercalcemia type 1; *AIP,* associated with familial isolated pituitary adenomas; *RET,* typically associated with MEN 2A and MEN 2B; and *MAX*, a rare cause of hereditary paraganglioma-pheochromocytoma syndrome. Consequently, multigene panel testing has become an important component in the diagnostic evaluation of patients suspected of harboring a pathogenic *MEN1* variant. This is important because many of the aforementioned monogenic diseases have different management guidelines that correspond with their respective features. In patients who continue to exhibit a negative genotype following the extensive testing protocols described above, it is conceivable that yet unidentified genes may be responsible for the MEN 1 phenocopy. Finally, the possibility of coincidental sporadic occurrence of 2 manifestations with no underlying germline pathogenic variant should not be overlooked, particularly as the sensitivity of cross-sectional imaging continues to improve.

Recent Controversies in Surgical Strategies for Treating MEN 1–Related PHPT

PHPT is the most common, and typically the earliest, manifestation of MEN 1. In pediatric patients with MEN 1 who are undergoing prospective surveillance screening, 75% to 80% have biochemical evidence of PHPT by 21 years of age, although symptomatic disease is not typically seen before the third decade of life.[4] In addition to a younger age of onset, MEN 1–related PHPT differs from sporadic disease in a number of aspects. The former is characterized by asymmetric and asynchronous multigland involvement, in contrast to sporadic disease that is largely attributable to a single adenoma. Moreover, the female preponderance seen in sporadic PHPT is absent in MEN 1–related PHPT. Furthermore, while serum calcium and PTH elevations tend to be milder, patients with MEN 1–related PHPT have more severe bone mineral loss and kidney complications than what is observed in their counterparts with sporadic PHPT.

The diagnosis of MEN 1–related PHPT, as with sporadic disease, is made biochemically with the demonstration of hypercalcemia in association with inappropriately elevated PTH levels. Given the multiglandular nature of parathyroid involvement, the utility of preoperative imaging localization studies (eg, ultrasonography, ^{99m}Tc sestamibi scintigraphy, and/or CT) in MEN 1 is less well defined than in sporadic PHPT. An exception to this arises in the setting of persistent or recurrent disease where a "target" is required for reoperation. Nonetheless, some surgeons routinely use these modalities prior to index parathyroidectomy for evaluation of possible ectopic/supernumerary parathyroid glands (which occur in 7%-10% of cases) and concomitant thyroid pathology. A novel development in this area has been the application of PET imaging using radiolabeled choline analogues for parathyroid adenoma localization in MEN 1. For example, in a recent multicenter French study of 71 patients with MEN 1, ^{18}F-fluorocholine PET/CT offered superior detection of multiglandular and ectopic disease compared with conventional imaging (sestamibi and ultrasonography), with the highest sensitivity reported in cases of persistent/recurrent PHPT.[8] However, routine use of this modality is limited by cost, availability, and the requirement for an onsite cyclotron when radiotracers with short half-lives (eg, ^{11}C-choline or ^{11}C-methione) are used.

Indications for surgery for MEN 1–related PHPT largely mirror those for sporadic

disease. These include symptoms related to hypercalcemia and, in asymptomatic patients, serum calcium concentration greater than 1 mg/dL (>0.25 mmol/L) above the upper normal limit; skeletal involvement (T-score of ≤−2.5 at any site or a vertebral fracture); or kidney involvement (estimated glomerular filtration rate or creatinine clearance <60 mL/min per 1.73 m^2, presence of nephrocalcinosis or nephrolithiasis, or 24-hour urinary calcium excretion >250 mg/24 h [>6.25 mmol/24 h] in women or >300 mg/24 h [>7.5 mmol/24 h] in men).[9] An additional indication for parathyroidectomy, particularly in patients with MEN 1, is the presence of medically refractory peptic ulcer disease due to concomitant gastrinoma. In these cases, hypercalcemia can exacerbate the hypergastrinemia, and parathyroidectomy markedly reduces gastrin secretion. In the absence of these indications, there is no clear consensus regarding the optimal timing of surgery, particularly in the pediatric population. While some clinicians favor early intervention to reduce the number of years that a patient is at risk of developing bone and kidney sequelae (which may be more severe than in sporadic disease), others argue that the deferral of surgery avoids the devastating possibility of postsurgical hypoparathyroidism during a time when skeletal maturation is incomplete (ie, in children and adolescents), with the hope that fewer procedures will be required throughout a patient's lifetime for recurrent disease. Whether early parathyroidectomy reduces morbidity and mortality in patients with MEN 1 remains to be determined.

The choice of extent of index surgery for MEN 1–related PHPT involves a trade-off between resecting enough abnormal parathyroid tissue to achieve durable eucalcemia while leaving enough residual tissue to avoid rendering a patient chronically hypoparathyroid. Total parathyroidectomy with autotransplant of fragments of parathyroid tissue into the forearm or neck, or subtotal parathyroidectomy with resection of 3 to 3 and one-half glands, are both recommended as procedures of choice in the most recent clinical practice guidelines.[2] However, in recent years, total parathyroidectomy has fallen out of favor due to unacceptably high rates of permanent hypoparathyroidism, and most surgeons currently perform subtotal resections. Although the risk of hypoparathyroidism is reduced with subtotal parathyroidectomy, it is not completely obviated, which has led some groups to perform more conservative resections, involving either removal of a single abnormal-appearing gland or unilateral clearance of all parathyroid tissue with ipsilateral thymectomy. Proponents of these techniques (collectively termed "less-than-subtotal parathyroidectomy") argue that the increased risks of persistent and recurrent PHPT are offset by a reduced incidence of chronic hypoparathyroidism. Interestingly, in the study highlighted earlier, in which 71 patients with MEN 1 underwent localization with 18F-fluorocholine PET/CT, those with only 1 or 2 foci of disease were selected for less-than-subtotal parathyroidectomy, although postoperative outcomes for this group were not reported.[8] Nonetheless, in a recent study of approximately 200 patients with MEN 1 who had PHPT, those who underwent less-than-subtotal parathyroidectomy were actually found to have a higher rate of long-term hypoparathyroidism compared with those treated with subtotal parathyroidectomy (9% vs 7%), which was explained by the higher proportion of reoperations in the former group due to persistence/recurrent disease.[10] Thus, subtotal parathyoidectomy appears to provide the optimal balance between maximizing disease-free survival and avoiding prolonged hypoparathyroidism. Concomitant transcervical thymectomy is also recommended at the time of surgery to address the possibility of ectopically located parathyroid tissue in the thymus and to reduce the future risk of thymic NETs (with the caveat that only part of the thymus is resectable transcervically and therefore this risk is not completely abrogated).

MEN 1–related PHPT is characterized by high rates of disease recurrence regardless of operative approach. For patients with recurrent symptomatic PHPT who have previously undergone subtotal parathyroidectomy, ultrasound-guided ethanol injection has been used at the author's institution for ablation of enlarged parathyroid glands. This technique has been shown to have a favorable safety profile and achieved normocalcemia in 75% of patients in one study for a mean duration of 25 months.[11] In situations where reoperation is indicated (eg, after less-than-subtotal parathyroidectomy), but the patient is not a surgical candidate, cinacalcet, an allosteric modulator of the calcium-sensing receptor, has been shown to be effective in reducing calcium and PTH levels in small MEN 1 series. However, its ability to prevent bone and kidney sequelae associated with PHPT has not been established.

Emerging Strategies in the Detection and Management of MEN 1–Related DP-NETS

DP-NETs are highly prevalent in MEN 1 and occur in up to 80% of patients by 80 years of age. They currently represent the most common cause of MEN 1–related mortality due to their malignant potential. These tumors may secrete excess quantities of hormones that produce distinct clinical syndromes or can be functionally silent (while still secreting hormonally inactive peptides such as pancreatic polypeptide, chromogranin A, and neurotensin). Management of MEN 1–related DP-NETs is challenging due to their multifocal nature, which may be further complicated by the synchronous occurrence of both functioning and nonfunctioning tumors in the same patient. The main objectives of treatment are alleviating hormonal hypersecretion (in the case of functional tumors) and mitigating the risk of distant metastases, while minimizing intervention-related morbidity and mortality.

Nonfunctioning Pancreatic NETs
Due to the increased sensitivity of imaging modalities, nonfunctioning pancreatic NETs are now the most frequently diagnosed DP-NET, and have been reported to occur as early as ages 12

to 14 years in asymptomatic children with MEN 1.[4] The most recent clinical practice guidelines recommend annual testing of biochemical tumor markers, including fasting glucagon, chromogranin A, and pancreatic polypeptide. However, recent evidence indicates that the diagnostic accuracy of these markers is low and their use is therefore no longer recommended. Thus, imaging currently forms the cornerstone of diagnosis of nonfunctioning pancreatic NETs. Endoscopic ultrasonography is the most sensitive modality, but it is operator dependent, invasive, and may miss clinically significant lesions in the pancreatic tail. MRI is generally preferred over CT for screening purposes, due to better sensitivity and lack of ionizing radiation, although the latter is still useful for operative planning. A recent development in this area has been the increased application of functional imaging using ^{68}Ga-labeled somatostatin analogues. For instance, in a study of 58 patients with MEN 1, ^{68}Ga-DOTANOC PET/CT detected 3 times as many pancreatic NETs as conventional imaging and led to a change in clinical management in almost 50% of cases, either in the form of intensified follow-up or referral for surgical treatment.[12]

When should intervention be considered for MEN 1–related nonfunctioning pancreatic NETs? Current guidelines suggest surgical resection for tumors measuring greater than 10 mm or those that exhibit significant growth during follow-up (ie, doubling of tumor size over a 3- to 6-month interval and exceeding 10 mm).[2] This is based on multi-institutional data that demonstrate that tumor diameter correlates with metastatic risk. Conversely, more recent evidence suggests that nonfunctioning pancreatic NETs smaller than 20 mm in diameter are generally indolent, and a "watch-and-wait" strategy had been advocated in the absence of marked progression. However, distant metastasis of lesions below the 20 mm threshold can still occur, and noninvasive biomarkers for the prediction of aggressive behavior are urgently needed to facilitate decision-making for individual patients. Several single-center studies have reported certain *MEN1*

genotypes that portend a more aggressive course of DP-NETs, including pathogenic variants that disrupt the interaction between menin and the transcription factor JunD or nonsense/frameshift variants. However, none of these reported genotype-phenotype correlations have been independently validated and therefore this information cannot currently be used to guide individualized treatment decisions. Promising recent developments in disease stratification include the use of plasma-based metabolic and proteomic profiling to identity polyamines and circulating protein signatures associated with disease progression in MEN 1–related DP-NETs.[13] However, these techniques also require prospective validation before routine clinical adoption.

Gastrinomas

Gastrin-secreting NETs (gastrinomas) are the most common type of functioning DP-NET seen in persons with MEN 1 and are often multifocal and duodenal in origin. They occur in approximately 30% to 50% of affected individuals and are typically diagnosed in the third decade of life. Despite their small size, local lymph node metastases are reported in up to 80% of patients but do not appear to have a negative impact on survival. Hypersecretion of gastrin, if unopposed, leads to excessive gastric acid secretion with subsequent peptic ulceration and gastrointestinal bleeding (ZES).

Establishing the diagnosis of gastrinoma in patients with MEN 1 can be challenging. Although the gold standard diagnosis involves demonstration of a fasting serum gastrin concentration greater than 10 times the upper normal limit in the presence of a gastric pH of 2 or less, these criteria are seldom used in routine clinical practice due to unreliable gastrin assays and limited availability of secretin, which is required for stimulation testing to confirm the diagnosis in the two-thirds of cases where the serum gastrin is elevated but less than 10 times the upper normal limit. Furthermore, assessment of gastric acidity requires cessation of proton-pump inhibitors, which can be potentially risky in a patient who truly has ZES. To address this, modern diagnostic criteria for ZES in persons with MEN 1 on proton-pump inhibitor therapy have been proposed that incorporate symptomatology, biopsy results, and findings on somatostatin receptor PET-CT.[14] However, these criteria have not yet been validated.

Before the introduction of proton-pump inhibitors, ZES was the primary cause of death in persons with MEN 1. Currently, high-dosage proton-pump inhibitor therapy is effective in controlling acid hypersecretion in most patients. Therefore, unlike other functioning MEN 1–related NETs, the role of surgical intervention for gastrinomas is to prevent metastatic disease, although the timing and extent of intervention remain controversial. This is because very few patients are cured without aggressive surgery due to the multiplicity of tumors in the duodenum, their small size, and frequent metastasis to surrounding lymph nodes. This, coupled with the favorable prognosis for patients with small gastrinomas (<2-3 cm), creates uncertainty about the survival benefit of routine surgery in this context.

Insulinomas

Insulinomas are the second most common functioning DP-NET in persons with MEN 1. They represent the initial manifestation of the syndrome in approximately 10% of cases and have been reported in children as young as 5 or 6 years.[4] Although most are solitary, multifocal insulinomas can be found in 30% of patients and may be distributed throughout the pancreas. Most insulinomas (>90%) are benign and patients typically present with Whipple's triad, which consists of hypoglycemic symptoms, a plasma glucose concentration less than 55 mg/dL (<3.0 mmol/L), and resolution of symptoms after glucose administration. Early recognition of the sympathoadrenal symptoms (eg, palpitations, diaphoresis) and neuroglyopenic symptoms (eg, confusion, irritability) associated with hypoglycemia is of utmost importance, particularly in children and adolescents, who may be erroneously diagnosed with behavioral

disorders. Thus, current guidelines advise insulinoma screening starting at age 5 years with careful history taking and annual fasting glucose measurement.[2] Since almost all patients with MEN 1–related insulinoma are symptomatic, obtaining an accurate history often provides stronger diagnostic clues than fasting glucose checks, which can be challenging in young children. Nonetheless, the diagnosis is established with a 72-hour fast and demonstration of inappropriately elevated plasma insulin, C-peptide, and/or proinsulin in the setting of hypoglycemia and a negative antidiabetes medication screen.

Once the biochemical diagnosis of insulinoma is made, preoperative localization is required for operative planning. This can be difficult in the presence of other concomitant functioning and nonfunctioning DP-NETs that may also be seen on ultrasonography, CT, and/or MRI. In these cases, more invasive techniques such as selective intra-arterial calcium stimulation and hepatic venous sampling can be used to help regionalize the source of insulin excess. Recently, ^{68}Ga-exendin-4 PET/CT has been shown to have a sensitivity of 84.6% and specificity of 100% in the diagnosis of insulinoma in a small cohort of patients with MEN 1.[15] This technique takes advantage of the high expression of GLP-1 receptors on the surface of insulinoma cells and may be helpful in differentiating insulinomas from other concurrent DP-NETs when used in conjunction with other cross-sectional imaging modalities. However, widespread use is currently limited by lack of availability outside of a small number of European centers.

Surgery is the mainstay of treatment of insulinomas and requires a more nuanced approach in MEN 1 compared with sporadic lesions because of the possibility of multifocal disease and the aforementioned difficulties with localization. Enucleation may be feasible for small, solitary insulinomas (ie, <2 cm) that do not closely abut the main pancreatic duct, and it provides high rates of symptom resolution with minimal risk of pancreatic exocrine insufficiency. For lesions located in the pancreatic head that are not amenable to enucleation, a pancreatoduodenectomy (Whipple procedure) is typically indicated. However, this procedure is associated with relatively high rates of morbidity, particularly in MEN 1 cohorts. In patients who are poor operative candidates, recent advances in interventional gastroenterology have enabled adjunctive therapies, such as endoscopic ultrasound-guided ethanol ablation, to be used. Additionally, at the author's institution, if enucleation of a pancreatic head insulinoma is not achievable based on intraoperative assessment, then intraoperative ultrasound-guided ethanol ablation is offered in lieu of pancreatoduodenectomy. This novel approach is primarily driven by patients' preference to avoid the morbidity associated with pancreatoduodenectomy for a benign, albeit debilitating, disease process. In a small series of patients with both MEN 1 and sporadic insulinomas, endoscopic ultrasonography and intraoperative ultrasound-guided ethanol injections were associated with hypoglycemia resolution rates of 69%, while the remaining patients experienced improvement in the severity and frequency of their symptoms.[16] For patients with multifocal insulinomas, combined resections are performed, which most commonly entail distal pancreatectomy with enucleation of any pancreatic head lesions. Although these extensive procedures offer high hypoglycemia cure rates, they may also lead to new-onset diabetes in more than 25% of patients.

Other Functional DP-NETs

Functional DP-NETs, other than gastrinomas and insulinomas, are rare in MEN 1 and occur in 1% to 3% of patients. These include VIPomas, somatostatinomas, and glucagonomas. The classification of a tumor as "functional" is based on elevated hormone levels coupled with a corresponding clinical syndrome. In the absence of a syndrome, tumors are classified as hypersecretory rather than functional. This distinction is important because elevated glucagon levels in a patient with MEN 1–related DP-NETs do not indicate glucagonoma syndrome if the characteristic signs and symptoms of necrolytic migratory erythema, diabetes mellitus, and weight loss are absent.

VIPomas present with symptoms of watery diarrhea, hypokalemia, achlorhydria, and dehydration, while somatostatinomas may present with diabetes mellitus, diarrhea, steatorrhea, and cholelithiasis. In cases of these rare functional DP-NETs, surgical intervention is typically recommended in the absence of distant metastatic disease.

New Perspectives on MEN 1–Related Pituitary Adenomas

Pituitary adenomas occur in about 40% of persons with MEN 1 and are the first manifestation of disease in 13% of patients. As with their sporadic counterparts, MEN 1–related pituitary adenomas show a predilection towards women. They may occur at any age but are most commonly diagnosed in the fourth decade of life, with MRI being the imaging study of choice. Prolactinomas are the most frequent subtype, followed by nonfunctioning adenomas and, in less than 10% of cases, somatotropinomas, ACTH-secreting adenomas, and gonadotropin-secreting adenomas.[17] In contrast to other MEN 1–related tumors, multiple pituitary adenomas are rare. While earlier reports of MEN 1–related pituitary adenomas suggested that these tumors were more aggressive and resistant to treatment compared with their sporadic counterparts, more recent cohorts (published since the most recent clinical practice guidelines) have not supported this claim.[17] Indeed, most lesions detected by prospective screening appear to be functioning and functioning microadenomas that are indolent during follow-up, with macroadenomas accounting for one-third of tumors.

Treatment strategies for MEN 1–related pituitary adenomas are similar to those used for sporadic tumors, with dopamine agonists as first-line therapy for prolactinomas. When tumors are unresponsive to medical therapy or when there is mass effect with compression of the optic nerves and/or chiasm, management is transsphenoidal surgery or radiation as second-line therapy. ACTH- and gonadotropin-secreting tumors are treated with surgery as first-line therapy.

Clinical Case Vignettes

Case 1

A 25-year-old woman with a genetic diagnosis of MEN 1 is found to have the following laboratory values during routine biochemical testing:

> Serum calcium = 11.3 mg/dL (8.6-10.2 mg/dL) (SI: 2.83 mmol/L [2.15-2.55 mmol/L])
> Serum PTH = 95 pg/mL (15-65 pg/mL) (SI: 95 ng/L [5-65 ng/L])
> 25-Hydroxyvitamin D = 30 ng/mL (20-100.2 ng/mL) (SI: 74.9 nmol/L [50-250 nmol/L])

A surveillance abdominal CT reveals the presence of two 5-mm right kidney stones, but no other significant abnormalities. She currently has no symptoms. She takes no regular home medications.

Which of the following is the most appropriate management?

A. Observe, with a plan to measure calcium, PTH, and 25-hydroxyvitamin D in 12 months

B. Start cinacalcet

C. Consult an experienced parathyroid surgeon

D. Refer for genetic testing for CASR pathogenic variants

E. Request selective parathyroid venous sampling

Answer: C) Consult an experienced parathyroid surgeon

This patient has a biochemical diagnosis of PHPT and fulfills 2 criteria for surgery: serum calcium concentration more than 1 mg/dL (>0.25 mmol/L) above the upper normal limit and kidney involvement with evidence of nephrolithiasis on imaging. Therefore, referral to an experienced parathyroid surgeon (Answer C) would be appropriate and observation (Answer A) is incorrect. Cinacalcet (Answer B) has been used to treat patients with recurrent symptomatic MEN 1–related PHPT who are not surgical candidates or who decline an operation. This would not be appropriate as first-line therapy in this case. This patient already has a confirmed genetic diagnosis of MEN 1 and therefore referral for genetic testing

for *CASR* pathogenic variant analysis (Answer D) is not indicated. Selective parathyroid venous sampling (Answer E) is an invasive method of parathyroid localization that has been used in the context of recurrent sporadic PHPT when imaging is unrevealing. It is not indicated in this scenario.

Case 1 (continued)

The patient is evaluated by a parathyroid surgeon who requests a ^{99m}Tc sestamibi scan. This reveals a possible area of uptake in the region of the right inferior parathyroid gland with no evidence of ectopic parathyroid tissue. The patient is counseled regarding the risks and benefits of surgery and agrees to undergo parathyroidectomy.

Which of the following operative approaches achieves the best balance between maximizing duration of eucalcemia while minimizing the risk of prolonged hypoparathyroidism?

A. Total parathyroidectomy with parathyroid autotransplantation

B. Subtotal (3 and one-half gland) parathyroidectomy

C. Focused right inferior parathyroidectomy

D. Right-sided unilateral clearance

E. Total parathyroidectomy without parathyroid autotransplantation

Answer: B. Subtotal (3 and one-half gland) parathyroidectomy

In a recent series of 194 patients with MEN 1–related PHPT, subtotal parathyroidectomy (Answer B) achieved the best balance between disease-free survival (152 months) and rates of long-term hypoparathyroidism (7%).[10] Although disease-free survival was longer (210 months) after total parathyroidectomy with autotransplantation (Answer A), this approach was associated with a high incidence of prolonged hypoparathyroidism (40%). Focused resections (Answer C) and unilateral clearance (Answer D) fall under the umbrella of less-than-subtotal parathyroidectomy. These procedures were associated with significantly worse disease-free survival (60 months) and a higher rate of prolonged hypoparathyroidism (9%) compared with subtotal parathyroidectomy. This latter finding may seem surprising, as the purported benefit of less-than-subtotal resection is that the risk of hypoparathyroidism is minimized. However, this approach results in a higher frequency of reoperation for persistent/recurrent disease, which is associated with a higher risk of complications including prolonged hypoparathyroidism. Parathyroidectomy without parathyroid autotransplantation (Answer E), although curative, would guarantee permanent hypoparathyroidism and is therefore not recommended.

Case 2

A 35-year-old woman presents to the emergency department with a 12-month history of intermittent episodes of lethargy, confusion, and difficulty concentrating. She has a family history of MEN 1 on her father's side but has declined genetic testing herself and has not undergone surveillance screening. She has no other relevant medical history. Her symptoms are alleviated with consumption of food but have become progressively more challenging to control over the past weeks.

Laboratory test results on initial evaluation:

> Blood glucose = 42 mg/dL (70-99 mg/dL) (SI: 2.3 mmol/L [3.9-5.5 mmol/L])
> Pregnancy test, negative

She is admitted to the general medicine floor, and intravenous dextrose infusion is started, with prompt relief of her symptoms.

Which of the following is the best next step for establishing the cause of this patient's symptoms?

A. CT of the abdomen and pelvis

B. MRI of the abdomen and pelvis

C. Somatostatin receptor PET/CT

D. 72-Hour fast

E. Endoscopic ultrasonography

Answer: D) 72-hour fast

This patient is likely to have MEN 1, although this should be confirmed with genetic testing. Her symptoms are consistent with fulfilling the Whipple triad, which raises suspicion for the diagnosis of insulinoma. The diagnosis can be established by demonstrating inappropriately high serum insulin concentrations during a spontaneous or provoked episode of hypoglycemia, for example, during a 72-hour fast (Answer D). Imaging with CT (Answer A), MRI (Answer B), and/or endoscopic ultrasonography (Answer E) would be reasonable diagnostic tests *after* the biochemical diagnosis of insulinoma has been established and would also be indicated as part of MEN 1 surveillance screening. Somatostatin receptor imaging (Answer C) in the form of ^{68}Ga DOTATATE PET/CT is an option when conventional imaging studies do not identify a lesion, although insulinomas express variable levels of subtype 2 somatostatin receptors and may be less likely to be detected with this modality.

Case 2 (continued)

The patient undergoes a supervised fast, which is terminated after 2 hours when she develops neuroglycopenic symptoms and her plasma glucose concentration drops to 48 mg/dL (SI: 2.66 mmol/L). Insulin and C-peptide are measured at the time of hypoglycemia and both are nonsuppressed. Screening for oral hypoglycemic drugs is negative. CT of the abdomen and pelvis with intravenous contrast reveals a 2-cm mass within the parenchyma of the body of the pancreas in close proximity to the main pancreatic duct (*Figure 2, arrow, following page*). No other lesions are seen within the pancreas and the rest of the scan is unremarkable.

Figure 2. 2-cm Mass Within the Parenchyma
of the Body of the Pancreas

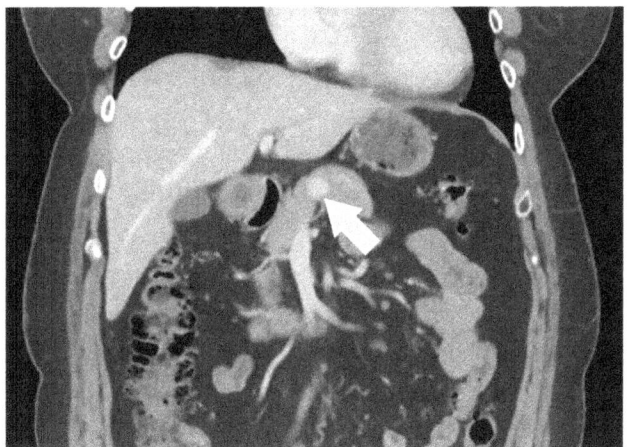

[Color—Print (Color Gallery page CG40) or web & ePub editions]

Which is the most appropriate definitive management for this patient?

A. Distal pancreatectomy

B. Pancreatoduodenectomy (Whipple procedure)

C. Enucleation

D. Ultrasound-guided ethanol injection

E. Initiate diazoxide

Answer: A) Distal pancreatectomy

The diagnosis of insulinoma in this patient has been established and the lesion has been localized on cross-sectional imaging. Therefore, surgical resection is the definitive treatment of choice in this patient. Based on the location of the tumor within the body of the pancreas, distal pancreatectomy (Answer A) would be the most appropriate operation.

Enucleation (Answer C) would not be feasible in this case given the lesion's proximity to the main pancreatic duct and its location deep within the parenchyma.

Pancreatoduodenectomy (Answer B) would be indicated for lesions in the pancreatic head that are not amenable to enucleation, although ultrasound-guided ethanol injection (Answer D) has also been used for benign insulinomas where the decision is made to avoid the morbidity associated with an extensive resection.

Diazoxide (Answer E) can sometimes be used for controlling hyperglycemia in patients who decline surgery or are not operative candidates, but this would not be definitive management.

Case 3

A 41-year-old man with known MEN 1 has a history of PHPT (treated with subtotal parathyroidectomy 5 years ago) and ZES (treated with duodenotomy and excision of multiple duodenal gastrinomas 10 years ago). He presents with concerns of progressively worsening diarrhea and epigastric discomfort despite maximal proton-pump inhibitor therapy.

Laboratory test results:

Serum gastrin = 9787 pg/mL (<100 pg/mL)
(SI: 9787 ng/mL [<100 ng/mL])

An image from upper gastrointestinal endoscopy is shown (*Figure 3*).

Figure 3. Upper Gastrointestinal Endoscopy

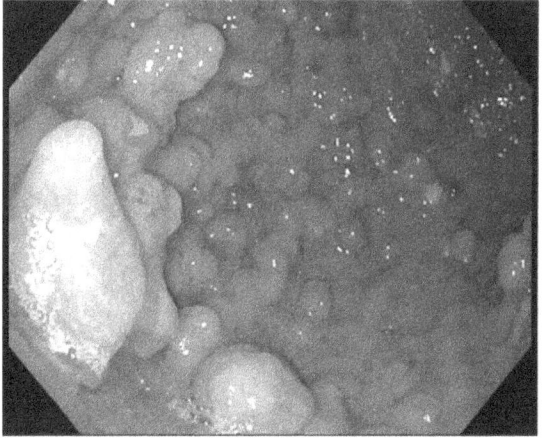

[Color—Print (Color Gallery page CG40) or web & ePub editions]

Which of the following does this patient's endoscopy findings represent?

A. Type 1 gastric NETs

B. Type 2 gastric NETs

C. Type 3 gastric NETs

D. Type 4 gastric NETs

E. Duodenal gastrinomas

Answer: B) Type 2 gastric NETs

This patient's history and presenting features are suspicious for recurrent ZES, and the endoscopy photograph shows multifocal type 2 gastric NETs (Answer B). Type 2 gastric NETs arise in the context of sustained hypergastrinemia in MEN 1 and ZES, which stimulates enterochromaffin-like cell hyperplasia.

Type 1 gastric NETs (Answer A) are associated with chronic atrophic gastritis, which is not the cause of hypergastrinemia in this patient.

Type 3 gastric NETs (Answer C) are usually large solitary lesions which are sporadic and not associated with specific syndromes, and type 4 gastric NETs (Answer D) do not exist.

Duodenal gastrinomas (Answer E) may be the underlying cause of ZES in this patient, but they are not depicted in the endoscopy images.

Key Learning Points

- Emerging data suggest that patients with MEN 1 without detectable *MEN1* germline pathogenic variants (or other genes that can present with an MEN 1–like phenotype), exhibit a less aggressive disease course, prompting considerations for a tailored, less intensive surveillance strategy.

- Primary hyperparathyroidism is the most common MEN 1 manifestation, for which subtotal parathyroidectomy offers the optimal balance between achieving eucalcemia while minimizing the risk of postoperative prolonged hypoparathyroidism.

- Surgical intervention for MEN 1–related nonfunctioning pancreatic neuroendocrine tumors is indicated for tumors 20 mm or larger; however, tumors smaller than this may still metastasize and there are currently no reliable validated biomarkers for the prediction of aggressive behavior.

- Effective management of functioning DP-NETs in MEN 1 requires a multifaceted approach. This involves not only accurate diagnosis and tumor localization, but also weighing the benefits of surgical intervention against potential complications and the challenge of multifocality.

- Pituitary tumors in MEN 1 are mostly microadenomas that may not be as aggressive as previously thought when compared with their sporadic counterparts.

References

1. Brandi ML, Agarwal SK, Perrier ND, Lines KE, Valk GD, Thakker RV. Multiple endocrine neoplasia type 1: latest Insights. *Endocr Rev.* 2021;42(2):133-170. PMID: 33249439

2. Thakker RV, Newey PJ, Walls GV, et al. Clinical practice guidelines for multiple endocrine neoplasia type 1 (MEN1). *J Clin Endocrinol Metab.* 2012;97(9):2990-3011. PMID: 22723327

3. Brandi ML, Gagel RF, Angeli A, et al. Guidelines for diagnosis and therapy of MEN type 1 and type 2. *J Clin Endocrinol Metab.* 2001;86(12):5658-5671. PMID: 11739416

4. Shariq OA, Lines KE, English KA, et al. Multiple endocrine neoplasia type 1 in children and adolescents: clinical features and treatment outcomes. *Surgery.* 2022;171(1):77-87. PMID: 34183184

5. Pieterman CRC, Hyde SM, Wu S-Y, et al. Understanding the clinical course of genotype-negative MEN1 patients can inform management strategies. *Surgery.* 2021;169(1):175-184. PMID: 32703679

6. de Laat JM, van der Luijt RB, Pieterman CRC, et al. MEN1 redefined, a clinical comparison of mutation-positive and mutation-negative patients. *BMC Med.* 2016;14(1):182. PMID: 27842554

7. Carvalho RA, Urtremari B, Jorge AAL, et al. Germline mutation landscape of multiple endocrine neoplasia type 1 using full gene next-generation sequencing. *Eur J Endocrinol.* 2018;179(6):391-407. PMID: 30324798

8. Gauthé M, Dierick-Gallet A, Delbot T, et al. (18)F-fluorocholine PET/CT in MEN1 patients with primary hyperparathyroidism. *World J Surg.* 2020;44(11):3761-3769. PMID: 32681321

9. Bilezikian JP, Khan AA, Silverberg SJ, et al; International Workshop on Primary Hyperparathyroidism. Evaluation and management of primary hyperparathyroidism: summary statement and guidelines from the Fifth International Workshop. *J Bone Miner Res.* 2022;37(11):2293-2314. PMID: 36245251

10. Shariq OA, Abrantes VB, Lu LY, et al. Primary hyperparathyroidism in patients with multiple endocrine neoplasia type 1: Impact of genotype and surgical approach on long-term postoperative outcomes. *Surgery.* 2024;175(1):8-16. PMID: 37891063

11. Singh Ospina N, Thompson GB, Lee RA, Reading CC, Young WF Jr. Safety and efficacy of percutaneous parathyroid ethanol ablation in patients with recurrent primary hyperparathyroidism and multiple endocrine neoplasia type 1. *J Clin Endocrinol Metab.* 2015;100(1):E87-E90. PMID: 25337928

12. Kostiainen I, Majala S, Schildt J, et al. Pancreatic imaging in MEN1—comparison of conventional and somatostatin receptor positron emission tomography/computed tomography imaging in real-life setting. *Eur J Endocrinol.* 2023;188(5):421-429. PMID: 36943311

13. Fahrmann JF, Wasylishen AR, Pieterman CRC, et al. Blood-based proteomic signatures associated with MEN1-related duodenopancreatic neuroendocrine tumor progression. *J Clin Endocrinol Metab.* 2023;108(12):3260-3271. PMID: 37307230

14. Metz DC, Cadiot G, Poitras P, Ito T, Jensen RT. Diagnosis of Zollinger-Ellison syndrome in the era of PPIs, faulty gastrin assays, sensitive imaging and limited access to acid secretory testing. *Int J Endocr Oncol.* 2017;4(4):167-185. PMID: 29326808

15. Antwi K, Nicolas G, Fani M, et al. 68Ga-exendin-4 PET/CT detects insulinomas in patients with endogenous hyperinsulinemic hypoglycemia in MEN-1. *J Clin Endocrinol Metab.* 2019;104(12):5843-5852. PMID: 31298706

16. Sada A, Ramachandran D, Oberoi M, et al. Ethanol ablation for benign insulinoma: intraoperative and endoscopic approaches. *J Surg Res.* 2024;293:663-669. PMID: 37839097

17. Le Bras M, Leclerc H, Rousseau O, et al. Pituitary adenoma in patients with multiple endocrine neoplasia type 1: a cohort study. *Eur J Endocrinol.* 2021;185(6):863-873. PMID: 34636744

ENDO 2024
COLOR GALLERY CONTENTS

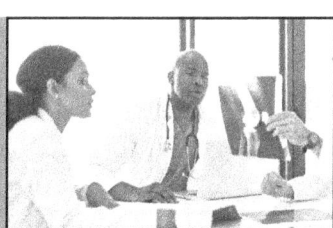

ADIPOSE TISSUE, APPETITE, OBESITY, AND LIPIDS

ADRENAL

BONE AND MINERAL METABOLISM

CARDIOVASCULAR ENDOCRINOLOGY

DIABETES MELLITUS AND GLUCOSE METABOLISM

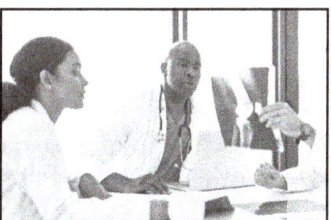

ADIPOSE TISSUE, APPETITE, OBESITY, AND LIPIDS

Primer on Weight-Loss Medications
Nasreen Alfaris, MD, MPH

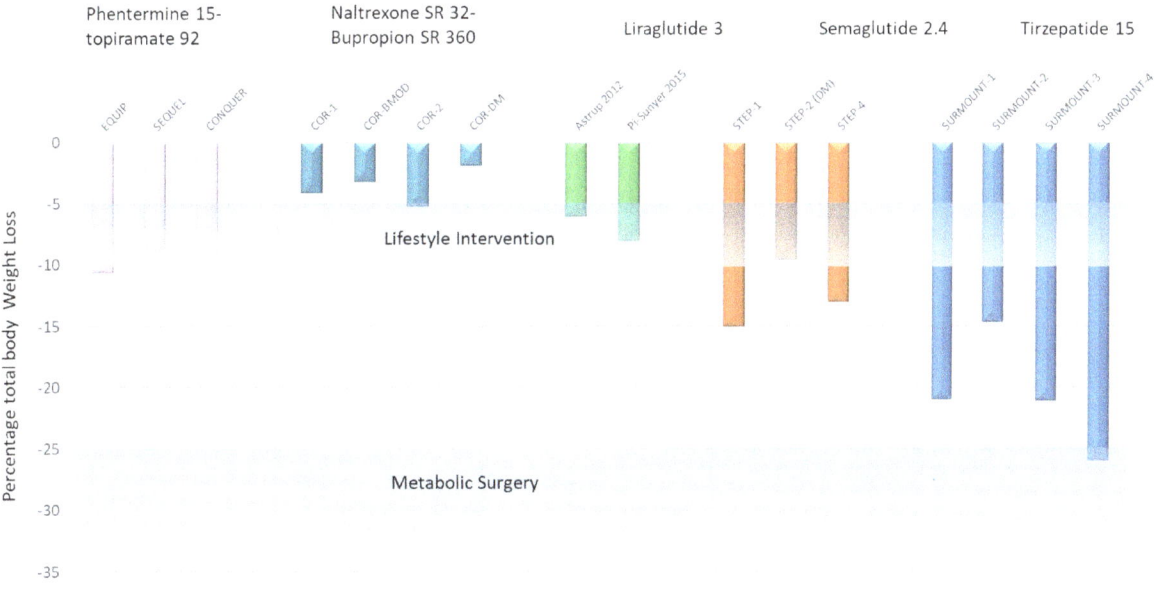

Practical Approach to Patients With Metabolic Dysfunction-Associated Steatotic Liver Disease
Kenneth Cusi, MD

	NAFLD	Other benefits	Contraindications	Side effects
Pioglitazone (91–9591–95)	Improves steatohepatitis; improves liver fibrosis in some studies (92, 94)	Cardiometabolic benefit	Caution if history of osteoporosis	Lower-extremity edema (5%-8%)
		Prevents development of T2D	Avoid if history of heart failure or bladder cancer	Dose-dependent weight gain: 15 mg/d: 1%-2% 30-45 mg/d: 3%-5%
GLP-1 receptor agonists (78, 102, 103) (liraglutide, semaglutide)	Liraglutide and semaglutide ameliorate inflammation and progression of fibrosis	Cardiometabolic benefit	Cholelithiasis	Gastrointestinal side effects
		Weight loss	Pancreatitis (?)	
			At risk of medullary thyroid cancer	
Dual GIP-GIP-1 receptor agonist (tirzepatide) (107)	Reduces steatosis	Weight loss	At risk of medullary thyroid cancer	Gastrointestinal side effects
SGLT2 inhibitors (111–113111–113)	Reduces steatosis (unknown effect on steatohepatitis)	Cardiometabolic benefit	CKD (eGFR 20-30 depending on SGLT2i)	Genital infections
		Prevention of ESRD		Volume depletion, hypotension Diabetic ketoacidosis (rare)
Metformin (1, 19, 109)	No effect on steatohepatitis	Cardiometabolic benefit	CKD (eGFR < 30)	Gastrointestinal side effects
			Heart failure	B_{12} deficiency
			Cirrhosis	Risk of lactic acidosis (rare)
DPP-4 inhibitors (108, 109)	No effect on steatosis (unknown if steatohepatitis benefit)	Weight neutral	Pancreatitis	
Insulin (114, 115)	Reduces steatosis (unknown effect on steatohepatitis)	Cardiometabolic benefit (controversial)	Caution in patients at high risk of hypoglycemia	Hypoglycemia (more in patients with cirrhosis)

Abbreviations: CKD, chronic kidney disease; DPP-4, dipeptidyl dipetidaase-4; eGFR, estimated glomerular filtration rate; ESRD, end-stage renal disease; GIP, glucose-dependent insulinotropic polypeptide; GLP-1, glucagon-like peptide 1; NAFLD, nonalcoholic fatty liver disease; SGLT2i, sodium glucose cotransporter 2 inhibitor; T2D, type 2 diabetes.

Reprinted from Belfort-DeAguiar R et al. *J Clin Endocrinol Metab*, 2023; 108(2): 483-495. © The Authors. Published by Oxford University Press on behalf of the Endocrine Society.[17]

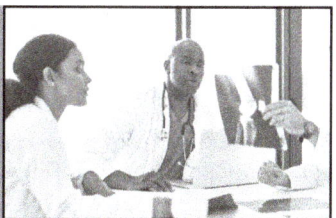

ADIPOSE TISSUE, APPETITE, OBESITY, AND LIPIDS

Primer on Weight-Loss Medications
Nasreen Alfaris, MD, MPH

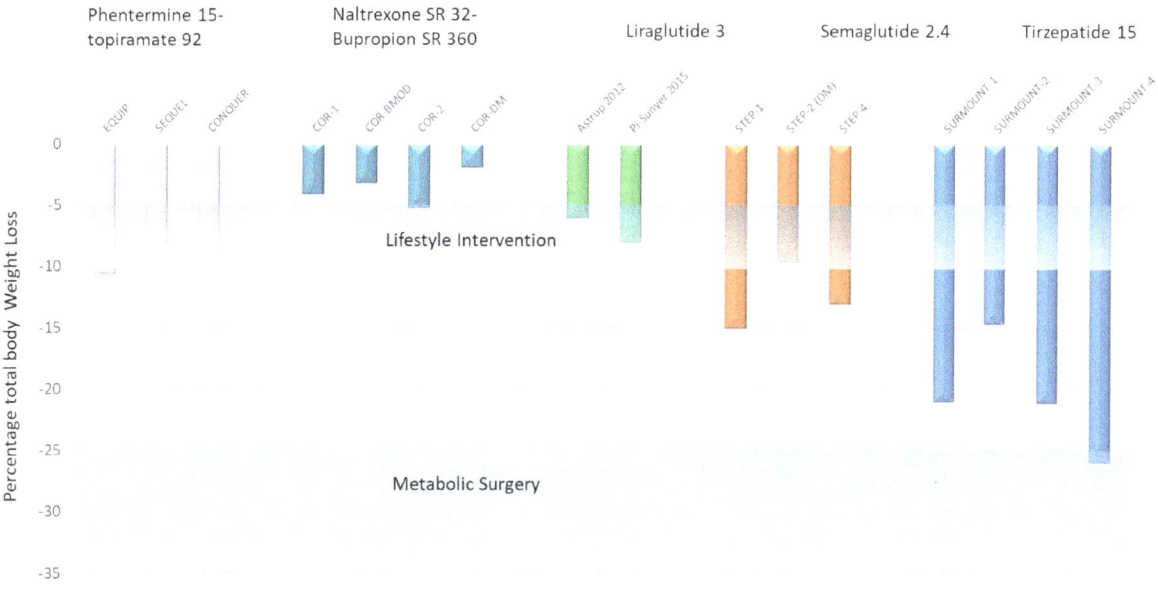

Figure. Percentage Total Body Weight Loss in RCTs of Approved AOMs.

Practical Approach to Patients With Metabolic Dysfunction-Associated Steatotic Liver Disease
Kenneth Cusi, MD

	NAFLD	Other benefits	Contraindications	Side effects
Pioglitazone (91–9591–95)	Improves steatohepatitis; improves liver fibrosis in some studies (92, 94)	Cardiometabolic benefit	Caution if history of osteoporosis	Lower-extremity edema (5%-8%)
		Prevents development of T2D	Avoid if history of heart failure or bladder cancer	Dose-dependent weight gain: 15 mg/d: 1%-2% 30-45 mg/d: 3%-5%
GLP-1 receptor agonists (78, 102, 103) (liraglutide, semaglutide)	Liraglutide and semaglutide ameliorate inflammation and progression of fibrosis	Cardiometabolic benefit	Cholelithiasis	Gastrointestinal side effects
		Weight loss	Pancreatitis (?) At risk of medullary thyroid cancer	
Dual GIP-GIP-1 receptor agonist (tirzepatide) (107)	Reduces steatosis	Weight loss	At risk of medullary thyroid cancer	Gastrointestinal side effects
SGLT2 inhibitors (111–113111–113)	Reduces steatosis (unknown effect on steatohepatitis)	Cardiometabolic benefit	CKD (eGFR 20-30 depending on SGLT2i)	Genital infections
		Prevention of ESRD		Volume depletion, hypotension Diabetic ketoacidosis (rare)
Metformin (1, 19, 109)	No effect on steatohepatitis	Cardiometabolic benefit	CKD (eGFR < 30)	Gastrointestinal side effects
			Heart failure Cirrhosis	B_{12} deficiency Risk of lactic acidosis (rare)
DPP-4 inhibitors (108, 109)	No effect on steatosis (unknown if steatohepatitis benefit)	Weight neutral	Pancreatitis	
Insulin (114, 115)	Reduces steatosis (unknown effect on steatohepatitis)	Cardiometabolic benefit (controversial)	Caution in patients at high risk of hypoglycemia	Hypoglycemia (more in patients with cirrhosis)

Abbreviations: CKD, chronic kidney disease; DPP-4, dipeptidyl dipetidaase-4; eGFR, estimated glomerular filtration rate; ESRD, end-stage renal disease; GIP, glucose-dependent insulinotropic polypeptide; GLP-1, glucagon-like peptide 1; NAFLD, nonalcoholic fatty liver disease; SGLT2i, sodium glucose cotransporter 2 inhibitor; T2D, type 2 diabetes.

Reprinted from Belfort-DeAguiar R et al. *J Clin Endocrinol Metab*, 2023; 108(2): 483-495. © The Authors. Published by Oxford University Press on behalf of the Endocrine Society.[17]

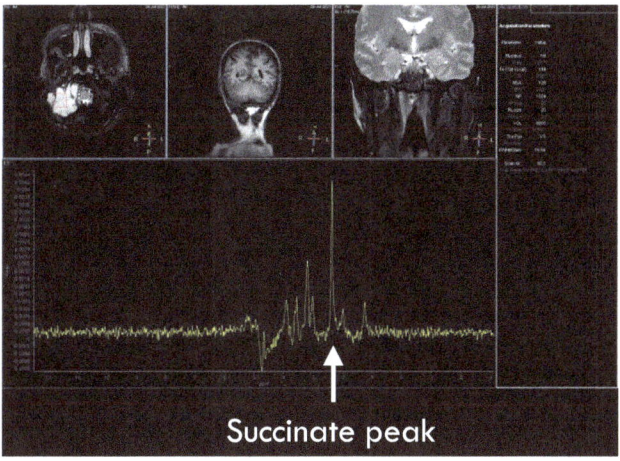

BONE AND MINERAL METABOLISM

Primary Hyperparathyroidism in Pregnancy
Dalal S. Ali, MD, MSc, and Aliya A. Khan, MD

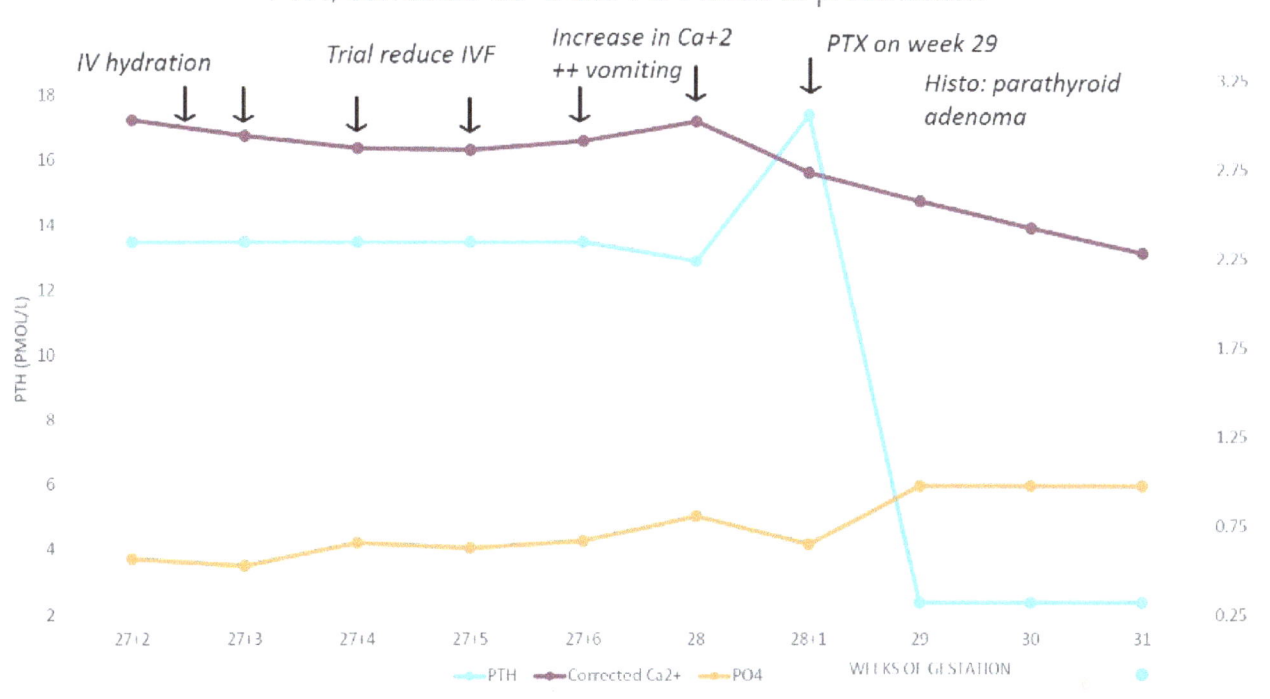

Bone Health in the Orthopedic Surgery Population

Alexandra N. Krez, BA, and Emily M. Stein, MD, MS

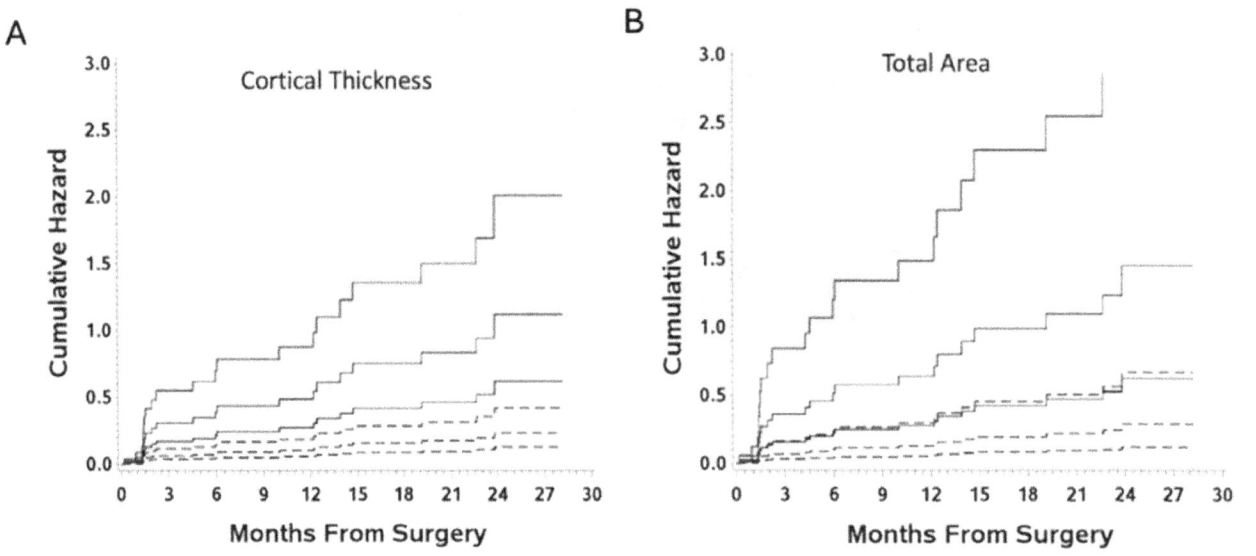

Panel A, Participants grouped according to tertiles of cortical thickness with black line ≥1.7 mm, blue line 1.2-1.7 mm, and red line ≤1.2 mm. Panel B, Participants grouped according to tertile of total area with black line ≥712 mm, blue line 620-712 mm, and red line 430-620 mm. Solid line represents hazard for patients who had fusions involving ≥6 levels, and dashed lines represent hazard for patients who had fusions involving <6 levels. Reprinted with permission from Dash AS et al. Osteoporos Int, 2023; 35(3): 551–560. © International Osteoporosis Foundation and Bone Health and Osteoporosis Foundation. Published by Springer Nature.[5]

Spinal Fusion Surgery

in the Orthopaedic Surgery Population

Risk Factors for Poor Bone Quality and Post-Operative Complications

Age> 50 years old

History of fragility fracture

Prior failed spinal surgery

Current tobacco use

Vitamin D deficiency

Alcohol use (≥ 3 units/d)

Chronic kidney disease (≥ stage 3)

Diabetes

Chronic glucocorticoid use

Evaluation

Medical history with a focus on medical conditions and medications that cause secondary bone loss, fragility fractures and falls

Dual x-ray absorptiometry at the spine, hip and 1/3 radius (if available)

Consider spine CT measurements of vBMD

Check serum 25-hydroxyvitamin D

Management

Address modifiable risk factors: smoking cessation, limit alcohol use, maintain a healthy weight, and home interventions to reduce fall risk (if indicated)

Maintain a daily calcium intake between 1000 to 1200 mg from diet and supplements

Vitamin D supplementation to maintain 25OHD level of ~ 30 ng/ml

For patients with osteoporosis or at high risk:
Consider anabolic agents (teriparatide). If anabolic agents are contra-indicated or their use is limited by cost, anti-resorptive agents can be considered

Radius Tibia

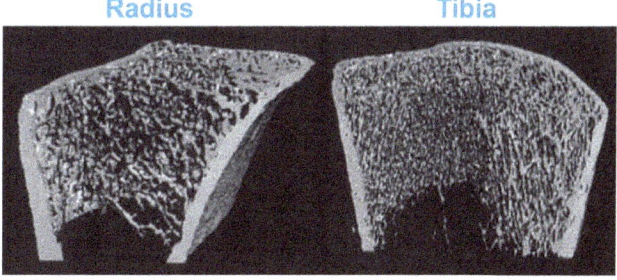

CARDIOVASCULAR ENDOCRINOLOGY

Cardiovascular Outcomes With New Diabetes Medications

Jane E. B. Reusch, MD, and Layla Abushamat, MD, MPH

Risk Factor	ABCs goals for many adults	Less stringent ABCs goals
A1C	<7.0%	<8.0%
Blood Pressure	<130/80 mmHg	<140/90 mmHg
Cholesterol, non-HDL	<130 mg/dL	<160 mg/dL
Smoking, current	Nonsmoker	Nonsmoker
Percentage meeting all ABCs goals	11.1 (8.1–14.9)	36.8 (31.8–42.1)

Notes: ABCs = A1C, blood pressure, cholesterol, and smoking. CI = confidence interval. Estimates are crude percentages and 95% confidence intervals. Data source: 2017–2020 National Health and Nutrition Examination Survey.

Centers for Disease Control and Prevention. National Diabetes Statistics Report website. https://www.cdc.gov/diabetes/data/statistics-report/index.html.[4]

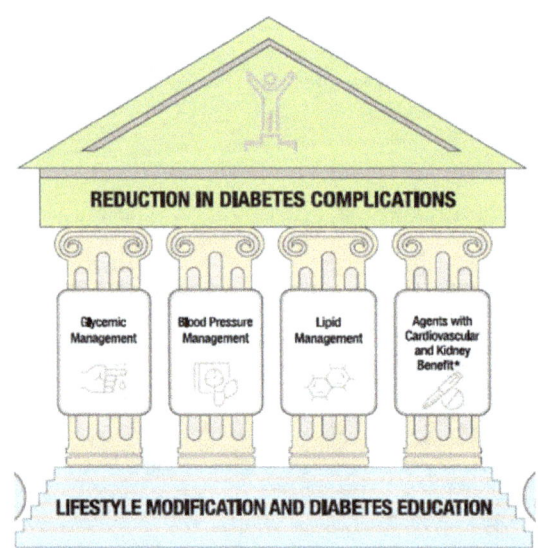

Reprinted from American Diabetes Association Professional Practice Committee. 10. Cardiovascular disease and risk management: Standards of Medical Care in Diabetes—2022. Diabetes Care, 2022; 45(Suppl. 1): S144–S174. © by the American Diabetes Association.[5]

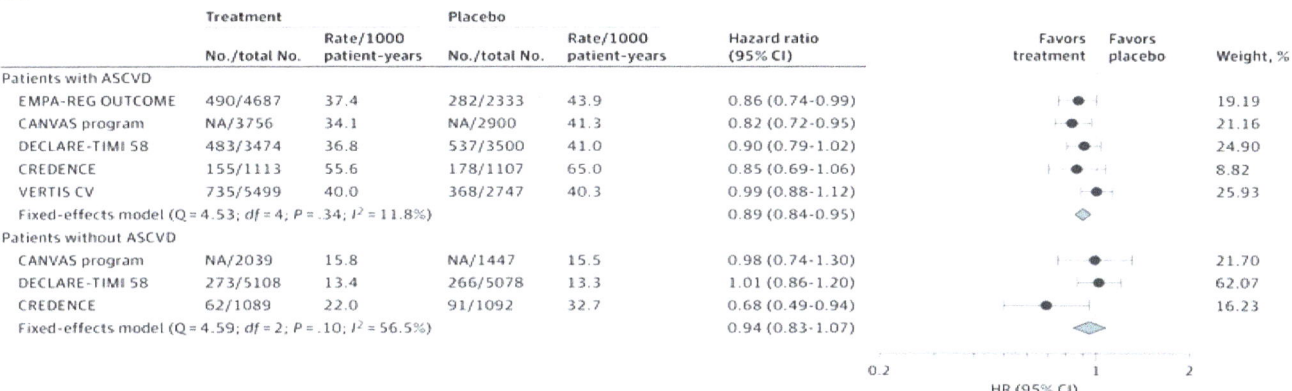

A Overall MACEs

	Treatment		Placebo						
	No./total No.	Rate/1000 patient-years	No./total No.	Rate/1000 patient-years	Hazard ratio (95% CI)		Favors treatment	Favors placebo	Weight, %
EMPA-REG OUTCOME	490/4687	37.4	282/2333	43.9	0.86 (0.74-0.99)				15.72
CANVAS program	NA/5795	26.9	NA/4347	31.5	0.86 (0.75-0.97)				20.12
DECLARE-TIMI 58	756/8582	22.6	803/8578	24.2	0.93 (0.84-1.03)				32.02
CREDENCE	217/2202	38.7	269/2199	48.7	0.80 (0.67-0.95)				10.92
VERTIS CV	735/5499	40.0	368/2747	40.3	0.99 (0.88-1.12)				21.23
Fixed-effects model (Q = 5.22; df = 4; P = .27; I^2 = 23.4%)					0.90 (0.85-0.95)				

B MACEs by ASCVD status

	Treatment		Placebo						
	No./total No.	Rate/1000 patient-years	No./total No.	Rate/1000 patient-years	Hazard ratio (95% CI)		Favors treatment	Favors placebo	Weight, %
Patients with ASCVD									
EMPA-REG OUTCOME	490/4687	37.4	282/2333	43.9	0.86 (0.74-0.99)				19.19
CANVAS program	NA/3756	34.1	NA/2900	41.3	0.82 (0.72-0.95)				21.16
DECLARE-TIMI 58	483/3474	36.8	537/3500	41.0	0.90 (0.79-1.02)				24.90
CREDENCE	155/1113	55.6	178/1107	65.0	0.85 (0.69-1.06)				8.82
VERTIS CV	735/5499	40.0	368/2747	40.3	0.99 (0.88-1.12)				25.93
Fixed-effects model (Q = 4.53; df = 4; P = .34; I^2 = 11.8%)					0.89 (0.84-0.95)				
Patients without ASCVD									
CANVAS program	NA/2039	15.8	NA/1447	15.5	0.98 (0.74-1.30)				21.70
DECLARE-TIMI 58	273/5108	13.4	266/5078	13.3	1.01 (0.86-1.20)				62.07
CREDENCE	62/1089	22.0	91/1092	32.7	0.68 (0.49-0.94)				16.23
Fixed-effects model (Q = 4.59; df = 2; P = .10; I^2 = 56.5%)					0.94 (0.83-1.07)				

Reprinted from McGuire DK et al. JAMA Cardiol, 2021; 6(2):148–158.[7]

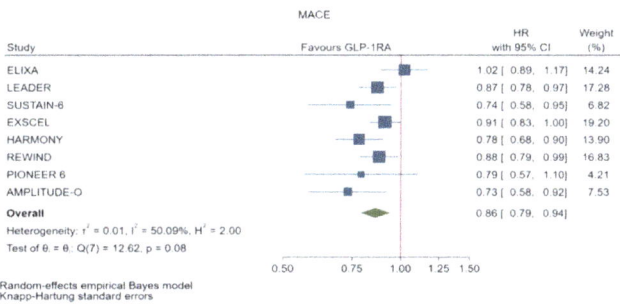

Reprinted from Giugliano D et al. Cardiovasc Diabetol, 2021; 20(1): 189.[8]

Figure 4. Forest Plot of a Meta-Analysis of the 6 Cardiovascular Outcomes Trials With GLP-1 Receptor Agonists on MACE in Patients With or Without CVD. 80

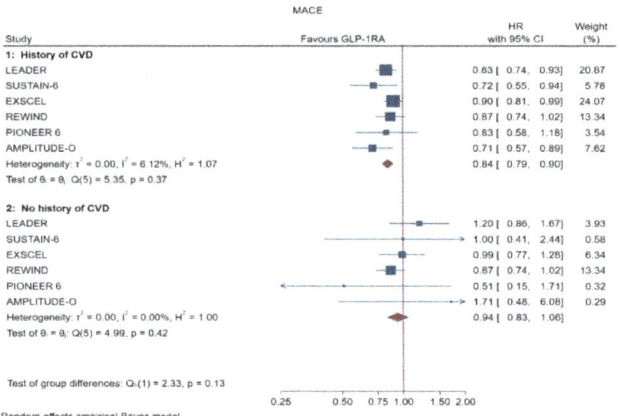

Patients with a history of CVD (top) and patients without such a history (bottom). Reprinted from Giugliano D et al. *Cardiovasc Diabetol*, 2021; 20(1): 189.[8]

Treatment of Primary Aldosteronism

Anand Vaidya, MD, MMSc

Figure 1. Pathophysiology of Primary Aldosteronism 88

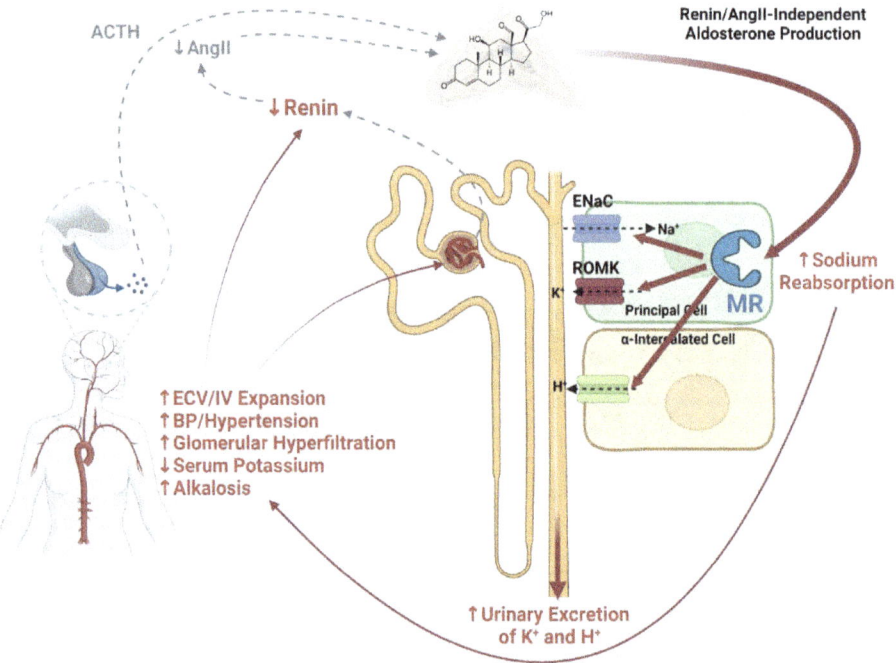

Abbreviations: ACTH, adrenocorticotropic hormone; Ang II, angiotensin II; BP, blood pressure; ECV, extracellular volume; ENaC, epithelial sodium channel; H+, hydrogen; IV, intravascular; K+, potassium; MR, mineralocorticoid receptor; Na+, sodium; ROMK, renal outer medullary potassium channel. Aldosterone is physiologically regulated by the renin-angiotensin system, adrenocorticotropic hormone, and potassium. In primary aldosteronism, one or both adrenal glands contain foci of dysregulated aldosterone synthase capable of producing aldosterone independent of stimuli by angiotensin II and/or adrenocorticotropic hormone. This excess aldosterone production activates the MR in principal cells even in volume-expanded states wherein renin and angiotensin II are suppressed, resulting in inappropriate sodium reabsorption via ENaC along with a commensurate excretion of potassium and hydrogen ions. This vicious cycle can induce the clinical manifestations of elevated blood pressure and hypertension, glomerular hyperfiltration, hypokalemia, and metabolic alkalosis. Created with biorender.com. Reprinted from Hundemer GL et al, *Endocrine Reviews*, 2024; 45(1): 69–94. © The Endocrine Society.[1]

Figure 2. Medical Treatments for Primary Aldosteronism

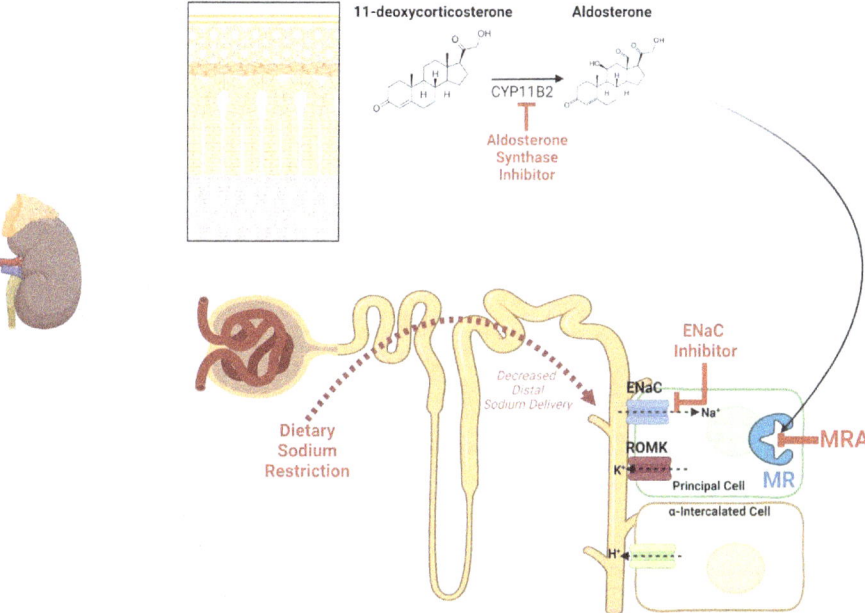

Abbreviations: ENaC, epithelial sodium channel; H+, hydrogen; K+, potassium; MR, mineralocorticoid receptor; MRA, mineralocorticoid receptor antagonist; Na+, sodium; ROMK, renal outer medullary potassium channel. Dietary sodium restriction leads to volume contraction, decreased glomerular filtration, and decreased sodium delivery to the distal nephron thereby limiting aldosterone-MR-ENaC-mediated sodium reabsorption. MR antagonists prevent the interaction between aldosterone and the MR in the principal cell, thereby preventing ENaC-mediated sodium reabsorption. ENaC inhibitors directly block ENaC-mediated sodium reabsorption. Aldosterone synthase inhibitors block CYP11B2-mediated conversion of 11-deoxycorticosterone to aldosterone in the adrenal cortex. Created with biorender.com. Reprinted from Hundemer GL et al, *Endocrine Reviews*, 2024; 45(1): 69–94. © The Endocrine Society.[1]

Figure 3. Biomarkers of Optimal Medical Therapy in Primary Aldosteronism.

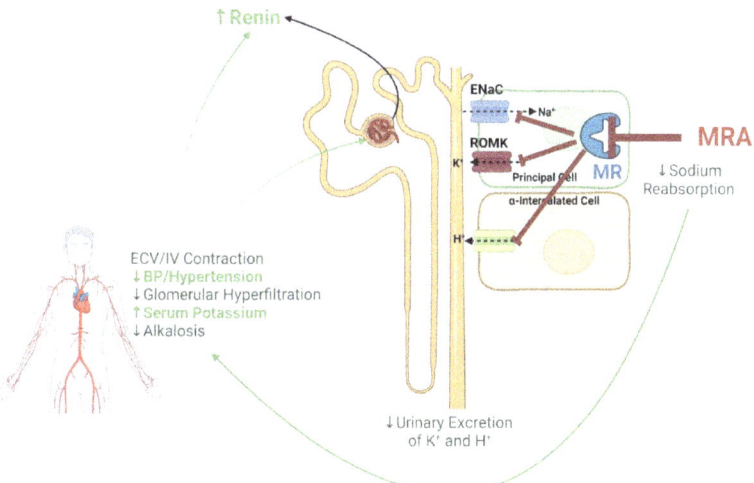

Abbreviations: BP, blood pressure; ECV, extracellular volume; ENaC, epithelial sodium channel; H+, hydrogen; IV, intravascular; K+, potassium; MR, mineralocorticoid receptor; MRA, mineralocorticoid receptor antagonist; Na+, sodium; ROMK, renal outer medullary potassium channel. Through blockade of the interaction between aldosterone and the MR in the principal cell of the distal nephron, MR antagonists decrease ENaC-mediated sodium reabsorption. This, in turn, results in decreased volume expansion along with decreased potassium and hydrogen ion urinary excretion. If the degree of MR blockade is sufficient to cause intravascular volume contraction and relative kidney hypoperfusion, renin will rise due to secretion from the juxtaglomerular cells. Thus, a rise in renin along with a lowering of blood pressure and normalization of serum potassium serve as biomarkers of adequate MR blockade in primary aldosteronism. In bold are the key biomarkers that reflect optimized medical therapy in primary aldosteronism: normalization of blood pressure, normalization of serum potassium, and a rise in renin. Created with biorender.com. Adapted from Hundemer GL et al, *Endocrine Reviews*, 2024; 45(1): 69–94. © The Endocrine Society.[1]

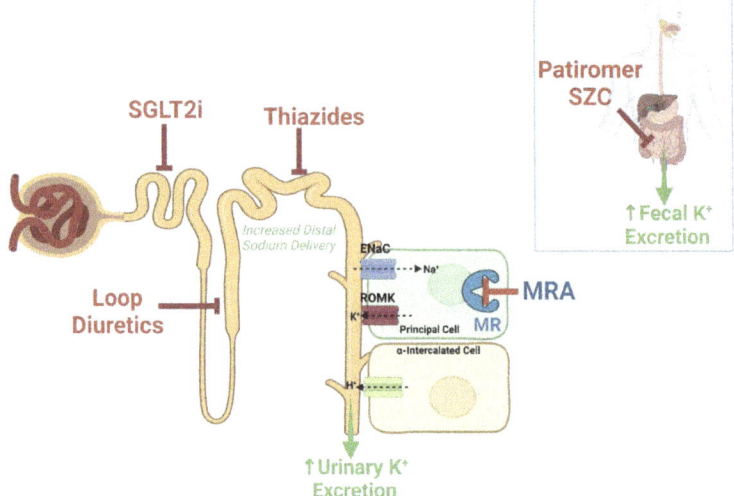

Abbreviations: ENaC, epithelial sodium channel; H+, hydrogen; K+, potassium; MR, mineralocorticoid receptor; MRA, mineralocorticoid receptor antagonist; Na+, sodium; ROMK, renal outer medullary potassium channel; SGLT2i, sodium-glucose cotransporter-2 inhibitor; SZC, sodium zirconium cyclosilicate. SGLT-2 inhibitors (via blockade of SGLT-2 in the proximal tubule), loop diuretics (via blockade of the Na+-K+-Cl- cotransporter along the thick ascending loop of Henle), and thiazide diuretics (via blockade of the sodium-chloride symporter in the distal convoluted tubule) all cause increased urinary distal sodium delivery and reabsorption, which enhances the electronegative charge in the tubular lumen thereby driving urinary potassium excretion in the collecting duct. Patiromer and sodium zirconium cyclosilicate serve to bind potassium in the gastrointestinal tract, thereby increasing fecal potassium excretion. Created with biorender.com. Reprinted from Hundemer GL et al, *Endocrine Reviews*, 2024; 45(1): 69–94. © The Endocrine Society.[1]

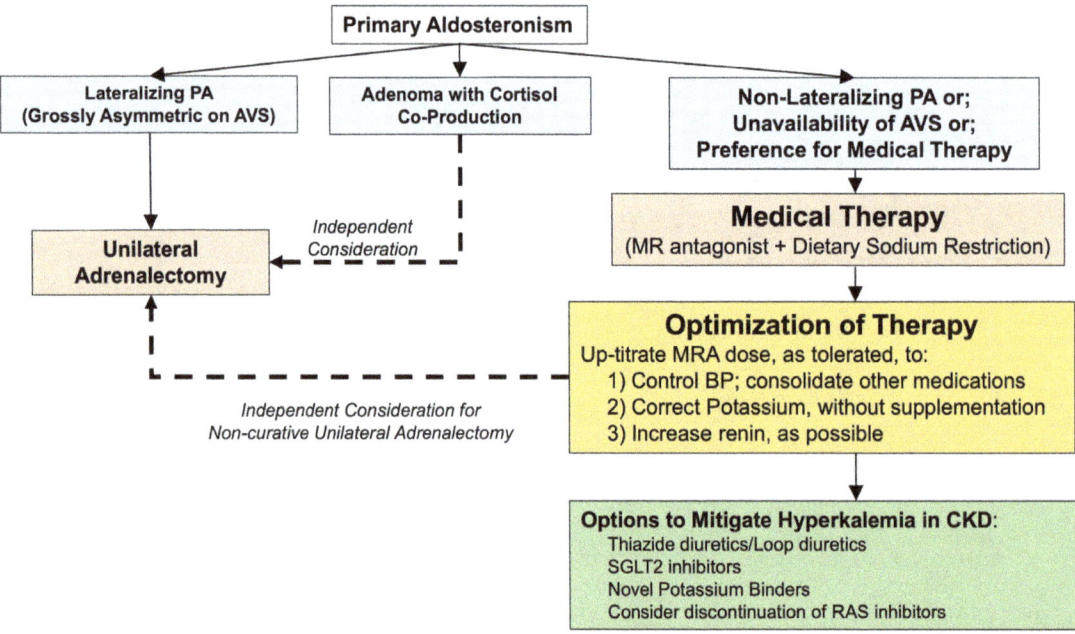

Abbreviations: AVS, adrenal vein sampling; BP, blood pressure; HTN, hypertension; K+, potassium; MRA, mineralocorticoid receptor antagonist; PA, primary aldosteronism; RAS, renin-angiotensin system; SGLT2, sodium-glucose cotransporter-2. For patients with lateralizing PA, unilateral adrenalectomy is the standard recommendation. Unilateral adrenalectomy should also be considered for patients with an adenoma with cortisol co-production. For patients with nonlateralizing PA, those for whom AVS is not available, or those with lateralizing PA who have declined surgical treatment, we suggest treating with MR antagonist therapy and dietary sodium restriction. To optimize MR antagonist therapy, we recommend up-titrating the dose as tolerated with the goals of normalizing blood pressure (and ideally reducing other antihypertensive medications in the process), normalizing serum potassium without the use of potassium supplementation (if applicable), and achieving a rise in renin as a biomarker of restoration of normal renin-angiotensin system activity. If hyperkalemia becomes a barrier to MR antagonist up-titration, addition of a potassium-wasting diuretic (thiazide or loop), an SGLT-2 inhibitor, a novel potassium binder (patiromer or sodium zirconium cyclosilicate), and/or discontinuing renin-angiotensin system inhibitors should be considered. If a case of PA is severe enough and refractory to maximal medical therapy, unilateral adrenalectomy may be considered for disease attenuation (rather than disease cure). Reprinted from Hundemer GL et al, *Endocrine Reviews*, 2024; 45(1): 69–94. © The Endocrine Society.[1]

What's New in Diabetes Technology?

Grazia Aleppo, MD

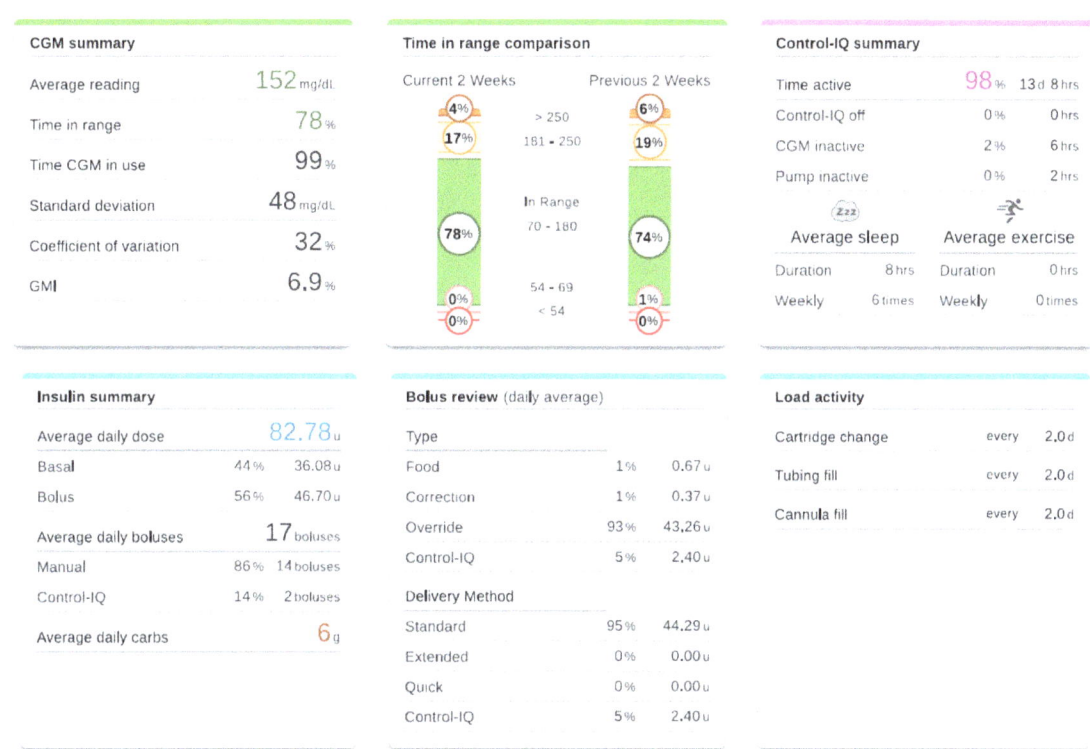

Dashboard shows average glucose levels, GMI, time-in-range, and use of Control IQ in the upper panels. Lower panels show the insulin summary with basal insulin delivered by the algorithm, bolus doses, number of boluses per day, and average daily grams of carbohydrate entered. Bolus review shows how the user has used the bolus (whether by bolus calculator or otherwise) and the average cartridge change (number of days).

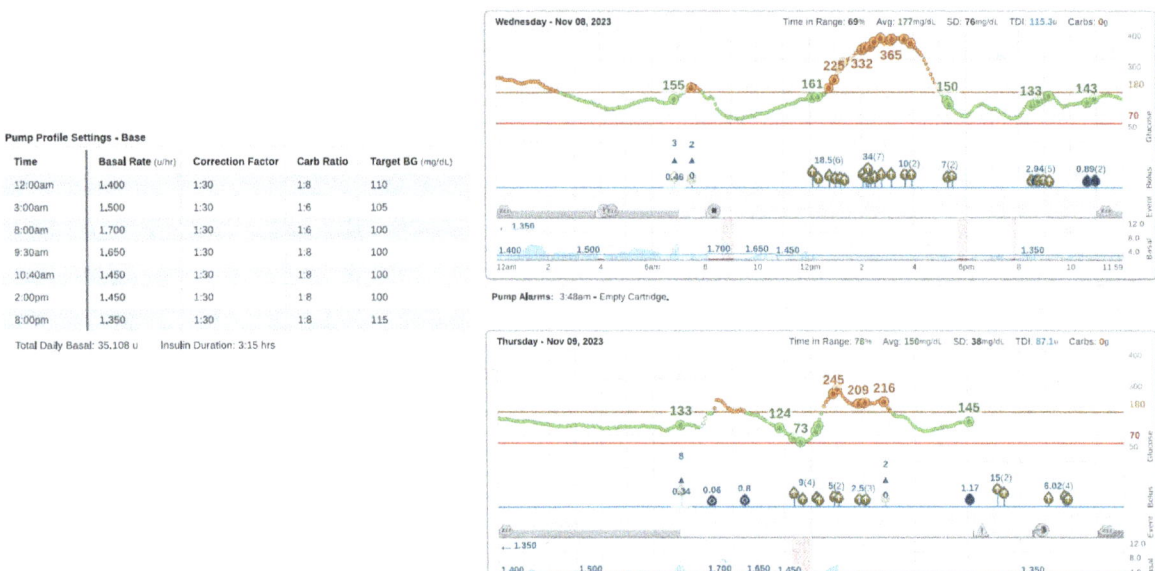

Pump Profile Settings - Base

Time	Basal Rate (u/hr)	Correction Factor	Carb Ratio	Target BG (mg/dL)
12:00am	1.400	1:30	1:8	110
3:00am	1.500	1:30	1:6	105
8:00am	1.700	1:30	1:6	100
9:30am	1.650	1:30	1:8	100
10:40am	1.450	1:30	1:8	100
2:00pm	1.450	1:30	1:8	100
8:00pm	1.350	1:30	1:8	115

Total Daily Basal: 35.108 u   Insulin Duration: 3:15 hrs

The left panel shows the pump profile settings, with basal rates, correction factor, carbohydrate ratio, and target blood glucose. The right panel shows the daily views with information on the CGM data, the boluses entered by the user, and the basal insulin delivery information.

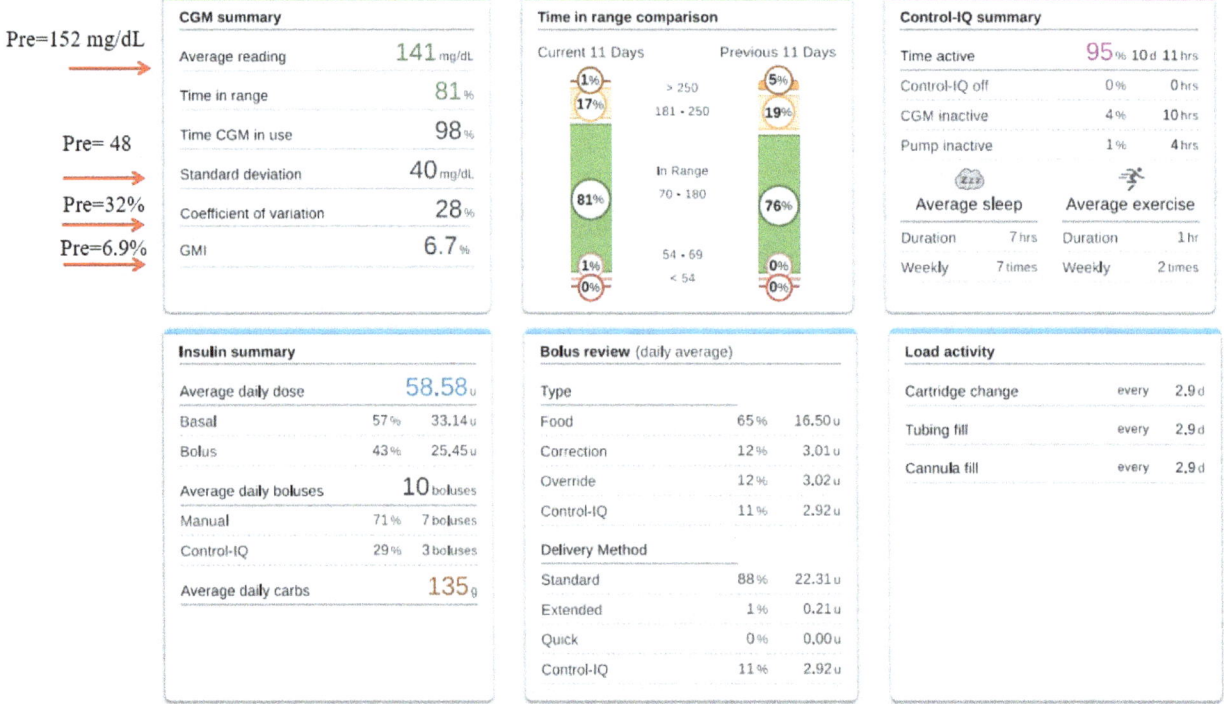

Pre=152 mg/dL

Pre= 48

Pre=32%

Pre=6.9%

CGM summary

Average reading	141 mg/dL
Time in range	81 %
Time CGM in use	98 %
Standard deviation	40 mg/dL
Coefficient of variation	28 %
GMI	6.7 %

Time in range comparison

Current 11 Days — Previous 11 Days

1%	> 250	5%
17%	181 - 250	19%
81%	In Range 70 - 180	76%
1%	54 - 69	0%
0%	< 54	0%

Control-IQ summary

Time active	95 %	10 d 11 hrs
Control-IQ off	0%	0 hrs
CGM inactive	4%	10 hrs
Pump inactive	1%	4 hrs

Average sleep		Average exercise	
Duration	7 hrs	Duration	1 hr
Weekly	7 times	Weekly	2 times

Insulin summary

Average daily dose		58.58 u
Basal	57%	33.14 u
Bolus	43%	25.45 u
Average daily boluses		10 boluses
Manual	71%	7 boluses
Control-IQ	29%	3 boluses
Average daily carbs		135 g

Bolus review (daily average)

Type		
Food	65%	16.50 u
Correction	12%	3.01 u
Override	12%	3.02 u
Control-IQ	11%	2.92 u
Delivery Method		
Standard	88%	22.31 u
Extended	1%	0.21 u
Quick	0%	0.00 u
Control-IQ	11%	2.92 u

Load activity

Cartridge change	every	2.9 d
Tubing fill	every	2.9 d
Cannula fill	every	2.9 d

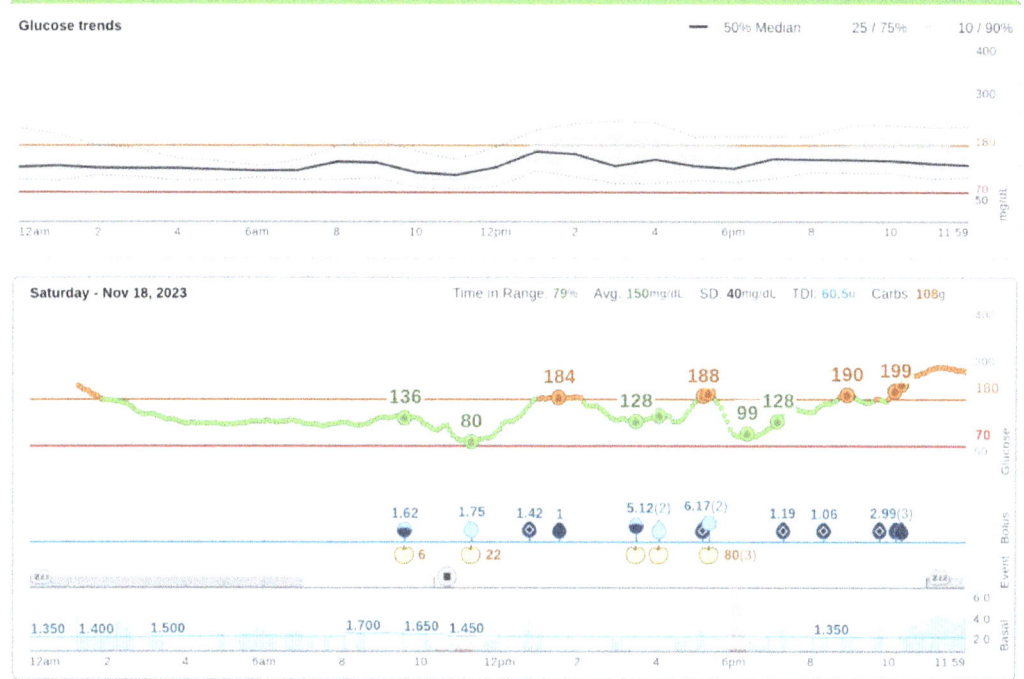

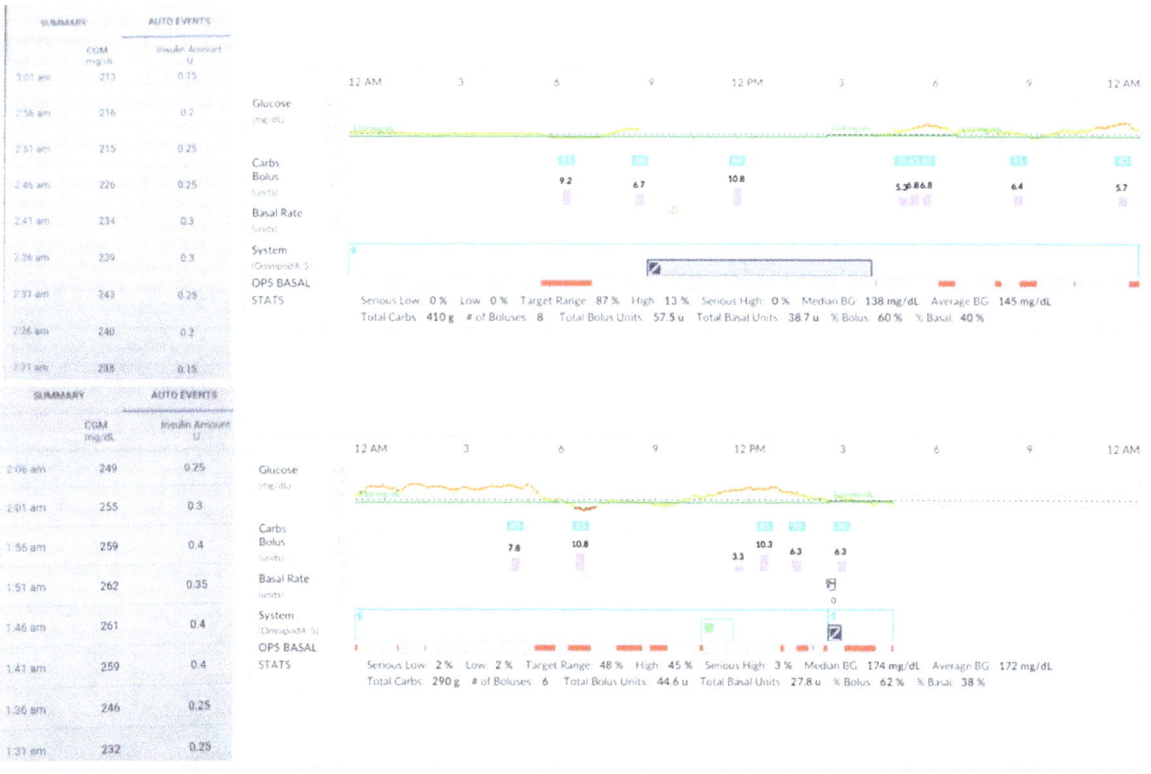

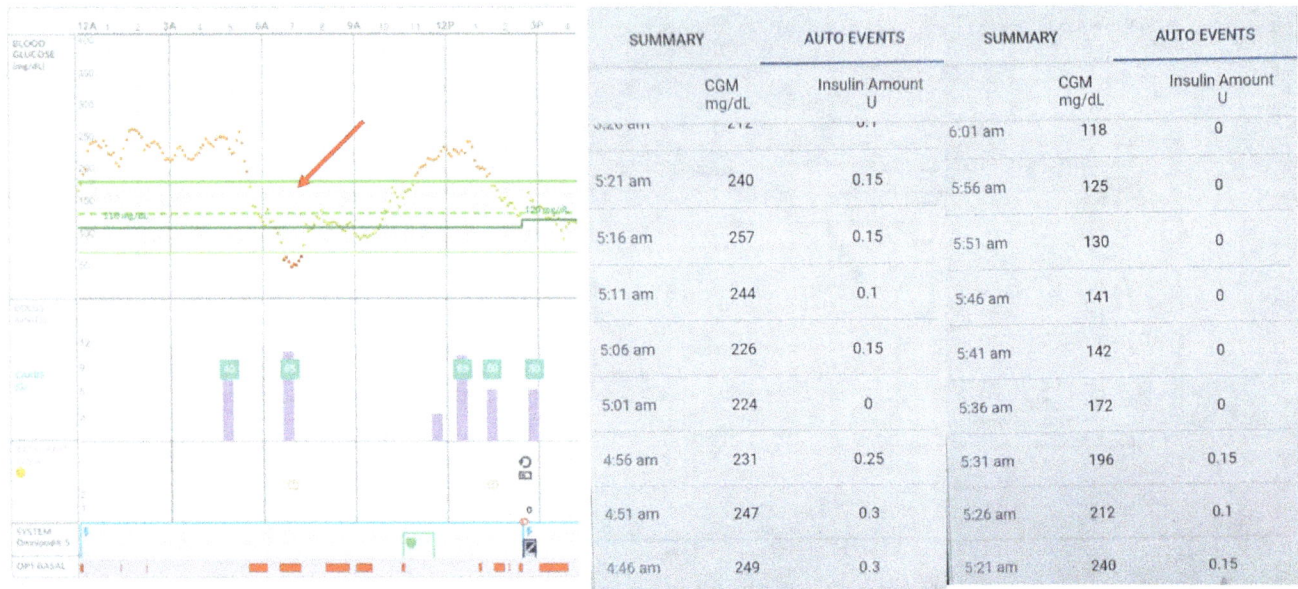

SUMMARY	AUTO EVENTS		SUMMARY	AUTO EVENTS
	CGM mg/dL	Insulin Amount U		CGM mg/dL	Insulin Amount U
5:20 am	212	0.1	6:01 am	118	0
5:21 am	240	0.15	5:56 am	125	0
5:16 am	257	0.15	5:51 am	130	0
5:11 am	244	0.1	5:46 am	141	0
5:06 am	226	0.15	5:41 am	142	0
5:01 am	224	0	5:36 am	172	0
4:56 am	231	0.25	5:31 am	196	0.15
4:51 am	247	0.3	5:26 am	212	0.1
4:46 am	249	0.3	5:21 am	240	0.15

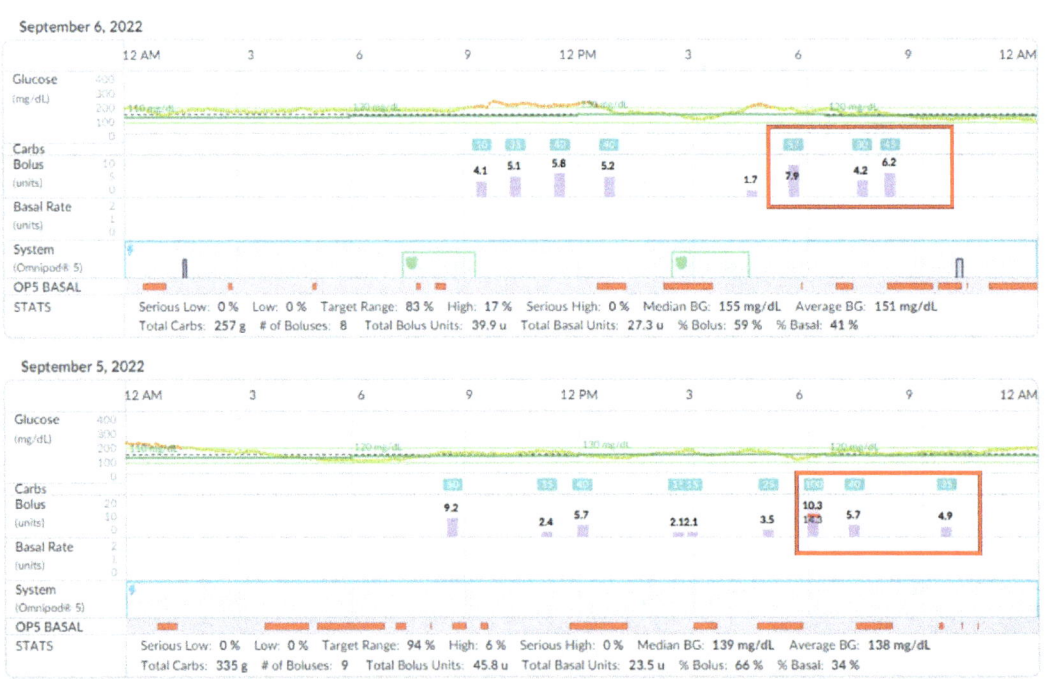

September 6, 2022

STATS — Serious Low: 0 % Low: 0 % Target Range: 83 % High: 17 % Serious High: 0 % Median BG: 155 mg/dL Average BG: 151 mg/dL
Total Carbs: 257 g # of Boluses: 8 Total Bolus Units: 39.9 u Total Basal Units: 27.3 u % Bolus: 59 % % Basal: 41 %

September 5, 2022

STATS — Serious Low: 0 % Low: 0 % Target Range: 94 % High: 6 % Serious High: 0 % Median BG: 139 mg/dL Average BG: 138 mg/dL
Total Carbs: 335 g # of Boluses: 9 Total Bolus Units: 45.8 u Total Basal Units: 23.5 u % Bolus: 66 % % Basal: 34 %

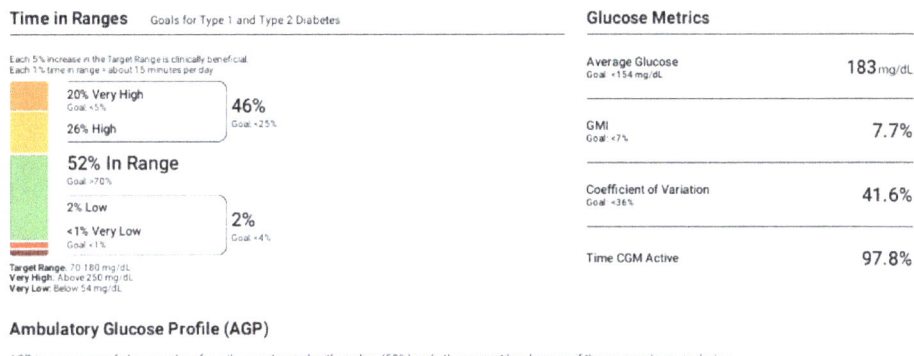

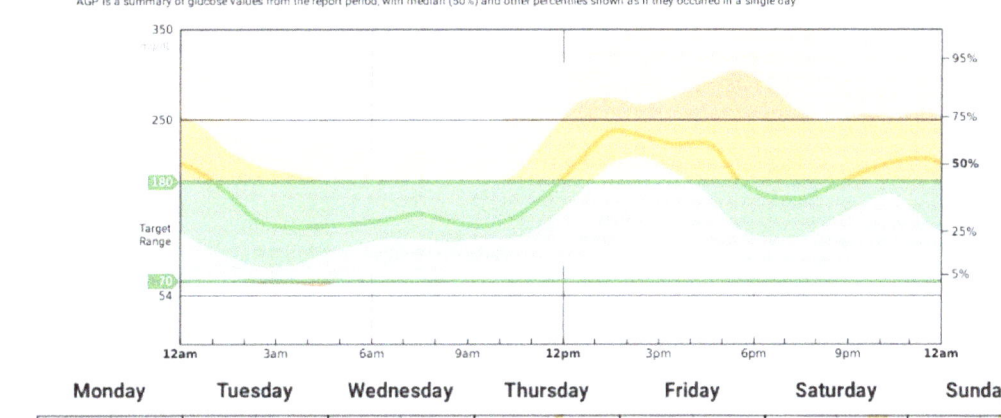

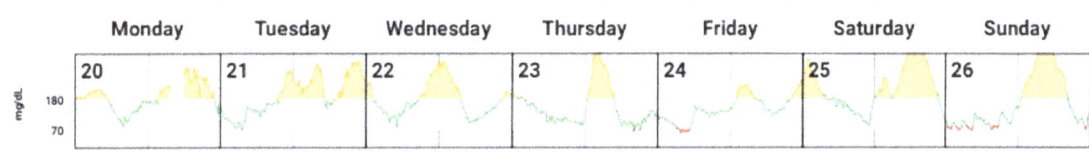

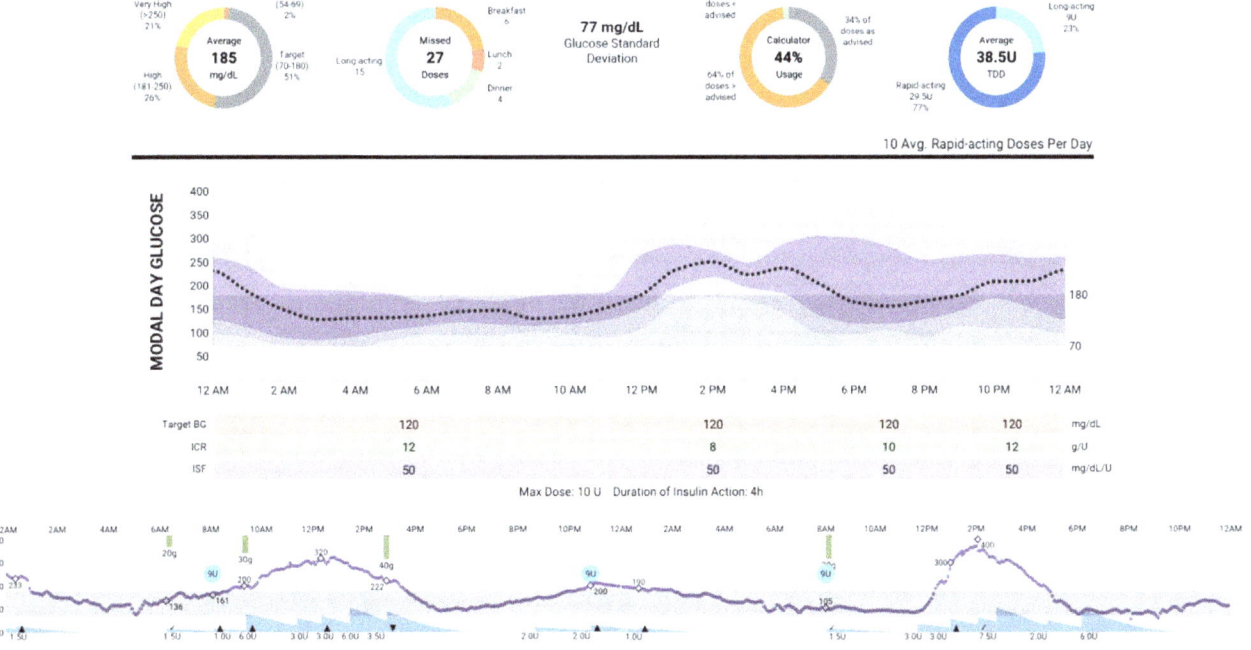

Addressing Social Determinants of Health in Routine Diabetes Care

A. Enrique Caballero, MD

Acculturation	Nutrition and Food Availability
Biology	Other Forms of Medicine
Clinicians' Cultural Awareness	Perception of Body Image
Depression and Emotional Distress	Quality of Life
Educational Level	Religion and Faith
Fears	Socioeconomic Status
Group Engagement/Family/Community Support	Technology
Health Literacy	Unconscious Bias
Intimacy/Sexual Dysfunction	Vulnerable Groups
Judging	Why? (Always get the patient's perspective)
Knowledge of the Disease	Xercise!
Language	You Are in Charge. (Patient-Centered Approach)
Medical Adherence	Zip it! (Let the Patient Talk!)

Caballero AE. Front Endocrinol (Lausanne), 2018; 9(479): 1-15. © by the Author. Published by Frontiers Media S.A.[6]

Diabetes and Varied Diets: Intermittent Fasting, Ketogenic Diets, and Holiday Fasting

Nancy Samir Elbarbary, MBBCh, MSc, MD, PhD

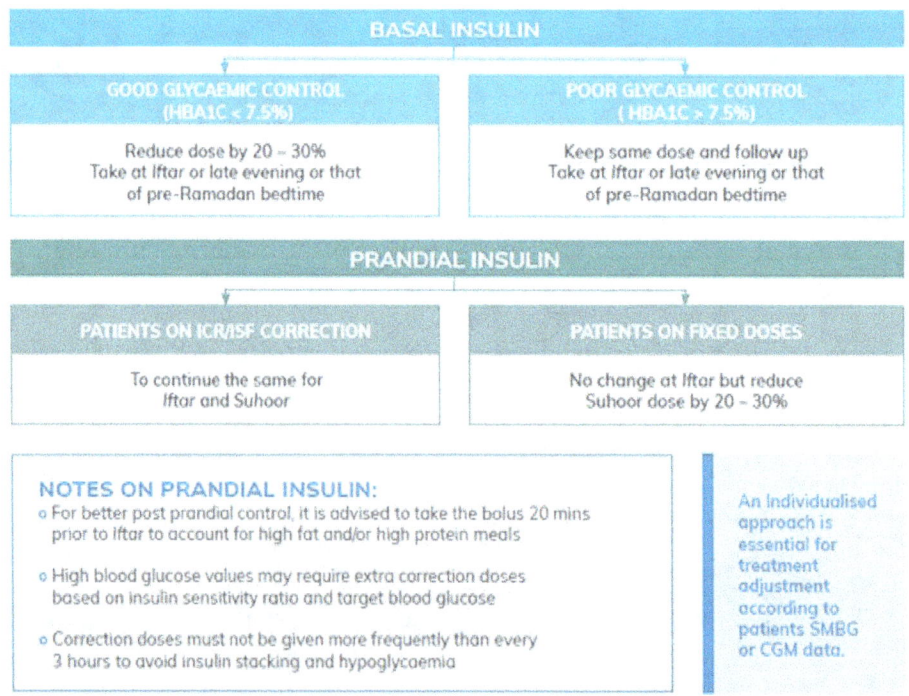

Adapted from Hassanein M et al. Diabetes Res Clin Pract, 2022; 185: 109185. © Elsevier B.V.

Figure 2. Schematic Adjustments of Insulin and/or Food Considerations During Fasting and Nonfasting Hours . . . 130

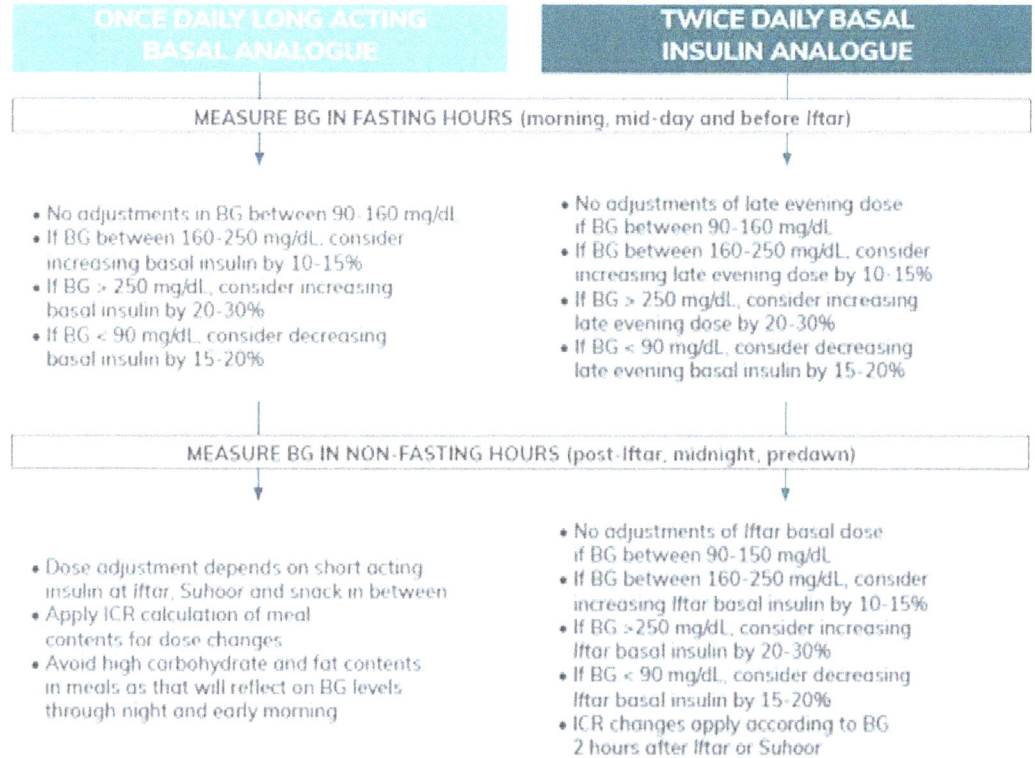

Reprinted from International Diabetes Federation & Diabetes and Ramadan, *Diabetes and Ramadan: Practical Guidelines 2021*, Chapter 9, "Management of Type 1 diabetes when fasting during Ramadan."

Figure 3. Basal and Bolus Insulin During Ramadan 130

BASAL INSULIN	BOLUS INSULIN
Reduce basal insulin by 20-35% in the last 4-5 hours before *Iftar* Increase dose by 10-30% after *Iftar* up to midnight	Prandial insulin bolus is calculated based on usual ICR and insulin sensitivity factor

NOTES ON BOLUS INSULIN:

- Bolus doses on insulin can be delivered in three different patterns:
    - Immediately, knows as standard or normal bolus
    - Slowly over a certain period of time (extended or square bolus)
    - A combination of the two, a combo or dual wave bolus

- Meals higher in fat content may need an extended or combo bolus as the rise in glucose following the meal will be delayed by the fat content

- It is recommended to use bolus calculators in determining carbohydrate and correction dosing to avoid insulin stacking and hypoglycaemia

Adapted from Hassanein M et al. *Diabetes Res Clin Pract*, 2022; 185: 109185. © Elsevier B.V.

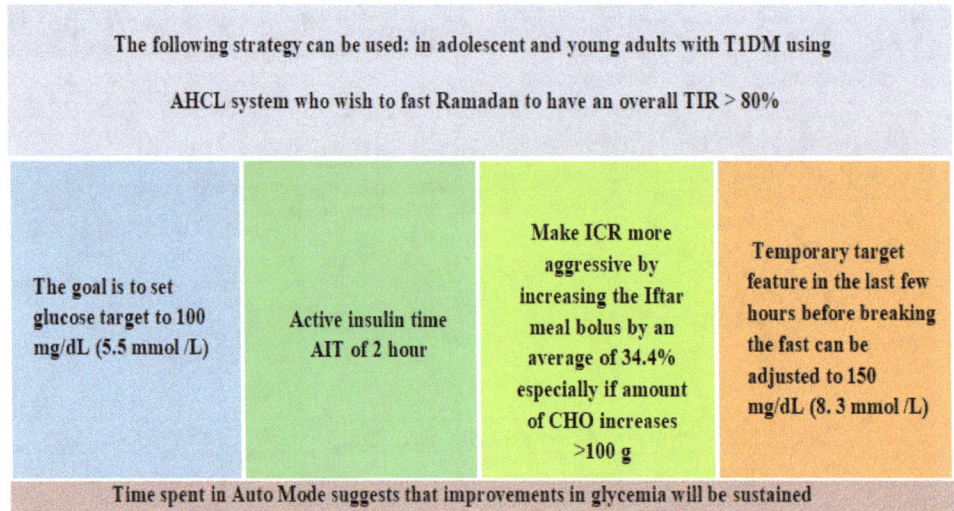

Reprinted from Elbarbary NS, Ismail EAR. Glycemic control during Ramadan fasting in adolescents and young adults with type 1 diabetes on MiniMed™ 780G advanced hybrid closedloop system: a randomized controlled trial. *Diabetes Res Clin Pract.* 2022;191:110045.[18]

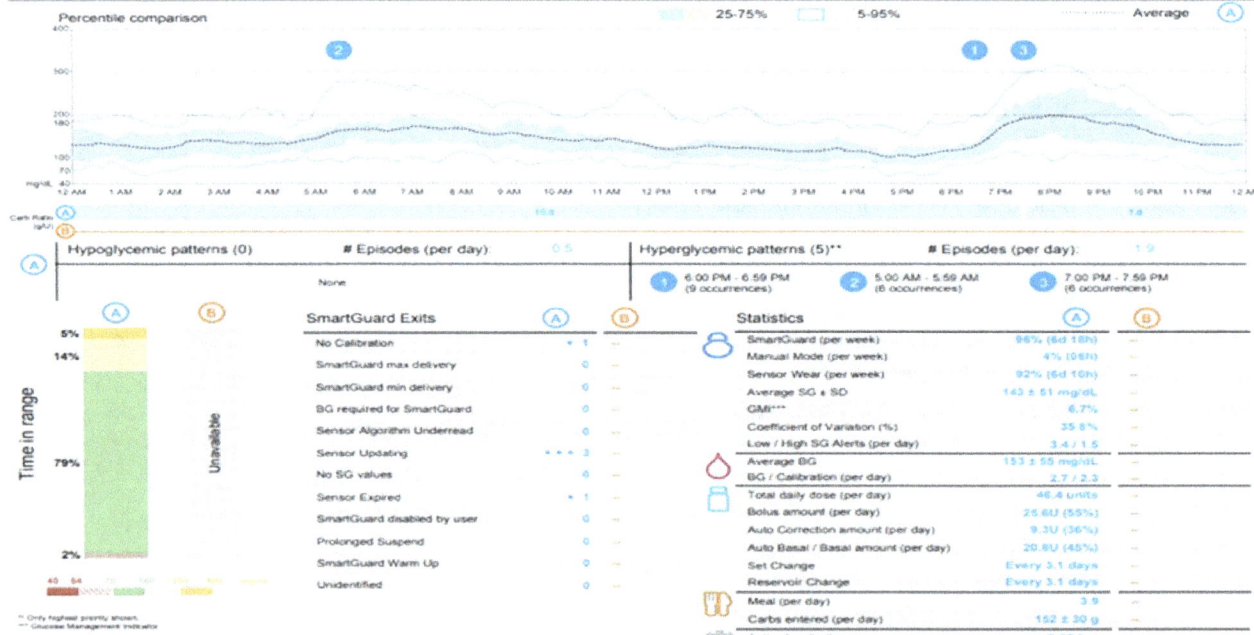

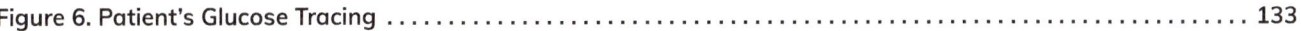
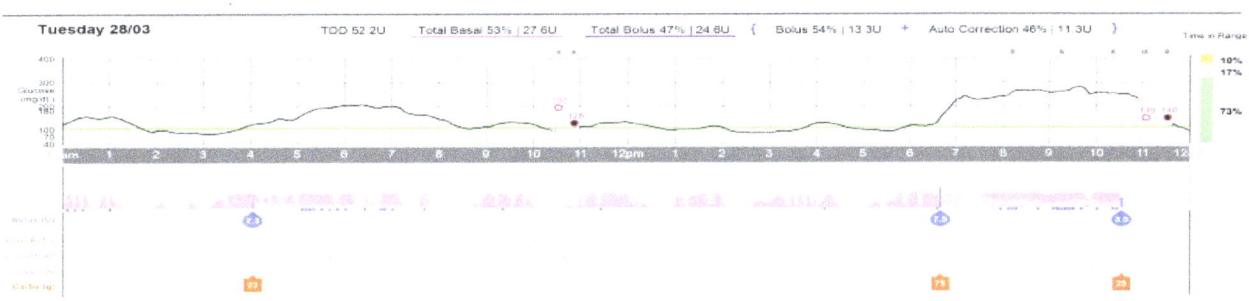

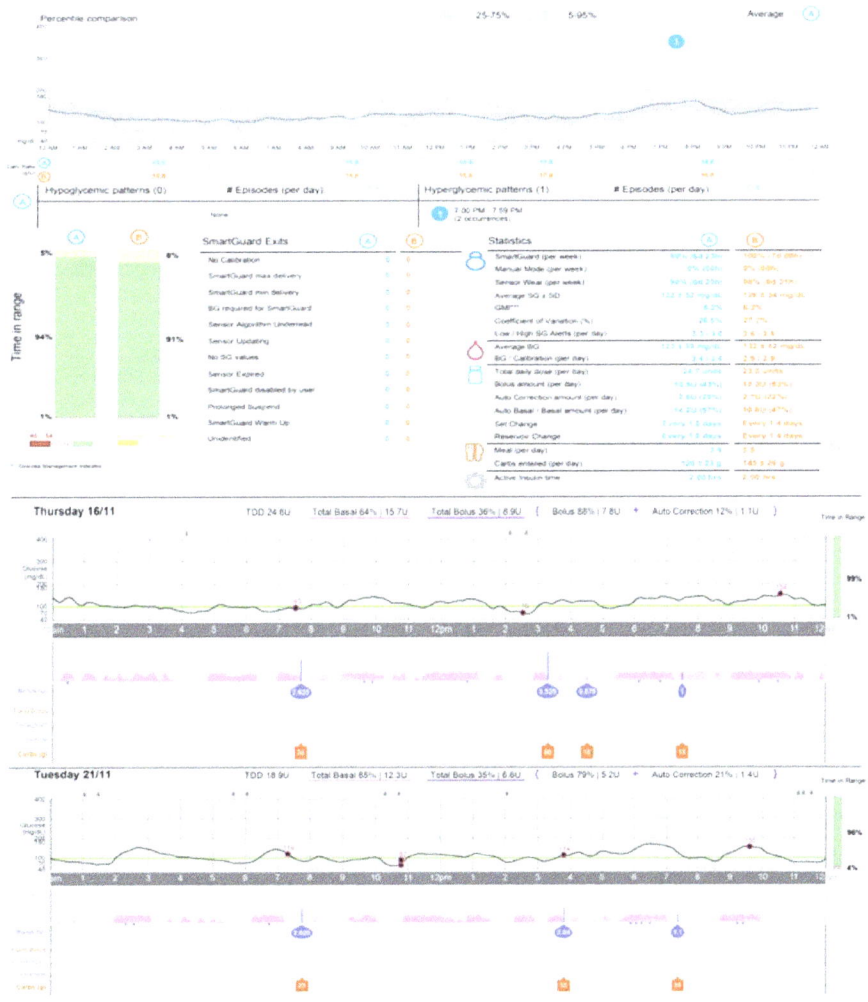

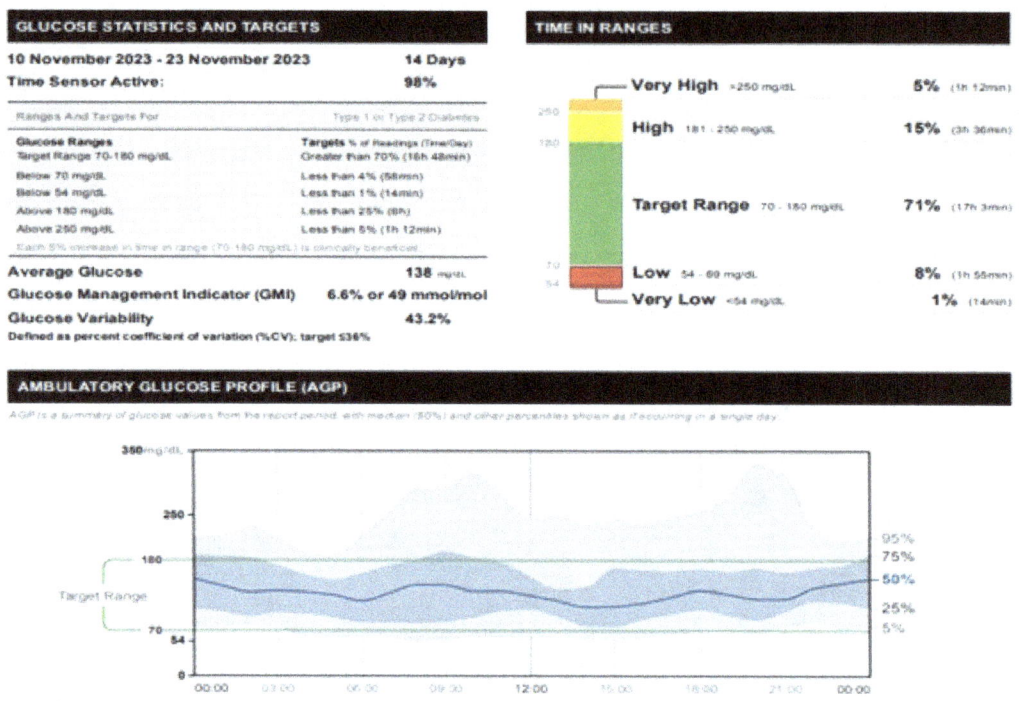

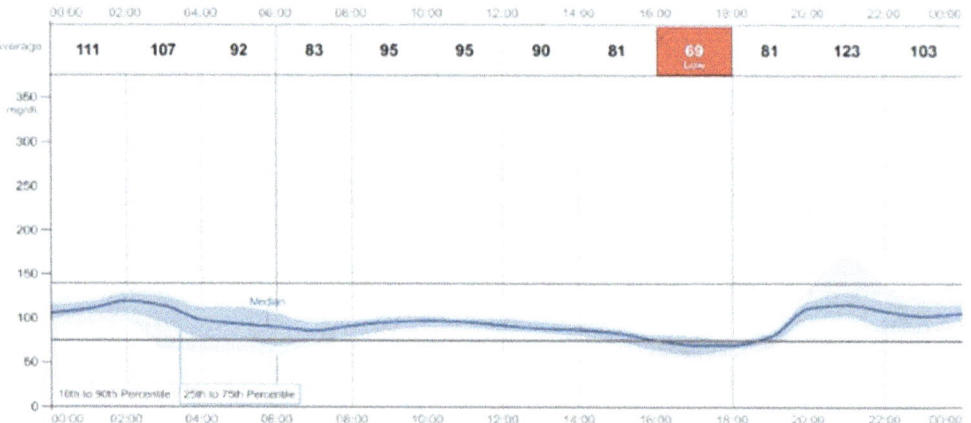

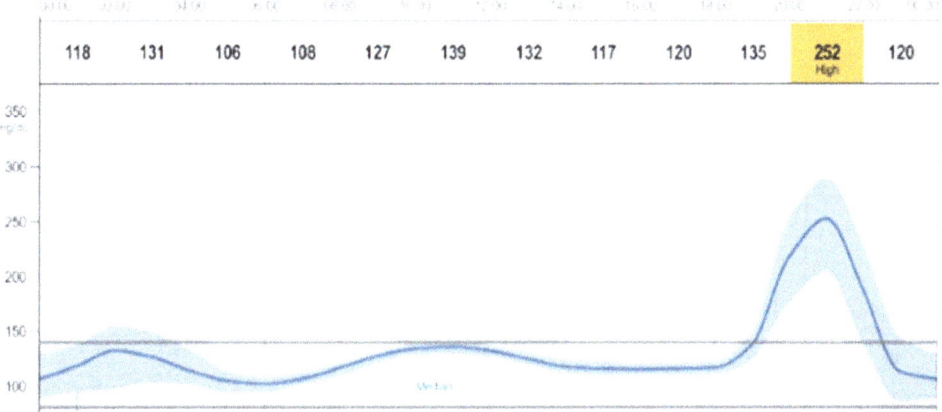

Diabetes and Pregnancy

Alon Y. Mazori, MD, and Carol J. Levy, MD, CDCES

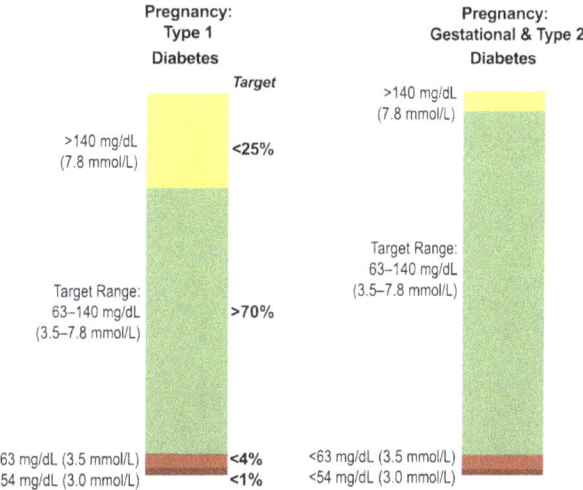

Reprinted from Battelino T et al. *Diabetes Care*, 2019; 42(8): 1593-1603. © by the American Diabetes Association.[11]

B Time in Target Glucose Range According to Time of Day

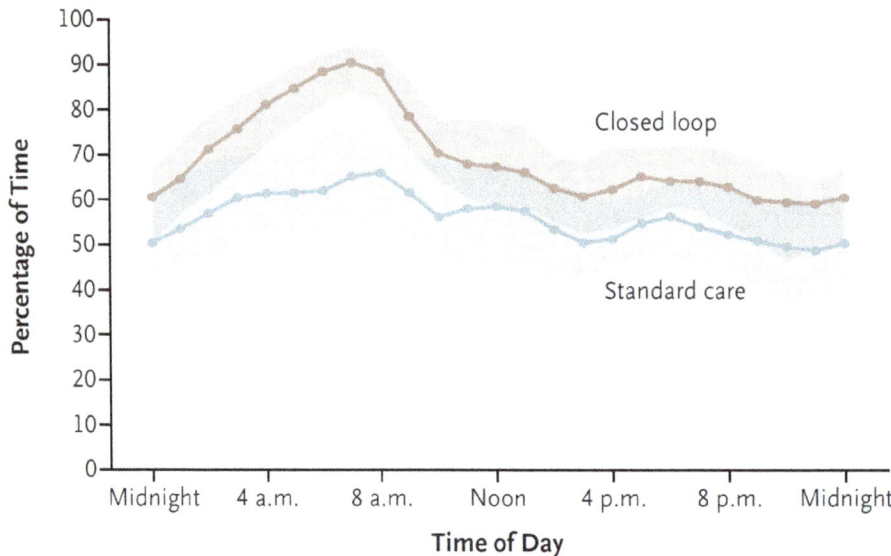

Panel B shows an envelope plot of time in the pregnancy-specific target glucose range, as measured by CGM, for each treatment group, according to the time of day, from 16 weeks' gestation until delivery. Shaded areas indicate the interquartile range. Reprinted with permission from Lee TTM et al. *N Engl J Med*, 2023; 389(17): 1566-78. © Massachusetts Medical Society.[14]

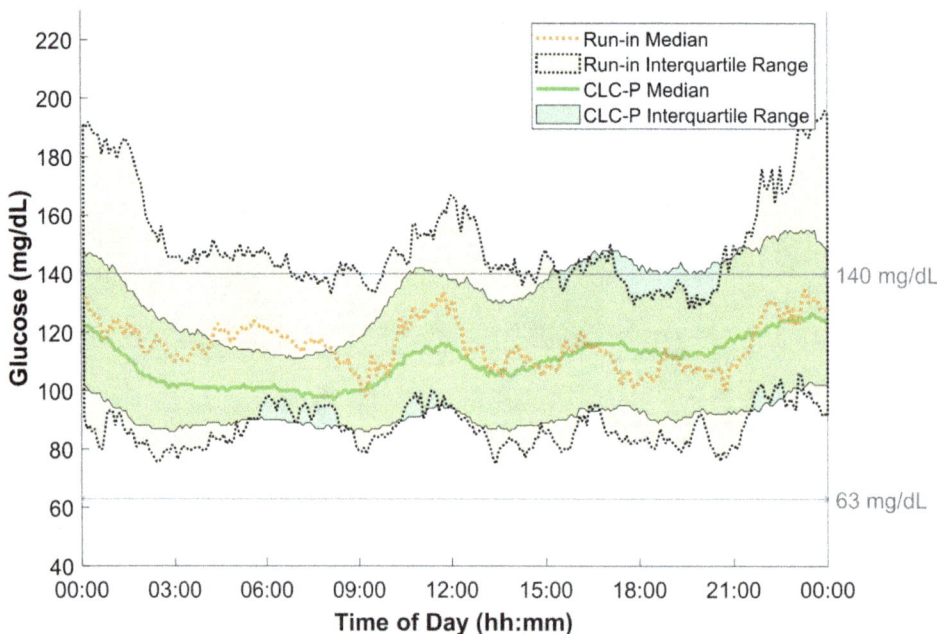

Comparison of glucose levels based on continuous glucose monitoring data between CLC-P (solid lines indicating median, and green shading indicating interquartile range) and run-in (dashed lines indicating median, and yellow shading indicating interquartile range). To convert values for glucose to millimoles per liter, multiply by 0.05551. Reprinted from Levy CJ et al. *Diabetes Care*, 2023; 46(7): 1425-1431. © by the American Diabetes Association.[15]

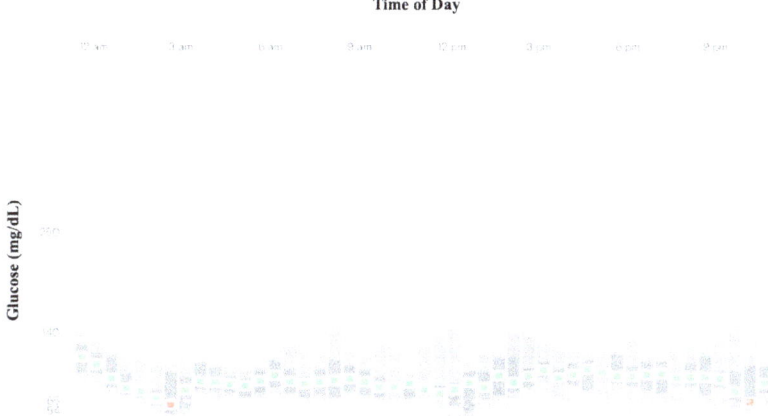

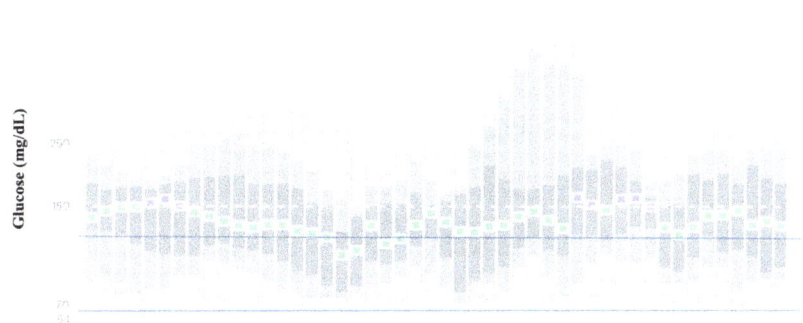

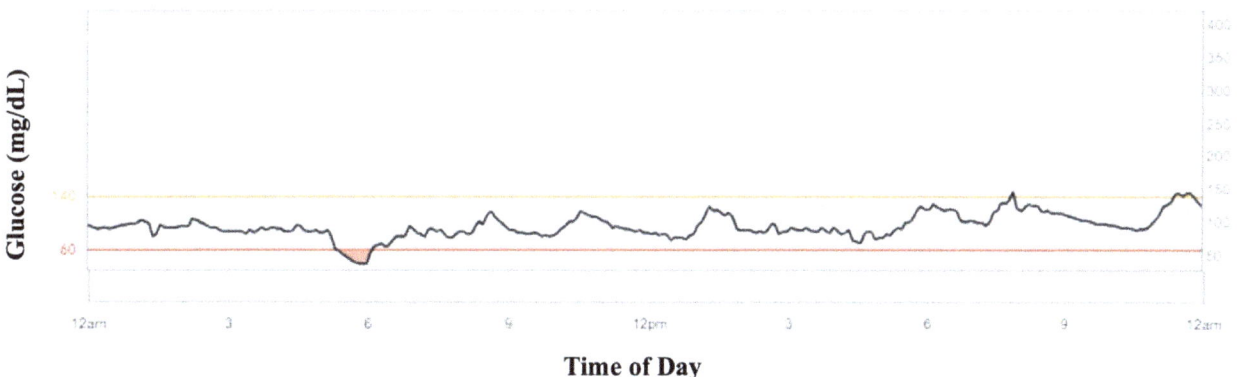

Radiation Therapy in the Management of Cushing Disease and Acromegaly

Moisés Mercado, MD

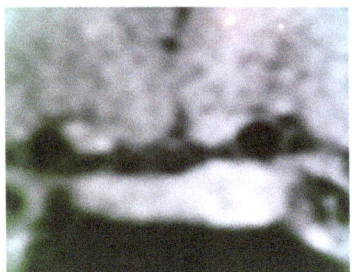

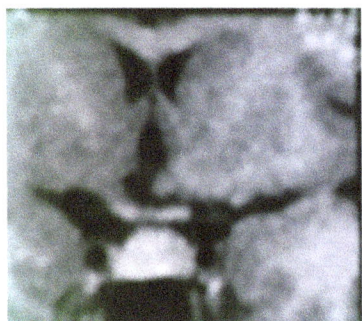

MRI showing a 1.8-cm lesion extending cephalically but without contacting the optic chiasm (distance between chiasma and tumor 4 mm).

Approach to the Patient With Hypoglycemia

Alia Munir, MBBCh, PhD

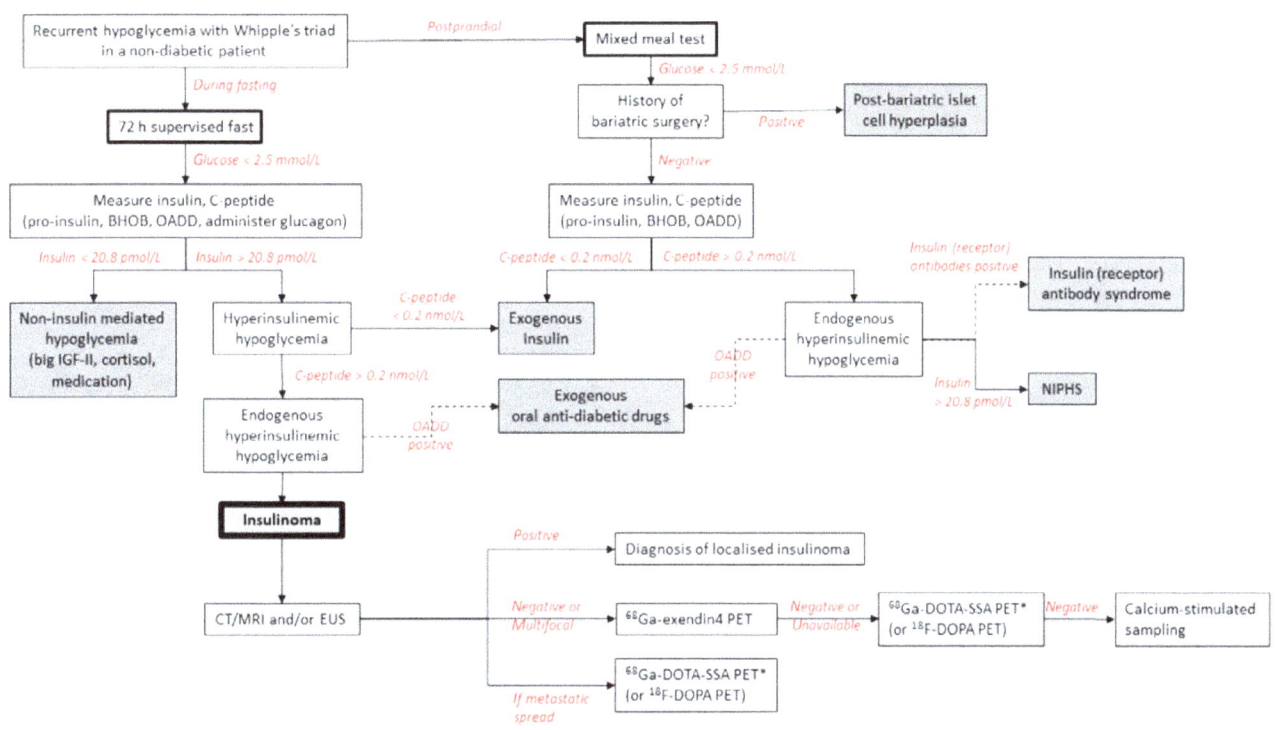

Reprinted from Hofland J et al. *J Neuroendocrinol*, 2023; 35(8): e13318. © The Authors. Published by John Wiley & Sons Ltd on behalf of the British Society for Neuroendocrinology.[4]

Time (min)	Glc mg/dl/mmol/L	Insulin pmol/L
0	81/ 4.5	30
30	117/ 6.4	348
60	85/ 4.8	317
120	70/ 3.8	225
150	63/ 3.5	150
180	60/ 3.3	83
210	55/ 3.1	49
240	60/ 3.3	50
270	65/ 3.6	67
300	63/ 3.5	31

Time	Glc (mg/dl/mmol/L) Criteria 2.2 mol/L	Insulin Nr 17.8-173 Criteria > 36 pmol/L	C-peptide pmol/L Nr 298-2350 Criteria >200pmol/L
10:00	65/3.6	50.2	391
15:15	45/2.5	49.8	417
18:00	62/3.4	43.3	414
21:00	40/2.3	38.2	401
02:00	38/2.1	36.1	322

Beta hydroxy butyrate 1.4 mmol/L
Sulphonylurea screen neg
IgG Insulin antibodies neg

Diagnostic Challenges and Individualized Management of Acromegaly

Elena V. Varlamov, MD, and Maria Fleseriu, MD

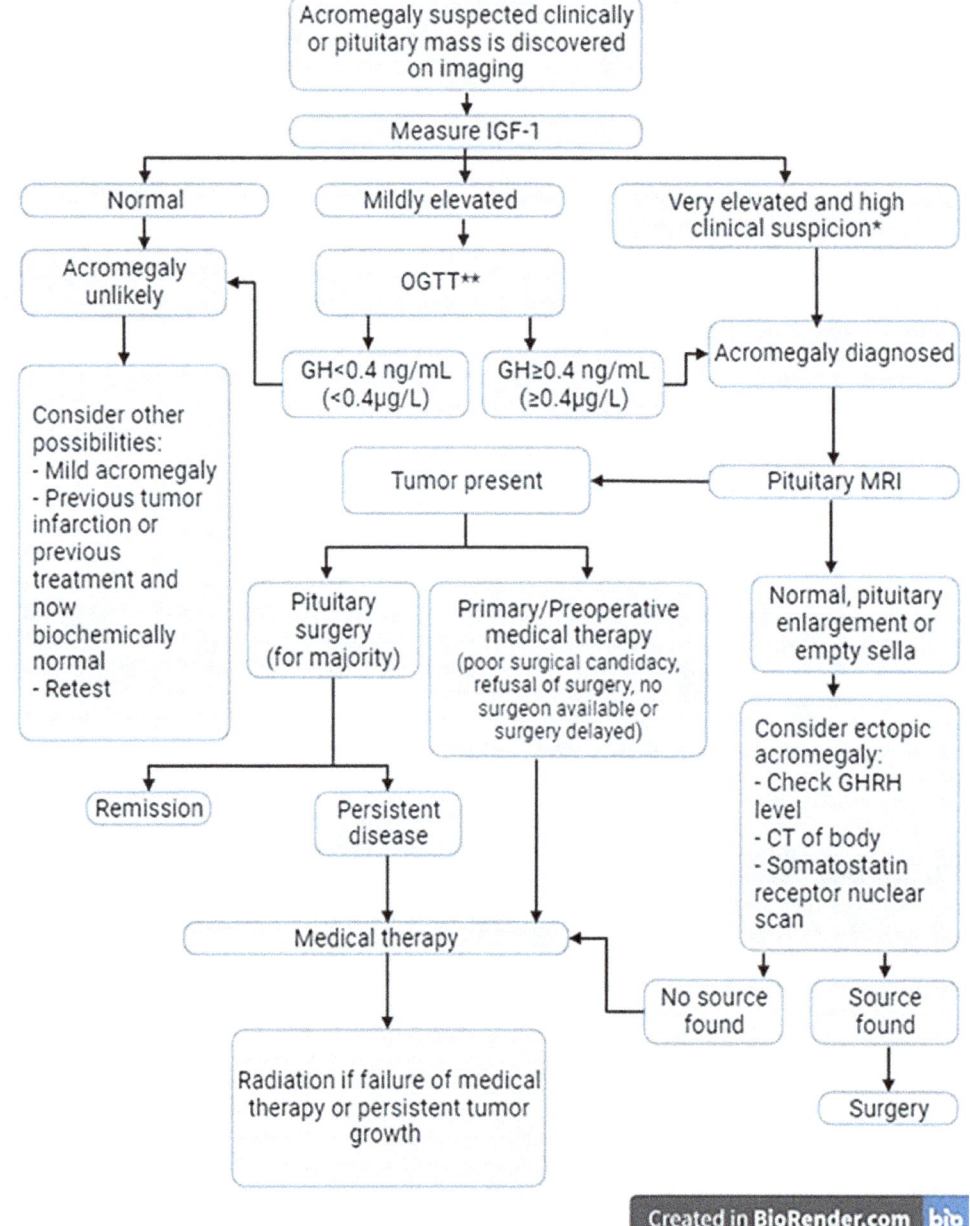

*Consensus[9] recommends IGF-1 >1.3 upper normal limit. **OGTT can show "suppressed" levels (GH <0.4 ng/mL [<0.4 μg/L]) in mild acromegaly and "unsuppressed" levels in patients on oral estrogen and occasionally in slim healthy adults.[9] Adapted from Fleseriu M et al. *Lancet Diabetes Endocrinol*, 2022; 10(11): 804-26. © Elsevier Ltd.[1]

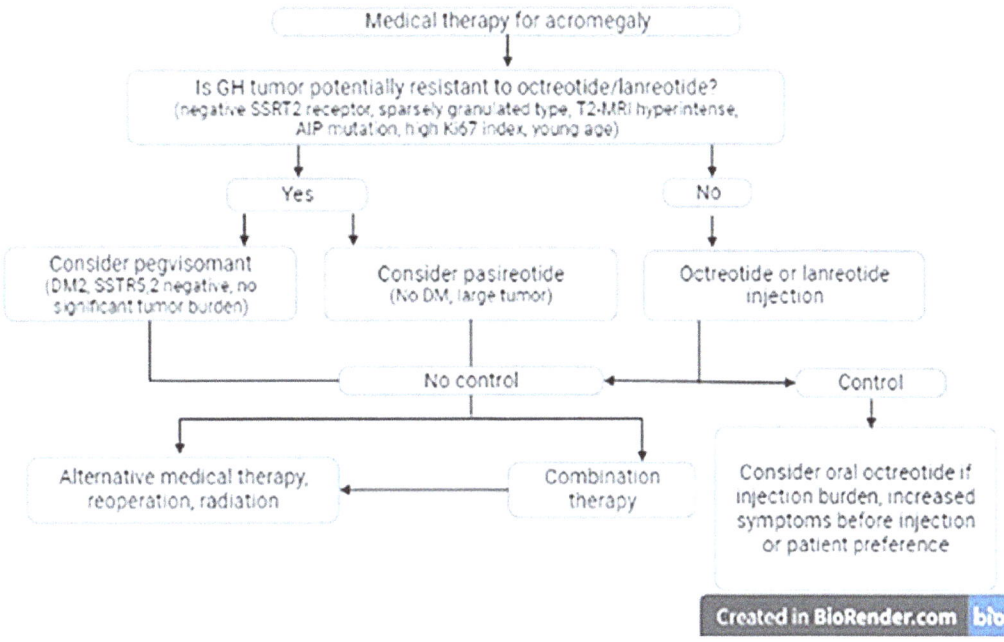

Reprinted from Ting Lim DS & Fleseriu M. *Endocr Pract*, 2022; 28(3): 321-332. © AACE. Published by Elsevier Inc.[7]

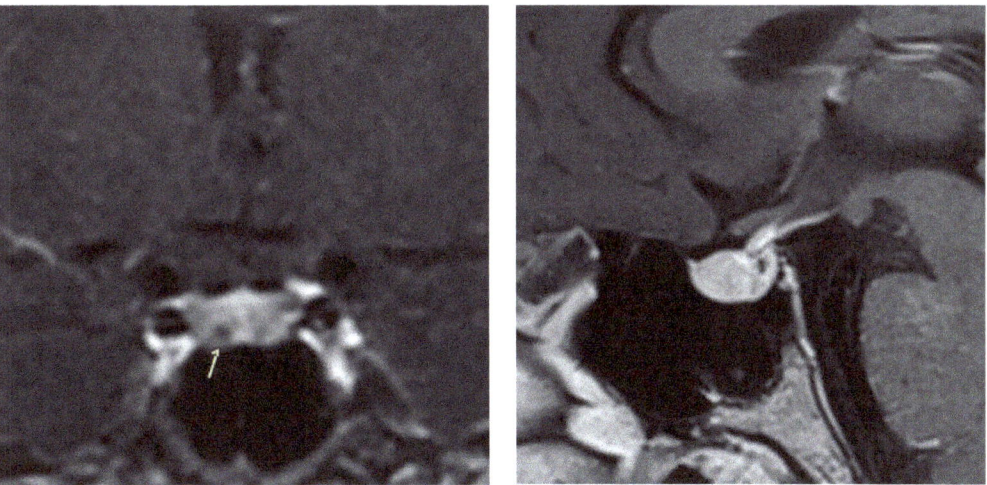

Coronal view   Sagittal view

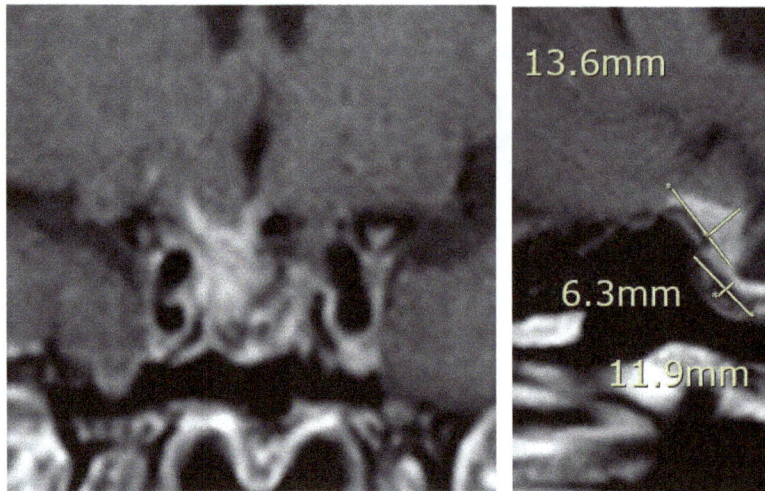

Coronal view   Sagittal view

What to Do? Add Salt, Water, Both, or Neither

Joseph G. Verbalis, MD

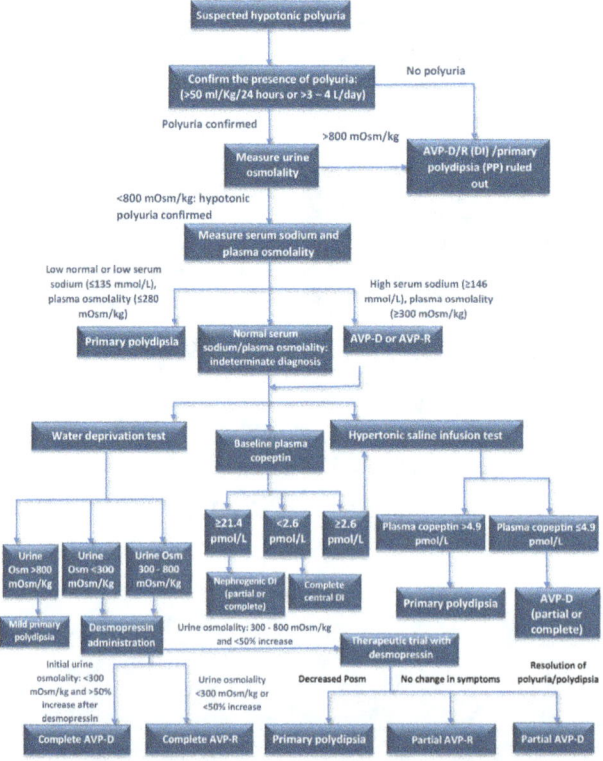

In the first step, polyuria should be confirmed; otherwise polyuria–polydipsia syndrome is excluded and genitourinary (GU) evaluation is needed. In case of polyuria and a urinary osmolality less than 800 mOsm/kg, serum sodium and plasma osmolality are measured. If these concentrations are in the normal range, further differentiation is done using either a classic water-deprivation test or a copeptin-based algorithm (if copeptin measurement is available). Adapted from Gubbi S et al. in Endotext (eds. Feingold KR et al.). © 2000-2024, MDText.com, Inc.

Figure 2. Algorithm for Evaluation and Treatment of Patients With Hypoosmolality **235**

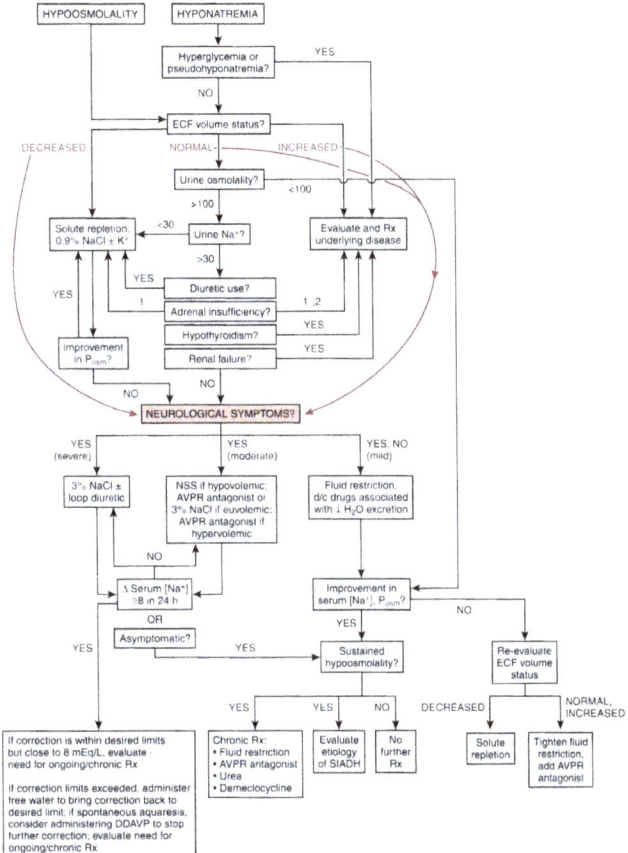

The dark red arrow in the center emphasizes that the presence of CNS dysfunction resulting from hyponatremia should always be assessed immediately, so that appropriate therapy can be started as soon as possible in significantly symptomatic patients, even while the outlined diagnostic evaluation is proceeding. Values for osmolality are in mOsm/kg H_2O, and those referring to serum [Na^+] are in mmol/L. Abbreviations: Δ, change (in concentration); 1°, primary; 2°, secondary; AVPR, arginine vasopressin receptor; d/c, discontinue; DDAVP, desmopressin; ECF, extracellular fluid volume; Posm, plasma osmolality; Rx, treatment; SIADH, syndrome of inappropriate antidiuretic hormone secretion. Reprinted from Verbalis JG. Hyponatremia and hypoosmolar disorders. In National Kidney Foundation's Primer on Kidney Diseases, 8th edition, edited by Gilbert SJ & Weiner DE. Elsevier Saunders, Philadelphia: 62-70, 2023.

PEDIATRIC ENDOCRINOLOGY

Challenges for Pediatric and Adult Endocrinologists in the Diagnosis and Management of Individuals With a Variant in Sex Development

Martine Cools, MD, PhD

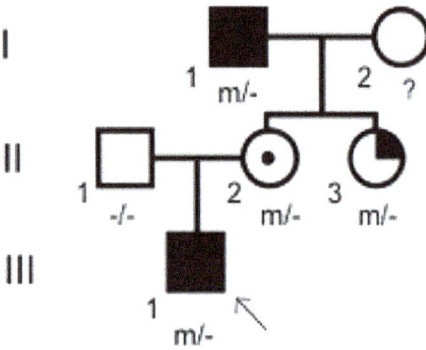

Test	Result	Age-specific reference	SI
Platelet count (10E3/μL)	684	217-497	684 10E9/L
LH (mU/mL)	8.7	1-9	8.7 IU/L
FSH (mU/L)	5.3	1.5-12	5.3 IU/L
Testosterone (ng/dL)	184	NA	6.38 nmol/L
Androstenedione (ng/dL)	89	22-122	3.1 nmol/L
DHT	54	30-120	1.83 nmol/L
AMH (μg/L)	61	62-130	435 pmol/L

Baetens D et al. *Orphanet J Rare Dis*, 2014; 9: 209. BioMed Central Ltd., part of Springer Nature.[15]

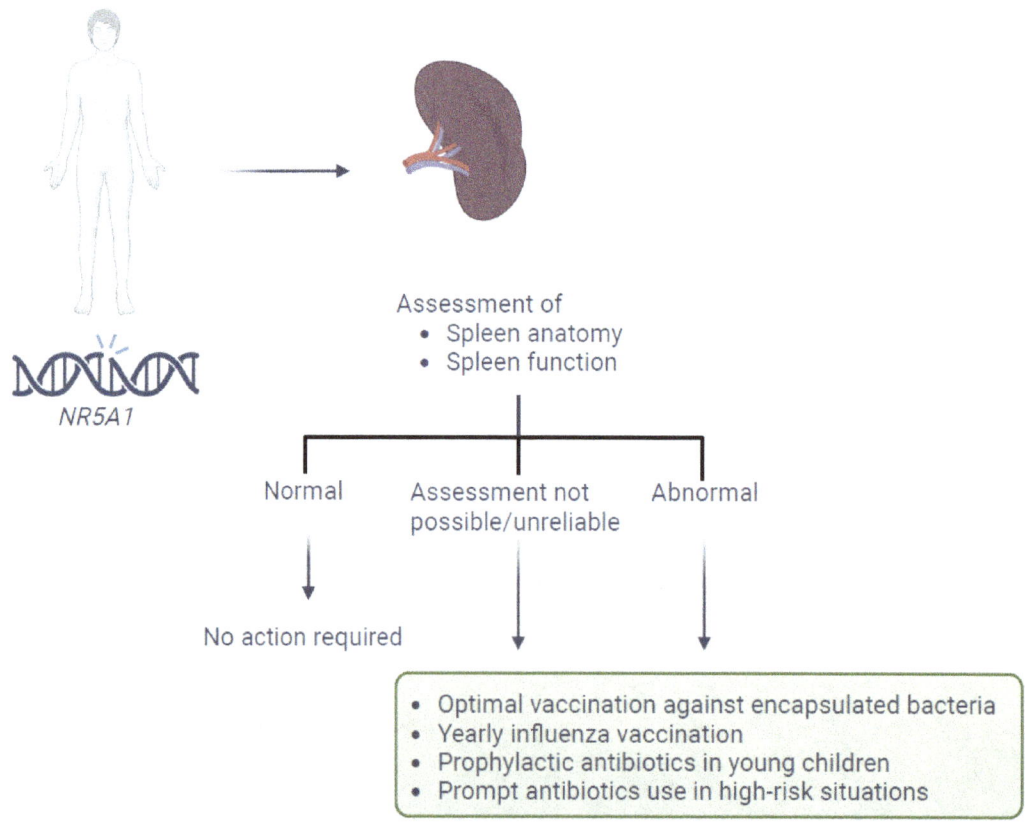

Reprinted with permission from Cools M et al. *European Journal of Endocrinology*, 2024; 190(1): 34-43. © The Authors. Published by Oxford University Press on behalf of European Society of Endocrinology.[9]

Managing Menopause

Margaret E. Wierman, MD

Figure. Intergroup Difference in the Number of Events per 5 Years of Women Aged 50 to 59 Years Enrolled in the WHI Trials **319**

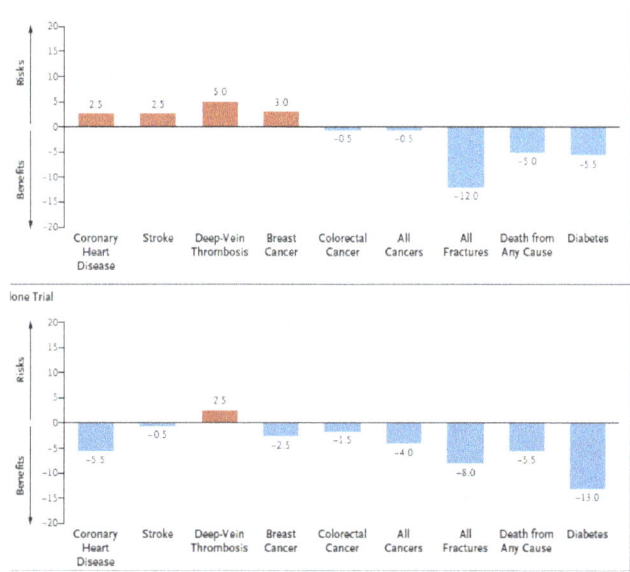

Reprinted with permission from Mason JE and Kaunitz AM. *N Engl J Med*, 2016; 374(9): 803-806. © Massachusetts Medical Society.[3]

Weird Thyroid Function Test Results

Trevor E. Angell, MD

Figure. Cartoon Schema of Thyroid Hormone Physiology. **331**

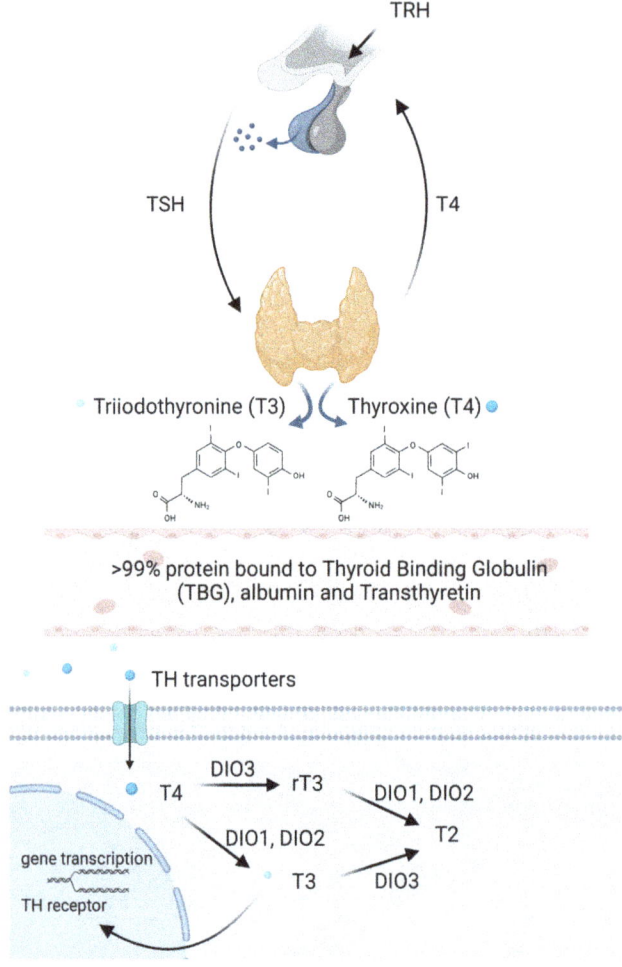

Abbreviations: DIO1, deiodinase type 1; DIO2, deiodinase type 2; DIO3, deiodinase type 3; TH, thyroid hormone; TSH, thyroid stimulating hormone; TRH, thyrotropin releasing hormone.

Challenging Thyroid Nodules

Amanda La Greca, MD, and Sarah E. Mayson, MD

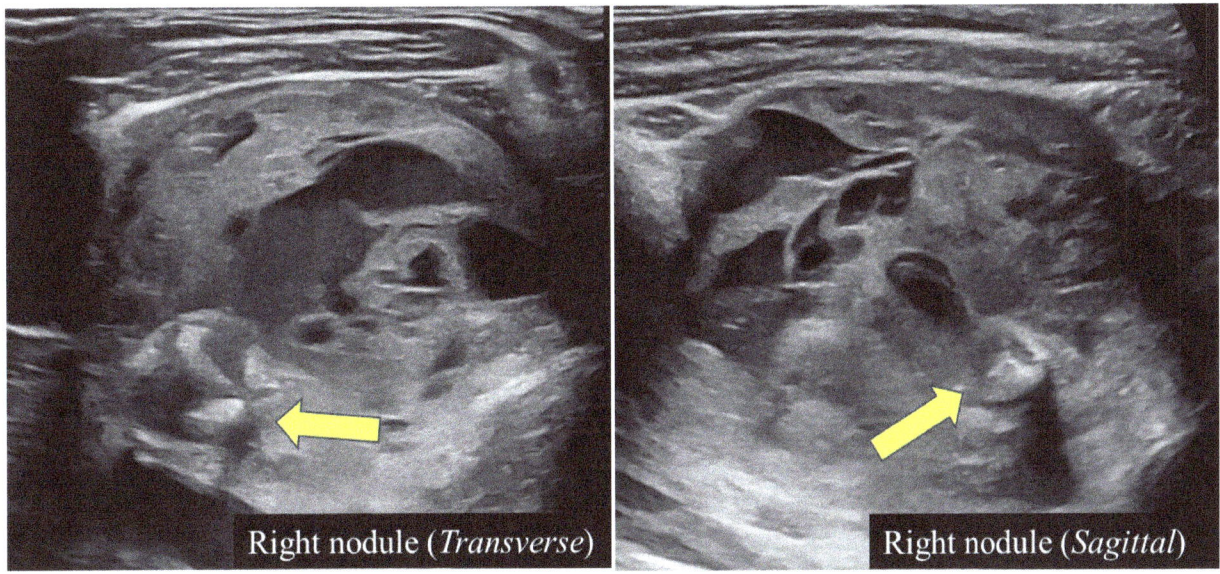

Yellow arrows indicate macrocalcifications inferiorly and posteriorly within the nodule.

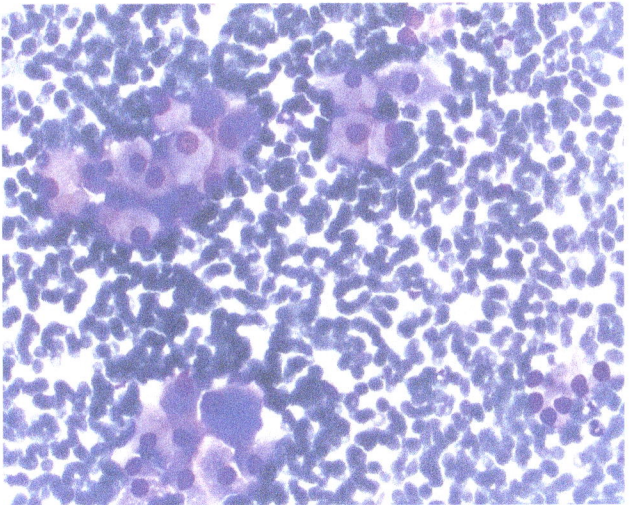

Figure 6. Ultrasound Image Showing Tumor Thrombus in the Left Internal Jugular Vein

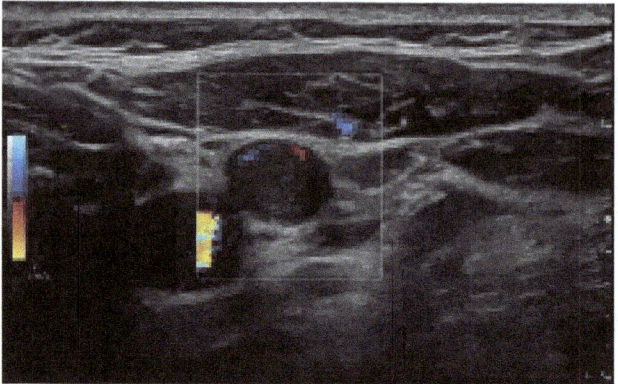

Left neck zone III trans

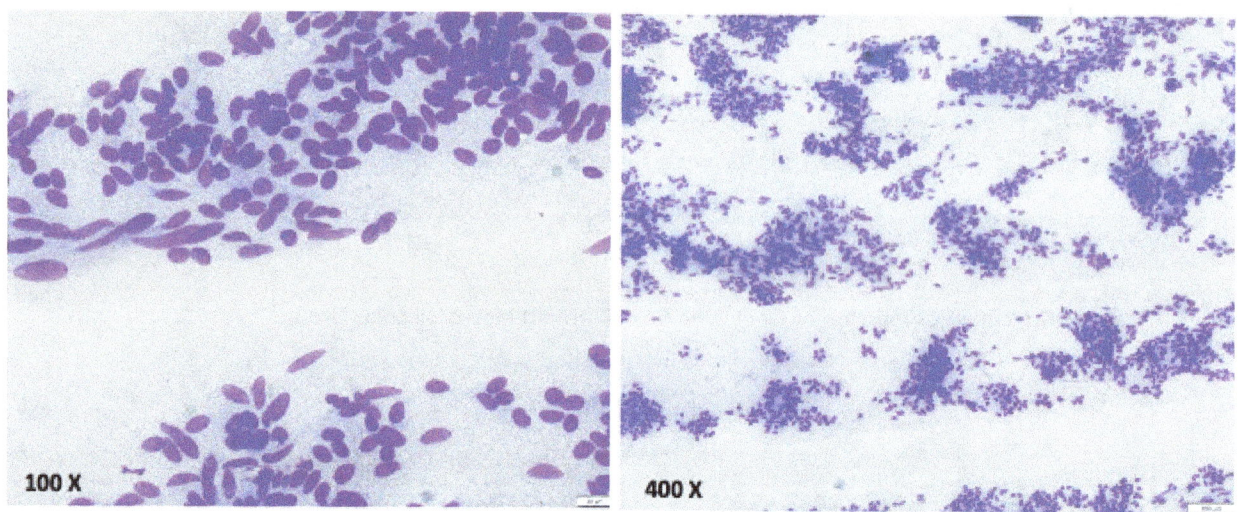

100 X   400 X

Hypercellular aspirate with numerous noncohesive spindle-shaped cells. The nuclei are elongated with granular chromatin and inconspicuous nucleoli.

Complex Hyperthyroidism Cases

Layal Chaker, MD, PhD, and Robin Peeters, MD, PhD

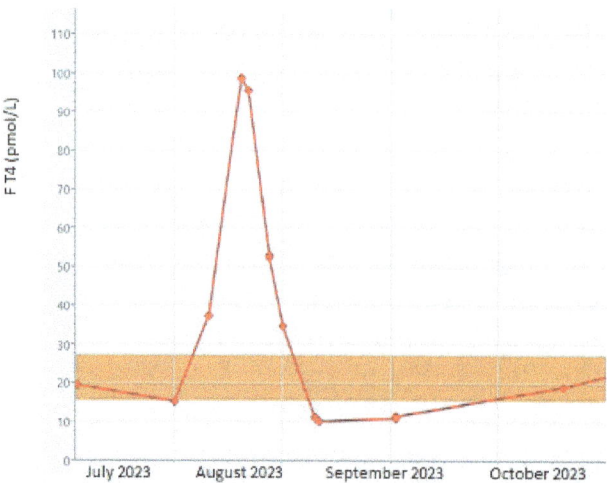

Lobectomy for Thyroid Cancer: Update on Indications, Risk Assessment, and Follow-up Strategy
Eyal Robenshtok, MD

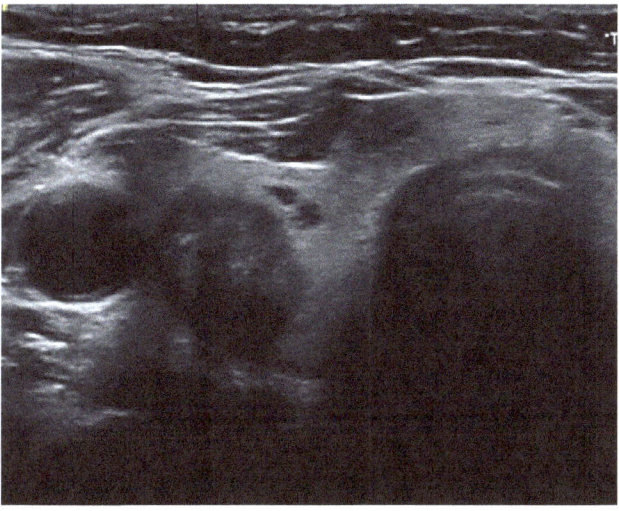

TUMOR BIOLOGY

What's New in Diagnosis and Management of Multiple Endocrine Neoplasia Type 1?
Omair A. Shariq, MD, MS

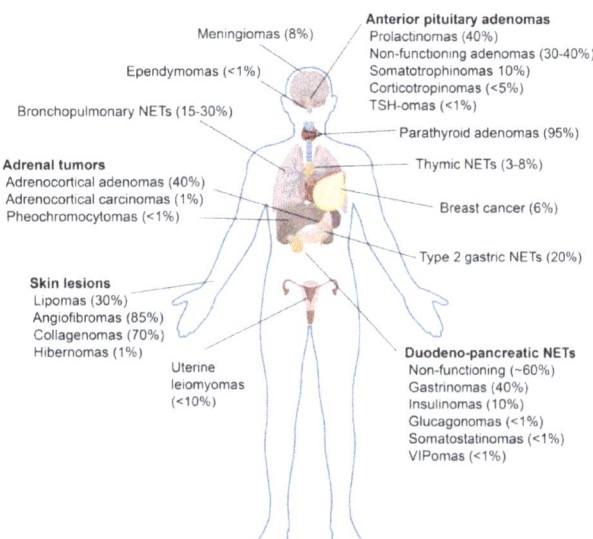

Percentages indicate estimated lifetime penetrance of each tumor type.

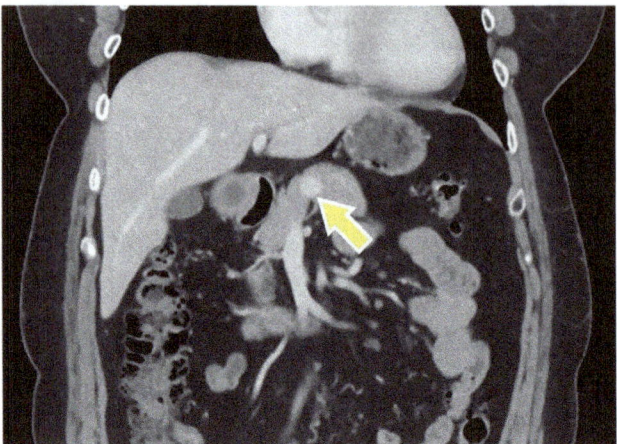

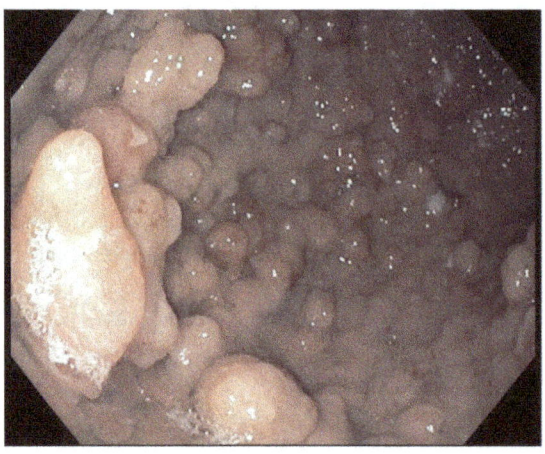

www.ingramcontent.com/pod-product-compliance
Lightning Source LLC
Chambersburg PA
CBHW080410190526
45161CB00003B/187